Current Progress in Pharmaceutical Sciences

Current Progress in Pharmaceutical Sciences

Editor: Erica Helmer

FOSTER ACADEMICS
www.fosteracademics.com

www.fosteracademics.com

FOSTER ACADEMICS

Cataloging-in-Publication Data

Current progress in pharmaceutical sciences / edited by Erica Helmer.
p. cm.
Includes bibliographical references and index.
ISBN 978-1-63242-512-6
1. Pharmacology. 2. Drugs--Research. 3. Pharmacy. I. Helmer, Erica.
RM300 .C87 2017
615.1--dc23

Foster Academics,
118-35 Queens Blvd., Suite 400,
Forest Hills, NY 11375, USA

ISBN 978-1-63242-512-6 (Hardback)

Printed and bound in China.

Contents

Preface

Pharmaceutical science studies the development and effects of general, preventive and other types of medicine. This book on pharmaceuticals explores the various branches that come under pharmaceutical care and diagnosis. This book outlines the processes and applications of pharmaceutical science in detail. It elucidates the concepts and innovative models around prospective developments with respect for this field. The book presents researches and studies performed by experts across the globe. It will provide comprehensive knowledge to the readers. This book, with its detailed analyses and data, will prove immensely beneficial to professionals and students involved in this area at various levels.

Significant researches are present in this book. Intensive efforts have been employed by authors to make this book an outstanding discourse. This book contains the enlightening chapters which have been written on the basis of significant researches done by the experts.

Finally, I would also like to thank all the members involved in this book for being a team and meeting all the deadlines for the submission of their respective works. I would also like to thank my friends and family for being supportive in my efforts.

Editor

1

Three-component synthesis of pyrano[2,3-*d*]-pyrimidine dione derivatives facilitated by sulfonic acid nanoporous silica (SBA-Pr-SO_3H) and their docking and urease inhibitory activity

Ghodsi Mohammadi Ziarani[1*†], Sakineh Faramarzi[1], Shima Asadi[1], Alireza Badiei[2], Roya Bazl[3] and Massoud Amanlou[3*†]

Abstract

Background: A straightforward and efficient method for the synthesis of pyrano[2,3-*d*]pyrimidine diones derivatives from the reaction of barbituric acid, malononitrile and various aromatic aldehydes using SBA-Pr-SO_3H as a nanocatalyst is reported.

Results: Reactions proceed with high efficiency under solvent free conditions. Urease inhibitory activity of pyrano[2,3-*d*]pyrimidine diones derivatives were tested against Jack bean urease using phenol red method. Three compounds of **4a**, **4d** and **4l** were not active in urease inhibition test, but compound **4a** displayed slight urease activation properties. Compounds **4b**, **4k**, **4f**, **4e**, **4j**, **4g** and **4c** with hydrophobic substitutes on phenyl ring, showed good inhibitory activity (19.45-279.14 μM).

Discussion: The compounds with electron donating group and higher hydrophobic interaction with active site of enzyme prevents hydrolysis of substrate. Electron withdrawing groups such as nitro at different position and meta-methoxy reduced urease inhibitory activity. Substitution of both hydrogen of barbituric acid with methyl group will convert inhibitor to activator.

Keywords: SBA-Pr-SO_3H, Barbituric acid, Pyrano[2,3-*d*]pyrimidine diones, Multicomponent reaction (MCRs), Urease inhibitory

Introduction

Pyran derivatives are ordinary structural subunits in a variety of important natural products, including carbohydrates, alkaloids, polyether antibiotics, pheromones, and iridoids [1]. Uracil and its fused derivatives, such as pyrano[2,3-*d*]pyrimidines, pyrido[2,3-*d*]pyrimidines or pyrimido[4,5-*d*]pyrimidines are well recognized by synthesis as well as biological chemists.

These annelated uracils have received considerable attention over the past years due to their wide range of biological activity. Compounds with these ring systems have diverse pharmacological properties such as antiallergic [2], antihypertensive [3], cardiotonic [4], bronchiodilator [5], antibronchitic [6], or antitumour activity [7]. The synthesis of the mentioned compounds containing a pyran and an uracil ring poses significant synthetic challenges. Therefore, for the preparation of these complex molecules large efforts have been directed towards the synthetic manipulation of uracils. As a result, a number

* Correspondence: gmziarani@hotmail.com; amanlou@tums.ac.ir
†Equal contributors
[1]Department of Chemistry, Alzahra University, Vanak Square, P.O. Box 19938939973, Tehran, Iran
[3]Drug Design and Development Research Center and Department of Medicinal Chemistry, Faculty of Pharmacy, Tehran University of Medical Sciences, Tehran, Iran
Full list of author information is available at the end of the article

of reports have described in literature [8-12] which usually require drastic conditions, long reaction times and complex synthetic pathways and the yields are poor. Thus new routes for the synthesis of these molecules have attracted considerable attention in search for a rapid entry to these heterocycles.

The general procedures for the preparation of pyrano [2,3-*d*] pyrimidine-2,4(1H,3H)-diones include the reaction of arylidenemalononitriles with barbituric acid under traditional hot reaction conditions [13,14] or microwave irradiation [15]. In these methods the arylidenemalononitriles are previously derived from malononitrile and aldehydes. Recently, direct condensation of aldehydes, malononitrile and barbituric acid in aqueous media has been reported under ultrasound irradiation [16], or catalyzed by diammonium hydrogen phosphate [17].

Different catalysts such as *L*-proline [18], *N*-methylmorpholine [19], [BMIm]BF_4 [20], 1,4-dioxane [13,21], $H_{14}[NaP_5W_{30}O_{110}]$ [22] and [K $Al(SO_4)_2$] [23] under heating also 3-deoxy-D-arabino-heptulosonate 7-phosphate (DAHP) [17] and *L*-proline [24] under room temperature condition have been researched for the synthesis of pyrano[2,3-*d*]pyrimidine diones derivatives. In addition, Et_3N was examined under microwave irradiation [25]. The catalyst free procedures for the preparation of the pyrano pyrimidine diones were also investigated using microwave irradiation [15], ultrasonic [16], heating with water [26] and ball-milling technique [27].

Mesoporous materials are a special type of nanomaterials with ordered arrays of uniform nanochannels. These materials have important applications in a wide variety of fields such as separation, catalysis, adsorption, advanced nanomaterials, etc [28-33]. SBA-15 has many advantages such as: largest pore-size mesoporous material with highly ordered hexagonally arranged meso-channels, with thick walls, adjustable pore size from 3 to 30 nm, and high hydrothermal and thermal stability [34-38], therefore it is expected to be an useful catalyst in the synthesis of organic compounds.

The surface of SBA-15 was modified by acidic functional groups (e.g., $-SO_3H$) to prepare nano-solid acid catalyst which can use in the synthesis of various heterocyclic compounds [35]. Recently, we have also reported the use of this catalyst for the synthesis of quinoxaline derivatives [39], polyhydroquinolines [40], triazoloquinazolinones and benzimidazoquinazolinones [41].

Moreover, to the best of our knowledge there is no report on the use of these materials as nanoreactors in the synthesis of pyrano pyrimidine diones derivatives. In the present work, we report our results on the research of convenient and green way for the synthesis of pyrano [2,3-*d*]pyrimidine diones derivatives using SBA-Pr-SO_3H as a nanocatalyst and their urease inhibitory activity was investigated.

Material and methods

Gc-Mass analysis was performed on a Gc-Mass model: 5973 network mass selective detector, Gc 6890 Agilent. IR spectra were recorded from KBr disk using a FT-IR Bruker Tensor 27 instrument. Melting points were measured by using the capillary tube method with an electro thermal 9200 apparatus. The ^{1}H-NMR (250 MHZ) was run on a Bruker DPX, 250 MHZ. Nitrogen adsorption and desorption isotherms were measured at -196°C using a Japan Belsorb II system after the samples were vacuum dried at 150°C overnight. Surface areas were calculated by the Brunauer-Emmett-Teller (BET) method, and pore sizes were calculated by the Barrett-Joyner-Halenda (BJH) method. Thermogravimetry analysis (TGA) was carried out in Perkin Elmer Pyris Diamond instrument from ambient temperature to 800°C using 20°C/min ramp rate.

Preparation of catalyst

Synthesis and functionalization of SBA-15

The nanoporous compound SBA-15 was synthesized and functionalizaed according to our previous report and the modified SBA-15-Pr-SO_3H was used as nanoporous solid acid catalyst in the following reactions [40-43].

General procedure for the preparation pyrano[2,3-*d*] pyrimidine diones

The SBA-Pr-SO_3H (0.02 g) was activated in vacuum at 100°C and then after cooling to room temperature, barbituric acid (0.265 g, 2 mmol), 4-nitrobenzaldehyde (0.362 ml, 2.4 mmol) and malonitrile (0.132 g, 2 mmol) was added to the catalyst in a reaction vessel (Scheme 1). The reaction mixture was heated for 15 min in bath oil at 140°C. After the completion of reaction as indicated

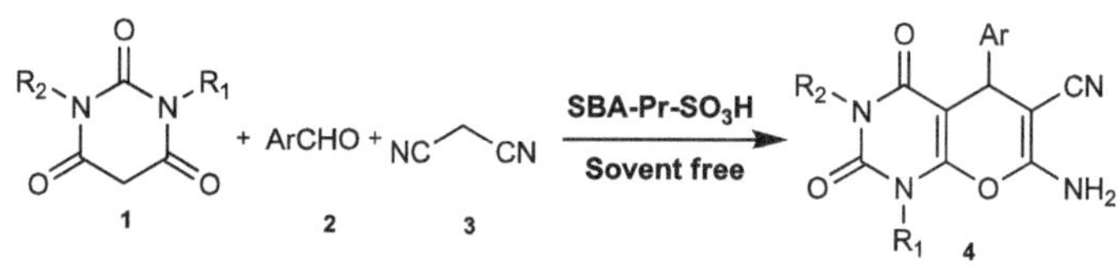

Scheme 1 Three-component synthesis of pyrano[2,3-*d*]pyrimidine dione derivatives.

Table 1 Optimization of the reaction conditions in the synthesis of 4i

Entry	Solvent	Time	Yield (%)	Catalyst
1	H_2O	7 h	32	SBA-Pr-SO_3H
2	EtOH	5 h	31	SBA-Pr-SO_3H
3	EtOH (1:1)/H_2O	6 h	28	SBA-Pr-SO_3H
4	CH_3CN	5 h	50	SBA-Pr-SO_3H
5	neat (140°C)	15 min	90	SBA-Pr-SO_3H
6	neat (140°C)	20 min	30	-

[a] Reaction conditions: barbituric acid (2 mmol), 4-nitrobenzaldehyde (2.4 mmol), malonitrile (2 mmol) and catalyst (0.02 g).
[b] Isolated yields.

by TLC, the generated solid was recrystallized in DMF and ethanol to afford pure product **4**. The resulting solid product was solved in DMF, and then filtered for removing the unsolvable catalyst and then the filtrate was cooled to afford the pure product as a solid. The spectroscopic and analytical data for selected compounds are presented in the following part. The catalyst was washed subsequently with acetonitrile, diluted acid solution, distilled water and then acetone, dried under vacuum and re-used for several times without loss of significant activity.

Spectral data for product

7-Amino-6-cyano-5-(3-methylphenyl)-5H-pyrano[2,3-d] pyrimidine-2,4(1H,3H)-diones **4f:** IR (KBr): υ_{max}= 3411 and 3320 (NH_2), 2961 and 2740 (CN), 1733 and 1700 (C=O) cm^{-1}. ^1H NMR (250 MHz, $CDCl_3$): δ = 2.47 (s, 3H, CH_3), 4.13 (s, 1H, CH), 6.95-7.17 (m, 6H, ArH & NH_2), 11.09 (s, 1H, NH) 12.00 (s, 1H, NH) ppm. Mass (m/z): 296 (M^+), 285, 149 (100).

7-Amino-6-cyano-5-(3-methoxylphenyl)-5H-pyrano[2,3-d] pyrimidine-2,4(1H,3H)-diones **4h:** IR (KBr): υ_{max}= 3183 and 2834 (NH_2), 2246 and 2200 (CN), 1690 and 1538 (C=O), 1459, 1375 cm^{-1}. ^1H NMR (250 MHz, $CDCl_3$): δ

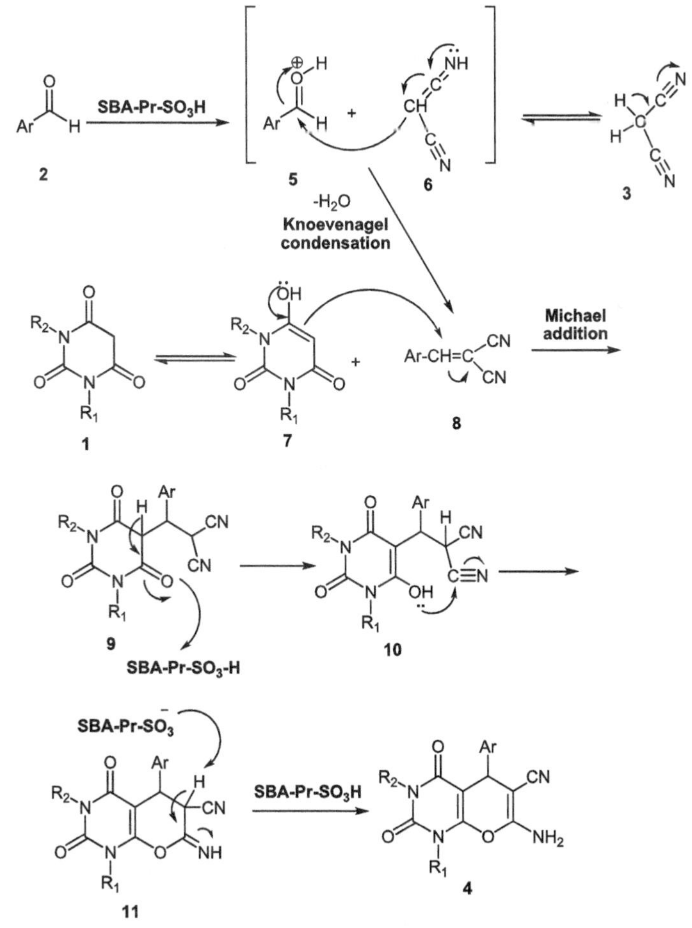

Scheme 2 Plausible mechanism for the formation of pyrano[2,3]pyrimidine dione derivatives 4.

Table 2 Synthesis of pyrano[2,3-*d*]pyrimidine diones derivatives 4 under optimized conditions

Entry	Ar	R_1, R_2	Product Structure[a]	Time (min)	Yield[b] (%)	M.p. (°C) Found	M.p. (°C) Reported
1	Ph	Me, Me	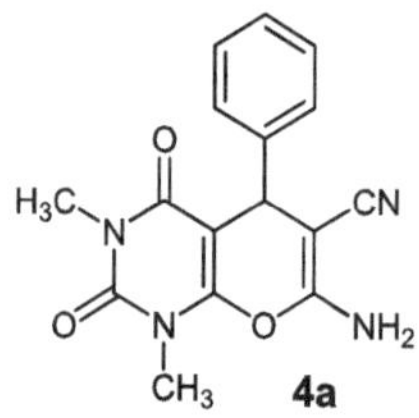 **4a**	5	65	236–238	260–262 [26]
2	2,4-$(Cl)_2$-Ph	H, H	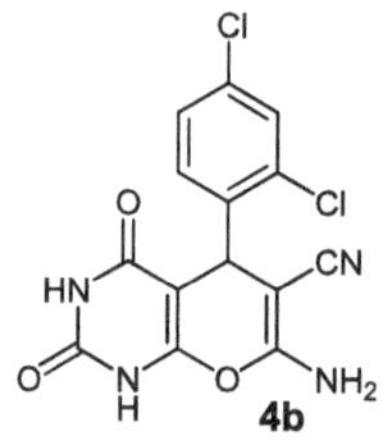 **4b**	20	61	242–243	243–246 [16]
3	4-Me-Ph	H, H	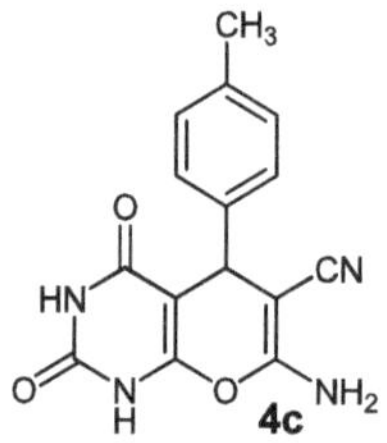 **4c**	25	62	226–227	225 [18]
4	3-NO_2-Ph	H, H	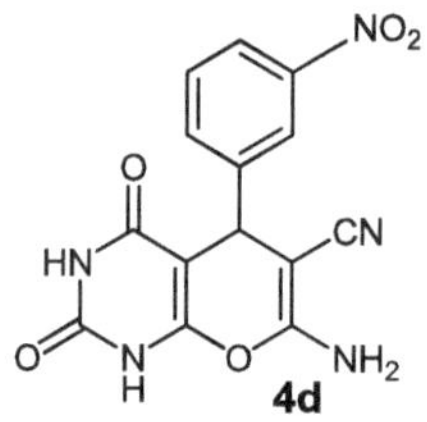 **4d**	15	80	255–226	255–257 [18]
5	4-Cl-Ph	H, H	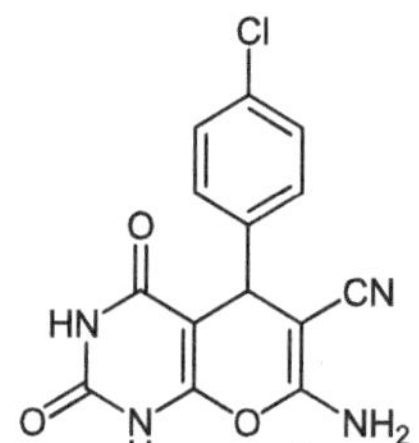 **4e**	45	30	234–235	234–237 [15]
6	3-Me-Ph	H, H	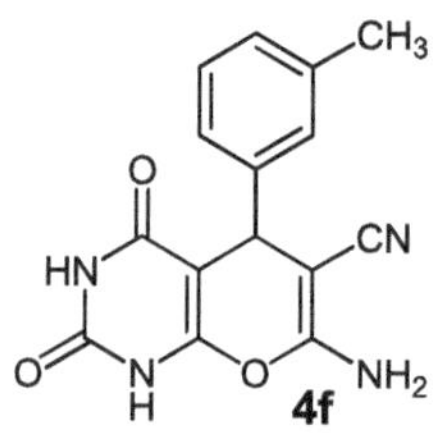 **4f**	30	80	224–225	–

Table 2 Synthesis of pyrano[2,3-*d*]pyrimidine diones derivatives 4 under optimized conditions *(Continued)*

7	4-OMe-Ph	H, H	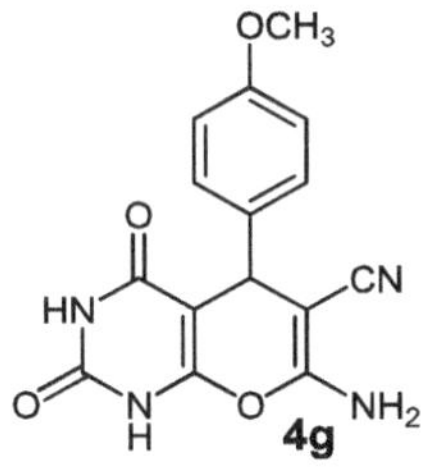 **4g**	35	71	280–284	280 [18]
8	3-OMe-Ph	H, H	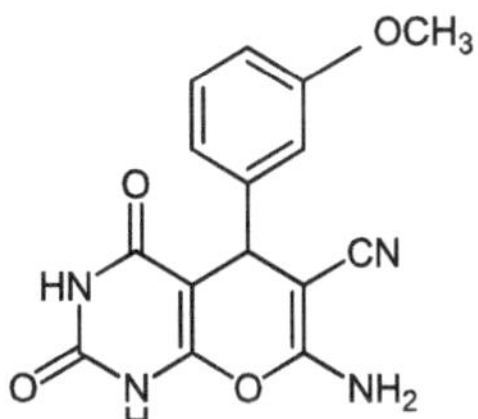 **4h**	10	75	200–206	-
9	4-NO_2-Ph	H, H	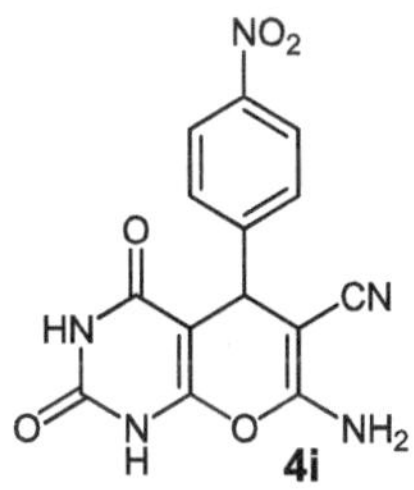 **4i**	15	90	227–228	227–229 [15]
10	4-Br-Ph	H, H	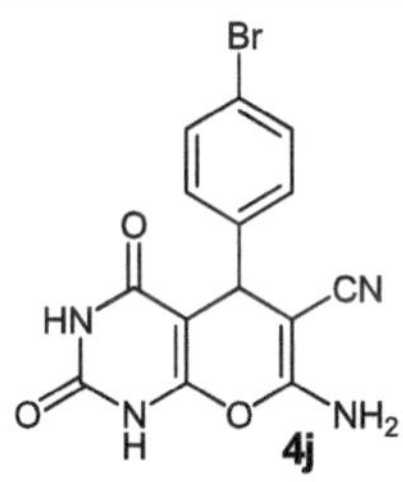 **4j**	15	81	235–236	229–230 [24]
11	2,6-$(Cl)_2$-Ph	H, H	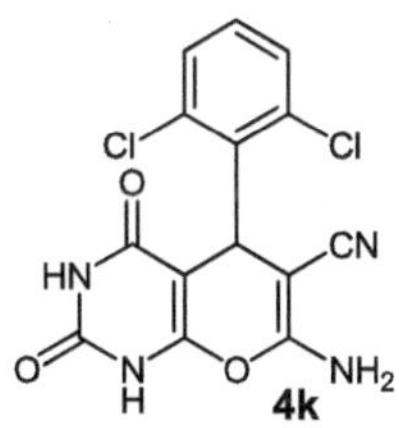 **4k**	15	72	227–228	-

Table 2 Synthesis of pyrano[2,3-*d*]pyrimidine diones derivatives 4 under optimized conditions *(Continued)*

12	4-OH-Ph	Me, Me	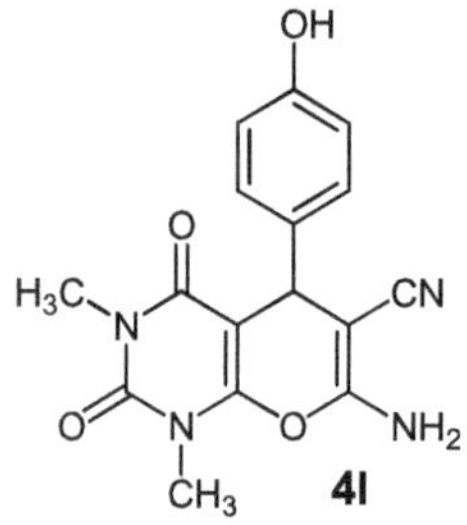 **4l**	20	70	289 (dec)	-

[a] All the compounds were characterized by IR, NMR, MS, and Mp.
[b] Isolated yields.

= 3.35 (s, 3H, OCH_3), 4.16 (s, 1H, CH), 6.96-7.78 (m, 4H, ArH), 8.48 (s, 2H, NH_2) 11.03 (s, 1H, NH), 11.77 (s, 1H, NH) ppm. Mass (m/z): 312 (M^+), 276, 230, 215.

7-Amino-6-cyano-5-(2,6-dichlorophenyl)-5H-pyrano [2,3-d]pyrimidinone **4k:** IR (KBr): υ_{max}= 3368, 3337, 3148 and 3038 (NH_2), 2930 and 2196 (CN), 1703 and 1664 (C=O), 1102, 1283, 763 cm^{-1}. ^1H NMR (250 MHz, $CDCl_3$): δ = 5.28 (s, 1H, CH), 7.94 (s, 2H, NH_2), 7.24- 7.36 (m, 5H, -ArH & NH_2), 11.05 (s, 1H, NH), 12.20 (s, 1H, NH) ppm. Mass (m/z): 352 (M^+), 316, 282, 267, 257, 191, 167, 122, 82.

7-Amino-6-cyano-1,3-dimethyl-5-(4-Hydroxyphenyl)-1,5-dihydro-pyrano[2,3-d]pyrimidine-2,4-dione **4l:** IR (KBr): υ_{max}= 3415, 3315, 3203 and 3020 (NH_2), 2192 (CN), 1688, 1659 and 1529 (C=O), 1348 cm^{-1}. ^1H NMR (250 MHz, $CDCl_3$): δ = 3.17 (s, 3H, CH_3), 3.40 (s, 3H, CH_3), 4.40 (s, 1H, CH), 6.83-8.25 (m, 6H, ArH, & NH_2) ppm. Mass (m/z): 326 (M^+), 327(M^{+1}), 306, 281, 149 (100).

Docking approach

AutoDockTools 1.5.4 (ADT) [44], Autogrid 4.2 [45] and Autodock 4.2 [45] were used to prepare input files, calculate grid box and docking experiments. A grid map consisted of 40 × 40 × 40 Å points around the active site was used. The center of the grid was set to the average coordinates of the two Ni^{2+} ions in the α chain of *H. pylori* urease (pdb ID: 3LA4). A Lamarckian genetic algorithm (LGA) was used for the conformational search. The reliability of the applied docking protocol was assessed by re-docking acetohydroxamic acid (AHA) into the active site of the *H. pylori* urease. Each Lamarckian

Table 3 Comparison of SBA-Pr-SO_3H and various catalysts in the synthesis of pyrano[2,3-*d*]pyrimidine diones derivatives 4

Entry	Catalyst	Solvent	Condition	Time	Yield	Year/Ref.
1	Et_3N	DMF	MW	10–12 min	65–70	2003 [25]
2	*L*-proline	EtOH	Reflux	30 min–12 h	80–92	2010 [18]
3	*N*-methylmorpholine	[bmim][PF_6]	70°C	15 min	85–89	2004 [19]
4	-	H_2O	MW	3–5 min	86–94	2004 [15]
5	$H_{14}[NaP_5W_{30}O_{110}]$	EtOH	Reflux	30–60 min	85–90	2010 [22]
6	-	1,4-dioxane/H_2O	80°C	18 min	65–87	1984 [13]
7	[BMIm]BF_4	[BMIm]BF_4	90°C	3–5 h	82–95	2005 [20]
8	-	H_2O	80°C	7.5–11 h	72–81	2007 [26]
9	-	1,4-dioxane/H_2O	Reflux	1–2 min	60–70	1997 [21]
10	*L*-proline	EtOH	r.t	30–150 min	68–88	2009 [24]
11	-	Ball-milling	r.t	15–90 min	94–99	2009 [27]
12	-	H_2O	US	1–3 h	62–78	2005 [16]
13	DAHP	EtOH	r.t	2 h	71–81	2008 [17]
14	[$KAl(SO_4)_2$]	H_2O	80°C	40–50 min	80–90	2010 [23]
15	SBA-Pr-SO_3H	-	140°C	5–45 min	91	This work

[BMIm]BF_4: 1-Butyl-3-methylimidazolium Tetrafluoroborate.
DAHP: 3-deoxy-D-arabino-heptulosonate 7-phosphate.

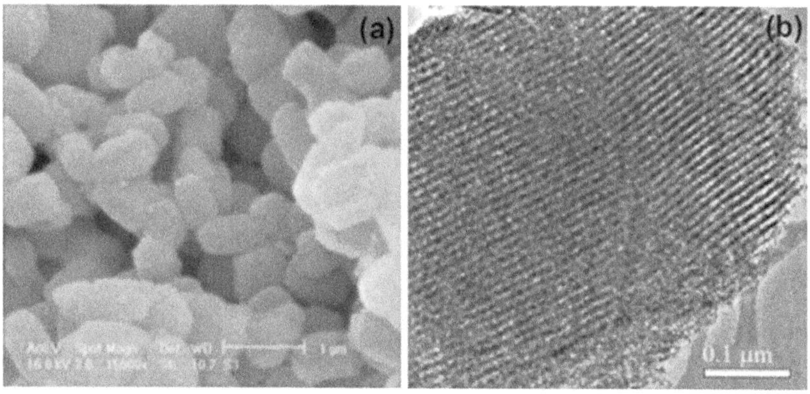

Figure 1 (a) SEM and (b) TEM images of SBA-Pr-SO_3H.

job consisted of 250 runs. The initial population was 150 structures, and the maximum number of energy evaluations and generations was 2.5×10^7. The other parameters were set to default values. The final structures were clustered and ranked according to the most favorable docking energy. This protocol was then similarly applied to all synthesized compounds [46].

Computational resources

The computational studies were carried out on a computer cluster comprising four sets of HP Prolient ML370-G5 tower servers equipped with two quad-core Intel Xeon E5355 processors (2.66 GHz) and 4 GB of RAM, running a Linux platform (SUSE 10.2).

Urease inhibitory assay

All the chemicals used were of analytical grade from Merck Co., Germany. All aqueous solutions were prepared in MilliQ (Millipore, USA) water. Jack-bean urease was obtained from Merck (5 units/mg). After proper dilution, the concentration of enzyme solution adjusts at 2 mg/ml which is determined by UV spectroscopy at $\lambda = 280$ nm. Urease activity was measured by rapid phenol red urease test contains phenol red 0.1% (w/v) and 100 mM urea in 10 mM phosphate buffer, pH 7.0. Based on this method, the colour change from yellow (pH 6.8) to bright pink (pH 8.2) of phenol red pH indicator as a result of urea hydrolysis to ammonia was measured. The urease activity of the synthesized compounds (10 μl in DMSO) was monitored spectrophotometrically at 560 nm after incubation at 37°C for 30 min [47].

Results and discussion

In this article, we want to report the use of SBA-Pr-SO_3H as a nano and green solid acid catalyst and nano- reactor in the synthesis of 7-amino-6-cyano-5-aryl-5H-pyrano [2,3-*d*]pyrimidinones by the Knoevenagel–Michael condensation reaction. The procedure consisted of the mixture of malonitrile, aromatic aldehydes, and barbituric acid derivatives. The reaction proceeded in high yields in the presence of SBA-Pr-SO_3H as catalyst at room temperature and solvent free conditions to obtain our desired products **4a-4l** (Scheme 1).

First the suitable conditions for the above transformation are examined with various solvents in different temperatures in the presence of SBA-Pr-SO_3H as nanocatalyst as shown in Table 1. The results revealed when the reaction proceeds in the absence of solvent, the desired product was obtained in high yield (90%) and very short reaction time. By increasing the temperature of the media to 130°C, the reaction time decreases to 15 minutes so the best reaction conditions were obtained (entry 5, Table 1). The same reaction was done without using any catalyst and a very low yield of product was obtained.

A reasonable mechanism for the formation of the product **4** is outlined in Scheme 2. First the oxygen of carbonyl group in benzaldehyde **2** was protonated and malonitrile **3** tautomerized to **6.** The Knoevenagel condensation of compounds **5** and **6** was occurred to form the cyano-olefin **8**. Subsequently, the tautomerized barbituric acid **7** endures nucleophilic attack to **8** and gives the Michael adduct **9.** The intermediate **9** tautomerizes in the presence of acidic catalyst to generate intermediate **10** which cyclizes to give compound **11** which subsequently tautomerized to afford the fully aromatized compound **4.**

Table 2 shows the obtained results in the reaction of a series of representative aldehydes with malononitrile and barbituric derivatives. The most derivatives were obtained in short reaction time ranging 5-45 minutes in high to very high yields. The effect of substituents on the aromatic ring did not show special effects in terms of yields under these reaction conditions.

Literature surveys revealed that various conditions have been employed in this reaction as demonstrated in Table 3.

Table 4 Urease inhibitory activities (IC_{50} in μM) and interaction energies (kcal mol^{-1}) of pyrano[2,3-*d*]pyrimidine diones derivatives 4

Entry	Product	Docking energy (kcal/mol)	IC_{50} (μM)	Structure
1	**4a**	−5.46	98.77	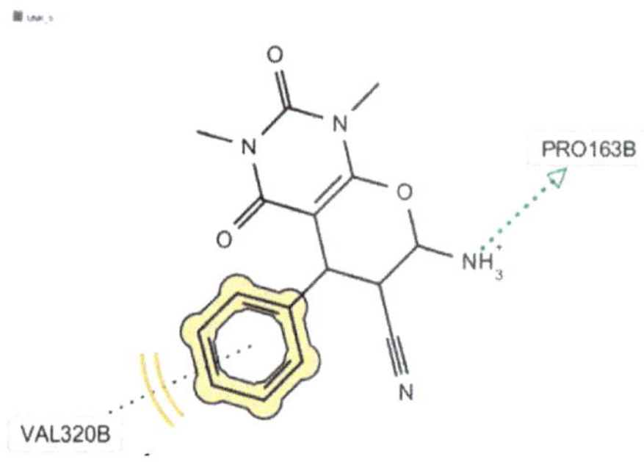
2	**4b**	−6.43	19.45	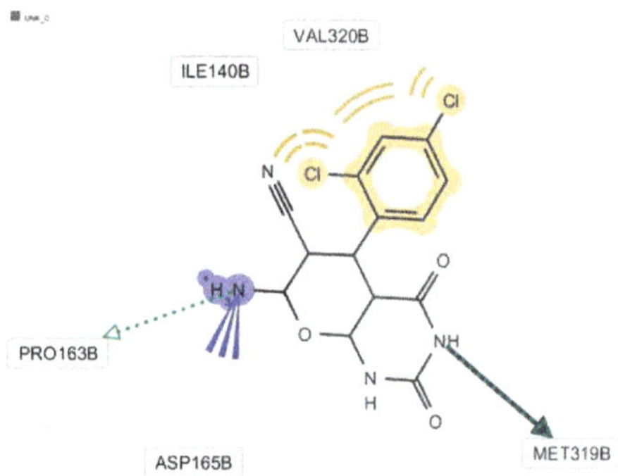
3	**4c**	−5.65	71.92	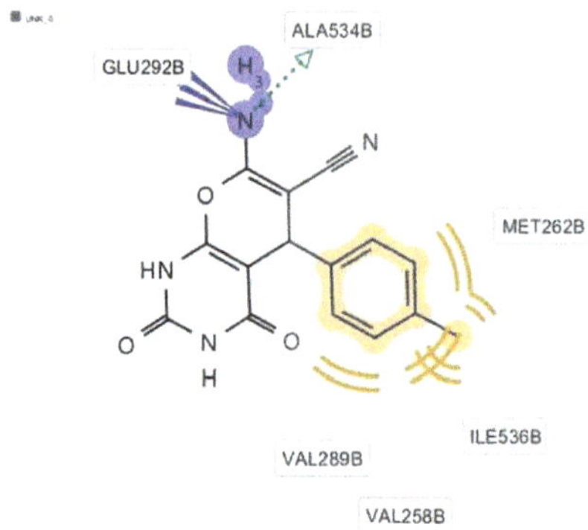
4	**4d**	−5.46	98.93	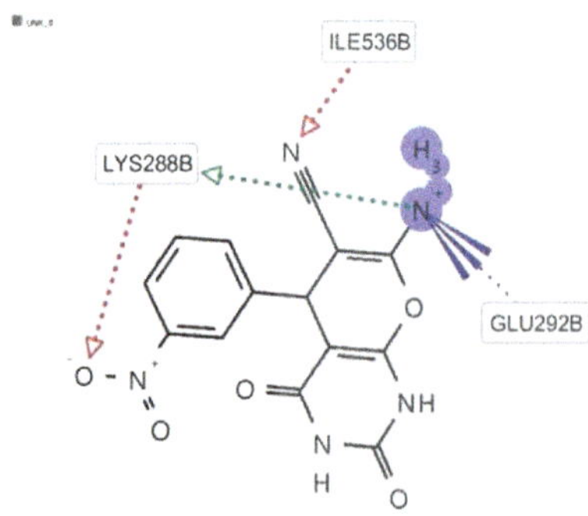

Table 4 Urease inhibitory activities (IC_{50} in μM) and interaction energies (kcal mol^{-1}) of pyrano[2,3-*d*]pyrimidine diones derivatives 4 *(Continued)*

5	**4e**	−5.87	49.65	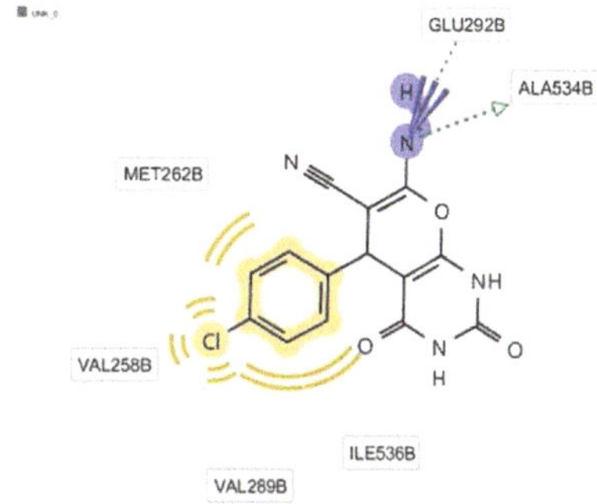
6	**4f**	−5.98	41.13	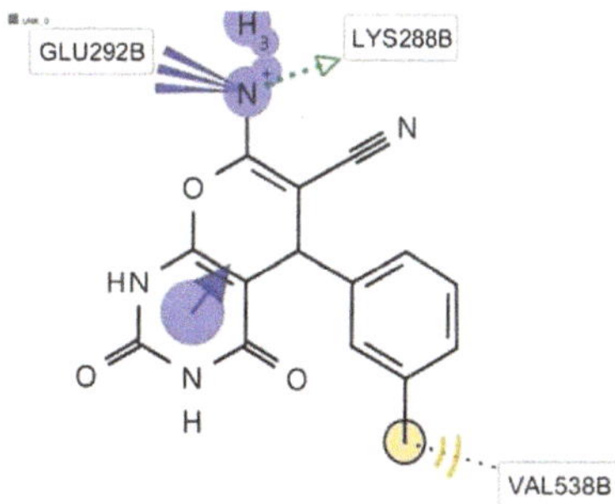
7	**4g**	−5.73	62.92	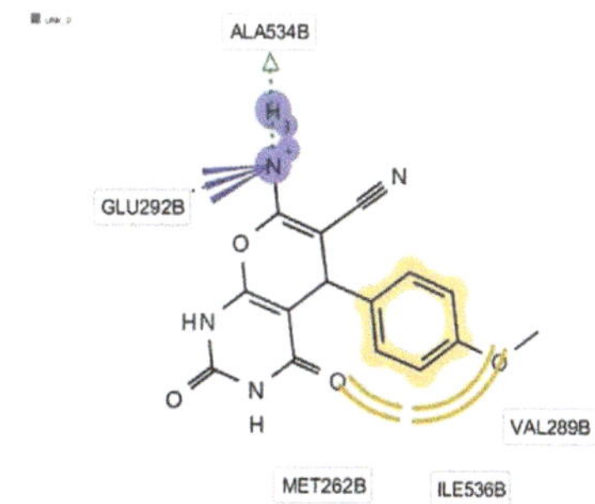
8	**4h**	−5.42	106.29	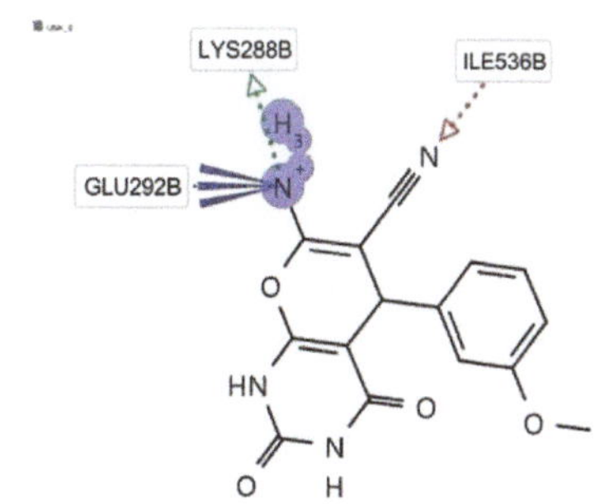

Table 4 Urease inhibitory activities (IC_{50} in μM) and interaction energies (kcal mol^{-1}) of pyrano[2,3-*d*]pyrimidine diones derivatives 4 *(Continued)*

9	**4i**	−4.85	279.14	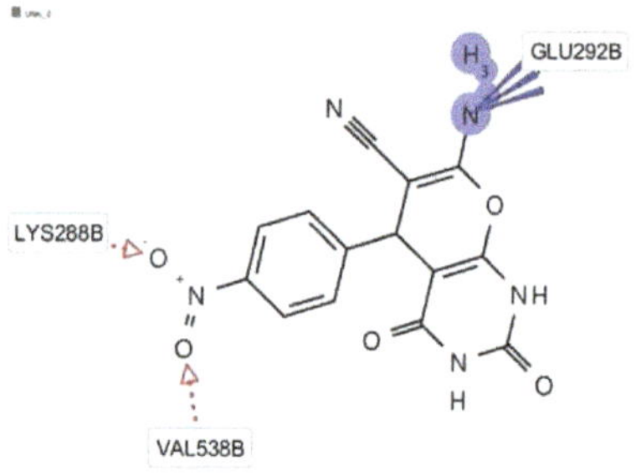
10	**4j**	−5.85	51.31	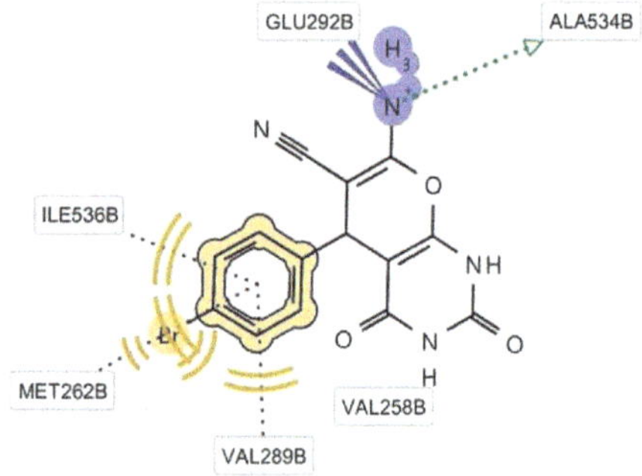
11	**4k**	−5.99	41.0	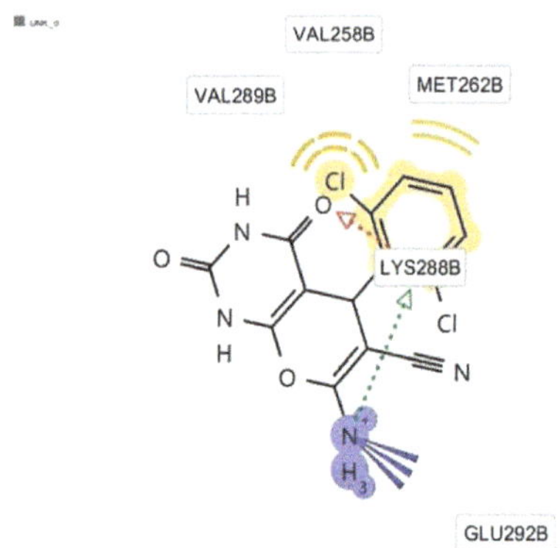

Table 4 Urease inhibitory activities (IC_{50} in μM) and interaction energies (kcal mol^{-1}) of pyrano[2,3-*d*]pyrimidine diones derivatives 4 *(Continued)*

12	**4l**	−5.41	107.62	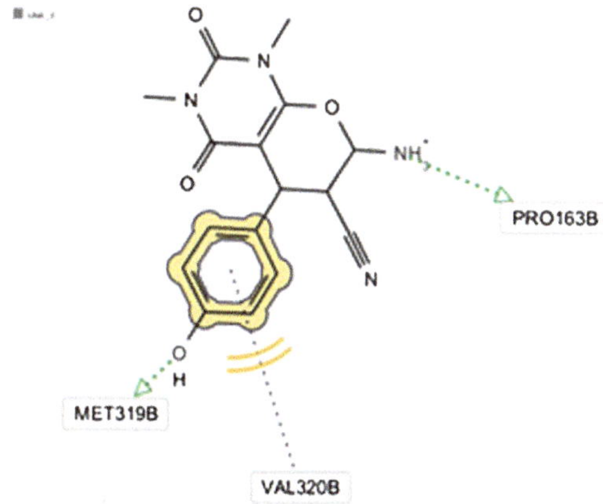
13		−3.98	21.0	Thiourea

[a] Green and red arrows are presented H-bond donor and acceptor interactions, respectively.
[b] Yellow areas are parts with hydrophobic interactions.
[c] Blue lines depict the electrostatic interactions.
[*] The IC_{50} values for activator.

The results illustrated that SBA-Pr-SO_3H was an efficient catalyst in the synthesis of these compounds.

Preparation of catalyst

Pure Nanoporous compound SBA-15 was synthesized according to the well-established method designed by Zhao & coworkers [42] with triblock poly(ethylene oxide)-b-poly(propylene oxide)-b-poly(ethylene oxide) copolymer (Pluronic, $EO_{20}PO_{70}EO_{20}$, P_{123}) as the template. The SBA-15 silica was functionalized with (3-mercaptopropyl) trimethoxysilane (MPTS) and then, the thiol groups were oxidized to sulfonic acid by hydrogen peroxide. Analyzing of the catalyst surface was performed by various methods such as TGA, BET and CHN methods which demonstrated that the propylsulfonic acids were immobilized into the pores. Calculating average pore diameter of the surface area was performed by the BET method and pore volume of SBA-Pr-SO_3H are 440 m^2 g^{-1}, 6.0 nm and 0.660 cm^3 g^{-1}, respectively, which are smaller than those of SBA-15 due to the immobilization of sulfonosilane groups into the pores [40]. The TGA analysis of SBA-Pr-SO_3H confirmed the amount of organic groups on SBA-15. The weight reduction of SBA-Pr-SO_3H in the temperature range between 200-600°C indicated that the amount of organic group was 1.2 mmol/g. SEM image of SBA-Pr-SO_3H (Figure 1a) shows uniform particles about 1μm. The same morphology was observed for SBA-15. It can be concluded that morphology of acid catalyst was saved without change during the surface modifications. On the other hand, the TEM image (Figure 1b) reveals the parallel channels, which resemble to the pores configuration of SBA-15. This indicates that the pore of SBA-Pr-SO_3H was not collapsed during two steps reactions.

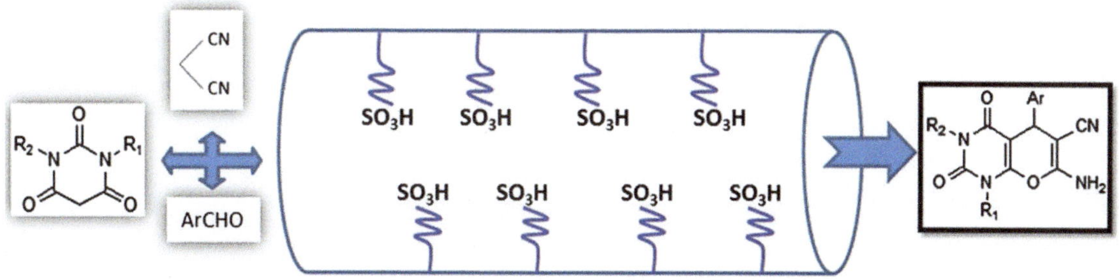

Figure 2 SBA-Pr-SO_3H act as a nano-reactor in this reaction.

The pyrano[2,3-*d*]pyrimidine diones structurally similar to barbituric acids. The antibacterial and urease inhibitory activity of barbituric acid derivatives were reported [46,48,49]. Many urease inhibitors have been synthesized and tested, but because of their toxicity and instability use of them in vivo is impossible [48-50]. Thus, the search is still on for finding strong and specific urease inhibitors.

As shown in Table 4, all prepared pyrano[2,3-*d*]pyrimidine diones are demonstrated different profile of activity. This might be due to similarity of synthesised compounds to substrate of enzyme. While compounds **4a, 4d** and **4l** were not active in urease inhibition test, compound **4a** displayed slight urease activation properties. Compounds **4b, 4k, 4f, 4e, 4j, 4g** and **4c** with hydrophobic substitutes on phenyl ring, show good inhibitory activity (Table 4). These compounds with electron donating group and subsequent hydrophobic interaction with active site of enzyme prevents the hydrolysis of substrate. Electron withdrawing groups such as nitro, 3-methoxy reduced urease inhibitory activity due to decreasing partial charge on nitrogen atoms of barbiturate moiety on pyrano[2,3-*d*] pyrimidine ring which is essential for inhibitory activity. Substitution of both hydrogen of barbituric acid with methyl groups will convert the inhibitor to activator.

Conclusions

In conclusion we have developed a nano-catalyzed multicomponent synthesis of pyrano pyrimidine diones in good to very good yields. In comparison with previous investigations (Table 3), we presented SBA-Pr-SO_3H as an efficient and active nano-reactor (Figure 2). Our method is simple as no special apparatus, reagents or chemicals, and work up are required, and the formed compound is filtered and purified just by simple crystallization. This synthesis is also advantageous in terms of atom economy as well as is devoid of any hazardous chemicals. The urease inhibitory activity of pyrano[2,3-*d*]pyrimidine dione derivatives were reported for first time.

Competing interest

The authors declare that they have no competing of interests related to this publication.

Authors' contributions

GMZ: Collaboration in design and identifying of the structures of target compounds, manuscript preparation. SF: Synthesis of the intermediates and some target compounds. SA: Synthesis of some target compounds and collaboration in identifying of the structures of target compounds. AB: Synthesis and characterization of nano catalyst. RB: Collaboration in docking study and evaluation of urease inhibitory test. MA: Collaboration in design of docking study, management of urease test and manuscript preparation. All authors read and approved the final manuscript.

Acknowledgements

We gratefully acknowledge for financial support from the Research Council of Alzahra University and University of Tehran and Tehran University of Medical Sciences.

Author details

[1]Department of Chemistry, Alzahra University, Vanak Square, P.O. Box 19938939973, Tehran, Iran. [2]School of Chemistry, College of Science, University of Tehran, Tehran, Iran. [3]Drug Design and Development Research Center and Department of Medicinal Chemistry, Faculty of Pharmacy, Tehran University of Medical Sciences, Tehran, Iran.

References

1. Tietze LF, Kettschau G: **In Topics in Current Chemistry**. In *Volume 189*. Edited by. Berlin: Springer; 1997:1–120.
2. Kitamura N, Onishi A: **Eur. Pat. 163599 (1984).** *Chem Abstr* 1984, **104:**186439.
3. Furuya S, Ohtaki T: **Pyridopyrimidine derivatives, their production and use. Eur Pat Appl EP 608565 (1994).** *Chem Abstr* 1994, **121:**205395w.
4. Heber D, Heers C, Ravens U: **Positive inotropic activity of 5-amino-6-cyano-1, 3-dimethyl-1, 2, 3, 4-tetrahydropyrido [2, 3-d] pyrim idine-2, 4-dione in cardiac muscle from guinea-pig and man. Part 6: compounds with positive inotropic activity.** *Die Pharmazie* 1993, **48:**537–541.
5. Coates WJ: **Pyrimidopyrimidine Derivatives. Eur Pat 351058.** *Chem Abstr* 1990, **113:**40711.
6. Sakuma Y, Hasegawa M, Kataoka K, Hoshina K, Yamazaki N, Kadota T, Yamaguchi H: **1, 10-Phenanthroline Derivatives. WO 91/05785 PCT Int. Appl., 1989 May 2.** *Chem Abstr* 1991, **115:**71646.
7. Broom AD, Shim JL, Anderson GL: **Pyrido [2,3-d] pyrimidines. IV. Synthetic studies leading to various oxopyrido [2,3-d] pyrimidines.** *J Org Chem* 1976, **41:**1095–1099.
8. Srivastava P, Saxena AS, Ram VJ: **An elegant approach towards the regioselective synthesis of deazalumazines through nucleophile induced ring transformation reactions of 6-aryl-3-cyano-4-methylthio-2h-pyran-2-ones.** *Synthesis* 2000, 541–544.
9. Hirota K, Kuki H, Maki Y: **Novel synthesis of pyrido[3,4-d]pyrimidines, pyrido[2,3-d]pyrimidines, and quinazolines via palladium-catalyzed oxidative coupling.** *Heterocycles* 1994, **37:**563–570.
10. Ahluwalia VK, Kumar R, Khurana K, Batla R: **A convenient synthesis of 1,3-diaryl-1,2,3,4,-tetrahydro-5,7,7-trimethyl-4-oxo-2-thioxo-7H-pyrano [2 ,3-d]pyrimidines.** *Tetrahedron* 1990, **46:**3953–3963.
11. Wamhoff H, Muhr J: **Reactions of uracils; 15. 7-Ethoxypyrimido[4,5-d] pyrimidines via a uracil-carbodiimide derivative and their products of aminolysis and pyrolysis.** *Synthesis* 1988, **11:**919–921.
12. Ahluvalia VK, Sharma HR, Tyagi R: **A novel one step synthesis of pyrano (2,3-d) pyrimidines.** *Tetrahedron* 1986, **42:**4045–4048.
13. Sharanin YA, Klokol GV: **Nitrile cyclization reactions. XVI. Reaction of arylidene drivatives of malononitrile and ethyl cyanoacetate with barbituric acid.** *Zh Org Khim* 1984, **20:**2448–2452.
14. Ibrahim MKA, El-Moghayar MRH, Sharaf MAF: **Activated nitriles in heterocyclic synthesis: a novel synthesis of pyrano[2,3-d]pyrimidine, pyrano[2,3-c]pyrazole, pyrano[2,3-d]thiazole, and thiazolo[3,2-a]pyridine drivatives.** *Indian J Chem Sect B* 1987, **26B:**216–219.
15. Gao Y, Tu S, Li T, Zhang X, Zhu S, Fang F, Shi D: **Effective synthesis of 7-amino-6-cyano-5-aryl-5H-pyrano[2,3-d]pyrimidine-2,4(1H,3H)-diones under microwave irradiation.** *Synth Commun* 2004, **34:**1295–1299.
16. Jin TS, Liu LB, Tu SJ, Zhao Y, Li TS: **Clean one-pot synthesis of 7-amino-5-aryl-6-cyano-1,5-dihydro-2H-pyrano[2,3-d]pyrimidine-2,4(3H)-diones in aqueous media under ultrasonic irradiation.** *J Chem Res* 2005, **3:**162–163.
17. Balalaie S, Abdolmohammadi S, Bijanzadeh HR, Amani AM: **Diammonium hydrogen phosphate as a versatile and efficient catalyst for the one-pot synthesis of pyrano[2,3-d]pyrimidinone derivatives in aqueous media.** *Mol Divers* 2008, **12:**85–91.
18. Heravi MM, Ghods A, Bakhtiari K, Derikvand F: **Zn[(L)proline]2: an efficient catalyst for the synthesis of biologically active pyrano[2,3-d]pyrimidine derivatives.** *Synth Commun* 2010, **40:**1927–1931.
19. Shestopalov AA, Rodinovskaya LA, Shestopalov AM, Litvinov VP: **One-step synthesis of substituted 4,8-dihydropyrano[3,2-*b*]pyran-4-ones.** *Russ Chem Bull* 2004, **53:**724–725.
20. Yu J, Wang H: **Green synthesis of pyrano[2,3--d]--pyrimidine derivatives in ionic liquids.** *Synth Commun* 2005, **35:**3133–3140.

21. Zoorob HH, Abdelhamid M, El-Zahab MA, Abdel-Mogib M, AMA I: 1, 3-Dimethylpyrimidoheterocycles as antibacterial agents. *Arzneim Forsch* 1997, **47:**958–962.
22. Heravi MM, Ghods A, Derikvand F, Bakhtiari K, Bamoharram FF: H_{14} [$NaP_5W_{30}O_{110}$] catalyzed one-pot three-component synthesis of dihydropyrano[2,3-c]pyrazole and pyrano[2,3-d]pyrimidine derivatives. *J Iran Chem Soc* 2010, **7:**615–620.
23. Mobinikhaledi A, Foroughifar N, Bodaghi Fard MA: Eco-friendly and efficient synthesis of pyrano[2,3-d] pyrimidinone and tetrahydrobenzo[b] pyran derivatives in water. *Synth React Inorg, Met-Org, Nano-Met Chem* 2010, **40:**179–185.
24. Bararjanian M, Balalaie S, Movassagh B, Amani AM: One-pot synthesis of pyrano[2,3-d]pyrimidinone derivatives catalyzed by L-proline in aqueous media. *J Iran Chem Soc* 2009, **6:**436–442.
25. Devi I, Kumar BSD, Bhuyan PJ: A novel three-component one-pot synthesis of pyrano[2,3-*d*]pyrimidines and pyrido[2,3-*d*]pyrimidines using microwave heating in the solid state. *Tetrahedron Lett* 2003, **44:**8307–8310.
26. Shaabani A, Samadi S, Rahmati A: One-pot, three-component condensation reaction in water: an efficient and improved procedure for the synthesis of pyran annulated heterocyclic systems. *Synth Commun* 2007, **37:**491–499.
27. Mashkouri S, Naimi-Jamal MR: Mechanochemical solvent-free and catalyst-free one-pot synthesis of pyrano[2,3-d]pyrimidine-2,4(1H,3H)-diones with quantitative yields. *Molecules* 2009, **14:**474–479.
28. Kresge CT, Leonowicz ME, Roth WJ, Vartuli JC, Beck JS: Ordered mesoporous molecular sieves synthesized by a liquid crystal template mechanism. *Nature* 1992, **359:**710–712.
29. Tanev PT, Pinnavaia TJ: A neutral templating route to mesoporous molecular sieves. *Science* 1995, **267:**865–867.
30. Tanev PT, Chibwe M, Pinnavaia TJ: Titanium-containing mesoporous molecular sieves for catalytic oxidation of aromatic compounds. *Nature* 1994, **368:**321–323.
31. Bagshaw SA, Pinnavaia TJ: Templating of mesoporous molecular sieves by nonionic polyethylene oxide surfactants. *Science* 1995, **268:**1242–1244.
32. Attard GS, Glyde JC, Goliner CG: Liquid-crystalline phases as templates for the synthesis of mesoporous silica. *Nature* 1995, **378:**366–368.
33. Huo QS, Leon R, Petroff PM, Stucky GD: Mesostructure design with gemini surfactants: supercage formation in a three-dimensional hexagonal array. *Science* 1995, **268:**1324–1327.
34. Zhao DY, Feng JP, Huo QS, Melosh N, Fredrickson GH, Chmelka BF, Stucky GD: Triblock copolymer syntheses of mesoporous silica with periodic 50 to 300 angstrom pores. *Science* 1998, **279:**548–552.
35. Zhao DY, Huo QS, Feng JP, Chmelka BF, Stucky GD: Nonionic triblock and star diblock copolymer and oligomeric surfactant syntheses of highly ordered, hydrothermally stable, mesoporous silica structures. *J Am Chem Soc* 1998, **120:**6024–6036.
36. Zhao DY, Sun JY, Li QZ, Stucky GD: Morphological control of highly ordered mesoporous silica SBA-15. *Chem Mater* 2000, **12:**275–279.
37. Newalkar BL, Komarneni S, Katsuki H: Rapid synthesis of mesoporous SBA-15 molecular sieve by a microwave–hydrothermal process. *Chem Commun* 2000, **23:**2389–2390.
38. Madhugiri S, Dalton A, Gutierrez J, Ferraris JP, Balkus KJ: Electrospun MEH-PPV/SBA-15 composite nanofibers using a dual syringe method. *J Am Chem Soc* 2003, **125:**14531–14538.
39. Mohammadi Ziarani G, Badiei A, Haddadpour M: Application of sulfonic acid functionalized nanoporous silica (SBA-Pr-SO_3H) for one-pot synthesis of quinoxaline derivatives. *Int J Chem* 2011, **3:**87–94.
40. Mohammadi Ziarani G, Badiei A, Khaniania Y, Haddadpour M: One Pot synthesis of polyhydroquinolines catalyzed by sulfonic acid functionalized SBA-15 as a New nanoporous acid catalyst under solvent free conditions. *Iran J Chem Chem Eng* 2010, **29:**1–10.
41. Mohammadi Ziarani G, Badiei A, Aslani Z, Lashgari N: Application of sulfonic acid functionalized nanoporous silica (SBA-Pr-SO_3H) in the green one-pot synthesis of triazoloquinazolinones and benzimidazoquinazolinones. *Arabian J Chem.* in press doi:10.1016/j.arabjc.2011.06.020.
42. Zhao DHQ, Feng J, Chmelka BF, Stucky GD: Nonionic triblock and star diblock copolymer and oligomeric sufactant syntheses of highly ordered, hydrothermally stable, mesoporous silica structures. *J Am Chem Soc* 1998, **120:**6024–6036.
43. Mohammadi Ziarani G, Badiei A, Shakiba Nahad M, Hassanzadeh M: Application of SBA-Pr-SO_3H in the synthesis of benzoxazole derivatives. *Eur J Chem* 2012, **3:**433–436.
44. Sanner MF: Python: a programming language for software integration and development. *J Mol Graph Model* 1999, **17:**57–61.
45. Morris GM, Huey R, Lindstrom W, Sanner MF, Belew RK, Goodsell DS, Olson AJ: AutoDock4 And AutoDockTools4: automated docking with selective receptor flexibility. *J Comput Chem* 2009, **30:**2785–2791.
46. Azizian H, Nabati F, Sharifi A, Siavoshi F, Mahdavi M, Amanlou M: Large-scale virtual screening for the identification of new helicobacter pylori urease inhibitor scaffolds. *J Mol Model* 2012, **18:**2917–2927.
47. Quintana-Guzman EM, Schosinsky-Nevermann K, Arias-Echandy M, Davidovich Rose H: Comparative study of urease tests for helicobacter pylori detection in gastric biopsies. *Rev Biomed* 1999, **10:**145–151.
48. Chandrashekhar C, Latha K, Vagdevi H, Vaidya V: Synthesis and antimicrobial activity of chalcones of naphtho [2, 1-b] furan condensed with barbituric acid. *Der Pharma Chemica* 2011, **3:**329–333.
49. Yan Q, Cao R, Yi W, Chen Z, Wen H, Ma L, Song H: Inhibitory effects of 5-benzylidene barbiturate derivatives on mushroom tyrosinase and their antibacterial activities. *Eur J Med Chem* 2009, **44:**4235–4243.
50. Khan KM, Ali M, Wadood A, Khan M, Lodhi MA, Perveen S, Choudhary MI, Voelter W: Molecular modeling-based antioxidant arylidene barbiturates as urease inhibitors. *J Mol Graphics Modell* 2011, **30:**153–156.

2

Effect of folic acid on bone metabolism: a randomized double blind clinical trial in postmenopausal osteoporotic women

Pooneh Salari[1*], Mohammad Abdollahi[2], Ramin Heshmat[3], Hamidreza Aghaei Meybodi[3] and Farideh Razi[3]

Abstract

Background: In spite of several studies, the impact of homocysteine level and folic acid supplementation on bone metabolism is yet to be recognized. In this registered clinical trial (IRCT2014042217385N1), we aimed to find out the power of 6-month folic acid supplementation on homocysteine level and bone metabolism.

Methods: Forty postmenopausal osteoporotic women (50 to 87 years) were enrolled in the study. All participants were randomized to receive folic acid 1 mg (n = 17) or placebo (n = 14). At baseline, 3 months, and finally 6 months post intervention, the level of homocysteine, vitamin B12, and bone biomarkers were measured.

Results: Both groups were similar at baseline. The homocysteine decreased in both groups but statistically non-significant ($P > 0.05$). The changes of the serum level of vitamin B12, osteocalcin, and β cross laps were significant between groups after 6 months ($P \leq 0.05$).

Conclusion: The trend of changes of bone biomarkers after 6 months folic acid supplementation shows that homocysteine concentration and/or folic acid supplementation have impact on the rate of bone metabolism. However, further investigations by larger sample size and differentiating age and gender are still needed to clarify the exact role of folate, homocysteine and vitamin B12.

Keywords: Homocysteine, Folic acid, BMD, Bone biomarkers, Osteoporosis, Clinical trial

Introduction

Osteoporosis, the senile chronic disease is mainly caused by estrogen deficiency, while, environmental and lifestyle factors as well as metabolic and genetic disorders are contributing. As a chronic senile inflammatory disease, it is believed that osteoporosis has common pathophysiological basis with cardiovascular diseases [1]. Hyperhomocysteinemia is considered as an independent risk factor for several chronic senile diseases and conditions including cardiovascular diseases, and Alzheimer disease [2,3]. As the number of devastating consequences in osteoporotic patients is increasing worldwide, determining the possible risk factors and their elimination is crucial. Keeping this in mind, recent studies have shown the possible role of platelets, inflammation, and homocysteine as well as the role of specific medications in the common pathophysiologic pathway of cardiovascular diseases and osteoporosis [4-10]. Accordingly, the role of hyperhomocysteinemia in the pathogenesis of osteoporosis has been considered as a focal point. Serum concentration of homocysteine is inversely related to those of vitamin B12 and folic acid [11]. From one point during menopause the serum level of homocysteine is increased and from the other point hyperhomocysteinemia is linked with risk of fracture. Folate supplementation may modify the serum concentration of homocysteine, and of greater importance may affect fracture risk, because high homocysteine levels increase the risk of fracture [12]. To our knowledge, there is no enough data about the effect of folate supplementation and homocysteine lowering therapy on bone metabolism and fracture risk. Our previous systematic review showed the possible impact of high homocysteine level on bone quality via induction of osteoclast related bone resorption [3]. With all these in mind, the exact role of homocysteine

* Correspondence: poonehsalari@gmail.com
[1]Medical Ethics and History of Medicine Research Center, Tehran University of Medical Sciences, 23# 16 Azar Ave, Keshavarz Blvd, 1417633114 Tehran, Iran
Full list of author information is available at the end of the article

level and folic acid supplementation in regulation of bone metabolism is yet to be elucidated. Based on the implication of bone biomarkers in determination of bone metabolism in osteoporotic patients in a short period of time we aimed to examine the effect of folic acid supplementation on serum level of homocysteine and bone metabolism in postmenopausal osteoporotic women in a randomized, double-blind, placebo-controlled study. For this purpose, we selected key indicators such as bone specific alkaline phosphatase (BALP) from enzymes, osteocalcin (OC) from bone protein markers, β cross laps (CTX) and pyridinoline (PYD) from collagenous bone resorption markers to evaluate bone metabolism. All selected bone biomarkers are easily changed within 3–6 months treatment and usually used for monitoring effectiveness of treatment. Furthermore measuring OC and CTX both together is considered as a reasonable choice for evaluating bone degradation and synthesis [13].

Methods

Subjects

Forty postmenopausal osteoporotic women who referred to the Diabetes and Metabolic Disorders Clinic were enrolled in the double blind randomized clinical trial. Osteoporosis was diagnosed by the mean of dual energy X-ray absorptimetry (Hologic®) at femur neck and lumbar vertebrae in all participants. Osteoporosis was defined on the basis of WHO criteria as having BMD ≥ 2.5 SD below the normal mean for young adult women or T-sore ≤ −2.5. Participants profile including age, age at menopause, habit of smoking, alcohol consumption, past medical history and use of medications were collected. Participants with a history of cancer, acute infection, endocrinology diseases, taking medications affecting bone metabolism, such as corticosteroids, gonadotropin releasing hormone (GnRH) analogues, anticonvulsant drugs, heparin, aluminum containing antacids, thyroid hormones and anti-osteoporosis medications were excluded (Table 1). The study was registered in the Iranian Registry of Clinical Trials with the code of IRCT2014042217385N1.

The study was approved by the Ethics Committee of the Endocrinology and Metabolism Research Institute of Tehran University of Medical Sciences. All participants signed the written informed consent after receiving complete information about the study and their contribution.

Table 1 Exclusion criteria

Exclusion criteria	
Cancer	Medications:
Acute infection	Corticosteroids
Endocrinologic diseases	Gonadotropin releasing hormone (GnRH) and its analogues Antiosteoporotic medications (bisphosphonates, calcium and vitamin D, teriparatide, calcitonin, etc)
Taking medications affecting bone metabolism	Anticonvulsants
	Heparin
	Aluminum containing antacids
	Thyroid hormones
	Selective serotonin reuptake inhibitors (SSRIs)

Experimental design

All participants were randomly assigned to folic acid or placebo. The patients' assignments were double blind. The method of randomization was simple. Because of few dose–response studies, the most proper dose of folic acid to lower homocysteine concentration is not fully clarified. In a dose–response trial, no significant relation was observed in reduction of homocysteine level when various doses of folic acid were used [8]. Also, the Homocysteine Lowering Trialists Collaboration meta-analysis showed no significant dose-dependent response in the dose range (800–2000 μg/day) of folic acid [14]. Noteworthy, pharmacological doses of folic acid (5 mg/day) may increase the risk of adverse effects [15]. Therefore, present study was designed to administer folic acid at dose of 1 mg/day as a supplement (Figure 1).

Both folic acid and placebo tablets were completely similar in taste, texture and appearance and were produced by Rooz Daru Company (Iran). All participants were asked to inform the clinic in the case of any change in their lifestyle, medication or occurrence of any side effect. Over the study period, in each visit, the patients were asked to feel free to exit from the study if they did not comply with the described protocol.

Laboratory studies

Blood and urine samples were taken at baseline and after 3 and 6 months. All samples were collected in the early morning and fasting condition. Blood samples were centrifuged at 10000 × g for 10 min and kept in the fridge at −70°C until analysis. Serum levels of bone biomarkers including OC, BALP, homocysteine, vitamin B12 and urinary concentrations of PYD and β cross laps were measured. Serum OC and β cross laps were quantified by N-MID®Osteocalcin ELISA and Urine BETA CrossLaps® ELISA Immuno Diagnostic Systems (IDS) (Germany), respectively. Urinary PYD and serum level of BALP were measured by MICROVUE PYD EIA® and MICROVUE BAP EIA® Kits from QUIDEL Corporation (Germany), respectively. Serum level of homocysteine was quantified with enzymatic assay by Axis Shield® and serum level of vitamin B12 was measured by the method of chemiluminescence By Diasorin Liaison®. Intra- and inter-assay coefficients of variation (CV) were 2.2% and 5.1% for osteocalcin, 3.9% and 6.9% for β cross

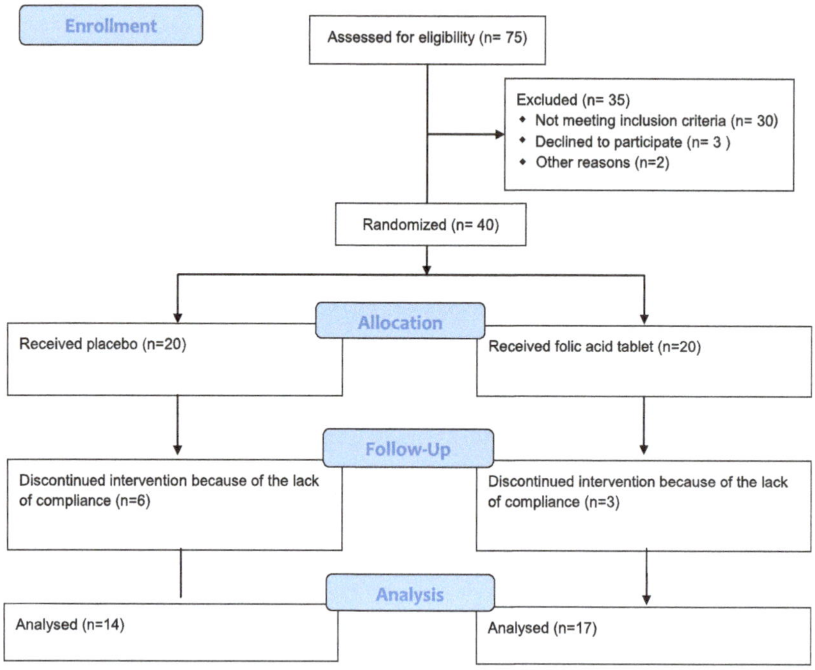

Figure 1 Consort flowchart.

laps, 11.2% and 9.9% for PYD, 7.6% and 5.8% for BALP, and 4.4% and 2.2% for homocysteine.

Statistical analysis

The StatsDirect version 3.0.117 was used for statistical analysis. Data are expressed as mean ± SD. Normal distribution of data was confirmed by Kolmogorov-Smirnov test. Baseline values and values after supplementation were compared using T-test. Comparison between groups before and after supplementation was performed using General Linear Model (repeated measure) test. The Pearson correlation test was used for correlations. $P \leq 0.05$ was considered significant.

Results

The study performed on 40 postmenopausal women, of those 31 participants completed the study (response rate = 77.5%). Three participants from the treatment group and 6 participants from the control group withdrew the study because of lack of compliance (Figure 1). Table 2 shows the demographic data of all participants. No lifestyle or medication change as well as side effect was recorded. The distribution of data was normal. No statistically significant difference was found between groups at baseline (Table 2). The average baseline homocysteine and vitamin B12 levels were 12.77 μmol/L and 605.72 pg/ml, respectively. The average baseline level of BALP, OC and CTX was 30.5 U/L, 15.48 ng/ml, and 2.74 (μg/mmol Cr), respectively which were in the normal range. The average baseline urinary PYD level of 43.27 (μg/mmol Cr) was higher than normal level.

Table 3 presents the biochemical results after supplementation. The serum level of homocysteine decreased in both groups along the study. No significant change was found in each group ($P = 0.22$ in treatment group versus $P = 0.26$ in the control group) and between groups at 6 months ($P = 0.06$).

In the treatment group, the serum level of vitamin B12 decreased in the first three months followed by an increase after 6 months, while in the control group it decreased during the study period. No significant change in the serum level of vitamin B12 was found in each group ($P = 0.189$ and $P = 0.173$). After 6 months serum concentration of vitamin B12 was significantly lower in the control group compared with the treatment group ($P = 0.01$) (Table 3).

The serum level of OC showed a non-significant increase and a decrease in the control group ($P = 0.460$) and treatment groups, respectively ($P = 0.384$). After 6 months, serum level of OC was significantly higher in the control group compared with the treatment group ($P = 0.034$; Table 3).

The serum level of BALP showed a non-significant increase in the treatment ($P = 0.614$) and control ($P = 0.326$) groups. No significant difference was observed between groups after 6 months ($P = 0.543$; Table 3).

Table 2 Demographic data and baseline characteristics of study participants

	Normal values	Treatment group (17)	Control group (14)	*P* value
Age (yr)		63.8 ± 8.1	64.2 ± 7.3	0.870
BMI (kg/m^2)		25.2 ± 4.5	26.7 ± 3.1	0.290
Age at menopause (yr)		48.8 ± 4.6	46.6 ± 4.7	0.196
Lumbar BMD (g/cm^2)		0.67 ± 0.16	0.71 ± 0.06	0.370
Femoral BMD		0.59 ± 0.07	0.60 ± 0.06	0.709
Lumbar T-score		−3.11 ± 0.43	−3.01 ± 0.62	0.615
Femoral T-score		−2.32 ± 0.63	−2.29 ± 0.46	0.832
Homocysteine (μmol/L)	5-20	11.70 ± 6.63	14.07 ± 3.60	0.242
Vit B12 (Pg/ml)	160-970	745.70 ± 623.07	435.75 ± 245.25	0.091
OC (ng/ml)	12.8-55.0	15.34 ± 6.94	15.66 ± 9.99	0.916
BALP (U/L)	14.2-42.7	29.94 ± 11.02	31.17 ± 11.90	0.767
UPYD (μg/mmol cr)	16.0-37.0	42.99 ± 11.67	43.61 ± 11.14	0.882
U β cross laps (μg/mmol cr)	0.73-7.07	2.45 ± 1.58	3.10 ± 1.75	0.285

All data are presented as Mean ± SD. Yr = year; BMI = body mass index; BMD = bone mineral density; Vit B12 = vitamin B12; OC = osteocalcin; BALP = bone alkaline phosphatase; UPYD = urine pyridinium cross links; U β cross laps = urine β cross laps.

The urinary levels of PYD and β cross laps non-significantly increased in both groups, more prominently in the control group (Table 3). After 6 months, the increase in the level of β cross laps in the control group was higher than that of treatment group ($P = 0.01$).

Baseline level of PYD and BALP in the control group was inversely correlated with BMD and T-score of the lumbar spine ($r = -0.53$, $P = 0.05$) and ($r = -0.59$, $P = 0.02$), respectively. In the control group, the level of β cross laps at baseline and after 6 months showed a negative correlation with BMD and T-score of the lumbar spine ($r = -0.61$, $P = 0.02$) and ($r = -0.61$, $P = 0.01$), respectively. In addition homocysteine concentration at the end of the study was inversely correlated with BMD and T-score of femur ($r = -0.65$, $P = 0.01$) and ($r = -61$, $P = 0.01$), respectively.

Discussion

In this study we aimed to evaluate the effect of folate supplementation on homocysteine level and bone metabolism in postmenopausal osteoporotic women. In addition we presumed correlations between homocysteine, bone biomarkers and bone specific characteristics including BMD and T score. For this purpose we measured each participant's BMD and T-score of the femur and lumbar spine as well as bone biomarkers. In fact measuring femoral BMD has been considered as the standard of choice for osteoporosis because this site

Table 3 Statistics for serum concentrations of bone biomarkers in both groups in the study period

	Treatment group (N = 17)			*P* value	Control group (N = 14)			*P* value
	Baseline	3 months	6 months		Baseline	3 months	6 months	
Homocysteine (μmol/L)	11.70 ± 6.63	11.52 ± 4.47	10.17 ± 4.09	0.226	14.07 ± 3.60	14.50 ± 4.78	13.21 ± 4.54	0.266
CI 95%	8.55-14.85	9.40-13.65	8.23-12.12		12.18-15.96	11.99-17.00	10.83-15.59	
Vit B12 (Pg/ml)	745.70 ± 623.07	517.17 ± 260.77	655.17 ± 460.18	0.189	435.75 ± 245.25	375.50 ± 475.02	235.42 ± 57.96	0.173
CI 95%	449.51-1041.89	393.21-641.14	436.42-873.94		307.69-564.23	126.66-624.33	205.70-265.79	
OC (ng/ml)	15.34 ± 6.94	14.10 ± 6.13	13.84 ± 4.87	0.384	15.66 ± 9.99	16.71 ± 9.92	17.70 ± 10.03	0.460
95% CI	12.03-18.64	11.18-17.02	11.53-16.16		10.43-20.90	11.51-21.91	12.44-22.96	
BALP (U/L)	29.94 ± 11.02	30.82 ± 9.66	31.74 ± 9.30	0.614	31.17 ± 11.90	32.14 ± 14.35	34.46 ± 15.10	0.326
95% CI	24.70-35.19	26.23-35.42	27.33-36.17		24.94-37.41	24.62-39.66	26.55-42.37	
UPYD (μg/mmol cr)	42.99 ± 11.67	47.18 ± 9.99	46.61 ± 17.60	0.369	43.61 ± 11.14	45.11 ± 11.04	51.26 ± 15.56	0.107
95% CI	37.44-48.54	42.43-51.93	38.25-54.99		37.78-49.45	39.32-50.90	43.11-59.41	
U β cross laps (μg/mmol cr)	2.45 ± 1.58	2.43 ± 1.22	2.77 ± 1.86	0.358	3.10 ± 1.75	3.25 ± 1.92	3.68 ± 2.40	0.398
95% CI	1.70-3.20	1.85-3.01	1.90-3.66		2.18-4.03	2.24-4.27	2.42-4.94	

All data are presented as Mean ± SD. CI = confidence interval; Vit B12 = vitamin B12; OC = osteocalcin; BALP = bone alkaline phosphatase; UPYD = urine pyridinium cross links; U β cross laps = urine β cross laps.

shows the fracture risk similar or higher than that of other sites [16].

Our results showed that supplementation with 1 mg folic acid non-significantly decreases homocysteine level; however reduction of homocysteine in the treatment group was more than control group. According to the Table 1, the mean homocyteine level of all participants at baseline was higher than 10 μmol/L which is a mild elevation [17]. There are several studies which indicate significant homocysteine lowering effect of folic acid in doses 400–800 μg per day [18-20]. It is noteworthy to consider that participants of those studies were supplemented with different doses of vitamin B12 (9–1000 μg/day) in addition to folic acid. We suppose that lack of significant effects of folic acid supplementation on homocysteine level is because of mildly elevated values of homocysteine and normal levels of vitamin B12 in both groups at the baseline. Our thought is in agreement with that of Homocysteine Lowering Trialists Collaboration [14]. In addition to serum homocysteine level, folate status may be affected. There is a report that in healthy older adults with normal serum folate level, folic acid supplementation cannot reduce homocysteine level while in those with low serum folate supplementation it may lower homocysteine concentration [21]. It should be noted that in our study and most of other studies, blood samples were taken in the fasting state while a study indicated that about 50% of participants show hyperhomocysteinemia after methionine load [22]. Therefore it is suggested that fasting blood sample lacks enough sensitivity for measuring serum homocysteine. Likewise racial differences which affect polymorphism of the methylenetetrahydrofolate reductase (MTFHR) gene may affect homocysteine metabolism and should be taken into account in future studies.

In the control group the hemocysteine level at the end of the study was negatively correlated with BMD and T score of femur at baseline ($r = -0.65$, $P = 0.01$). Although several studies indicated significant higher levels of homocysteine in osteoporotic women and its inverse relationship with BMD of total femur [23-25] or the risk of fracture [26,27], other investigations did not confirm the association between homocysteine and BMD and/or bone markers [28,29]. This is because of a weak correlation between homocysteine and BMD that failed to be detected in small sample size. A dose–response relationship between homocysteine concentration and bone loss in men and premenopausal women has been reported [30]. In a case–control study in the Women's Health Initiative Observational Study, the modest association of high homocysteine levels with increased risk of hip fracture was found [12]. On the other hand, a high level of homocysteine or low level of vitamin B12 and folate were not found as the risk factors of vertebral fractures in postmenopausal women. However, the relationship between levels of homocysteine and vitamin B12 and low BMD was recognized [31]. In a cohort study, association of high homocysteine concentration and higher bone loss over 4 years in postmenopausal women was found [32].

Our data showed significant difference in the serum level of vitamin B12 after 6 months and its serum level was significantly lower in the control group at the end of the study ($P = 0.01$).

Vitamin B12 acts as a cofactor for transformation of homocysteine to methionine. So both folic acid and vitamin B12 may reduce serum homocysteine. Vitamin B12 seems to be involved in osteoblast activity and formation of bone [33], and inhibits osteoclast function [34]; however, the exact mechanism of vitamin B12 in influencing bone density is not fully understood.

According to the Framingham Osteoporosis Study, serum level of vitamin B12 less than 250 pg/ml is considered as vitamin B12 deficiency and is associated with lower BMD [35]. The participants in our study had normal serum level of vitamin B12 and after 6 months its mean interestingly reached 233.45 pg/ml in the control group.

We found no correlation between vitamin B12 and bone markers or BMD which is in agreement with other study which showed no relationship between vitamin B12 supplementation and level of BALP in Mexican women [36].

It was found that vitamin B12 and folate are correlated with BMD in postmenopausal women and the possibility of involvement of a mechanistic link was suggested [37].

We observed non-significant increase and decrease in the level of OC in the control and treatment groups, respectively; however we found a significant difference between groups. To date no study has evaluated the pattern of alteration of OC in relation to homocysteine.

The level of BALP over the study period showed non-significant increase in both groups, more profoundly in the control group.

Homocysteine interacts with lysyl oxidase in collagen post-translational modifications and cross linking. Therefore it influences formation of the cross-link [38]. In addition to bone formation markers, bone resorption markers including PYD and β cross laps were assessed in the present study. Our results showed parallel non-significant increase in the levels of both PYD and β cross laps in both groups. Furthermore the level of β cross laps was significantly higher in the control group. According to the higher level of all measured bone biomarkers in the control group after 6 months, it is suggested that folic acid supplementation reduces serum level of homocysteine which follows by suppression of bone metabolism. However because of small sample size, the power of our study does not permit to prove our hypothesis. Not only our study but also studies with longer duration up to 2 years could not show a significant effect of folic acid supplementation on bone markers [34,39]. Despite a significant reduction of homocysteine levels with folic acid and vitamin B12 supplementation, no significant impact of vitamin B supplementation on bone markers was found in another study while the final level of CTX and alkaline phosphatase was higher in the control group [17]. In contrast, a study reported a strong correlation between homocysteine and serum c-terminal telopeptide (CTx) levels [40]. The results of a recent longitudinal study showed a positive correlation between homocysteine and total alkaline phosphatase. It was concluded that increase in BALP after hyperhomocysteinemia is the result of induction of bone regeneration after bone resorption [29]. Those results may support our results from this point of view.

Regarding the small sample size and enrolment of patients from one referral center limits extrapolation of the results of the study. Although we asked the participants to follow their routine lifestyle in the study period, our information about their lifestyle is lacking. Noteworthy to consider, all of the participants had mildly elevated serum level of homocysteine which may affect their response to supplementation; also none of the participants were taking calcium and/or vitamin D or other type of supplement.

Our study presents that level of all of the biochemical bone markers showed the highest increase in the control group versus the treatment group in the study period and the changes in OC, and β cross laps were significant between groups. Our hypothesis is that serum level of homocysteine, folate supplementation and serum level of vitamin B12 may have a preventive effect on bone metabolism and inversely affect bone metabolism and its rate, however because of the limited sample size, the potency of our study is not enough to be extrapolated. Therefore further investigations about the impact of folic acid supplementation on the rate of bone metabolism in men and women from different ages with larger sample size is highly recommended.

Competing interests
The authors declare that they have no competing interests.

Authors' contribution
PS: Study design, preparing the medication, performing the study, statistical analysis and drafting the manuscript; MA: Contribution in study design, performing the study, revising the manuscript; RH: Collaboration in performing the study, statistical analysis and revising the manuscript; HRAM: Contribution in study design, performing the study and revising the draft; FR: Laboratory analysis and revision of the draft. All authors read and approved the final manuscript.

Acknowledgement
The research project financially supported by Endocrinology and Metabolism Research Institute and Diabetic Research Center of Tehran University of Medical Sciences and the authors would like to thank them. Also the authors would like to thank Dr Keshtkar, Miss Shirazi and Dr Ghorbani for their great help and assistance. Also we gratitude all study participants.

Author details
[1]Medical Ethics and History of Medicine Research Center, Tehran University of Medical Sciences, 23# 16 Azar Ave, Keshavarz Blvd, 1417633114 Tehran, Iran. [2]Faculty of Pharmacy and Pharmaceutical Sciences Research Center, Tehran University of Medical Sciences, Tehran, Iran. [3]Endocrinology and Metabolism Research Institute, Tehran University of Medical Sciences, Tehran, Iran.

References
1. Salari P, Abdollahi M: **A comprehensive review of the shared roles of inflammatory cytokines in osteoporosis and cardiovascular diseases as two common old people problem: actions toward development of new drugs.** *Int J Pharmacol* 2011, **7**(5):552–567.
2. Wald DS, Law M, Morris JK: **Homocysteine and cardiovascular disease: evidence on causality from a meta-analysis.** *Br Med J* 2002, **325**:1202–1206.
3. Seshadri S, Beiser A, Selhub J, Jacques PF, Rosenberg IH, D'Agostino RB, Wilson PW, Wolf PA: **Plasma homocysteine as a risk factor for dementia and Alzheimer's disease.** *N Engl J Med* 2002, **346**:476–483.
4. Salari P, Abdollahi M: **Association of hyperhomocysteinemia with osteoporosis: a systematic review.** *Therapy* 2008, **5**(2):215–222.
5. Salari P, Abdollahi M: **The role of platelets in bone remodeling.** *Inflamm Allergy Drug Target* 2010, **9**:393–399.
6. Salari P, Abdollahi M: **Controversial effects of non-steroidal anti-inflammatory drugs on bone: a review.** *Inflamm Allergy Drug Target* 2009, **8**:169–175.
7. Salari Sharif P, Asalforoush M, Ameri F, Larijani B, Abdollahi M: **The effect of n-3 fatty acids on bone biomarkers in Iranian postmenopausal osteoporotic women: a randomized clinical trial.** *AGE* 2010, **32**:179–186.
8. Salari Sharif P, Abdollahi M: **A systematic review on the relation between use of statins and osteoporosis.** *Int J Pharmacol* 2011, **7**(2):180–188.
9. Salari Sharif P, Abdollahi M: **A systematic review on the relationship between β-blockers and bone health.** *Int J Pharmacol* 2010, **6**(5):577–583.
10. Abdollahi M, Larijani B, Rahimi R, Salari P: **Role of oxidative stress in osteoporosis.** *Therapy* 2005, **2**(5):787–796.
11. Brattstrom L: **Vitamins as homocysteine-lowering agents.** *J Nutr* 1996, **126**:S1276–S1280.
12. LeBoff MS, Narweker R, LaCroix A, Wu L, Jackson R, Lee J, Bauer DC, Cauley J, Kooperberg C, Lewis C, Thomas AM, Cummings S: **Homocysteine levels and risk of hip fracture in postmenopausal women.** *J Clin Endocrinol Metab* 2009, **94**:1207–1213.
13. Leeming DJ, Alexandersen P, Karsdal MA, Qvist P, Schaller S, Tankó LB: **An update on biomarkers of bone turnover and their utility in biomedical research and clinical practice.** *Eur J Clin Pharmacol* 2006, **62**:781–792.
14. Homocysteine Lowering Trialists Collaboration: **Lowering blood homocysteine with folic acid based supplements: meta-analysis of randomized trials.** *BMJ* 1998, **316**:894–898.
15. Van Wijngaarden JP, Dhonukshe-Rutten RA, Van Schoor NM, van der Velde N, Swart KM, Enneman AW, Van Dijk SC, Brouwer-Brolsma EM, Zilikens MC, Van Meurs JB, Brug J, Uitterlinden AG, Lips P, De Groot LC: **Rationale and design of the B-PROOF study, a randomized controlled trial on the effect of supplemental intake of vitamin B12 and folic acid on fracture incidence.** *BMC Geriatric* 2011, **11**:80.
16. Kanis JA, McCloskey EV, Johansson H, Oden A, Melton LJ III, Khaltaev N: **A reference standard for the description of osteoporosis.** *Bone* 2008, **42**:467–475.
17. Jacques PF, Selhub J, Bostom AG, Wilson PWF, Rosenberg IH: **The effect of folic acid fortification on plasma folate and total homocysteine concentrations.** *N Engl J Med* 1999, **340**:1449–1454.
18. Keser I, Ilich JZ, Vrkic N, Giljevic Z, Colic Baric I: **Folic acid and vitamin B12 supplementation lowers plasma homocysteine but has no effect on serum bone turnover markers in elderly women: a randomized, double-blind, placebo-controlled trial.** *Nutr Res* 2013, **33**:211–219.
19. Wolters M, Hermann S, Hahn A: **Effect of multivitamin supplementation on the homocysteine and methylmalonic acid blood concentrations in women over the age of 60 years.** *Eur J Nutr* 2005, **44**:183–192.
20. Lewerin C, Nilsson-Ehle H, Matousek M, Lindstedi G, Steen B: **Reduction of plasma homocysteine and serum methylmalonate concenttrations in apparently healthy elderly subjects after treatment with folic acid, vitamin B12 and vitamin B6: a randomized trial.** *Eur J Clin Nutr* 2003, **57**:1426–1436.

21. Anderson CAM, Jee SH, Charleston J, Narrett M, Appel LJ: **Effects of folic acid supplementation on serum folate and plasma homocysteine concentrations in older adults: a dose–response trial.** *Am J Epidemiol* 2010, **172:**932–941.
22. Van der Driend R, Biesma DH, Banga JD: **Postmethionine-load homocysteine determination for the diagnosis of hyperhomocysteinemia and efficacy of homocysteine lowering treatment regimens.** *Vasc Med* 2001, **7:**29–33.
23. Bozkurt N, Erdem M, Yilmaz E, Erdem A, Biri A, Kubatova A, Bozkurt M: **The relationship of homocysteine B12 and folic acid with the bone mineral density of the femur and lumbar spine in Turkish postmenopausal women.** *Arch Gynecol Obstet* 2009, **280:**381–387.
24. Bucciarelli P, Martini G, Martinelli I, Ceccarelli E, Gennari L: **The relationship between plasma homocysteine levels and bone mineral density in post-menopausal women.** *European J Intern Med* 2010, **21:**301–305.
25. Kuyumcu ME, Yesil Y, Oztürk ZA, Cınar E, Kızılarslanoglu C, Halil M, Ulger Z, Yesil NK, Cankurtaran M, Anoğul S: **The association between homocysteine (hcy) and serum natural antioxidants in elderly bone mineral densitometry (BMD).** *Arch Gerontol Geriatr* 2012, **55:**739–743.
26. Van Meurs JB, Dhonukshe-Rutten RA, Pluijm SM, van der Klift M, De Jonge R, Lindemans J, De Groot LC, Hofman A, Witteman JC, Van Leeuwen JP, Breteler MM, Lips P, Pols HA, Uitterlinden AG: **Homocysteine levels and the risk of osteoporotic fracture.** *N Eng J Med* 2004, **350:**2033–2041.
27. McLean RR, Jacques PF, Selhub J, Tucker KL, Samelson EJ, Broe KE, Hannan MT, Cupples LA, Kiel DP: **Homocysteine as a predictive factor for hip fracture in older persons.** *N Eng J Med* 2004, **350:**2042–2049.
28. Holstein JH, Herrmann M, Splett C, Hermann W, Garcia P, Histing T, Klein M, Kurz K, Siebel T, Pohlemann T, Menger MD: **Hyper homocysteinemia is not associated with reduced bone quality in humans with hip osteoarthritis.** *Clin Chem Lab Med* 2010, **48:**821–827.
29. Rumbak I, Zizic V, Sokolić L, Cvijetićc S, Kajfež R, Barić IC: **Bone mineral density is not associated with homocysteine level, folate and vitamin B12 status.** *Arch Gyneol Obstet* 2012, **285:**991–1000.
30. Kim BJ, Koh JM, Ahn SH, Lee SH, Kim EH, Bae SJ, Kim HK, Choe JW, Lim KH, Pyun KH, Kim TH, Kim SY, Kim GS: **High serum total homocysteine levels accelerates hip bone loss in healthy premenopausal women and men.** *Bone* 2013, **52:**56–62.
31. Maghraoui AE, Ghozlani I, Mounach A, Rezqi A, Oumghar K, Achemlal L, Bezza A, Ouzzif Z: **Homocysteine folate and vitamin B12 levels and vertebral fracture risk in postmenopausal women.** *J Clin Densitometr* 2012, **15:**328–333.
32. Zhu K, Beilby J, Dick IM, Devine A, Soós M: **The effects of homocysteine and MTHFR genotype on hip bone loss and fracture risk in elderly women.** *Osteoporos Int* 2009, **20:**1183–1191.
33. Kim GS, Kim CH, Park JY, Lee KU, Park CS: **Effects of vitamin B12 on cell proliferation and cellular alkaline phosphatase activity in human bone marrow stromal osteoprogenitor cells and UMR106 osteoblastic cells.** *Metabolism* 1996, **45:**1443–1446.
34. Herrmann M, Schmist J, Umanskaya N, Colaianni G, Al Marrawi F, Widmann T, Zallone A, Wildemann B, Herrmann W: **Stimulation of osteoclast activity by low B-vitamin concentrations.** *Bone* 2007, **41:**584–591.
35. Tucker KL, Hannan MT, Qiao N, Jacques PF, Selhub J, Cupples LA, Kiel DP: **Low plasma vitamin B12 associated with lower bone mineral density: the Framingham osteoporosis study.** *J Bone Miner Res* 2005, **20:**152–158.
36. Shahab-Ferdows S, Anaya-Loyola MA, Vergara-Castañeda H, Rosado JL, Keyes WR, Newman JW, Miller JW, Allen LH: **Vitamin B-12 supplementation of rural Mexican women changes biochemical vitamin B-12 status indicators but does not affect hematology or a bone turnover marker.** *J Nutr* 2012, **142:**1881–1887.
37. Haliloglu B, Aksungar FB, Ilter E, Peker H, Akm FT, Ozekier U: **Relationship between bone mineral density bone turnover markers and homocysteine folate and vitamin B12 levels in postmenopausal women.** *Arch Gynecol Obstet* 2010, **281:**663–668.
38. Liu G, Nellaiappan K, Kagan HM: **Irreversible inhibition of lysyl oxidase by homocysteine thiolactone and its selenium and oxygen analogues. Implications for homocystinuria.** *J Biol Chem* 1997, **272:**32370–32377.
39. Herrmann M, Umanskaya N, Traber L, Schmidt-Gayk H, Menke W, Lanzer G, Lenhart M, Peter Schmidt J, Herrmann W: **The effect of B-vitamins on biochemical bone turnover markers and bone mineral density in osteoporotic patients: a 1-year double blind placebo controlled trial.** *Clin Chem Lab Med* 2007, **45:**1785–1792.
40. Gerdhem P, Iwaska KK, Isakkson A, Pettersson K, Väänänen HK, Obrant KJ, Akesson K: **Associations between homocysteine bone turnover BMD mortality and fracture risk in elderly women.** *J Bone Miner Res* 2007, **22:**127–134.

3

Synthesis, *in vitro* aerobic and hypoxic cytotoxicity and radiosensitizing activity of novel metronidazole tethered 5-fluorouracil

Khosrou Abdi[1,2], Ali Khalaj[2,4*], Seyed Nasser Ostad[3], Navid Lamei[4] and Mohammad Reza Khoshayand[5]

Abstract

Background and the purpose of the study: Several 2, 4-dinitrophenyl and 2,4-dinitrophenylamine tethered 5-FU (5-fluorouracil) compared to their components have shown minimal or no cytotoxicity to HT-29 cell line under aerobic conditions but high cytotoxicity and radiosensitizing effects under hypoxic conditions. In the present study the cytotoxicity and radiation potentiation of three novel analogues of these compounds by replacing 2,4-dinitrophenyl moiety with 2-methyl-5-nitroimidazole, a known radiosensitizer and cytotoxic agent was investigated.

Methods: Tethered compounds **7–9** were prepared by the reaction of 1-(*t*-butoxycarbonyl)-5-fluorouracil **6** with metronidazole esters **2–4** followed by removal of the *t*-butoxycarbonyl protecting group. Cytotoxicity of compounds in HT-29 cells with or without radiation were determined by 3-(4,5-Dimethylthiazol-2-yl)-2,5-diphenyltetrazolium bromide (MTT), propidium iodide (PI)-digitonin and clonogenic assays.

Results: Tethered compounds **7–9** induced time-and concentration–dependent cytotoxicity under hypoxia but had no significant effect under aerobic conditions. These compounds also showed selective and concentration- dependent radiosensitization effects under hypoxic conditions.

Conclusion: Tethered compounds **7–9** compared to 5-FU **5** showed minimal cytotoxicities under aerobic and selective radiosensitizing activities under hypoxic conditions. Also effects of these compounds were higher than those of metronidazole **1** which is a known cytotoxin and radiosensitizer under hypoxic conditions.

Keywords: Cytotoxicity, Radiosensitizing, Metronidazole, 5-Fluorouracil, MTT& PI-digitonin assays

Introduction

Oxygen as a radiosensitizer increases the effects of radiation by the formation of free radicals that damage DNA [1]. Electron affinic nitroaromatic and nitroheterocyclic compounds act like oxygen by formation of nitro radical anion through one electron reduction and are solid tumor targeting agents because of the presence of hypoxic cells in these tumors due to insufficient blood supply [2]. The cytotoxicity of these compounds under hypoxia has also been attributed to an increase in the oxidative damage of DNA, formation of hydroxyl compounds under deoxygenated conditions, and suppression of intracellular radioprotectors of sulfhydryl compounds [3]. Under aerobic conditions where the initially reduced species can be readily re-oxidized by molecular oxygen, the cytotoxicity of these compounds has been attributed to the parent nitro compounds, or bio-activation by NADPH: quinine oxidoreductase (DT diaphorase) which can act as an oxygen insensitive reductase [4].

Nitroimidazoles [1,2] specifically 2- and 5-nitro derivatives are known as cytotoxin and radiosensitizer toward hypoxic cells and have been subject of many clinical studies. However these compounds have shown limited therapeutic impact on radiotherapy due to clinical problems that includes dose-limiting side effects such as neurotoxicity [5]. Additionally several hybrid or dual functional agents have been described in which nitroimidazoles are attached through a linker unit to cytotoxic nitrogen mustards, [1,2,6] and aziridine moieties

* Correspondence: akhalaj@tums.ac.ir
[2]Department of Medicinal Chemistry, Tehran University of Medical Sciences, Tehran 14174, Iran
[4]Drug Design & Development Research Center, Tehran University of Medical Sciences, Tehran 14174, Iran
Full list of author information is available at the end of the article

[1,2,7] which have shown higher cytotoxicity and enhanced radiosensitizing activity than those of the corresponding counterparts in both aerobic and hypoxic cells. In these compounds cellular reduction of the nitro group to more electron donating species activate the nitrogen of the cytotoxic group by the release of electron through the aromatic ring and generate reactive alkylating species [7].

Previously, results of our study on *in vitro* aerobic cytotoxicity of 2, 4-dinitrophenylamine tethered 5-FU through three carbon atoms in HT-29 cell line with and without radiation showed that the compound unlike its components has no cytotoxicity but is radiosensitizer [8]. Since in the tested compound 5-FU is not a leaving group, it was reasoned that the aerobic cytotoxicity of the reported 2,4-dinitrophenylamine mustard [6] and 2,4-dinitrophenyl aziridine [7] are due to their alkylating moieties.

Also results of our investigations on 2,4-dinitrobenzyl, 2,4-dinitrobenzoyl, 3,5-dinitrobenzoyl and 2,4-dinitrophenacetyl derivatives of 5-FU showed that with exception of 3,5-dinitrobenzoyl derivatives other compounds have selective- cytotoxicity and radiosensitization effects under hypoxic conditions [9]. Since the IC_{50} values of compounds which showed selective cytotoxicity were not different significantly it was concluded that they have similar mechanism of action and might produce the same reactive species [9].

In continuation of our investigations on this type of bifunctional compounds [8-11] in the present study the cytotoxicity and radiosensitization effects of three novel analogues of these compounds by replacing 2,4-dinitrophenyl moiety with 2-methyl-5-nitroimidazole (metronidazole), a known radiosensitizer and cytotoxic agent [2,12] was investigated. This manuscript describes cytotoxicities and radiosensitizing activities of metronidazole tethered 5-FU through ethyl and labile ester groups which was hypothesized upon *in vivo* hydrolysis to generate active metabolites which might have synergistic actions.

Materials and methods

Chemistry

Metronidazole **1**, 5-FU **5**, di-*t*-butoxydicarbonate $(Boc)_2O$, triethylamine, sodium hydride and other chemicals and solvents not listed here were from Merck Chemical Co. (Merck, Germany). Thin layer chromatography was carried out using Kieselge l60, 230–400 mesh, (Merck, Germany) to monitor the progress of reactions. Melting points were determined on a MEL-270 Sibata melting point apparatus and are uncorrected. ^{1}HNMR spectra were recorded on 500 MHz a Bruker (Germany), using DMSO-d_6 or $CDCl_3$ as solvent. Chemical shifts (δ) are reported in ppm relative to TMS as internal standard. Mass spectra were obtained on a Finningan TSQ-70 (USA) instrument. Infrared spectra were recorded on a Nicolet Magna IR-550 (USA) spectrometer. All compounds were characterized by the above techniques. Analytical and spectroscopic data for the known compounds were consistent with the reported literature values and data only for new compounds are presented.

Synthesis of 2-(2-Methyl-5-nitro-1H-imidazole-1-yl) ethyl-2-chloroacetate (3)

To a solution of metronidazole **1** (3.9 g, 24 mmol) in 100 ml of anhydrous dichloromethane was added 1.9 ml (24 mmol) triethylamine at temperature below 5°C and after stirring for 30 min the solution was treated with 3.2 ml (40 mmol) of chloroacetyl chloride dropwise within 5 min and then the resulting solution was stirred at room temperature overnight. The mixture was filtered and the residue after evaporation of the solvent was subjected to flash chromatography using Pet-ether: EtOAC as eluting solvent (80:20) to give 7.9 g (64%) of the compound **3**. mp 80-82°C; ^{1}H NMR (DMSO-d_6): δ 8.01 (s, 1H-imidazole), 4.61 (t, J = 5.12 Hz, 2H, CH_2-O), 4.48 (t, J = 5.12Hz, 2H, CH_2-N), 4.35 (s, 2H, CH_2-Cl), 2.18 (s, 3H, CH_3); FT-IR (KBr): 1720 (C = O), 1546, 1350 (NO_2) cm^{-1}.

Synthesis of 2-(2-Methyl-5-nitro-1H-imidazole-1-yl) ethyl-3-chloropropanoate (4)

The reaction of metronidazole **1** (3.9 g, 24 mmol) with 3.85 ml (40 mmol) of 3-chloropropionyl chloride under above conditions for the preparation of the ester **3** but purification of the product by crystallization from Pet-ether: EtOAC instead of flash chromatography gave 4.1 g (71%) of the ester **4**. mp 89-93°C;^{1}H NMR (DMSO-d_6): δ 8.01 (s, 1H-imidazole), 4.58 (t, J = 5.10 Hz, 2H, CH_2-O), 4.40 (t, J = 5.10 Hz, 2H, CH_2-N), 3.7 (t, J = 5.3 Hz, 2H, CH_2-Cl), 2.5 (t, J = 5.3 Hz, 2H, CH_2-C = O), 2.18 (s, 3H, CH_3); FT-IR (KBr): 1729 (C = O), 1540, 1345 (NO_2) cm^{-1}.

General procedure for the synthesis of tethered compounds 7–9

To a stirred solution of 225 mg (1 mmol) of 1-(*t*-butoxycarbonyl)-5-FU **6** [13] in 10 ml of anhydrous DMF in a round bottom flask which was kept in an ice bath was added 30 mg (1.25 mmol) of sodium hydride within 10 min and after stirring for 30 min at 5°C the mixture was then treated with a solution of 1 mmol of metronidazole esters **2-4** in 10 ml of anhydrous DMF and the mixture stirred at room temperature for 18 h. The mixture was then diluted with the same volume of water, extracted with ethyl acetate (3×20 ml), and the organic layer was dehydrated using anhydrous sodium sulfate. Evaporation of ethyl acetate gave an oily residue which was dissolved in 10 ml of methanol, treated with 0.42 g potassium carbonate and the obtained mixture was stirred at room temperature for 1 h. After evaporation of the solvent under reduced pressure, the residue was dissolved in water-ethyl acetate mixture (1:1), the organic layer was separated and dehydrated using anhydrous sodium sulfate and then evaporated under reduced pressure. For the preparation of compound **7**, the residue after evaporation of the solvent was purified by flash chromatography using Pet-ether: EtOAC as eluting solvent (70:30) to give 100 mg (35%) of the product. For the preparation of compounds **8** and **9**, residues were crystallized from Hexan-EtOAC to give 310 mg (92%) and 330 mg (93%) of the pure products respectively.

5-fluoro-3-(2-(2-methyl-5-nitro-1H-imidazol-1-yl)ethyl) pyrimidine-2,4(1H,3H)-dione(7)

mp 185-189°C; ^{1}HNMR ($CDCl_3$): δ 7.9 (s, 1H-imidazol), 7.8 (d, 1H, CH = CF), 4.0 (t, CH_2), 3.9 (t, CH_2), 2.4 (s, 3H, CH_3); FT-IR (KBr): 3108 (NH), 1722, 1671 (C = O), 1550, 1350 (NO_2) cm^{-1}; MS: m/z 81(100%), 130 (78%), 238 (39%), 155(24%).

2-(2-methyl-5-nitro-1H-imidazol-1-yl)ethyl 2-(5-fluoro-2,6-dioxo-2,3-dihydropyrimidin-1(6H)-yl)-acetate(8)

mp 231–234°C; ^{1}H NMR (DMSO-d_6): δ 7.99 (s, 1H-imidazole), 7.93 (d, J = 8.5 Hz, 1H, CH = CF), 4.65 (t, J = 5.02 Hz, 2H, CH_2-O), 4.42 (s, 2H, CH_2-C = O), 3.98 (t, J = 5.02 Hz, 2H, CH_2-N), 2.42 (s, CH_3); FT-IR (KBr): 3131 (NH), 1725, 1656 (C = O), 1542, 1349 (NO_2) cm^{-1}; MS: m/z 341 (7%), 296 (23%), 212 (80%), 171(74%), 130 (100%), 126 (42%).

2-(2-methyl-5-nitro-1H-imidazol-1-yl) ethyl 2-(5-fluoro-2,6-dioxo-2,3-dihydropyrimidin-1(6H)-yl)-propanoate(9)

mp 247-250°C; ^{1}H NMR (DMSO-d_6): δ 8.01 (s, 1H-imidazole), 7.98 (d, J = 8.5Hz, 1H, CH = CF), 4.57 (t, J = 5.05 Hz, 2H, CH_2-O), 4.39 (t, J = 5.05 Hz, 2H, CH_2-N), 3.78 (t, J = 6.8 Hz, 2H, CH_2-N), 2.70 (t, J = 6.8 Hz, 2H, CH_2-C = O), 2.44 (s, CH_3); FT-IR (KBr): 3124 (NH), 1721, 1652 (C = O), 1547, 1350 (NO_2) cm^{-1}; MS: m/z 355 (5%), 309 (21%), 226 (86%), 185(75%), 171 (42%), 130 (100%), 126 (59%).

In vitro cytotoxicity

Materials HT-29 cells, originally derived from human colorectal carcinoma were obtained from Pasteur Institute (Tehran, Iran). Fetal Bovine Serum (FBS), Penicillin/ Streptomycin 100X, Trypsin-EDTA 10X and Trypan blue were from Biosera (England). RPMI 1640 from Gibco (England), MTT and PI from Sigma (USA) and Digitonin from Merck (Germany) were used in this study.

Cell culture HT-29 cells were grown as an attached monolayer in RPMI 1640 supplemented with 10% fetal bovine serum, penicillin (50 unit/ml), and streptomycin (50 μg/ml). Cells were routinely grown in tissue culture flasks and kept in a humidified atmosphere of 5% CO_2 and 95% air at 37°C [14].

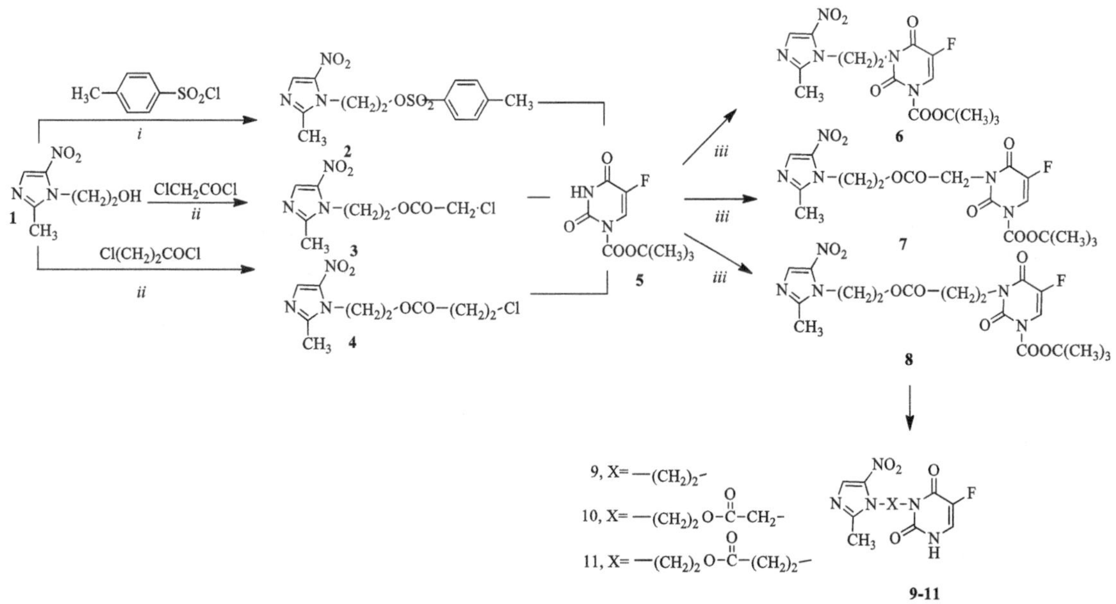

Scheme 1 Reagent and conditions for the synthesis of compounds 7–9. (i) Pyridine <15°C, (ii) CH_2Cl_2, triethylamine, r. t, (iii) 4-DMAP/CH_3CN, (iv) DMF, NaH, 80°C, (v) CH_3OH, K_2CO_3.

Methods of assay

Cytotoxicity of 5-FU**5**, metronidazole **1**, and tethered compounds **7–9** against HT-29 cells under both aerobic and hypoxic conditions were determined by measurement of the percentage of cell survivals using MTT [15] and PI-digitonin [16,17] and clonogenic forming assays [18]. Cells were seeded at the density of 10^4 cells/well in 96-well culture dishes and incubated for 4 h. Stock solutions of the tested compounds in DMSO at concentrations of 50 mmol which were prepared prior to the experiments diluted with culture media and at concentrations of 6.25-400 μmol/ml added to each well of plates. Cells in the control wells were treated with the same volume of medium which contained DMSO at concentration equal to those which were used in incubations treated with the tested compounds. Cell incubations were kept at 37°C under either air by purging with 95% nitrogen and 5% CO_2 or hypoxia in sealed GasPack jar by using Anoximat (Netherland) and an anaerobic chamber GasPak Jar (Merck, Germany) and GasPak pluss (Merck, Germany) [19] for 3 or 48 h. After removal of the supernatant of the culture medium, wells were washed with phosphate buffer saline (PBS), and the numbers of live cells were determined by following methods.

MTT assay

25 μl of the reagent (5 mg/ml in PBS) was added to each well, cell cultures were incubated for 4 h at 37°C and then the precipitated formazan was dissolved in 100 μl of DMSO and its absorbance was read in Elisa reader at 550 nm and a background wavelength of 690 nm. Survival was scored by the ratio of the absorbance of the treated cells to untreated cells with the tested compounds (control) and is expressed as percentage of the cell survival [15].

PI-digitonine assay

20 μl of a 1.53 mmol solution of PI in PBS for a final concentration of 30 μmol was added to each well, cell cultures were incubated for 60 min at 37°C and then the initial fluorescence intensity from the dead cells was measured in a multi-well plate reader, (BioTek, Synergy HT, USA) with 530-nm excitation and 645-nm emission filters. Then digitonin (600 nmol) was added to each well to permeabilize all cells and label all nuclei with PI and after 30 min incubation, the fluorescence intensity was measured again to obtain a value corresponding to the total number of cells. The percentage of dead cells was calculated as the proportion of fluorescence intensity of the dead cells to that of total cells multiplied by 100 and percentage of the cell viability was calculated by subtracting the percentage of dead cells from 100% [16].

The IC_{50} values for both MTT and PI-digitonine assays were determined from cell survival curves in which the percentages of cells that survived were plotted as a function of the concentration of the tested compounds.

Clonogenic forming assay

The medium of the cell cultures after treatment with the tested compounds and/or irradiation under aerobic or hypoxic conditions were first separated to remove the tested compounds, and washed with PBS. Cells were seeded in 6-well plates at concentration of 5×10^3 cells per well and maintained at 37°C for 14 days. The cells were then fixed in methanol, colonies which were formed stained with crystal violet and those containing more than 50 cells were scored. The number of colonies of treated and untreated dishes with the tested compounds were compared and expressed as the percentage of survival by clonogenic assay [18]. Clonogenic survival curves were constructed by plotting percent of survivals in response to different concentrations of the tested compounds.

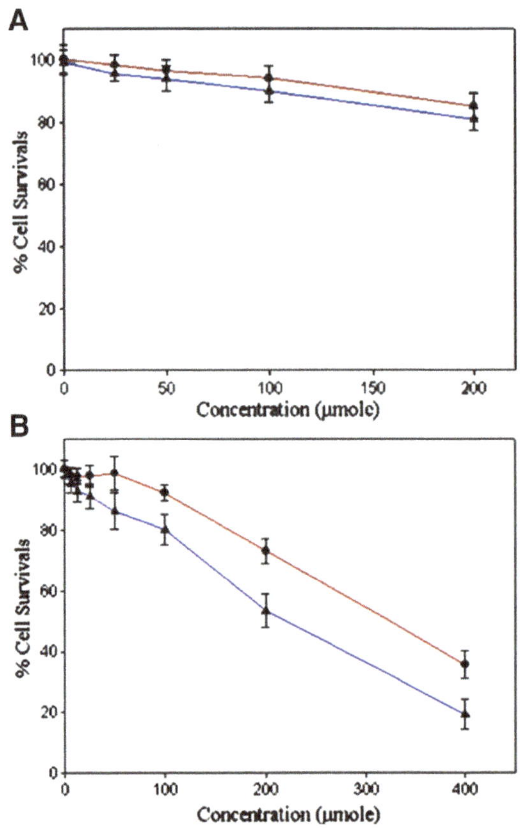

Figure 1 Clonogenic survival of incubation of HT-29 cell line with different concentration of compound 7 after 3 h (A) and 48 h (B) under aerobic (•) and hypoxic (▲) conditions. Data points were obtained from three independent experiments, and the standard deviations are given for each point. (Mean ± SD each set of experiments was performed in triplicates).

Table 1 Cytotoxicity and radiosensitization of metronidazole 1, 5-fluorouracil 5, and tethered compounds 7-9

Compound	IC_{50} (μmole)				SER					
	MTT assay[a]		PI assay[b]		Concentration (μmole)					
					25		50		100	
	Aerobic	Hypoxic	Aerobic	Hypoxic	Aerobic	Hypoxic	Aerobic	Hypoxic	Aerobic	Hypoxic
1	338 ± 12	265.9 ± 19	311 ± 16	250 ± 23	1.07 ± 0.06	1.26 ± 0.02	1.15 ± 0.09	1.69 ± 0.08	1.27 ± 0.02	2.06 ± 0.06
5	93 ± 9	89 ± 7	88 ± 7	84 ± 5	1.09 ± 0.06	1.04 ± 0.04	1.12 ± 0.09	1.18 ± 0.11	1.16 ± 0.11	1.12 ± 0.06
7	330 ± 16	240 ± 14	318 ± 20	230 ± 11	1.11 ± 0.11	1.41 ± 0.06	1.19 ± 0.05	1.85 ± 0.05	1.25 ± 0.010	2.17 ± 0.11
8	309 ± 25	232.1 ± 21	296 ± 18	229 ± 19	1.07 ± 0.03	1.51 ± 0.12	1.13 ± 0.08	1.95 ± 0.12	1.31 ± 0.12	2.26 ± 0.16
9	304 ± 18	234 ± 11	299 ± 14	224 ± 25	1.13 ± 0.06	1.43 ± 0.07	1.22 ± 0.10	1.79 ± 0.05	1.33 ± 0.05	2.13 ± 0.08

[a]3-(4,5-Dimethylthiazol-2-yl)-2,5-diphenyltetrazolium bromide.
[b]Propidium Iodide-Digitonin assay.

Radiosensitizing activity

Irradiation

HT-29 cells at 37°C under hypoxic or aerobic conditions were incubated with the tested compounds at concentrations of 25, 50, and 100 μmol for 3 h and then at room temperature were exposed to 4 different doses of radiation (2, 4, 8 and 12 Gy) at the dose rate of 1.67 Gy/min and Source Surface Distance (SSD) = 80 cm^2 by a ^{60}Co source (Theratron 780 MDS – Nordion).

Radiosensitivity measurement

Radiosensitivity of the tested compounds were determined through measurement of the cell growth inhibition using clonogenic assay [18]. Results are presented in terms of Sensitization Enhancement Ratio (SER) which were calculated from the equation SER = Do untreated cells/ Do treated cells, where Do values represent radiation dose that leads to 37% cell survival [20]. Do values were obtained from the survival curves of irradiation in the presence and absence of the tested compounds.

Statistical analyses

For the cell survival and cell death assays each experiment was repeated three times and results are mean ± SD of three independent experiments. Statistical analysis was performed using Sigmaplot 12 (Systat Software Inc.) for window and descriptive statistics are shown as arithmetic mean ± standard deviation. Independent samples' t-test was used to investigate the mean differences between irradiated and un-irradiated cells treated with the tested compounds and for comparison of more than two groups, Holm-Sidak multiple comparison test followed by one way analysis of variance (One way ANOVA) were performed and p value smaller than 0.05 was considered statistically significant.

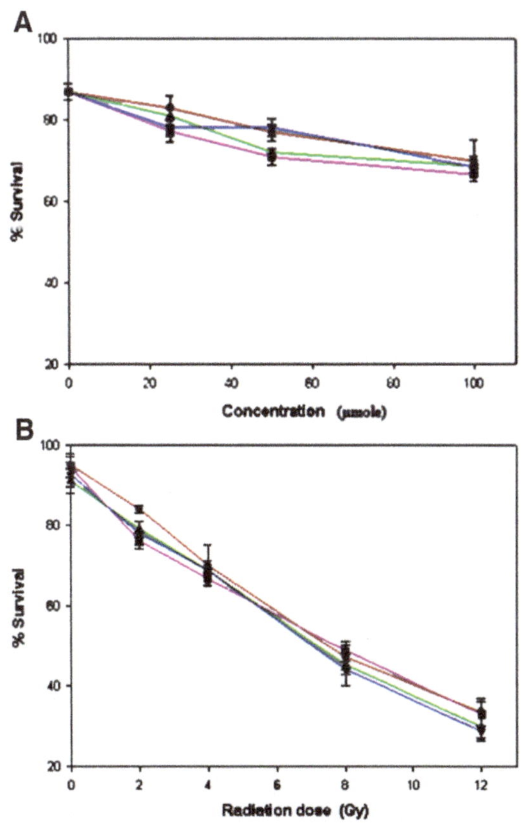

Figure 2 Clonogenic cell survival of HT-29 cells under aerobic conditions, (A): upon exposure to 4 Gy gamma-irradiation after incubation with different concentration (25, 50, 100 μmole) of metronidazole 1 and tethered compounds 7–9 for 3 h, (B): upon exposure to different doses (2, 4, 8 and 12 Gy) of radiation after incubation with 50 μmol of metronidazole 1 and tethered compounds 7–9 for 3 h. Each data points were obtained from three independent experiments, and the standard deviations are given for each point. (Mean ± SD).

Results and discussion

Tethered compounds **7–9** were prepared by the reaction of 1-(*t*-butoxycarbonyl)-5-FU **6** [13] with p-toluenesulfonic,

2-chloroacetic and 3-chloropropionic acid esters of metronidazole **1** (compounds **2–4**, Scheme 1) respectively in DMF in the presence of sodium hydride followed by removal of *t*-butoxycarbonyl group in methanolic potassium carbonate. Esters **3, 4** were obtained by the reported method for the preparation of the ester **2** [21] through the reaction of metronidazole **1** with 2-chloroacetyl chloride, and 3-chloropropionyl chloride respectively in pyridine.

Effects of different concentrations of 5FU **5**, metronidazole **1**, and tethered compounds **7**–**9** for different incubation periods on viability and proliferation of HT-29 cells were determined by MTT (15), PI-digitonin [16,17], and clonogenic assays (18). The tested compounds inhibited HT-29 cell proliferation in a time dependent manner and as it is shown for the compound **7** (Figure 1A) cell survival at 3 h after incubation were similar ($p > 0.05$) but after 48 h were significantly different ($p < 0.05$). IC_{50} values were assessed from cell survival curves in which the percentage of cells that survived after 48 h incubation were plotted as a function of the concentration of tested compounds (Table 1). Results of this study showed that IC_{50} values of each compound for the cell survival under aerobic or hypoxic conditions determined either by MTT or by PI-digitonin assays are not different significantly ($p > 0.05$) from each other and results of these tests which are seldom unanimous [12] were in good agreement.

While tethered compounds **7**–**9** under hypoxic conditions exhibited remarkable concentration–dependent cytotoxicity (Figure 1B), these compounds under aerobic conditions were not or were slightly cytotoxic whereas at concentrations up to 100 μmol could reduce viabilities of HT-29 cells only to less than 10% (Figure 1B). Consistent with these results the IC_{50} values of these compounds were significantly lower ($p < 0.05$) under hypoxic (232.1±21-240±14) compared to aerobic (304±18-330±16) conditions suggesting that compounds have hypoxia-selective cytotoxicity.

The radiosensitizing activities of all tested compounds were determined by measurement of the cell growth inhibition using a standard colony formation method following exposure of incubations with different concentrations of the tested compounds to different doses of the radiation [18]. Results are presented in term of Sensitization Enhancement Ratio (SER) which were obtained from the survival curves of irradiation in the presence and absence of the tested compounds for 37% survival respectively (20). The radiosensitization effects of compounds **7**–**9** at various concentrations under aerobic conditions were not different significantly ($p > 0.05$) (Figure 2A) and at a given concentration only increase in the dose of radiation resulted in decrease in the cell survival (Figure 2B). However under hypoxic conditions (Figures 3) radiosensitization effects of these compounds increased significantly with

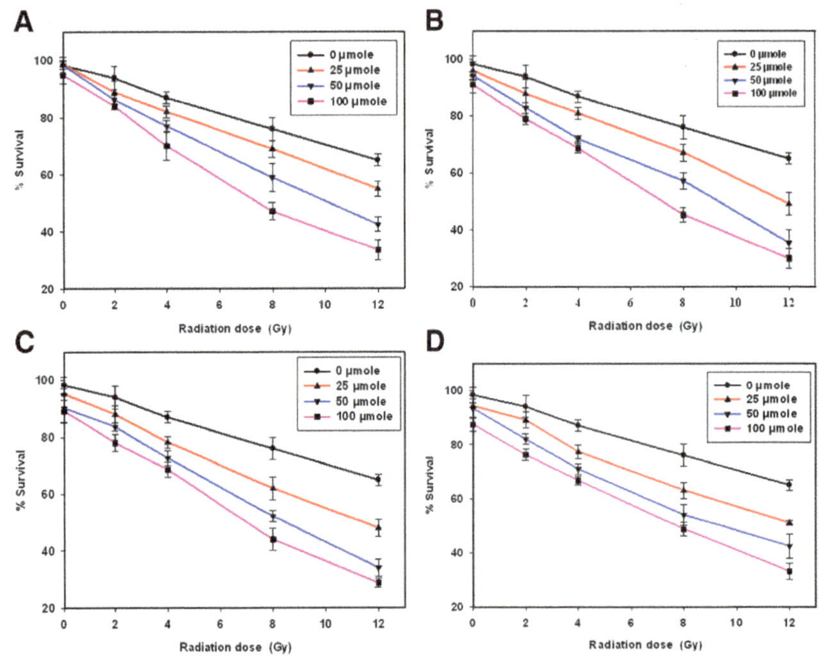

Figure 3 Clonogenic cell survival of HT-29 cells upon exposure to different doses of Gamma-radiation (2, 4, 6, 8 and 12 Gy) after incubation for 3 h with different concentrations (0, 25, 50 and 100 μmole) of metronidazole 1 and tethered compounds 7–9 under hypoxic conditions. Data points were obtained from three independent experiments, and the standard deviations are given for each point. (Mean ± SD, each set of experiments was performed in triplicates).

increase in their concentrations as well as the dose of radiation ($p < 0.05$) These results were further supported by their SER values (Table 1) which under hypoxic conditions were concentration- dependent and relative to aerobic conditions were significantly higher ($p < 0.05$). The SER values of tethered compound **7–9** under aerobic conditions at all concentrations were lower and under hypoxic conditions at concentrations of 50 and 100 μmol were higher than 1.6 which is the minimum required value [22] for an *in vitro* radiosensitizing activity, indicating that these compounds have hypoxia-selective radiosensitization effects. From the results of this study it appears that the functional groups and the length of the linker chain have no contribution on *in vitro* effects of tethered compounds **7–9** since cytotoxities and radiosensitizing activities of these compounds under either hypoxic or aerobic conditions were not significantly different from each other.

Conclusion

While the cytotoxicity of 5-FU **5** against HT-29 cell line under aerobic and hypoxic conditions were not different significantly and this compound at all concentrations showed no radiosensitizing activity, tethered compounds **7–9** showed higher cytotoxicities and selective radiosensitizing activities under hypoxic conditions. Also effects of these compounds relative to metronidazole **1** which is a known cytotoxin and radiosensitizer were comparable under aerobic but higher under hypoxic conditions. Further exploration of these compounds through modification of the linker chain might result in compounds which their uses in conjunction with tumor radiotherapy have greater toxicity to tumor than normal tissues.

Abbreviations

5 FU: 5- fluorouracil; MTT: 3-(4,5-Dimethylthiazol-2-yl)-2,5-diphenyltetrazolium bromide; PI: Propidium Iodide; SER: Sensitization enhancement ratio; PBS: Phosphate buffer saline; FBS: Fetal bovine serum.

Competing interests

The authors declare that they have no competing interests.

Authors' contributions

KA: Designer of the project, corresponding author of the manuscript.
AK: Determination of cytotoxicity and radiosensitizing activity of the tested compounds. OS-N: Supervisor for the determination of the cytotoxocity and radiosensitizing activity of the tested compounds. LN: Synthesis of the tethered compounds. KMR: supervising statistical analyses. All authors read and approved the final manuscript.

Acknowledgements

This research was supported by deputy of research and drug design & development research center of Tehran University of Medical Sciences (TUMS).

Author details

[1]Department Radiopharmacy, Tehran University of Medical Sciences, Tehran 14174, Iran. [2]Department of Medicinal Chemistry, Tehran University of Medical Sciences, Tehran 14174, Iran. [3]Department of Toxicology & Pharmacology, Tehran University of Medical Sciences, Tehran 14174, Iran. [4]Drug Design & Development Research Center, Tehran University of Medical Sciences, Tehran 14174, Iran. [5]Department of Drug and Food Control, Faculty of Pharmacy, Tehran University of Medical Sciences, Tehran 14174, Iran.

References

1. Nagasawa H, Uto Y, Kirk KL, Hori H: **Design of hypoxia-targeting drugs as new cancer chemotherapeutics.** *Biol Pharm Bull* 2005, **29:**2335–2342.
2. Wardman P: **Chemical radiosensitizers for use in radiotherapy.** *Clin Oncol* 2007, **19:**397–417.
3. Tao C, Desai NP, Soon-Shiong P, Sandford PA: **Dual functional cytotoxic/radiosensitizer compounds and methods for the preparation thereof.** *PCT Int Appl WO 96 40,091. Chem Abstr* 1996, **126:**131664n.
4. Palmer BD, Wilson WR, Pullen SM, Denny WA: **Hypoxia-selective antitumor agents. 5. Synthesis of water-soluble nitroaniline mustards with selective cytotoxicity for hypoxic mammalian cells.** *J Med Chem* 1990, **35:**3214–3222.
5. Parrick J, Porssa P, Davies LK, Dennis MF, Patel KB, Stratford MRK, Wardman P: **Targeting radiosensitizers to DNA by minor groove binding: nitroarenes based on netropsin and distamycin.** *Bioorg Med Chem Lett* 1993, **3:**1697–1702.
6. Lee HH, Palmer BD, Wilson WR, Denny WA: **Synthesis and hypoxia-selective cytotoxicity of A 2-nitroimidazole mustard.** *Bioorg Med Chem Lett* 1998, **8:**1741–1744.
7. Ahmed L, Jenkins TC, Walling JM, Stratford IJ, Sheldon PW, Adams GE, Fielden EM: **Analogues of RSU-1069: radiosensitization and toxicity *in vitro* and *in vivo*.** *Int J Radiat Oncol* 1986, **12:**1079–1081.
8. Khalaj A, Doroudi AR, Ostad SN, Khoshayand MR, Babai M, Adibpour N: **Synthesis, aerobic cytotoxicity, and radiosensitizing activity of novel 2,4-dinitrophenylamine tethered 5-fluorouracil and hydroxyurea.** *Bioorg Med Chem Lett* 2006, **16:**6034–6038.
9. Abdi K, Khalaj A, Ostad SN, Khoshayand MR: **Cytotoxicity and radiosensitising activity of synthesized dinitrophenyl derivatives of 5-fluorouracil.** *DARU J Pharm Sci* 2012, **20:**1–9. Doi: 10.1186/1560-8115-20-3.
10. Abdi K, Nafisi S, Manouchehri F, Bonsaii M, Khalaj A: **Interaction of 5-Fluorouracil and its derivatives with bovine serum albumin.** *J Photochem Photobiol B* 2012, **107:**20–26.
11. Khalaj A, Abdi K, Ostad SN, Khoshayand MR, Lamei N, Nedaie HA: **Synthesis, *in vitro* cytotoxicity and radiosensitizing activity of novel 3-[(2,4-dinitrophenylamino)alkyl]derivatives of 5-fluorouracil.** *Chem Biol Drug Des.* in press.
12. Ramalho TC, Franca TCC, Cortopassi WA, Goncalves AS, da Saliva AWS, da Cunha EFF: **Topology and dynamics of the interaction between 5-nitroimidazole radiosensitizers and duplex DNA studied by a combination of docking, molecular dynamic simulations and NMR spectroscopy.** *J Mol Struct* 2011, **992:**65–71.
13. Jaime-Figueroa S, Zamilpa A, Guzman A, Morgans DJ: **N-3-Alkylation of uracil and derivatives via N-1-Boc protection.** *Synthetic Commun* 2001, **31:**3747–3757.
14. Freshney RI: *Culture of animal cells: a manual of basic technique.* 6th edition. New York: Wiley-Blackwell; 2010.
15. Mosmann T: **Rapid colorimetric assay for cellular growth and survival: application to proliferation and cytotoxicity assays.** *J Immunol Methods* 1983, **65:**55–63.
16. Puttonen KA, Lehtonen S, Lampela P, Mannisto PT, Raasmaja A: **Different viabilities and toxicity types after 6-OHDA and Ara-C exposure evaluated by four assays in five cell lines.** *Toxicol In Vitro* 2008, **22:**182–189.
17. Zhang L, Mizumoto K, Sato N, Ogawa T, Kusumoto M, Niiyama H, Tanaka M: **Quantitative determination of apoptotic death in cultured human pancreatic cancer cells by propodium iodide and digitonin.** *Cancer Lett* 1999, **142:**129–137.
18. Franken NP, Rodermond HM, Stap J, Haveman J, van Bree C: **Clonogenic assay of cells *in vitro*.** *Nat Protoc* 2006, **1:**2315–2319.
19. Naito M, Hashimoto C, Masui S, Tsuruo T: **Caspase-independent necrotic cell death induced by a radiosensitizer, 8-nitrocaffeine.** *Cancer Sci* 2004, **95:**361–366.
20. Cariveau MJ, Stackhouse M, Cui X, Tiwari K, Waud W, Secrist JA, Xu B: **Clofarabine acts as radiosensitizer *in vitro* and *in vivo* by interfering with DNA damage response.** *Int J Radiation Oncol Biol* 2008, **70:**213–220.

21. Trivedi MN, Gabhe SY, Vachhani UD, Patel RB, Shah CP: **Synthesis of some 2-methyl-5-nitroimidazole derivatives as potential antimicrobial agents.** *J Chem Pharm Res* 2011, **3**:313–319.
22. Nakae T, Uto Y, Tanaka M, Shibata H, Nakata E, Tominaga M, Maezawa H, Hashomoto T, Kirk KL, Nagasawa H, Hori H: **Design, synthesis, and radiosensitizing activities of sugar-hybrid hypoxic cell radiosensitizers.** *Bioorg Med Chem Lett* 2008, **16**:675–682.

4

Raloxifene adjunctive therapy for postmenopausal women suffering from chronic schizophrenia: a randomized double-blind and placebo controlled trial

Gilda Kianimehr[1], Farzad Fatehi[2], Sara Hashempoor[3], Mohammad-Reza Khodaei-Ardakani[3], Farzin Rezaei[4], Ali Nazari[4], Ladan Kashani[5] and Shahin Akhondzadeh[6*]

Abstract

Background: Cumulative evidence from epidemiological, preclinical and clinical studies suggests estrogens may have psychoprotective effects in schizophrenic patients. Selective Estrogen Receptor Modulators could have therapeutic benefits in schizophrenia for both sexes without being hazardous to gynecological tissues or having feminizing effects. Few studies have been conducted regarding the effects of raloxifene on postmenopausal women suffering from schizophrenia. We conducted this placebo-controlled trial to compare the add-on effect of raloxifene to risperidone versus risperidone with placebo.

Methods: This was an 8-week, parallel-group, placebo-controlled trial undertaken at two universities affiliated psychiatric Hospitals in Iran. Forty-six postmenopausal women with the definite diagnosis of schizophrenia were enrolled in the study. Patients received risperidone (6 mg/day in 3 divided doses) combined with either placebo (N = 23) or 120 mg/day of raloxifene (N = 23) for 8 weeks. Patients were assessed by a psychiatrist at baseline and at 2 and 8 weeks after the start of medical therapy. Efficacy was defined as the change from baseline to endpoint in score on Positive and Negative Syndrome Scale (PANSS).

Results: For PANSS scores, the main effect comparing two types of intervention was not significant [F (1, 48) = 1.77, p = 0.18]. For positive subscale scores, there was marginal significant interaction between intervention type and time [F (2, 47) = 2.93, p = 0.06] and there was substantial main effect for time [F (2, 47) = 24.39, p = 0.001] within both groups showing reduction in positive subscale scores across the three time periods. In addition, the main effect comparing two types of intervention was significant [F (1, 48) = 3.78, p = 0.02]. On the other hand, for negative subscale scores, the main effect comparing two types of intervention was not significant [F (1, 48) = 1.43, p = 0.23]. For general subscale scores, the main effect comparing two types of intervention was not significant [F (1, 48) = 0.03, p = 0.86].

Conclusions: According to our findings, raloxifene as an adjunctive treatment to risperidone was only superior in improvement of positive symptoms and it was not effective in treating negative and general psychopathology symptoms.

Trial registration: The trial was registered at the Iranian registry of clinical trials: IRCT201205131556N42

Keywords: Schizophrenia, Menopause, Raloxifene, Selective estrogen receptor modulators

* Correspondence: S.akhond@neda.net
[6]Psychiatric Research Center, Roozbeh Psychiatric Hospital, Tehran University of Medical Sciences, South Kargar Street 13337, Tehran, Iran
Full list of author information is available at the end of the article

Background

Cumulative evidence from epidemiological, preclinical and clinical studies suggests estrogens may provoke psychoprotective effects in schizophrenic patients [1]. In addition, Selective Estrogen Receptor Modulators (SERMs) could have therapeutic benefits on both sexes with schizophrenia without any hazard to gynecological tissues or feminizing effects [1]. There are several lines of evidence that support the estrogen hypothesis of schizophrenia [2]. Most antipsychotics cause prolactin-inducing effects, and ensuing negative feedback on estrogen levels [2]. Sex differences in the incidence, onset and course of schizophrenia have led to the hypothesis that estrogens play a protective role in the pathophysiology of this disorder [3]. Estrogen treatment may boost the recovery of schizophrenia in women. However, adverse effects on uterine and breast tissue and other physical side effects may limit the long-term therapeutic use of estrogen [4-6]. Raloxifene hydrochloride is a selective estrogen receptor modulator that acts as an estrogen antagonist in breast tissue and may have agonistic actions in the brain, potentially offering mental health benefits with few estrogenic side effects [4].

Prognosis and severity of schizophrenia is different between males and females and as a result, it is suggested that estrogen may play a role in the pathogenesis of schizophrenia [1,3]. sex differences is a fascinating aspect of schizophrenia, which have been described for nearly all features of the illness, including the peak age of onset, symptoms and treatment response [7]. Estradiol and some SERMs are neuroprotective in a variety of experimental models of neurodegeneration; they could lessen the inflammatory response of glial cells, decrease anxiety and depression, and endorse cognition. Moreover, they are able to modulate synaptic plasticity in the hippocampus of rodents [8]; however, long term estrogen application may cause significant complications especially in menopausal women. Therefore, administration of Selective Estrogen Receptor Modulators (SERMs) may reduce such side effects. Raloxifene is a SERM that has similar dopaminergic and serotonergic effects as estrogen. Few studies have been conducted regarding the effects of raloxifene on postmenopausal women suffering from schizophrenia [9,10]. However, the sample size of these studies was relatively small [9.10]. We conducted this placebo-controlled trial to compare the add-on effect of raloxifene to risperidone in comparison with risperidone and placebo.

Methods

Trial organization

This was an 8-week, parallel-group, placebo-controlled trial undertaken at two universities affiliated psychiatric Hospitals in Iran (Roozbeh and Razi Hospital) from June 2012 to December 2013. The trial protocol was approved by the Institutional Review Board (IRB) of Tehran University of Medical Science (Grant No: 17215) and was conducted in agreement with the Declaration of Helsinki and its subsequent revisions. The trial was registered at the Iranian registry of clinical trials (www.irct.ir; registration number: (IRCT201205131556N42). Written informed consent was obtained from all eligible patients and/or their legally authorized representatives. Patients were informed that they are free to withdraw from the study at any time without any influence on their relationship with their health care provider.

Study population

Forty-six postmenopausal women with the definite diagnosis of schizophrenia were enrolled in the study. The diagnosis of schizophrenia was made according to DSM-IV TR. Diagnosis was made based on a Structured Clinical Interview for DSM-IV-TR Axis I Disorders (SCID) and was confirmed with chart review and senior physician interview. Inclusion criteria were postmenopausal (be in postmenopause is defined as period of one year spontaneous amenorrhea, a serum FSH level of >20 and clinical symptoms such as hot flashes,...) women who met the diagnostic criteria for schizophrenia according to DSM IV-TR consisting of Positive and Negative Syndrome Scale (PANSS) [11] score above 60 and disease onset over 2 years. Exclusion criteria were the concurrent presence of neurologic or organic disorders; IQ lower than 70; illicit drug use in past 6 months, consumption of antipsychotic drugs in the previous week or a long-acting antipsychotic drug in previous 2 months, receiving any antidepressant and mood stabilizer drugs during the trial, former hormone replace therapy, electroconvulsive therapy in past 2 weeks; endocrine abnormality; hepatic or renal dysfunction; and history of thromboemboli, abnormal uterine bleeding or breast and uterine cancer, and stroke.

Study design

Forty-six postmenopausal women with DSM-IV-TR diagnosed chronic schizophrenia received risperidone (6 mg/day in 3 divided doses) (Janssen Pharmaceuticals, Toronto, Canada; 2 mg tablet) combined with either placebo (N = 23) or 120 mg/day of raloxifene (Eli Lilly) (N = 23) for 8 weeks. Patients were assessed by a psychiatrist at baseline and at 2 and 8 weeks after the start of medical therapy. Efficacy was defined as the change from baseline to endpoint in score on PANSS.

Outcome measurement

PANSS is one of the most important rating tools for computing symptom severity in patients with schizophrenia. It comprises 3 subscales (positive scale, negative scale, and general psychotherapy scale) with 30 items in total ranging in score between 1 and 7 which leads to a minimum total score of 30. PANSS has been used in a number of trials in Iran [12-15]. The mean decline in PANSS scale as well as subscales from baseline was regarded as the main outcome measure of response in schizophrenia to treatment. The scale was measured at baseline, week 2 and week 8. Efficacy will be defined as change from baseline to endpoint in score on PANSS. Adverse events were evaluated using a 25 –item checklist and Extra-pyramidal Symptoms Rating Scale (ESRS) [16].

Statistical analysis

SPSS software, version 20.0 for Windows, was used to analyze the data. Continuous data are presented as mean ± standard deviation (SD). We used Kolmogorov-Smirnov Z test to determine the normal distribution of all continuous variables and due to normal distribution of PNSS score and subscales (positive, negative, general), we used parametrical tests to analyze data. A mixed between-within subjects analysis of variance was conducted to assess the impact of two different interventions (Risperidone + Raloxifene, Risperidone + placebo) on patient scores on PANSS score, positive subscale, negative subscale, and general psychotherapy subscale, across three time periods (the start of study, week 2, and week 8).

Results

Figure 1 shows flow diagram of the patients. The mean age (±SD) of the raloxifene group was 61.96 ± 4.49 years versus 60.44 ± 5.28 years in the placebo group (non significant). Demographic data of the patients is presented in Table 1.

For PANSS scores, there was no significant interaction between intervention type and time [Wilks' Lambda = 0.89, F (2, 47) = 2.79, p = 0.07]. There was substantial main effect for time [Wilks' Lambda = 0.36, F (2, 47) = 42.56, p < 0.01] within both groups showing a reduction in PANSS scores across three time periods (Table 2, Figure 2). Furthermore, the main effect comparing two types of intervention was not significant [F (1, 48) = 1.77, p = 0.18].

For positive subscale scores, there was marginal significant interaction between intervention type and time [Wilks' Lambda = 0.89, F (2, 47) = 2.93, p = 0.06] and there was substantial main effect for time [Wilks' Lambda = 0.44, F (2, 47) = 24.39, p < 0.01] within both groups showing a reduction in positive subscale scores across the three time periods (Table 2, Figure 3). In addition, the main effect comparing two types of intervention was significant [F (1, 48) = 3.78, p = 0.02] suggesting superior effectiveness of Risperidone plus Raloxifene over Risperidone plus Placebo.

For negative subscale scores, there was no significant interaction between intervention type and time [Wilks' Lambda = 0.99, F (2, 47) = 0.12, p = 0.73]. There was

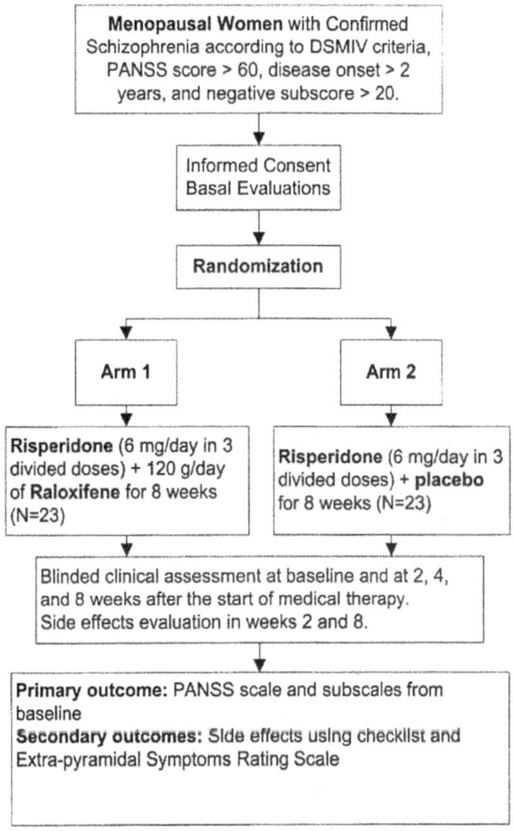

Figure 1 Trial flow diagram of adjunctive Raloxifene versus placebo.

substantial main effect for time [Wilks' Lambda = 0.46, F (2, 47) = 55.65, p < 0.01] within both groups showing a reduction in negative subscale scores across three time periods (Table 2, Figure 4). Additionally, the main effect comparing two types of intervention was not significant [F (1, 48) = 1.43, p = 0.23] suggesting no difference in effectiveness of the two therapies on negative subscale scores.

For general subscale scores, there was significant interaction between intervention type and time [Wilks' Lambda = 0.78, F (2, 47) = 6.78, p < 0.01]. There was substantial main effect for time [Wilks' Lambda = 0.34, F (2, 47) = 46.13, p < 0.01] within both groups showing a reduction in general subscale scores across the three time periods (Table 2, Figure 5). However, the main effect comparing two types of intervention was not significant [F (1, 48) = 0.03, p = 0.86] suggesting no difference in the effectiveness of the two therapies on general subscale scores.

Main adverse events included constipation (3 patients in Raloxifene group and 2 patients in placebo group), tremor (1 in each group), dry mouth (2 patients in raloxifene group), restless leg syndrome (1 patient in Raloxifene

Table 1 Demographic data of the raloxifene group versus the placebo group

		Risperidone + Raloxifene group (N = 25)	Risperidone + Placebo group (N = 25)	p-value
Age (±SD)		61.96 ± 4.49	60.44 ± 5.28	p > 0.05
Education	Illiterate	4 (36.36%)	7 (63.64%)	p > 0.05
	School	17 (51.52%)	16 (48.48%)	
	University	3 (50%)	3 (50%)	
Positive family history		13 (42%)	15 (60%)	p > 0.05
Age of onset		34.96 ± 11.69	29.40 ± 8.57	p > 0.05
Duration		17.24 ± 12.03	13.64 ± 12.41	p > 0.05
Previous treatment	Risperidone	7 (41.12%)	10 (58.88%)	p > 0.05
	Other atypical	3 (75.0%)	1 (25.0%)	
	Typical	11 (50.0%)	11 (50.0%)	
	Combination	4 (57.14%)	3 (42.86%)	
IQ	Normal	24 (52.17%)	22 (47.83%)	p > 0.05
	Borderline	1 (25.0%)	3 (75.0%)	

group), drowsiness (2 patients in placebo group), and loss of appetite (1 patient in placebo group). In addition, there was no ESRS difference between the two groups at weeks 2 and 8 [$F(1, 48) = 1.04$, $p = 0.30$].

Discussion

Adjunctive therapy and polypharmacy is used routinely for several chronic diseases. Medications with different mechanisms of action are used in polypharmacy. The use of adjunctive therapy in schizophrenia has been a major concern especially in recent years. The potential therapeutic efficacy of estrogens in schizophrenia is being identified and Selective Estrogen Receptor Modulators (SERMs) seem to be a better option in view of safety concerns. According to our findings, Raloxifene as an adjunctive treatment to risperidone was only superior for positive symptoms and it was not effective in treating negative and general psychopathology symptoms.

Recently, some studies have pointed to the adjunctive efficacy of raloxifene in improving schizophrenic symptoms [17]. In a 12-week, double-blind, randomized, placebo-controlled study [10], 33 postmenopausal women with schizophrenia were randomized to receive either adjuvant raloxifene (16 women) or adjuvant placebo (17 women) for three months. The addition of raloxifene produced significant differences in some aspects of memory and executive function in patients treated with raloxifene. In another 12-week, double-blind, randomized, placebo-controlled study, 33 postmenopausal women with schizophrenia and prominent negative symptoms were randomized to either adjunctive raloxifene or adjunctive placebo for 12 weeks [9]. The addition of raloxifene

Table 2 PANSS and subscale scores for the intervention type across three time periods

		Risperidone + Raloxifene (n = 25)	Risperidone + Placebo (n = 25)
	Time period	Mean ± SD	Mean ± SD
PANSS score	Week 0	105.52 ± 16.96	105.00 ± 11.68
	Week 2	89.08 ± 16.14	94.16 ± 19.78
	Week 8	68.32 ± 21.04	82.00 ± 26.14
Positive subscale	Week 0	25.76 ± 8.00	26.68 ± 7.04
	Week 2	20.92 ± 5.41	24.28 ± 6.33
	Week 8	14.32 ± 4.33	21.12 ± 7.07
Negative subscale	Week 0	28.04 ± 8.64	30.76 ± 9.09
	Week 2	24.88 ± 8.76	28.12 ± 10.88
	Week 8	19.60 ± 8.66	23.08 ± 12.08
General Psychopathology subscale	Week 0	50.44 ± 9.92	47.52 ± 6.46
	Week 2	43.56 ± 9.30	41.88 ± 9.76
	Week 8	34.56 ± 10.78	37.84 ± 11.89

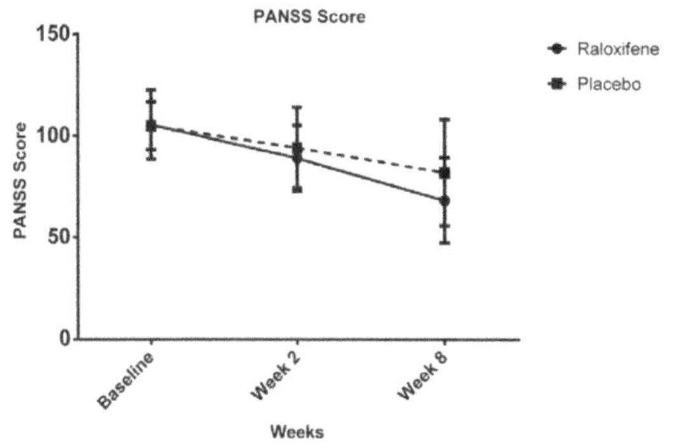

Figure 2 PANSS scores for the intervention type across three time periods (Raloxifene group: solid line, Placebo group: dashed line).

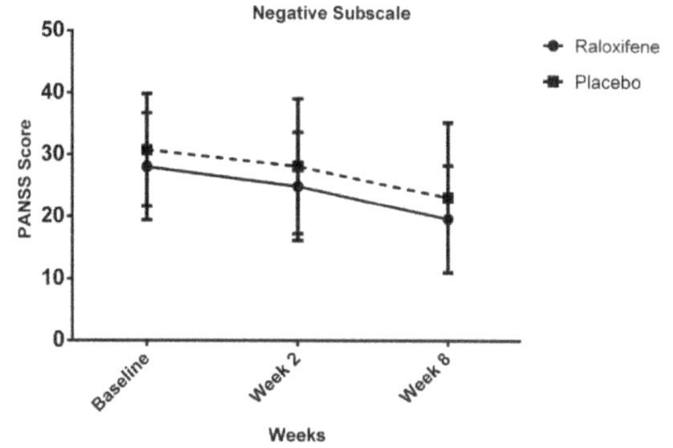

Figure 4 Negative subscale scores for the intervention type across three time periods (Raloxifene group: solid line, Placebo group: dashed line).

(60 mg/d) to regular antipsychotic treatment significantly reduced negative, positive, and general psychopathology symptoms compared to the placebo group.

In a randomized clinical trial [4], 35 postmenopausal women with schizophrenia received 120 mg/day adjunctive raloxifene compared to either adjunctive raloxifene HCl (60 mg/day) or placebo. A significantly greater recovery of total and general PANSS symptoms was noted in patients receiving 120 mg/day adjunctive raloxifene compared to either 60 mg/day adjunctive raloxifene HCl or placebo. In addition, adjunctive Raloxifene has been successfully used in single case reports for menstruating women suffering from resistant schizophrenia. A 29-year-old woman, with drug-resistant schizophrenia, experienced significant improvement in socio-occupational functioning, with reduction in symptom severity, over a 7-month follow-up period, [18].

It is significant that we encountered no adverse effects in the raloxifene group compared to the placebo group. The safer raloxifene profile compared with estrogenic compounds, makes it a preferred drug when adjunctive hormonal therapy of schizophrenia for post-menopausal women is considered. The lack of adverse effects on breast and uterine tissue is an imperative advantage of Raloxifene over estrogen [19].

The ovarian hormone 17β-estradiol acts in the central nervous system to regulate neuroendocrine events and reproduction. Estradiol controls gene expression, neuronal survival, neuronal and glial differentiation, and synaptic transmission and has anti-inflammatory, protective and reparative properties in the brain [20,21]. A number of studies seem to indicate that raloxifene acts on brain dopamine and serotonin systems in a way that is similar to that of conjugated estrogens [22].

It is proposed that conjugated estrogens may exercise their therapeutic potential either by modulating brain neurotransmission or through neuroprotective effects. On the other hand, the incidence of schizophrenia in men is consistently observed to be approximately 1.5 times higher than its in women [23] and there is a male predominance in incidence in the early twenties, but a

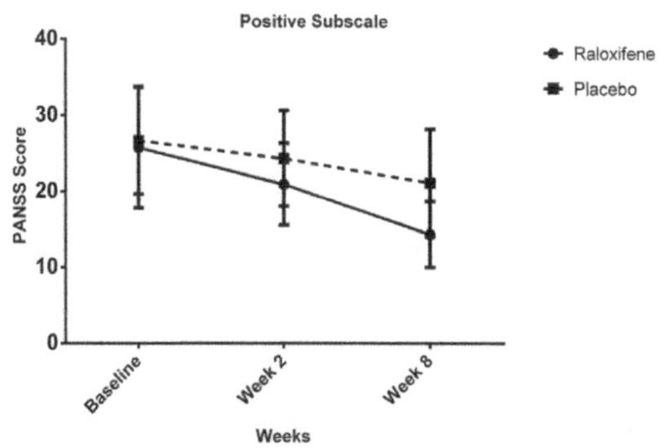

Figure 3 Positive subscale scores for the intervention type across three time periods (Raloxifene group: solid line, Placebo group: dashed line).

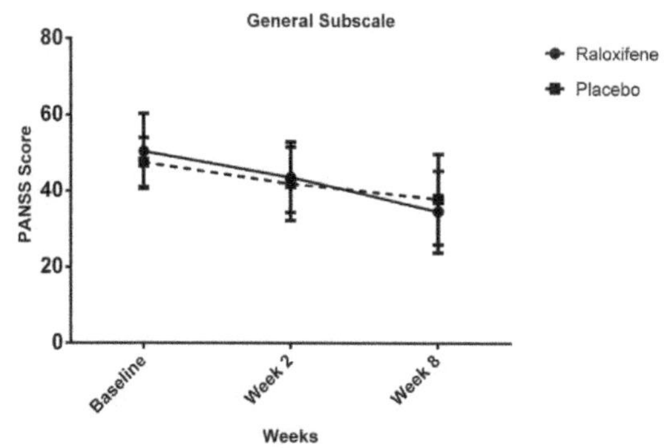

Figure 5 General Psychopathology subscale scores for the intervention type across three time periods (Raloxifene group: solid line, Placebo group: dashed line).

female predominance in older middle age [24]. Estrogen may have an impact on schizophrenia by several mechanisms. Short-term, it seems to have fast membrane effects by modifying functional activity in the dopaminergic synapse; for longer periods, it may appear to have genomic effects by altering synthesis at dopamine receptors. There is also evidence to suggest that estrogen alters serotonergic systems. Estrogen can also promote neuronal regeneration and block mechanisms of neuronal death [4]. In addition, numerous studies have described association between serotonin 1A receptor and major psychiatric disorders, such as schizophrenia and bipolar disorder [25]. Both serotonin and estrogen have been involved in modulation of mood and cognition. Even though substantial functional relations between estrogen and serotonin are recognized, the nature of their relationship has not been fully illuminated [26]. This study has some limitations which should be considered. The sample size was relatively small and the study course and follow-up period were relatively short. We did not measure the effect of raloxifene on menopausal symptoms as well. Furthermore, lack of cognitive assessments is another limitation of the present study.

Conclusions

In conclusion, it seems that according to our findings, raloxifene as an adjunctive treatment was shown to be superior to placebo in improving the positive symptoms in patients receiving risperidone. However, this drug did not show a benefit in treating the negative and general symptoms of schizophrenia when was added to risperidone therapy.

Abbreviations

SERMs: Selective estrogen receptor modulators; PNASS: Positive and negative syndrome scale.

Competing interests

No conflict of interest exists for any of the authors associated with the manuscript and there was no source of extra-institutional commercial funding. The funding organization had no role in the design and conduct of the study; in the collection, analysis, and interpretation of the data; or in the preparation, review, or approval of the manuscript and the decision to submit the paper for publication.

Authors' contributions

GK, SH and AN: Sample collection, FF: Statistical Analysis, Article writing, SA, LK, MK and FR: Designer and project manager, Article writing. All authors read and approved the final manuscript.

Acknowledgments

This study was supported by a grant from Tehran University of Medical Sciences to Prof. Shahin Akhondzadeh (Grant No: 17215). This study was Dr. Gilda Kianimehr's postgraduate thesis toward the Iranian Board of Psychiatry.

Author details

[1]Psychiatric Research Center, Roozbeh Hospital, Tehran University of Medical Sciences, Tehran 13337, Iran. [2]Shariati Hospital, Neurology Department, Tehran University of medical Sciences, Tehran, Iran. [3]Razi Psychiatric Hospital, University of Social Welfare and Rehabilitation, Tehran, Iran. [4]Qods Hospital, Kurdistan University of Medical Sciences, Sanandaj, Iran. [5]Infertility Ward, Arash Hospital, Tehran University of Medical Sciences, Tehran, Iran. [6]Psychiatric Research Center, Roozbeh Psychiatric Hospital, Tehran University of Medical Sciences, South Kargar Street 13337, Tehran, Iran.

References

1. Kulkarni J, Gavrilidis E, Worsley R, Hayes E: **Role of estrogen treatment in the management of schizophrenia.** *CNS Drugs* 2012, **26**(7):549–557.
2. Mortimer AM: **Relationship between estrogen and schizophrenia.** *Expert Rev Neurother* 2007, **7**(1):45–55.
3. Begemann MJ, Dekker CF, van Lunenburg M, Sommer IE: **Estrogen augmentation in schizophrenia: a quantitative review of current evidence.** *Schizophr Res* 2012, **141**(2–3):179–184.
4. Kulkarni J, Gurvich C, Lee SJ, Gilbert H, Gavrilidis E, de Castella A, Berk M, Dodd S, Fitzgerald PB, Davis SR: **Piloting the effective therapeutic dose of adjunctive selective estrogen receptor modulator treatment in postmenopausal women with schizophrenia.** *Psychoneuroendocrinology* 2010, **35**(8):1142–1147.
5. Akhondzadeh S, Nejatisafa AA, Amini H, Mohammadi MR, Larijani B, Kashani L, Raisi F, Kamalipour A: **Adjunctive estrogen treatment in women with chronic schizophrenia: a double-blind, randomized, and placebo-controlled trial.** *Prog Neuropsychopharmacol Biol Psychiatry* 2003, **27**(6):1007–1012.
6. Akhondzadeh S, Mokhberi K, Amini H, Larijani B, Kashani L, Hashemi L, Nejatisafa AA, Shafaei AR: **Is there a relationship between estrogen serum level and symptom severity throughout the menstrual cycle of patients with schizophrenia?** *Therapy* 2005, **2**(5):745–751.
7. Wu YC, Hill RA, Gogos A, van den Buuse M: **Sex differences and the role of estrogen in animal models of schizophrenia: interaction with BDNF.** *Neuroscience* 2013, **239**:67–83.
8. Velazquez-Zamora DA, Garcia-Segura LM, Gonzalez-Burgos I: **Effects of selective estrogen receptor modulators on allocentric working memory performance and on dendritic spines in medial prefrontal cortex pyramidal neurons of ovariectomized rats.** *Horm Behav* 2012, **61**(4):512–517.
9. Usall J, Huerta-Ramos E, Iniesta R, Cobo J, Araya S, Roca M, Serrano-Blanco A, Teba F, Ochoa S: **Raloxifene as an adjunctive treatment for postmenopausal women with schizophrenia: a double-blind, randomized, placebo-controlled trial.** *J Clin Psychiatry* 2011, **72**(11):1552–1557.
10. Huerta-Ramos E, Iniesta R, Ochoa S, Cobo J, Miquel E, Roca M, Serrano-Blanco A, Teba F, Ochoa S: **Effects of raloxifene on cognition in postmenopausal women with schizophrenia: A double-blind, randomized, placebo-controlled trial.** *Eur Neuropsychopharmacol* 2014, **24**(2):223–231.
11. Kay SR, Fiszbein A, Opler LA: **The positive and negative syndrome scale (PANSS) for schizophrenia.** *Schizophr Bull* 1987, **13**(2):261–276.
12. Farokhnia M, Azarkolah A, Adinehfar F, Khodaie-Ardakani MR, Hosseini SM, Yekehtaz H, Tabrizi M, Rezaei F, Salehi B, Sadeghi SM, Moghadam M, Gharibi F, Mirshafiee O, Akhondzadeh S: **N-acetylcysteine as an adjunct to risperidone for treatment of negative symptoms in patients with chronic schizophrenia: a randomized, double-blind, placebo-controlled study.** *Clin Neuropharmacol* 2013, **36**(6):185–192.
13. Farokhnia M, Sabzabadi M, Pourmahmoud H, Khodaie-Ardakani MR, Hosseini SM, Yekehtaz H, Tabrizi M, Rezaei F, Salehi B, Akhondzadeh S: **A double-blind, placebo controlled, randomized trial of riluzole as an adjunct to risperidone for treatment of negative symptoms in patients with chronic schizophrenia.** *Psychopharmacology (Berl)* 2014, **231**(3):533–542.
14. Khodaie-Ardakani MR, Mirshafiee O, Farokhnia M, Tajdini M, Hosseini SM, Modabbernia A, Rezaei F, Salehi B, Yekehtaz H, Ashrafi M, Tabrizi M, Akhondzadeh S: **Minocycline add-on to risperidone for treatment of negative symptoms in patients with stable schizophrenia: Randomized double-blind placebo-controlled study.** *Psychiatry Res* 2014, **215**(3):540–546.
15. Hosseini SM, Farokhnia M, Rezaei F, Gougol A, Yekehtaz H, Iranpour N, Salehi B, Tabrizi M, Tajdini M, Ghaleiha A, Akhondzadeh S: **Intranasal desmopressin as an adjunct to risperidone for negative symptoms of schizophrenia: A randomized, double-blind, placebo-controlled, clinical trial.** *Eur Neuropsychopharmacol* 2014, **24**(6):846–855.
16. Chouinard G, Margolese HC: **Manual for the Extrapyramidal Symptom Rating Scale (ESRS).** *Schizophr Res* 2005, **76**(2–3):247–265.
17. Kulkarni J, Gavrilidis E, Wang W, Worsley R, Fitzgerald PB, Gurvich C, Van Rheenen T, Berk M, Burger H: **Estradiol for treatment-resistant**

schizophrenia: a large-scale randomized-controlled trial in women of child-bearing age. *Mol Psychiatry* 2014, doi:10.1038/mp.2014.33.
18. Raveendranathan D, Shivakumar V, Jayaram N, Rao NP, Venkatasubramanian G: **Beneficial effects of add-on raloxifene in schizophrenia.** *Arch Womens Ment Health* 2012, **15**(2):147–148.
19. Chua WL, de Izquierdo SA, Kulkarni J, Mortimer A: **Estrogen for schizophrenia.** *Cochrane Database Syst Rev* 2005, **4:** CD004719.
20. Spencer JL, Waters EM, Romeo RD, Wood GE, Milner TA, McEwen BS: **Uncovering the mechanisms of estrogen effects on hippocampal function.** *Front Neuroendocrinol* 2008, **29**(2):219–237.
21. Vegeto E, Benedusi V, Maggi A: **Estrogen anti-inflammatory activity in brain: a therapeutic opportunity for menopause and neurodegenerative diseases.** *Front Neuroendocrinol* 2008, **29**(4):507–519.
22. Usall J, Coromina M, Araya S, Ochoa S: **Effect of raloxifene (a Selective Estrogen Receptor Modulator (SERM)) as coadjuvant to antidepressant treatment: a case report.** *Actas Esp Psiquiatr* 2011, **39**(5):334–336.
23. Welham J, Isohanni M, Jones P, McGrath J: **The antecedents of schizophrenia: a review of birth cohort studies.** *Schizophr Bull* 2009, **35**(3):603–623.
24. Abel KM, Drake R, Goldstein JM: **Sex differences in schizophrenia.** *Int Rev Psychiatry* 2010, **22**(5):417–428.
25. Kishi T, Okochi T, Tsunoka T, Okumura T, Kitajima T, Kawashima K, Yamanouchi Y, Kinoshita Y, Naitoh H, Inada T, Kunugi H, Kato T, Yoshikawa T, Ujike H, Ozaki N, Iwata N: **Serotonin 1A receptor gene, schizophrenia and bipolar disorder: an association study and meta-analysis.** *Psychiatry Res* 2011, **185**(1–2):20–26.
26. Amin Z, Canli T, Epperson CN: **Effect of estrogen-serotonin interactions on mood and cognition.** *Behav Cogn Neurosci Rev* 2005, **4**(1):43–58.

The immunological benefit of higher dose N-acetyl cysteine following mechanical ventilation in critically ill patients

Atabak Najafi[1], Mojtaba Mojtahedzadeh[1,2,3], Keyvan Haji Ahmadi[2], Mohammad Abdollahi[3], Maryam Mousavi[4], Legese Chelkeba[2,3], Farhad Najmeddin[2] and Arezoo Ahmadi[1*]

Abstract

Background: Sepsis complication is a major cause of death in multiple trauma critically ill patients. Defensin (cysteine rich anti-microbial peptides), as an important component of immune system, might play an important role in this process. There is also rising data on immunological effects of N-acetyl-cysteine (NAC), a commonly used anti-oxidant in oxidative stress conditions and glutathione (GSH) deficiencies. The aim of the present study was to evaluate the potential beneficial effects of NAC administration on multiple trauma patients with sepsis.

Methods: In a prospective, randomized controlled study, 44 multiple trauma critically ill patients who were mechanically ventilated and met the criteria of sepsis and admitted to the intensive care unit (ICU) were randomized into two groups . Control group received all standard ICU therapies and NAC group received intravenous NAC 3 gr every 6 hours for 72 hours in addition to standard therapies. Acute Physiology and Chronic Health Evaluation II (APACHE II) and Sequential Organ Failure Assessment (SOFA) scores, length of ICU stay, ICU mortality were recorded. Levels of serum Immunoglobulin M (IgM), Human β-Defensin 2 (HβD2) and GSH were assessed at baseline and 24, 72, 120 hours after intervention.

Results: During a period of 13-month screening, 44 patients underwent randomization but 5 patients had to be excluded. 21 patients in NAC group and 18 patients in control group completed the study. For both groups the length of ICU stay, SOFA score and systemic oxygenation were similar. Mortality rate (40% vs. 22% respectively, $p = 0.209$) and ventilator days (Mean ± SD 19.82 ± 19.55 days vs. 13.82 ± 11.89 days respectively, $p = 0.266$) were slightly higher for NAC group. IgM and GSH levels were similar between two groups ($p = 0.325$, 0.125 respectively), HβD2 levels were higher for NAC group (at day 3).

Conclusion: High dose of NAC administration not only did not improve patients' outcome, but also raised the risk of inflammation and was associated with increased serum creatinine.

Keywords: N-Acetyl, Cysteine (NAC), Glutathione (GSH), Human β Defensin 2 (HβD2), Immunoglobulin M (IgM), Multiple trauma, Sepsis

Background

Multiple trauma, a complex syndrome of injuries to various anatomical regions with defined intensity and subsequent systemic reactions [1]. Trauma is the major cause of death before the age of 45 in developed countries [2,3], claiming over 6 million kills annually around the world which is preventable in approximately 20% of cases [4,5]. Three pre-eminent causes of death in this patients are head trauma, hemorrhage and sepsis/Multi Organ Failure (MOF) [6]. Tissue ischemia induces Reactive Oxygen Species (ROS) production which in turn activates neutrophils and attracts them to the injury site. Extensive progression of this and other similar processes following trauma insult enhance the local inflammatory response to remote organs, resulting in the development of Systemic Inflammatory Response Syndrome (SIRS) [7-12]. In sepsis,

* Correspondence: aarezoo24@gmail.com
[1]Department of Anesthesiology and Critical Care Medicine, Sina Hospital, Faculty of Medicine, Tehran University of Medical Sciences, Tehran, Iran
Full list of author information is available at the end of the article

acute immunologic response and excessive release of pro-inflammatory cytokines [Interleukin 1(IL-1), Tumor Necrosis Factor α (TNF-α)] trigger target cells (leukocytes, endothelial cells, hepatocytes, lung and intestine epithelium) and induce cytokine, chemokine, ROS and proteolytic enzymes production [13-16].

It is obvious that patients with sepsis or multiple trauma require mechanical ventilation support. Due to the high concentration of inspired oxygen used, the probability of alveolar epithelial damage is high as the result of formation of free oxygen radicals. Some studies have suggested that the use of high doses of antioxidants in these patients could be beneficial [7].

Defensins are cysteine rich endogenous antimicrobial peptides which consist of to approximately 5% of total granulocyte proteins, following infection their levels in systemic circulation increases, defensins have a significant effect on a wide spectrum of microorganisms [17-19] and beyond that they also act as immunologic mediators [20]. Human β Defensin 2 (HβD2) is an inducible defensin, whose induction is impaired during sepsis [20,21].

NAC is a well-known anti-oxidant which is administered in various conditions where oxidative stress is present [22-24]. NAC is thiol containing compound that in addition to direct radical scavenging properties is a precursor for glutathione (GSH) synthesis [23,24]. NAC seems to have immunological effects (doses higher than 12 gram/day) that can affect different cytokines (IL-2, IL-4, IL-6, IL-10, TNF-α, NF-κB) [25,26] and phagocytic function [27]. NAC has received so much credit for its nephro-protective properties when used prior to radio-contrast media administration. The ischemia compounded by increased medullary O_2consumption may somewhat resemble ischemic acute tubular necrosis (ATN) in trauma and sepsis. Although near 10 Meta-Analyses has been published to justify its use many of these studies have significant pitfalls [25-27].

To our knowledge there are no studies about the effect of NAC as an antioxidant and/or immunomodulator in patients with SIRS/sepsis criteria following multiple trauma. Therefore, this study aimed to investigate HβD2 levels in multiple trauma patients with SIRS/sepsis and its potential correlation with progress and outcome of therapy, and to evaluate the effects of high dose NAC administration, in the early onset of sepsis during first hours to days after trauma, on immunologic responses and overall outcome. Furthermore, this study sought to examine the hypothesis that NAC administration can alter HβD2 levels either by immuno-modulatory activity or as a cysteine source.

Methods

Study design and patient population

Between March 2011 to April 2012, this prospective randomized clinical trial was conducted in general ICU of "Sina"and "Imam Khomeini" Hospital of Tehran University of Medical Sciences (TUMS), Iran. In all cases, informed consents were received from their legal guardian. The study protocol was approved by the ethical committee of TUMS. Our clinical trial was registered in Iranian Registry of Clinical Trial with code number of (IRCT 2014010716120 N1).

All the patients enrolled in the study had multiple trauma. The inclusion criteria were age older than 18 years, mechanical ventilation with FiO_2 more than 50%, an Acute Physiology and Chronic Health Evaluation (APACHE) II score greater than 15, suspected infection and at least two Systemic Inflammatory Response (SIRS) criteria (defined as the following conditions: body temperature > 38°C or < 36°C, heart rate > 90 beats/min, respiratory rate > 20 breath/min or $Paco_2$ < 32 mmHg, WBC >12,000 cells/mm^3, or < 4000 cells/mm^3, or > 10% immature [band] cells) diagnosed during the first 24 hours of ICU admission. Exclusion criteria for all patients were ages below 18 years, pregnancy, breast feeding, beyond 24 hours of sepsis diagnosis, Central Venous Pressure (CVP) > 18 mmHg, Systolic Blood Pressure < 90 mmHg or Mean Arterial Pressure (MAP) < 60 mmHg, Serum Creatinine ≥ 2 mg/dl, liver dysfunction (defined as the presence of hepatic cirrhosis or concentration of serum transaminases greater than third times the upper limit of normal range), history of myocardial infarction or heart failure (EF < 40%) and those received N-acetyl Cysteine (NAC) before initiation of study.

Patients were randomized via block randomization to receive one of the following treatments: standard treatment for sepsis (control group) and standard treatment plus NAC (intervention group) for 72 hours. Standard treatments for sepsis were implemented as following: early resuscitation within the first 6 hours of admission, appropriate diagnostic studies to ascertain causative organisms before starting antibiotics, early administration of broad-spectrum antibiotic therapy, reassessment of antibiotic therapy with microbiology and clinical data to narrow coverage, appropriate Volume resuscitation or vasopressor therapy, Mechanical ventilation adjusted to maintain SaO_2 > 95%, PaO_2 > 90 mmHg and $PaCO_2$ between 38 and 42 mmHg, appropriate analgesia and sedation provided for all patients, insulin treatment was administered to maintain glucose at < 200 mg/dl and appropriate prophylactic measures for deep vein thrombosis (DVT) and stress-related mucosal damage (SRMD). Patients in intervention group received intravenous NAC (Exir Pharmaceutical company, Tehran, Iran) 3gr in 250 ml 5% dextrose over 30 min every 6 hours for the first 72 hours of admission (Figure 1).

Demographic data and clinical information were obtained at the beginning. Monitoring parameters including MAP, heart rate, respiratory rate and CVP of each patient were recorded in the ICU flow sheets every

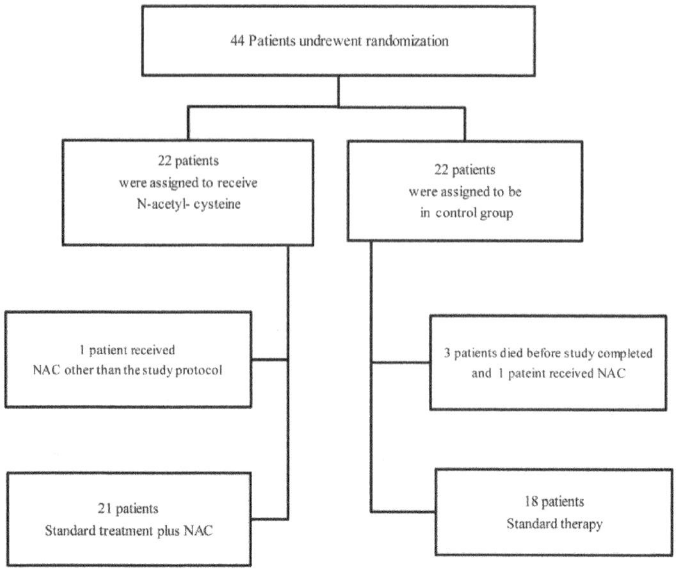

Figure 1 Enrollment and protocol study.

3 hours. Laboratory data including serum creatinine, Blood Urea Nitrogen (BUN), hemoglobin, platelet and white blood cell (WBC) counts, albumin, sodium and potassium were also collected daily during 5 days of study period.

Measurements

All patients had central venous catheter and arterial catheter for blood sampling. For all patients there were four scheduled time points to assess the level of IgM, GSH and HβD2. Blood samples were collected at baseline and 24, 72 and 120 hours after intervention and centrifuged at 3000 × g for 15 minutes to remove cells and cellular debris. The plasma stored at −80°C until the time of analysis. Levels of IgM, GSH and HβD2 were measured by commercially available enzyme-linked immunosorbent assay (ELISA) kits (CUSABIO® biotech co LTD, Wuhan Hubei, China) according to manufacturer instruction.

APACHE score was measured at the beginning and Sequential organ failure assessment (SOFA) score was calculated daily for 5 days. Length of ICU stay, ICU mortality and ventilator free days were recorded for all patients.

Statistical Analysis

All data were expressed as Mean ± SD. The unpaired *t* test for parametric data and Mann–Whitney test for nonparametric data were used to compare the differences between the treatment groups at each time point. Comparisons of the differences between the time points in each treatment group, repeated-measure one-way analysis of variance and nonparametric analysis of variance (Friedman test) were performed to analyze changes in levels of the biomarkers. The paired *t* test for parametric data and Wilcoxon rank sum test for nonparametric data were done to analyze changes in variables with 2 time points (at baseline and 24 hours after). P values less than 0.05 were considered statistically significant.

Results

Between March 2011 to April 2012, 44 consecutive patients who met the inclusion criteria were enrolled in the study. Five patients excluded from the study, three of them died before the end of the study and the other 2 patients received NAC dosage other than the study protocol. The remaining 39 patients were randomly assigned to NAC group and control group, each with 21 and 18 patients respectively. Demographic and baseline values for APACHE and SOFA scores have been summarized in Table 1. The differences in age and sex were not significant between two groups. ($p = 0.450$ and 0.204 respectively). Differences in baseline values for APACHE and SOFA scores were not statistically significant either (Table 1). Also the patients in each group were similar at baseline regarding to heart rate, MAP, temperature and Pao_2/Fio_2 (Table 1).

In comparison between two groups, in NAC group, ventilator days were longer (19.82 ± 19.55 vs. 13.82 ± 11.69 days), length of ICU stay was shorter (21.2 ± 20.71 vs. 27.72 ± 39.46 days) and mortality rate was higher (40% versus 22%), although the differences in ventilator days, length of ICU stay and mortality rate were not statistically significant ($p = 0.266$, $p = 0.545$, $p = 0.209$

Table 1 Demographic and baseline clinical characteristic of patients

	Control group	NAC group	P value
Age (years)	44.44 ± 17.684	40.14 ± 17.828	0.450
Male number	15	20	0.204
APACHE II	20.06 ± 5.162	21.05 ± 512	0.476
SOFA	7.28 ± 2.109	6.86 ± 1.457	0.468
GCS	7.28 ± 1.934	6.55 ± 1.143	0.145
MAP(mmHg)	92.72 ± 17.376	93.39 ± 14.467	0.899
HR(beat/min)	89.94 ± 18.005	97.09 ± 19.079	0.234
Temperature(°C)	37.339 ± 1.01	37.145 ± 0.965	0.536
PaO2/FiO2	196.607 ± 105.504	219.594 ± 123.307	0.529
SCr(mg/dl)	1.046±	1.053 ± 0.373	0.945

NAC: N-Acetylcysteine, APACHE: Acute Physiology and Chronic Health Evaluation, SOFA: Sequential Organ Failure Assessment, GCS: Glasgow Coma Scale, MAP: Mean Arterial Pressure, HR: Heart Rate.
Data shown as Mean ± SD. P values <0.05 consired significant.

respectively). Moreover, SOFA scores are associated with a trend towards a reduction in NAC group specially on day 3 but the trend was not statistically significant (Figure 2).

Pao_2:Fio_2 ratio improved in both groups (specially in the NAC group on day 3), although the difference was not significant (p = 0.567) (Figure 3). An upward trend in MAP, heart rate, WBC counts and Absolute Neutrophil Count (ANC) were shown in NAC group on day 1 through 5 after the start of NAC (Table 2). By means of paired *t*-test (before-after analysis) method, we had a significant decline in mean serum creatinine level between 1–3 days in control group (1.04 ± 0.25 versus 0.891 ± 0.253 p = 0.019). The mean serum creatinine level rose on day 1 through 3 in NAC group, however; this increase was not statistically significant (1.05 ± 0.373 versus 1.48 ± 2.87, p = 0.514). On day 5, creatinine levels reached similar levels in both groups (0.851 ± 0.205 Control group versus 0.920 ± 0.385 NAC group p = 0.502).

Furthermore the changes in the level of IgM (p = 0.325) and GSH (p = 0.125) were not significant among two groups but the mean serum levels of GSH were higher in NAC group (Table 3). Despite a non significant difference in HβD2 levels between two groups (p = 0.463), HβD2 levels are associated with a trend towards an increase in NAC group specially on day 3 (Figure 4).

Discussion

The aim of the current study was to focus on potential immunological effects of NAC administration in critical illness, we have also reassessed the antioxidant properties which had already been well established. In previous study, immunological effects of NAC were seen with doses relatively higher than usual dosage for antioxidant effects (higher than 9 gram/day) [25-27]. So we have administered 12 gram/day of NAC in our study. The previous study [24] reviewed the effects of NAC in a condition of GSH deficiency such as pulmonary disease and oxidative stress, they concluded that oral administration of NAC was a safe and beneficial supplement in setting of GSH deficiency. In other study conducted on piglets, it was observed that NAC has no significant effect on the total GSH level [28]. Another study investigated the effects of NAC (150 mg/kg bolus and then 12 mg/kg/day as continuous infusion for 3–5 days) on total antioxidant potential in 60 critically ill patients [29]. The need for inotropic support and mechanical ventilation and ICU stay did not vary significantly between NAC and placebo group. Also levels of total antioxidant potential remain unchanged during intervention. Other study evaluates the effects of NAC (150 mg/kg bolus followed by a continuous infusion of 12 mg/kg/hr from a minimum of 3 days up to a maximum of 5 days) for prevention of multisystem organ failure [30]. The mortality, the required days of inotropic support, mechanical ventilation, and intensive care did not significantly change between two groups.

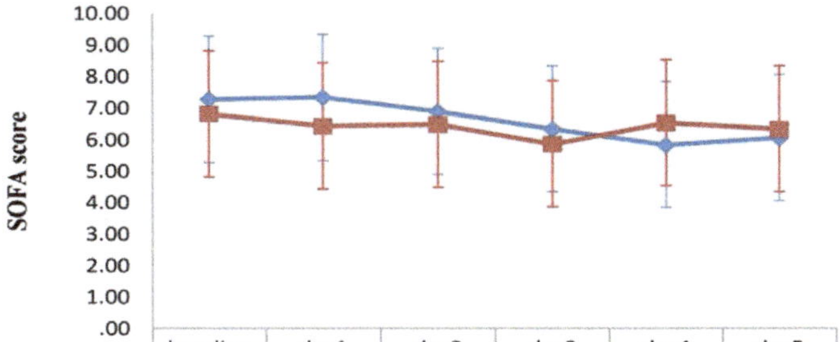

	baseline	day1	day2	day3	day4	day5
Control	7.28	7.33	6.89	6.33	5.83	6.06
NAC	6.81	6.43	6.48	5.86	6.52	6.33

Figure 2 Changes of patients SOFA score in different days of study. Difference between two groups is not significant (P=0.708). Figure shows mean SOFA score±SE.

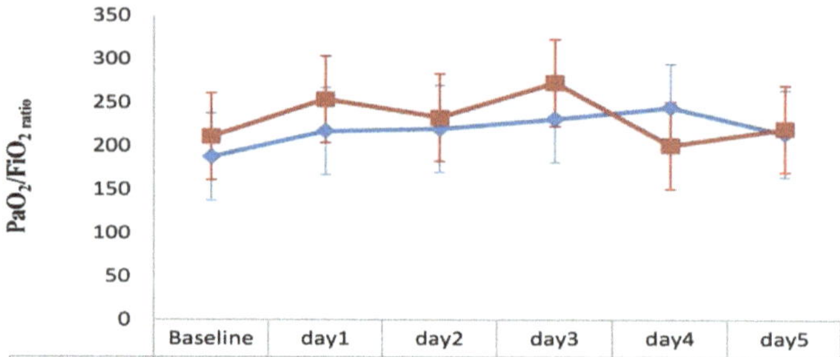

	Baseline	day1	day2	day3	day4	day5
Control	187.23	216.79	219.42	230.93	243.89	214.09
NAC	210.62	253.29	232.27	272.55	200.39	219.59

Figure 3 Changes of Pao_2/Fio_2 ratio in patients in different days of study. Difference between two groups is not significant (P = 0.567). Figure shows mean ±SE.

Furthermore, patients admitted after 24 hrs of hospital admission had a significantly worse mortality in the NAC group as well. Indeed, during 10 years ago several clinical randomized trials suggested that the beneficial impact of NAC were achieved if given early, due to attenuating inflammatory response by free radical scavenging effects, but if commenced in a later phase of sepsis, it may also worsen outcome, as a result of the impaired granulocyte – dependent bacterial killing [30-32]. Nevertheless, prophylactic NAC treatment failed to prevent postoperative organ dysfunction following major abdominal surgery [33].

The results of this study show that high doses of NAC (12 gram/day) for the first 72 hours in mechanically ventilated multiple trauma patients with sepsis patients (patients with sepsis diagnosis over 24 hour was excluded), do not significantly change in the total serum GSH level. Meanwhile in NAC group, the mean level of GSH is higher than control group, it is not along with any improvement in outcome. The ventilator day and mortality rate are higher in NAC group and it shows a negative impact on HR and MAP as well. Our data suggests reconsideration and conducts large sized trials in order to evaluate the efficacy of NAC as an anti-oxidant and a thiol group supplement for GSH deficiency. Further studies are recommended to conduct with focus on commencing NAC treatment in an earlier phase of sepsis, dosage and safety issues. In our study we have observed that NAC, which is often considered as a safe and well tolerated entity, is not as safe. Furthermore, in some circumstances its indication is questionable and present data are not satisfactory.

We have assessed systemic oxygenation and respiratory functions in terms of changes in PaO_2/FiO_2 ratio and the number of ventilator days. In other study administered 190 mg/kg/day NAC as continuous infusion for 3 days in 42 patients with established Acute Respiratory Distress Syndrome (ARDS) and compared it with placebo [34]. The mortality rate, the need for ventilator support and ICU stay and PaO2/FiO2 ratio did not differ significantly between both groups. In another randomized double-blind, placebo controlled clinical trial by Bernard et al. NAC 70 mg/kg every 8 hours was administered for ARDS patients for 10 days [35]. The number of days of acute lung injury decreased in NAC group, yet mortality rate did not change significantly between groups. In our study we encounter similar results. The analyses show no significant difference on day 1 through 5. Improvement in Pao2/Fio2 ratio is seen on day 5 in both groups. The number of ventilator days is longer for

Table 2 Changes of patients HR, MAP, WBC count, ANC in different days of study

		Base line	Day 1	Day 2	Day 3	Day 4	Day 5	P. value
HR	Control	89.94	90.67	87.89	84.67	86.56	89.00	0.040
	Intervention	96.43	97.19	97.81	100.86	97.67	94.19	
MAP	Control	91.18	80.29	87.47	85.12	83.71	82.53	0.042
	Intervention	94.48	89.29	92.05	94.33	90.95	89.95	
WBC count	Control	11726	10597	8930	7890	8117	89	0.06
	Intervention	13094	11791	10165	10874	11087	11191	
ANC	Control	10306.07	7737.73	7425.16	5804.00	5569.42	6732.95	0.001
	Intervention	10261.22	9507.84	8468.47	9800.79	9754.49		

MAP: Mean Arterial Pressure, HR: Heart Rate, ANC: Absolute Neutrophil Count.

Table 3 Changes of patients IgM and GSH level in different days of study

		Base line	Day1	Day3	Day5
IgM(mg/dl)	Control	35.28 ± 8.67	34.59 ± 8.87	32.00 ± 2.69	34.43 ± 5.69
	NAC	34.22 ± 6.38	33.35 ± 6.80	32.18 ± 6.28	31.64 ± 3.93
GSH(µg/dl)	Control	11.89 ± 8.95	11.05 ± 9.52	10.99 ± 7.20	9.26 ± 6.76
	NAC	15.9 ± 9.55	14.79 ± 12.89	15.35 ± 9.51	13.51 ± 6.76

NAC: N-AcetylCysteine, IgM: Immunoglobulin M, GSH: Gluthathione, Data are shown as Mean ± SD.

NAC group although the difference is not statistically significant. We can suggest that routine administration high dose of NAC has no effect on ventilator days and can be harmful.

Various studies have investigated the potential effect of NAC on immune system function in different setting (animal and human studies) and focused on diverse pathological conditions (ARDS, SIRS or sepsis, hepatic injury and etc.). For instance, in other study in critically ill patients with SIRS or sepsis noticed that, high doses of NAC (12, 18 gram/day) resulted in significantly improved phagocytic activity of neutrophils as compared with low doses of NAC. In contrast, they found that high dose NAC decreases respiratory burst and leads to impaired clearance of microorganisms [27].

Santiago and co-workers investigated NAC's effects on inflammatory response and reported that plasma IL-4 and IL-10 (anti-inflammatory cytokines) levels were higher in NAC treated group with respect to time of hepatic reperfusion, indicating a positive modulation effect of NAC on the anti inflammatory response mediated by this cytokines [25]. In in-vitro settings, NAC with similar concentrations above 25 mmol/L completely inhibited NF-κB signal. The trend was the same in in-vivo part of the study, Paterson and colleagues reported. A significant decrease in IL-8 levels in severe sepsis patients treated with NAC, while NAC had no effect on IL-6 levels as reported in that study [26]. Several studies evaluated the immune-modulating effects of NAC and its usage in sepsis, but the results were contradictory. Considerable amount of evidence showed that NAC administration suppressed neutrophils and macrophages activation, attenuating leukocyte–endothelial cell adhesion and inhibited TNF-α and IL-8 release [26,36-38]. Emet and co-workers reported that early NAC administration in severe sepsis did not affect cytokine levels [38,39].

In the current study, immune-modulating effect is evaluated by white blood cell count, absolute neutrophil count and serum IgM levels. In NAC group, WBC count and subsequently ANC are higher than control group which would be indicated more extensive inflammatory condition. The consistent tachycardia, elevated serum creatinine levels and higher 28 days mortality rate have observed in NAC group allegedly support these findings. IgM levels decrease from1 day through 5 in both groups. All patients are IgM deficient and NAC administration neither increase nor decrease IgM levels and it seems that no immune modulation properties are found in high doses of NAC.

Cysteine rich endogenous anti-microbial peptide HβD2 is an important component of immune system (Innate and adaptive) [20,40-43]. This study attempt to investigate whether HβD2 level can be accounted as a marker of SIRS or sepsis. In addition, the study also investigate whether NAC administration (as a cysteine source with probable immune-modulating properties) can elevate HβD2 levels

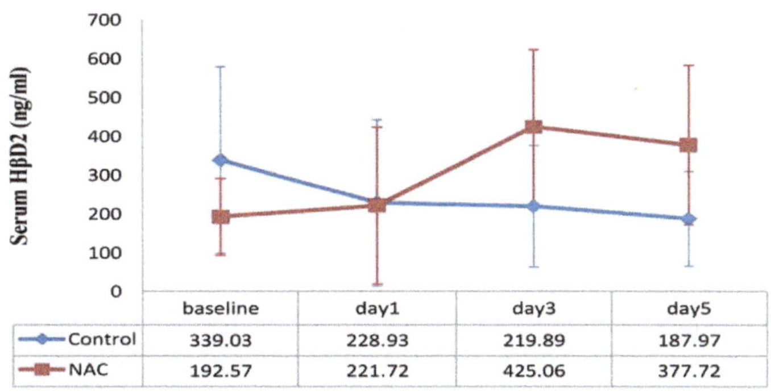

Figure 4 Changes in Serum HβD$_2$ in different days of study. Difference between two groups is not significant (P = 0.463). Figure shows mean±SE.

(HβD2 is known as an inducible one [44,45] among other defensins). Attributed roles to HβD2 in immune system are controversial, yet it is not clear whether HβD2 is an anti-inflammatory protective mediator during sepsis or vice versa. In other study, no difference was observed between survivors and non-survivors of severe sepsis and critical illness in terms of HβD2 levels. Ex-vivo inducible expression of HβD2 by peripheral blood cells was impaired in samples from patients with severe sepsis but this was not along with low levels of HβD2, interestingly HβD2 levels were significantly higher in patients with severe sepsis compared to non-septic critically ill and healthy controls. Which according to Chen et al., NF-κB was as crucial factor for activation of HβD2 gene. In conclusion Book and coworkers noted that up-regulation of HβD2 in sepsis occurred as a result of elevated pro-inflammatory cytokines (such as IL-1 and TNF) [46,47] and was an indicator of higher activity of inflammation and the availability of sources other than peripheral blood cells for HβD2 [21].

Circulating defensins were increased in non-neutropenic children with systemic infection and sepsis. Neutrophils were the major source of defensins, they served as a specific marker for PMN activation. Defensins were not associated with organ failure or poor outcome during sepsis, defensins released into systemic circulation is an indicator of host response to sepsis. These were observations from Thomas and colleagues in a study on levels of HβD2 and lactoferrin in children with severe sepsis, the reported range by them was 450 ng/ml (median) and 194–1032 (25%-75% range) for day 1, and 300 nano-gram/ml (median) and 75–681 (25%-75% range) [41].

We hypothesized that NAC as a cysteine rich source could increase HβD2 levels and our result has confirmed this hypothesis. According to the results of our study, HβD2 levels are associated with an upward trend in NAC and a downward trend in control group. The difference between means of the two groups, however were only noteworthy on day 3. Results indicate that NAC administration with such dosage may have induced HβD2 expression. Regarding the previous discussion on immune-modulating effect of NAC, the elevated HβD2 levels in response to NAC administration appears to be the consequence of profound cysteine source. In our survey, despite higher level of HβD2 in SIRS and sepsis, no potential benefits were found concerning SOFA score and outcome (evaluated based on 28 days mortality rate and ICU length of stay). In accordance with our results supposedly considered as a marker of inflammation in patients with sepsis, however, due to limitations of our study regarding sample size, difficulties in measuring other defensin subtypes with corresponding structure and lack of data on important cytokines like IL-1 and TNF, further studies are necessary in order to clarify HβD2 and other defensin activities and characterization of potential therapeutic or diagnostic targets.

One of the possible protective effects of NAC as a preventive in contrast induced nephropathy still remains undetermined. Based on various studies and meta -analyses NAC administration decreases the risk of contrast induced nephropathy [48-52]. In addition NAC may attenuate contrast induced nephropathy, as defined by albumin excretion, and seems to be independent of any effect on creatinine (NAC dosage: 500 mg IV prior to cardiac catheterization) [53].

Marenzi et al. suggested that NAC should have a protective effect solely when oxidative stress, induced by ischemia and reperfusion, is present (NAC dosage: 600 mg intravenous bolus before primary angioplasty and 600 mg orally twice daily for the 48 hours after angioplasty) [54]. Carbonell et al. found NAC's protect in the prevention of contrast induced nephropathy is based on reducing serum creatinine (SrCr) levels. The incidence of contrast induced nephropathy was significantly lower in NAC group but this effect was only valuable in high risk patients considering similar results that normal saline hydration produced in patients with normal renal function [55,56]. In conclusion Carbonell and coworkers recommend intravenous NAC prior to coronary angioplasty in high risk patients with SrCr ≥1.4 mg/dl, especially when hydration is impossible (NAC dosage: 600 mg every 12 hours IV) [56]. Macedo et al. in a study with focus on acute renal failure (ARF) associated with elective aortic aneurysm repair surgery, did not observe a change in ARF incidence and SrCr peak by NAC administration, in summary the study implied that potential beneficial effects of NAC in prevention of radiocontrast induced nephropathy should not be generalized to other insults applied to kidneys (NAC dosage: 1200 mg orally twice daily 24 hours before and 600 mg IV twice daily for 48 hours after) [57].

In chronic kidney disease (CKD) patients, some benefits has been observed by NAC, NAC reduces cardiovascular events in patients with stage 5 CKD and improves nitric oxide bioavailability (NAC dosage: Tepel et al., 600 mg Twice daily orally, Efrati et al. 1gr IV twice daily, 24 hours before and after angiography) [58,59]. Wittstock et al. demonstrated administration of NAC during dialysis session significantly improved arterial vascular reactivity in end stage CKD patients (NAC dosage: 5 gram IV during dialysis session) [60]. Contrary to that Renke et al. had reported, NAC had no effect on proteinuria and markers of tubular and renal fibrosis in non-diabetic CKD patients (NAC dosage: 1200 mg/day orally) [61].

In a study by Rosato and coworkers who evaluated the NAC effects on vascular system function in Systemic

Sclerosis patients, authors concluded that NAC improved vascular renal function in patients with low severity of disease (NAC dosage: 15 mg/kg/hour for 5 hours) [62].

Our study was not designed to assess how NAC affects the kidneys function, not to mention the fact that the dosage of NAC administered in this study was higher than dosages administered in studies on nephro-protective properties. Considering that rising in SrCr levels is noticeable. Using paired *t*-test (before after analysis) statistical method shows a significant increase in the mean of SrCr level in NAC group while at the same time the mean level of SrCr in control group is reduced. The mean level of SrCr during NAC administration have reached 1.48 mg/dl on day 3 and interestingly SrCr levels after discontinuation of NAC (on day 3) is decreased to its baseline (as low as 0.92 mg/dl). This may partially declare that high doses NAC administration is associated with progression towards acute kidney injury.

Conclusion

Considering adverse reactions observed in our study in terms of tachycardia, high blood pressure, leukocytosis and prolonged ventilator days and regarding the fact that no signs of improvement were observed in terms of mortality rate which was slightly higher for NAC group, high dosage of NAC is not recommended in critically ill patients with sepsis. NAC usage, even low dose, shall be administered with great caution in critically ill patients. Further studies on dosage and possible ceiling effect for NAC and re-evaluating safety of that, being conducted along with increased risk and extent of inflammatory profile. In this study no immuno-modulating effect associated with NAC was detected. According to SrCr variations during our study, we recommend to conduct further studies with adequate sample size to evaluate nephro-protective effects of NAC.

Competing interests

The authors declare that they have no competing interests.

Authors' contributions

MM: study design, patient selection, sample collection and handling, statistical analysis, analysis and interpretation of data, draft the manuscript and revising. KHA: study design, patient selection, sample collection and handling, analysis and interpretation of data, draft the manuscript and revising. MA: study design, sample analyzing via commercially available enzyme-linked immunosorbent assay kit, revised the manuscript. AN: study design, patient selection, sample collection and handling, draft the manuscript and revising. MM: study design. LCK: draft the manuscript and revising. FN: interpretation of data, revising the manuscript. AA: study design, patient selection, sample collection and handling, statistical analysis, analysis and interpretation of data, draft the manuscript and revising. All authors read and approved the final manuscript.

Acknowledgements

This work was supported by a grant from TUMS, Tehran, Iran. We thank Exir® pharmaceutical company for providing the drug. We also thank Dr. Alireza Ahmadvand and Maryam Baeeri for participating in this research.

Author details

[1]Department of Anesthesiology and Critical Care Medicine, Sina Hospital, Faculty of Medicine, Tehran University of Medical Sciences, Tehran, Iran. [2]Department of Clinical Pharmacy, Faculty of Pharmacy, Tehran University of Medical Sciences, Tehran, Iran. [3]Faculty of Pharmacy and Pharmaceutical Sciences Research Center, Tehran University of Medical Sciences, Tehran, Iran. [4]Department of Clinical Pharmacy, Faculty of Pharmacy, Mashhad University of Medical sciences, Mashhad, Iran.

References

1. Ertel W, Trentz O: **Polytrauma and multi-organ failure syndrome. Definition-pathophysiology-therapy.** *Zentralbl Chir* 1994, **119:**159.
2. Vyrostek SB, Annest JL, Ryan GW: **Surveillance for fatal and nonfatal injuries-United States, 2001.** *MMWR Surveill Summ* 2004, **53:**1–57.
3. Bardenheuer M, Obertacke U, Waydhas C, Nast-Kolb D: **Epidemiology of the severe multiple trauma-a prospective registration of preclinical and clinical supply.** *J Orthop Trauma* 2000, **14:**453.
4. Esposito TJ, Sanddal TL, Reynolds SA, Sanddal ND: **Effect of a voluntary trauma system on preventable death and inappropriate care in a rural state.** *J Trauma and Acute Care Surgery* 2003, **54:**663–670.
5. Brohi K, Singh J, Heron M, Coats T: **Acute traumatic coagulopathy.** *J Trauma* 2003, **54:**1127.
6. Homer T, Peter C, Frederick B: **Causes of death following multiple trauma.** *Curr Orthop* 2004, **18:**304–310.
7. Swain SD, Rohn TT, Quinn MT: **Neutrophil priming in host defense: role of oxidants as priming agents.** *Antioxid Redox Signal* 2002, **4:**69–83.
8. Martin P, D'Souza D, Martin J: **Wound healing in the PU. 1 null mouse—tissue repair is not dependent on inflammatory cells.** *Curr Biol* 2003, **13:**1122–1128.
9. Hietbrink F, Koenderman L, Rijkers G, Trauma L: **The role of the innate immune system.** *World J Emergency Surgery* 2006, **1:**15.
10. Power CP, Wang JH, Manning B: **Bacterial lipoprotein delays apoptosis in human neutrophils through inhibition of caspase-3 activity: regulatory roles for CD14 and TLR-2.** *J Immunol* 2004, **173:**5229–5237.
11. Echtenacher B, Hultner L, Mannel DN: **Cellular and molecular mechanisms of TNF protection in septic peritonitis.** *J Inflamm* 1996, **47:**85–89.
12. Cobb JP, O'Keefe GE: **Injury research in the genomic era.** *Lancet* 2004, **363:**2076–2083.
13. Vincent J-L, Sakr Y, Sprung CL: **Sepsis in European intensive care units: results of the SOAP study*.** *Crit Care Med* 2006, **34:**344–353.
14. Silva E, Pedro MA, Sogayar A: **Brazilian sepsis epidemiological study (BASES study).** *Crit Care* 2004, **8:**R251–R260.
15. Martin GS, Mannino DM, Eaton S, Moss M: **The epidemiology of sepsis in the United States from 1979 through 2000.** *N Engl J Med* 2003, **348:**1546–1554.
16. Angus DC, Pereira C, Silva E: **Epidemiology of severe sepsis around the world.** *Endocr Metab Immune Disord Drug Targets* 2006, **6:**207.
17. Milner SM, Bhat S, Buja M, Gulati S, Poindexter BJ, Bick RJ: **Expression of human β defensin 2 in thermal injury.** *Burns* 2004, **30:**649–654.
18. Burd RS, Furrer JL, Sullivan J, Smith AL: **Murine [BETA]-defensin-3 is an inducible peptide with limited tissue expression and broad-spectrum antimicrobial activity.** *Shock* 2002, **18:**461–464.
19. Ganz T, Lehrer RI: **Defensins.** *Pharmacol Ther* 1995, **66:**191–205.
20. Röhrl J, Yang D, Oppenheim JJ, Hehlgans T: **Human β-defensin 2 and 3 and their mouse orthologs induce chemotaxis through interaction with CCR2.** *J Immunol* 2010, **184:**6688–6694.
21. Book M, Chen Q, Lehmann LE: **Inducibility of the endogenous antibiotic peptide β-defensin 2 is impaired in patients with severe sepsis.** *Crit Care* 2007, **11:**R19.
22. Millea PJ: **N-acetylcysteine: multiple clinical applications.** *Am Fam Physician* 2009, **80:**265–269.
23. Kelly GS: **Clinical applications of N-acetylcysteine. Alternative medicine review.** *J Clinical Therapeutic* 1998, **3:**114.
24. Atkuri KR, Mantovani JJ, Herzenberg LA: **N-Acetylcysteine-a safe antidote for cysteine/glutathione deficiency.** *Curr Opin Pharmacol* 2007, **7:**355–359.
25. Santiago F, Bueno P, Olmedo C: **Effect of n-Acetylcysteine administration on intraoperative plasma levels of interleukin-4 and interleukin-10 in liver transplant recipients.** *Transplant Proc* 2008, **40:**2978–2980.
26. Paterson RL, Galley HF, Webster NR: **The effect of N-acetylcysteine on nuclear factor-[kappa] B activation, interleukin-6, interleukin-8, and**

intercellular adhesion molecule-1 expression in patients with sepsis*. *Crit Care Med* 2003, **31**:2574–2578.
27. Heller AR, Groth G, Heller SC: **N-acetylcysteine reduces respiratory burst but augments neutrophil phagocytosis in intensive care unit patients.** *Crit Care Med* 2001, **29**:272–276.
28. Lee TF, Jantzie LL, Todd KG, Cheung PY: **Postresuscitation N-acetylcysteine treatment reduces cerebral hydrogen peroxide in the hypoxic piglet brain.** *Intensive Care Med* 2008, **34**:190–197.
29. Molnar Z, MacKinnon K, Shearer E, Lowe D, Watson I: **The effect of N-acetylcysteine on total serum anti-oxidant potential and urinary albumin excretion in critically ill patients.** *Intensive Care Med* 1998, **24**:230–235.
30. Molnar Z, Shearer E, Lowe D: **N-Acetylcysteine treatment to prevent the progression of multisystem organ failure: A prospective, randomized, placebo-controlled study.** *Crit Care Med* 1999, **27**:1100–1104.
31. Spies CD, Reinhart K, Witt I: **Influence of N-acetlcycteine on direct indicators of tissue oxygenation in septicshock patients: Results from a prospective, randomized, double-blind study.** *Crit Care Med* 1994, **22**:1738–1746.
32. Ortolani O, Conti A, De Gaudio AR: **Protective effects of N-acetlcycteine and rutin on the lipid peroxidation of the lung epithelium during the adult respiratory syndrome.** *Shock* 2000, **13**:14–18.
33. Szakmany T, Marton S, Molnar Z: **Lack of effect of prophylactic N-acetlcycteine on postopertavie organdysfunction following major abdominal tumour surgery.** *Anaesth Intensive Care* 2003, **31**:267–271.
34. Domenighetti G, Suter PM, Schaller MD, Ritz R, Perret C: **Treatment with N -acetylcysteine during acute respiratory distress syndrome: a randomized, double-blind, placebo-controlled clinical study.** *J Crit Care* 1997, **12**:177–182.
35. Bernard GR, Wheeler AP, Arons MM: **A trial of antioxidants N-acetylcysteine and procysteine in ARDS.** *Chest* 1997, **112**:164–172.
36. Spapen H: **N-acetylcysteine in clinical sepsis: a difficult marriage.** *Crit Care* 2004, **8**:229–230.
37. Schmidt H, Schmidt W, Muller T, Bohrer H, Gebhard MM, Martin E: **N-acetylcysteine attenuates endotoxin-induced leukocyte-endothelial cell adhesion and macromolecular leakage in vivo.** *Crit Care Med* 1997, **25**:858–863.
38. Kharazmi A, Nielsen H, Schiøtz P: **N-acetylcysteine inhibits human neutrophil and monocyte chemotaxis and oxidative metabolism.** *Int J Immuno Pharmacology* 1988, **10**:39–46.
39. Emet S, Memis D, Pamukçu Z: **The influence of N-acetyl-L-cystein infusion on cytokine levels and gastric intramucosal pH during severe sepsis.** *Crit Care* 2004, **8**:229–230.
40. Yamaguchi Y, Ouchi Y: **Antimicrobial peptide defensin: Identification of novel isoforms and the characterization of their physiological roles and their significance in the pathogenesis of diseases.** *Proc Jpn Acad Ser B Phys Biol Sci* 2012, **88**:152.
41. Thomas NJ, Carcillo JA, Doughty LA, Sasser H, Heine RP: **Plasma concentrations of defensins and lactoferrin in children with severe sepsis.** *Pediatr Infect Dis J* 2002, **21**:34–38.
42. Shi Z, Zhao Z, Shu Q: **Protective effect of recombinant beta-defensin-2 on acute lung injury induced by sepsis in rats.** *Zhejiang da xue xue bao Yi xue ban J Zhejiang University Medical sciences* 2006, **35**:605.
43. Krisanaprakornkit S, Kimball JR, Weinberg A, Darveau RP, Bainbridge BW, Dale BA: **Inducible expression of human β-defensin 2 byFusobacterium nucleatum in oral epithelial cells: multiple signaling pathways and role of commensal bacteria in innate immunity and the epithelial barrier.** *Infect Immun* 2000, **68**:2907–2915.
44. Harder J, Bartels J, Christophers E, Schroder J: **A peptide antibiotic from human skin.** *Nature* 1997, **387**:861–61.
45. Liu K-X, Chen S-Q, Zhang H, Guo J-y, Li Y-S, Huang W-Q: **Intestinal ischaemia/reperfusion upregulates β-defensin-2 expression and causes acute lung injury in the rat.** *Injury* 2009, **40**:950–955.
46. Tsutsumi-Ishii Y, Nagaoka I: **Modulation of human β-defensin-2 transcription in pulmonary epithelial cells by lipopolysaccharide-stimulated mononuclear phagocytes via proinflammatory cytokine production.** *J Immunol* 2003, **170**:4226–4236.
47. Liu L, Roberts AA, Ganz T: **By IL-1 signaling, monocyte-derived cells dramatically enhance the epidermal antimicrobial response to lipopolysaccharide.** *J Immunol* 2003, **170**:575–580.
48. Tepel M, Van Der Giet M, Schwarzfeld C, Laufer U, Liermann D, Zidek W: **Prevention of radiographic-contrast-agent–induced reductions in renal function by acetylcysteine.** *N Engl J Med* 2000, **343**:180–184.
49. Kay J, Chow WH, Chan TM: **Acetylcysteine for prevention of acute deterioration of renal function following elective coronary angiography and intervention.** *JAMA* 2003, **289**:553–558.
50. Durham JD, Caputo C, Dokko J: **A randomized controlled trial of N-acetylcysteine to prevent contrast nephropathy in cardiac angiography.** *Kidney Int* 2002, **62**:2202–2207.
51. Duong MH, MacKenzie TA, Malenka D: **N-acetylcysteine prophylaxis significantly reduces the risk of radiocontrast-induced nephropathy: comprehensive meta-analysis.** *Catheter Cardiovasc Interv* 2005, **64**:471–479.
52. Birck R, Krzossok S, Markowetz F, Schnülle P, Van Der Woude FJ, Braun C: **Acetylcysteine for prevention of contrast nephropathy: meta-analysis.** *Lancet* 2003, **362**:598–603.
53. Levin A, Pate GE, Shalansky S: **N-acetylcysteine reduces urinary albumin excretion following contrast administration: evidence of biological effect.** *Nephrol Dial Transplant* 2007, **22**:2520–2524.
54. Marenzi G, Assanelli E, Marana I: **N-acetylcysteine and contrast-induced nephropathy in primary angioplasty.** *N Engl J Med* 2006, **354**:2773–2782.
55. Miner SE, Dzavik V, Nguyen-Ho P: **N-acetylcysteine reduces contrast-associated nephropathy but not clinical events during long-term follow-up.** *Am Heart J* 2004, **148**:690–695.
56. Carbonell N, Sanjuán R, Blasco M, Jordá Á, Miguel A: **N-acetylcysteine: short-term clinical benefits after coronary angiography in high-risk renal patients.** *Rev Esp Cardiol* 2010, **63**:12–19.
57. Macedo E, Abdulkader R, Castro I, Sobrinho AC, Yu L, Vieira JM: **Lack of protection of N-acetylcysteine (NAC) in acute renal failure related to elective aortic aneurysm repair-a randomized controlled trial.** *Nephrol Dial Transplant* 2006, **21**:1863–1869.
58. Tepel M, van der Giet M, Statz M, Jankowski J, Zidek W: **The antioxidant acetylcysteine reduces cardiovascular events in patients with End-stage renal failure a randomized, controlled trial.** *Circulation* 2003, **107**:992–995.
59. Efrati S, Dishy V, Averbukh M: **The effect of N-acetylcysteine on renal function, nitric oxide, and oxidative stress after angiography.** *Kidney Int* 2003, **64**:2182–2187.
60. Wittstock A, Burkert M, Zidek W, Tepel M, Scholze A: **N-acetylcysteine improves arterial vascular reactivity in patients with chronic kidney disease.** *Nephron Clin Pract* 2009, **112**:c184–c189.
61. Renke M, Tylicki L, Rutkowski P: **The effect of N-acetylcysteine on proteinuria and markers of tubular injury in Non-diabetic patients with chronic kidney disease.** *Kidney Blood Press Res* 2008, **31**:404–410.
62. Rosato E, Cianci R, Barbano B: **N-acetylcysteine infusion reduces the resistance index of renal artery in the early stage of systemic sclerosis.** *Acta Pharmacol Sin* 2009, **30**:1283–1288.

6

Synthesis, docking and acetylcholinesterase inhibitory assessment of 2-(2-(4-Benzylpiperazin-1-yl)ethyl)isoindoline-1,3-dione derivatives with potential anti-Alzheimer effects

Ahmad Mohammadi-Farani[1], Aram Ahmadi[2,4], Hamid Nadri[3] and Alireza Aliabadi[4*]

Abstract

Background: Alzheimer's disease (AD) as neurodegenerative disorder, is the most common form of dementia accounting for about 50-60% of the overall cases of dementia among persons over 65 years of age. Low acetylcholine (ACh) concentration in hippocampus and cortex areas of the brain is one of the main reasons for this disease. In recent years, acetylcholinesterase (AChE) inhibitors like donepezil with prevention of acetylcholine hydrolysis can enhance the duration of action of acetylcholine in synaptic cleft and improve the dementia associated with Alzheimer's disease.

Results: Design, synthesis and assessment of anticholinesterase activity of 2-(2-(4-Benzylpiperazin-1-yl)ethyl) isoindoline-1,3-dione derivatives showed prepared compounds can function as potential acetylcholinesterase inhibitor. Among 12 synthesized derivatives, compound 4a with *ortho* chlorine moiety as electron withdrawing group exhibited the highest potency in these series ($IC_{50} = 0.91 \pm 0.045$ μM) compared to donepezil ($IC_{50} = 0.14 \pm 0.03$ μM). The results of the enzyme inhibition test (Ellman test) showed that electron withdrawing groups like Cl, F and NO_2 can render the best effect at position *ortho* and *para* of the phenyl ring. But compound 4g with methoxy group at position 3(*meta*) afforded a favorable potency ($IC_{50} = 5.5 \pm 0.7$ μM). Furthermore, docking study confirmed a same binding mode like donepezil for compound 4a.

Conclusions: Synthesized compounds 4a-4l could be proposed as potential anticholinesterase agents.

Keywords: Synthesis, Phthalimide, Acetylcholinesterase (AChE), Anti-Alzheimer, Ellman test, Docking

Background

Alzheimer's disease (AD), is described by Dr. Alois Alzheimer in 1907 as a neurodegenerative disorder. AD as a disease of the central nervous system (CNS) characterized especially by premature senile mental deterioration. AD patients exhibit a significant decrease in cognitive ability and severe behavioral and psychological abnormalities such as irritability, anxiety and depression [1]. AD, one of the most diffuse neurodegenerative pathology among the elderly, causes a progressive impairment in functional performances and continuous reduction in cognitive activities and memory [2-7]. AD is the most common form of dementia accounting for about 50-60% of the overall cases of dementia among persons over 65 years of age, is a neurodegenerative alteration characterized by a low acetylcholine (ACh) in hippocampus and cortex [8]. AD is said to be the leading cause of dementia in elderly patients. Nowadays, with increase of the elderly population, the prevalence of AD is likely to increase. AD persons exert a decrease in mental functions and performances and consequently rendering them incapacitated and unable to perform normal daily activities. Elderly persons are the most common individuals afflicted with this disease. Unfortunately, the true nature or cause of the disease is still unknown and therefore, the development of effective anti-

* Correspondence: aliabadi.alireza@gmail.com
[4]Department of Medicinal Chemistry, Faculty of Pharmacy, Kermanshah University of Medical Sciences, Kermanshah, Iran
Full list of author information is available at the end of the article

alzheimer is one of the encouraging area in current medicinal chemistry researches [1].

Over two decades ago, several autopsy studies inside hippocampus revealed that the levels of the neurotransmitter acetylcholine in patients with Alzheimer's disease are importantly decreased [9]. Currently, the loss of cholinergic function is the only evidentiary finding responsible for cognitive decline. Hence, therapeutical development has focused on this theory. The loss of the basal forebrain cholinergic system is one of the most significant aspects of neurodegeneration in the brains of AD patients, and it is thought to play a central role in producing cognitive impairments [1,2,10,11]. Alzheimer's disease leads to a progressive decline of the cognitive function, executive function losses, memory deficits, and eventually to incapacitating dementia before death. In order to improve cholinergic neurotransmission, different strategies have been investigated including the increase of synthesis or pre-synaptic release of ACh, the stimulation of cholinergic post-synaptic muscarinic and nicotinic receptors, and the reduction of ACh synaptic degradation using AChE inhibitors (e.g., AChEIs or anticholinesterase agents) [12-19].

Acetylcholinesterase inhibitors have beneficial effects on cognitive, functional, and behavioral symptoms of AD. A recent review by the Quality Standard Subcommittee of the American Academy of Neurology investigated important issues in the management of dementia. The reviewers concluded that despite the small average degree of benefit of treatment with acetylcholinesterase inhibitors they should be the first-line treatment in patients with mild to moderate AD [4]. Four cholinesterase inhibitors tacrine, donepezil, rivastigmine, and galantamine are approved by the US Food and Drug Administration (FDA) and are currently in the market (Figure 1) [5].

According to the several reports about the efficacy of phthalimide derivatives in inhibition of AChE, [20-27] (Figure 2) in the current project, we focused on the design and synthesis of new anticholinesterase agents with phthalimide-based structure to reach more active analogs towards inhibition of AChE. Besides, we hope the new analogs to render lower side effects. Improving the pharmacokinetic properties of the designed compounds could be another aim of this study. In fact, phthalimide based compounds have similar pharmacophoric portions like indanone ring of the donepezil and are able to act as peripheral binding site inhibitor of AChE. We also investigated *in silico* binding mode of proposed ligands into the acetylcholinesterase enzyme in comparison with donepezil as reference drug by docking procedure.

Methods

Preliminary design

In the recent years, there are several reports about the potentiality of phthalimide derivatives as potent anticholinesterase agents. In fact, the phthalimide-based compounds can function as inhibitor of the peripheral binding site of AChE enzyme [20-27]. On the other hands, it is well-known in medicinal chemistry that piperazine ring can act as good bioisosteric replacement for piperidine moiety. According to the Figure 3, we designed a new series of donepezil-like analogues with replacement of the indanone and piperidine rings of the donepezil with

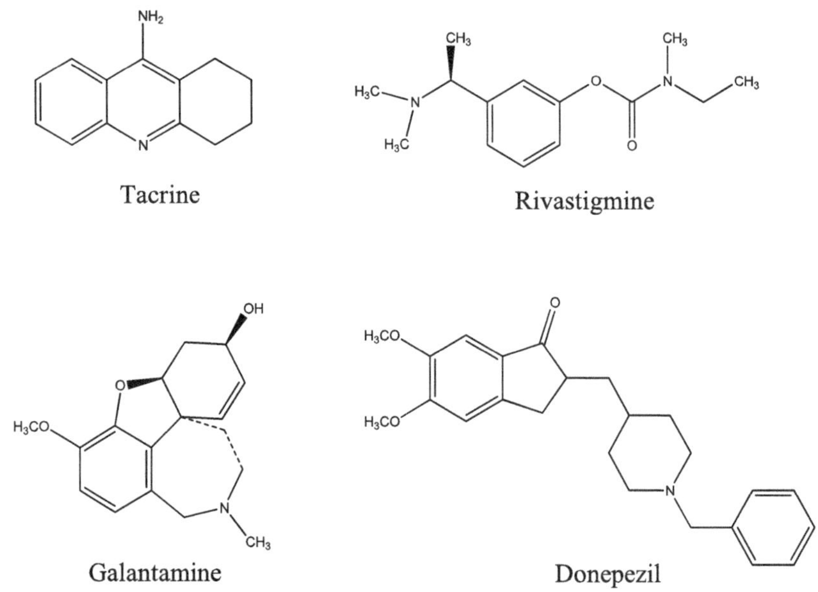

Figure 1 Structures of acetycholinesterase inhibitors in the market.

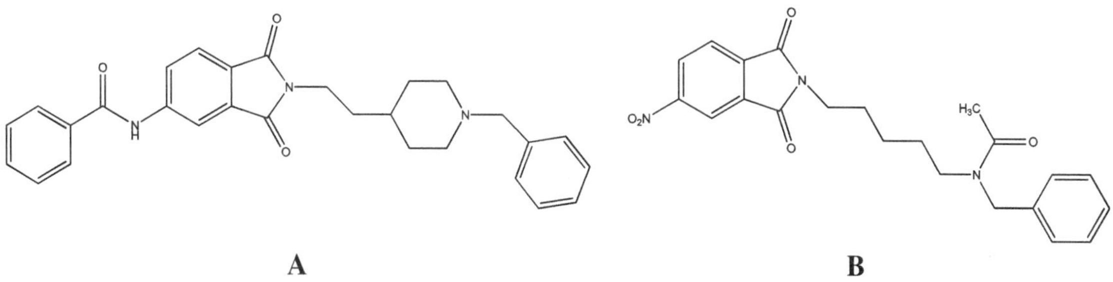

Figure 2 Two structures of phthalimide based anticholinesterase.

phthalimide (or isoindoline-1,3-dione) group and piperazine ring respectively. As illustrated in Figure 3, there are three distinct and critical portions in the structure of donepezil. Part A or peripheral binding site portion is necessary for binding to the AChE enzyme. The phenyl ring of the indanone moiety of donepezil participates in π-π stacking interaction with indole ring of Trp 279 in the active site of AChE. Part B is a linker region as well as an interacting part with Phe 330 in the active site of the AChE. According to the structure activity relationship (SAR) of donepezil-like analogs, the nitrogen atom of the piperidine ring is necessary for binding to the active site of the enzyme and removing of the nitrogen can be detrimental for anticholinesterase activity of the ligand. In fact, the charged nitrogen of the piperidine ring makes a cation-π interaction with Phe 330. Pat C or benzyl moiety unit plays its role through a π-π stacking interaction with indole ring of the Trp 84 [16]. Hence, in the designed compounds (Figure 3), the considering of these three pivotal portions of the donepezil was carried out and subsequently the synthesis of proposed compounds was done.

Chemistry

All chemical substances consisting starter materials, reagents and solvents were purchased from the commercial supplier like Merck and Sigma-Aldrich companies. The purity of the prepared compounds was proved by thin layer chromatography (TLC) using various solvents of different polarities. Merck silica gel 60 F_{254} plates were used for analytical TLC. Column chromatography was applied on Merck silica gel (70–230 mesh) for purification of intermediate and final compounds. ^{1}H-NMR spectra were recorded using a Bruker 400 MHz spectrometer in deutrated solvents, and chemical shifts are expressed as δ (ppm) with tetramethylsilane (TMS) as internal standard. The IR spectra were obtained on a Shimadzu 470 spectrophotometer using potassium bromide (KBr) disks. Melting points were determined

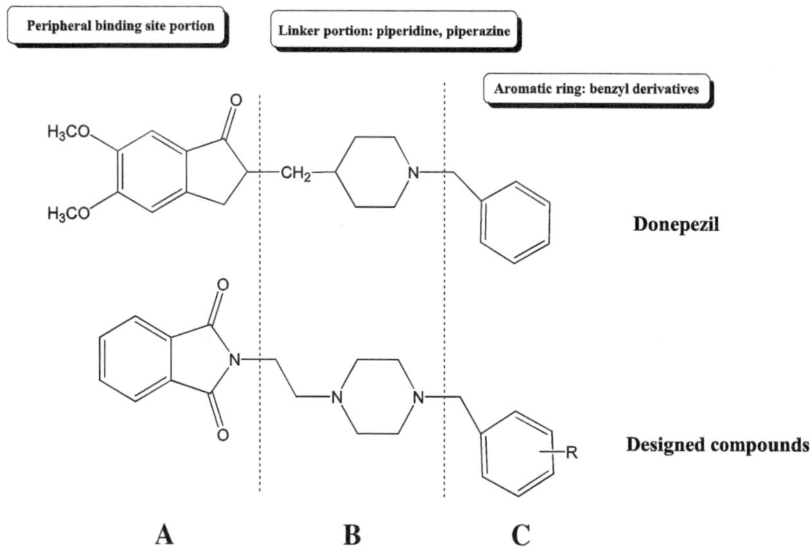

Figure 3 Design of new donepezil-like analogs based on the phthalimide structure.

using Electrothermal 9001 elemental analyzer apparatus and are uncorrected. The mass spectra were run on a Finigan TSQ-70 spectrometer (Finigan, USA) at 70 eV.

Synthesis of 2-(2-(piperazin-1-yl)ethyl)isoindoline-1,3-dione (3)

In a flask 3 g (20 mmol) of Phthalic anhydride, 2.6 ml (20 mmol) *N*-amnioethylpiperazine and 2.9 ml (20 mmol) triethylamine (Et_3N) were mixed in 40 ml of toluene solvent. The reaction mixture was refluxed for 24 hours and the termination of reaction and formation of the desired product was confirmed by thin layer chromatography. The discoloration of the reaction medium and formation of a yellow precipitate was also an indicator of the progress of the reaction. Then, toluene was evaporated under reduced pressure using rotary evaporator apparatus and the obtained yellow viscose and oily residue was washed several times by ethyl acetate (EtOAc) and diethyl ether (Et_2O) [28].

^1H NMR ($CDCl_3$, 400 MHz) δ (ppm): 2.37 (m, 4H, Piperazine), 2.54 (m, 4H, Piperazine), 3.22 (t, 2H, phthalimide-CH_2-$\underline{CH_2}$-piperazine), 3.44 (t, 2H, phthalimide-$\underline{CH_2}$-CH_2-piperazine), 4.73 (NH, Piperazine), 7.35-7.85 (m, 4H, Phthalimide). IR (KBr, cm^{-1}) ῡ: 3380, 3330, 3157, 3111, 2924, 1730, 1681, 1521, 1489, 1458, 1328, 1303, 1186, 1143, 1035, 910, 750, 710. MS (*m/z*, %): 259 (M^+, 10), 224 (30), 174 (30), 160 (60), 149 (85), 99 (100), 70 (70), 57 (65), 41 (40).

General procedure for synthesis of compounds 4a-4l:

In a flat-bottom flask equimolar quantities of compound 3 and appropriate derivative of benzyl chloride were added together in dichloromethane (CH_2Cl_2) solvent. The reaction mixture was stirred in room temperature overnight. Then, dichloromethane was evaporated under reduced pressure and the afforded residue was washed by diethyl ether and *n*-hexane. Methanol containing Hydrochloric acid gas was added to the residue to form the related hydrochloride salt of the product [29].

2-(2-(4-(2-Chlorobenzyl)piperazin-1-yl)ethyl)isoindoline-1,3-dione (4a)

^1H NMR (DMSO-d_6, 400 MHz) δ (ppm): 2.36 (m, 8H, Piperazine), 3.33 (t, 2H, CH_2-piperazine), 3.35 (s, 2H, -C $\underline{H_2}$-2-Chlorophenyl), 3.61 (t, 2H, -CH_2-Phthalimide), 7.25-7.32 (m, 2H, 2-Chlorophenyl), 7.34-7.44 (m, 2H, 2-Chlorophenyl), 7.46-7.87 (m, 4H, Phthalimide). MS (*m/ z*, %): 385 (M^++2, 2), 383 (M^+, 5), 225 (50), 223 (100), 160 (50), 125 (95), 89 (15), 70 (20). IR (KBr, cm^{-1}) ῡ: 3460, 3051, 2943, 2800, 2762, 1766, 1465, 1438, 1396, 1357, 1300, 1192, 1161, 1107, 1041, 921, 759, 717, 698.

2-(2-(4-(3-Chlorobenzyl)piperazin-1-yl)ethyl)isoindoline-1,3-dione (4b)

^1H NMR (DMSO-d_6, 400 MHz) δ (ppm): 2.34 (m, 4H, Piperazine), 3.35 (t, 2H, -CH_2-piperazine), 3.51 (s, 2H, -$\underline{CH_2}$-phenyl), 3.7 (t, 2H, -CH_2-phthalimide), 7.27-7.32 (m, H_2, H_5, 3-Chlorophenyl), 7.41 (d, 1H, *J* = 8 Hz, H_6-3-Chlorophenyl), 7.45 (d, *J* = 8 Hz, H_4-3-Chlorophenyl), 7.85 (m, 2H, H_5,H_6-phthalimide), 7.88 (m, 2H, H_4,H_7-phthalimide). IR (KBr, cm^{-1}) ῡ: 3160, 3113, 2924, 1710, 1681, 1533, 1521, 1489, 1458, 1327, 1303, 1186, 1143, 1037, 715.

2-(2-(4-(4-Chlorobenzyl)piperazin-1-yl)ethyl)isoindoline-1,3-dione (4c)

^1H NMR ($CDCl_3$, 400 MHz) δ (ppm): 2.2 (t, 2H, -N-CH_2-$\underline{CH_2}$-NH-, piperazine), 2.5 (t, 2H, -N-$\underline{CH_2}$-CH_2-NH-, Piperazine), 2.63 (t, 2H, phthalimide-CH_2-$\underline{CH_2}$-piperazine), 3.42 (s, 2H, -CH_2-phenyl), 3.8 (t, 2H, phthalimide-$\underline{CH_2}$-CH_2-piperazine), 7.23 (d, 2H, *J* = 8 Hz, $H_{2,6}$-4-chlorophenyl), 7.30 (d, 2H, *J* = 8 Hz, $H_{3,5}$-4-chlorophenyl phenyl), 7.76 (m, 4H, Phthalimide). IR (KBr, cm^{-1}) ῡ: 3400, 3380, 3135, 3111, 2927, 2812, 1703, 1681, 1533, 1521, 1489, 1456, 1328, 1305, 1186, 1143, 1035, 721, 707. MS (*m/z*, %): 384 (M^+ +1, 20), 383 (M^+, 18), 280 (20), 223 (100), 167 (30), 149 (90), 125 (90).

2-(2-(4-(2-Fluorobenzyl)piperazin-1-yl)ethyl)isoindoline-1,3-dione (4d)

^1H NMR (DMSO-d_6, 400 MHz) δ (ppm): 2.4 (m, 4H, piperazine), 3.1 (m, 4H, aliphatic), 3.8 (s, 2H, -CH_2-phenyl), 7.35 (m, 4H, 2-Fluorophenyl), 7.88 (m, 4H, Phthalimide). IR (KBr, cm^{-1}) ῡ: 3429, 2993, 2924, 2854, 1774, 1716, 1396, 1068, 1010, 721. MS (*m/z*, %): 368 (M^++1, 25), 313 (40), 285 (35), 257 (40), 236 (100), 152 (40), 111 (60), 97 (95), 83 (90), 69 (90), 57 (85), 43 (50).

2-(2-(4-(3-Fluorobenzyl)piperazin-1-yl)ethyl)isoindoline-1,3-dione (4e)

^1H NMR (DMSO-d_6, 400 MHz) δ (ppm): 3.37-3.87 (m, aliphatic), 3.99 (s, 2H, -CH_2-phenyl), 7.29 (d, 1H, *J* = 8 Hz, H_2-3-Fluorophenyl), 7.49 (m, 1H, H_6-3-Fluorophenyl), 7.66 (d, 1H, *J* = 8 Hz, H_5-3-Fluorophenyl), 7.68 (d, 1H, *J* = 8 Hz, H_3-3-Fluorophenyl), 7.86-7.88 (m, 4H, phthalimide). IR (KBr, cm^{-1}) ῡ: 3371, 2993, 2958, 2924, 2854, 1774, 1712, 1546, 1462, 1404, 1056, 972, 721.

2-(2-(4-(4-Fluorobenzyl)piperazin-1-yl)ethyl)isoindoline-1,3-dione (4f)

^1H NMR (DMSO-d_6, 400 MHz) δ (ppm): 3.99 (m, 12H, aliphatic), 3.96 (s, -CH_2-phenyl), 3.99 (t, 2H, -CH_2-phthalimide), 7.3 (t, 2H, *J* = 8 Hz, 4-Fluorophenyl), 7.58-7.73 (m, 4-Fluorophenyl), 7.83-7.88 (m, 4H, Phthalimide). IR (KBr, cm^{-1}) ῡ: 3367, 2997, 2854, 1774, 1716, 1604, 1512, 1462, 1400, 1056, 975, 721.

2-(2-(4-(3-Methoxybenzyl)piperazin-1-yl)ethyl)isoindoline-1,3-dione (4g)

^{1}H NMR (DMSO-d_6, 400 MHz) δ (ppm): 3.2-3.66 (m, aliphatic), 3.79 (s, 3H, -OCH_3), 3.97 (s, 2H, -CH_2-phenyl), 7.1-7.36 (m, 4H, 4-Methoxyphenyl), 7.58-7.66 (m, 4H, Phthalimide). IR (KBr, cm^{-1}) ῡ: 3371, 2993, 1774, 1716, 1612, 1462, 1435, 1400, 1381, 1269, 1056, 972, 906, 798, 721. MS (*m/z*, %): 379 (M^+, 15), 219 (100), 160 (30), 121 (80), 91 (20).

2-(2-(4-(4-Methoxybenzyl)piperazin-1-yl)ethyl)isoindoline-1,3-dione (4h)

^{1}H NMR (DMSO-d_6, 400 MHz) δ (ppm): 3.1-3.78 (m, aliphatic), 3.78 (s, 3H, -OCH_3), 4.4 (s, 2H, -CH_2-phenyl), 7.1 (dd, 4H, $J = 8$ Hz, 4-Methoxyphenyl), 7.43-7.58 (m, 4H, Phthalimide). IR (KBr, cm^{-1}) ῡ: 3429, 2978, 2935, 1778, 1716, 1612, 1516, 1462, 1435, 1400, 1235, 1184, 1072, 1029, 802, 725.

2-(2-(4-(2-Nitrobenzyl)piperazin-1-yl)ethyl)isoindoline-1,3-dione (4i)

^{1}H NMR (DMSO-d_6, 400 MHz) δ (ppm): 2.25-2.35 (m, 8H, Piperazine), 3.35 (t, 2H, -CH_2-piperazine), 3.66 (s, 2H, CH_2-phenyl), 3.68 (t, 2H, -CH_2-phthalimide), 7.4-7.66 (m, 4H, 2-Nitrophenyl), 7.83-7.89 (m, 4H, Phthalimide). IR (KBr, cm^{-1}) ῡ: 3155, 3111, 2956, 2922, 1681, 1521, 1489, 1458, 1327, 1303, 1188, 1141, 1035, 740, 717, 705. MS (*m/z*, %): 394 (M^+, 3), 377 (15), 259 (30), 235 (40), 234 (100), 200 (50), 160 (70), 130 (30), 99 (55), 78 (30) 56 (15).

2-(2-(4-(3-Nitrobenzyl)piperazin-1-yl)ethyl)isoindoline-1,3-dione (4j)

^{1}H NMR (DMSO-d_6, 400 MHz) δ (ppm): 2.51 (m, 4H, Piperazine), 3.53 (t, 2H, -CH_2-piperazine), 3.79 (s, -CH_2-phenyl), 3.85 (t, 2H, -CH_2-phthalimide), 7.6-7.66 (m, 2H, $H_{4,6}$-3-Nitrophenyl), 7.65 (s, 1H, H_2-3-Nitrophenyl), 7.75 (t, $J = 8$ Hz, 1H, H_5-3-Nitrophenyl), 7.85 (m, 2H, $H_{5,6}$-phthalimide), 7.88 (m, 2H, $H_{4,7}$-phthalimide). IR (KBr, cm^{-1}) ῡ: 3425, 2924, 2854, 1774, 1716, 1531, 1435, 1400, 1350, 1060, 806, 721.

2-(2-(4-(4-Nitrobenzyl)piperazin-1-yl)ethyl)isoindoline-1,3-dione (4k)

^{1}H NMR (DMSO-d_6, 400 MHz) δ (ppm): 2.3 (m, 8H, Piperazine), 3.33 (t, 2H, phthalimide-CH_2-$\underline{CH_2}$-piperazine), 3.56 (s, 2H, -CH_2-phenyl), 3.69 (t, 2H, phthalimide-$\underline{CH_2}$-CH_2-piperazine), 7.57 (d, 2H, $J = 8$ Hz, $H_{2,6}$-4-Nitrophenyl), 7.83-7.88 (m, 4H, Phthalimide), 8.19 (d, 2H, $J = 8$ Hz, $H_{3,5}$-4-Nitrophenyl). IR (KBr, cm^{-1}) ῡ: 3157, 3111, 2924, 1775, 1681, 1519, 1489, 1458, 1330, 1303, 1186, 1143, 1037, 750, 710. MS (*m/z*, %): 395 (M^++1, 10), 394 (M^+, 35), 235 (85), 234 (100), 191 (60), 174 (30), 160 (85), 90 (25), 70 (40).

2-(2-(4-Benzylpiperazin-1-yl)ethyl)isoindoline-1,3-dione (4l)

^{1}H NMR (DMSO-d_6, 400 MHz) δ (ppm): 2.51 (m, 4H, Piperazine), 3.55 (m, 8H, aliphatic), 3.99 (s, 2H, -CH_2-phenyl), 7.45-7.68 (m, 4H, phenyl), 7.85 (m, 4H, Phthalimide). IR (KBr, cm^{-1}) ῡ: 3414, 2997, 2924, 1774, 1712, 1635, 1431, 1396, 1064, 721. MS (*m/z*, %): 349 (10), 234 (20), 189 (100), 160 (35), 91 (90).

Anticholinesterase activity assay (Ellman test)

Lyophilized powder of acetylcholinesterase from electric eel source (AChE, E.C. 3.1.1.7, Type V-S, 1000 unit) was purchased from Sigma-Aldrich (Steinheim, Germany). 5,5'-Dithiobis-(2-nitrobenzoic acid), potassium dihydrogen phosphate, dipotassium hydrogen phosphate, potassium hydroxide, sodium hydrogen carbonate, and acetylthiocholine iodide were purchased from Fluka (Buchs, Switzerland). Compounds 4a-4l were dissolved in a mixture of 20 ml distilled water and 5 ml methanol and then diluted in 0.1 M KH_2PO_4/K_2HPO_4 buffer (pH 8.0) to afford a final concentration range. The Ellman test was carried out for assessment of the anticholinesterase activity of intended compounds *in vitro*. Prior to use, all solutions were adjusted to 25°C. To achieve 20-80% inhibition of AChE activity five different concentrations of each compound were tested. The assay solution consisted of a 0.1 M potassium phosphate buffer pH 8.0, with the addition of 0.01 M 5,50-dithio-bis(2-nitrobenzoic acid), 2.5 unit/mL of enzyme solution (AChE, E.C. 3.1.1.7, Type V-S, lyophilized powder, from electric eel) (Sigma Chemical). Compounds 4a-4l were added to the assay solution and preincubated at 25°C with the enzyme for 15 min followed by adding 0.075 M substrate (acetylthiocholine iodide). After rapid and immediate mixing the change of absorption was measured at 412 nm. In order to justify non enzymatic reaction assays were carried out with a blank containing all components except AChE.

The blank reading contained 3 ml buffer, 200 μl water, 100 μl DTNB and 20 μl substrate. The reaction rates were calculated, and the percent inhibition of test compounds was determined. Each concentration was analyzed in triplicate, and IC_{50} values were determined graphically from inhibition curves (log inhibitor concentration vs percent of inhibition). Spectrophotometric measurements were performed on a Cecil BioAquarius CE 7250 Double Beam Spectrophotometer [30].

Docking

ArgusLab 4.0 software was applied to perform molecular docking studies [31,32]. All intended ligands were constructed in arguslab workspace and all ligands 4a-4l were energy minimized by AM1 as semiemperical method. The pdb file of acetylcholinesterase enzyme in complex with donepezil (pdb code: 1EVE) was downloaded from brookhaven protein databank [33]. The geometry

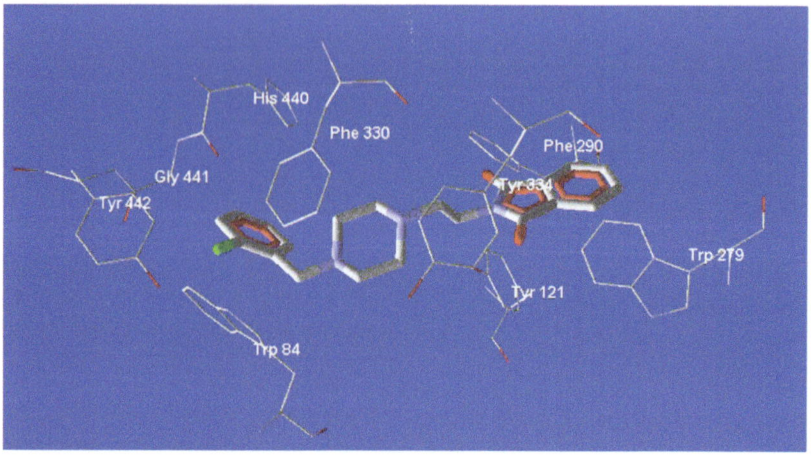

Figure 4 Docked molecule of compound 4a in the active site of AChE (PDB code: 1EVE). The principal amino acids (Trp 279, Phe 330, Trp 84) are evident in the nearby of the docked molecule.

optimization of structure of acetylcholinesterase enzyme was performed using universal force field (UFF) as a molecular mechanic method. The docking process was done for all ligands in the workspace of ArgusLab 4 software after defining the related groups for each ligand and also for related protein. The binding location of donepezil was defined as binding site for finding the best pose and conformation for all ligands. Binding mode and related interactions of all ligands were explored in Molegro molecular viewer software (Figure 4, Figure 5) [34].

Results and discussion

Chemistry

As summarized in the Scheme 1, all intermediate and final compounds 3 and 4a-4l were synthesized with an acceptable to high yield (ranging 61–96%) as listed in Table 1. Compound 3 was obtained through a Gabriel synthetic reaction. Reaction of phthalic anhydride with *N*-aminoethylpiperazine afforded the compound 3 with 61% yield. The reaction was carried out under reflux conditions in toluene solvent. Washing of yellowish oily product was done by ethyl acetate and *n*-hexane. A yellow powder was obtained after trituration. Obtained product was used for synthesis of 4a-4l derivatives. Room temperature stirring of equimolar quantities of compound **3** with appropriate benzyl chloride derivatives afforded 4a-4l derivatives. Dichloromethane was used as solvent and overnight stirring is necessary for achieving an acceptable yield. After evaporation, an oily residue was obtained. Methanolic hydrochloric acid was applied

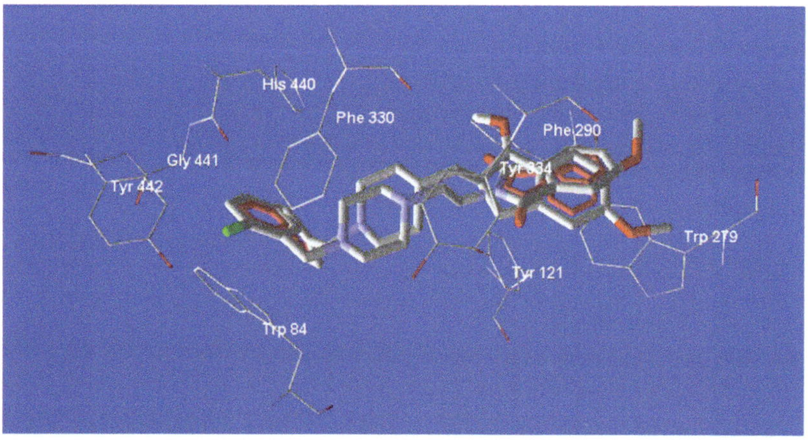

Figure 5 Superimposed structure of compound 4a with donepezil in the active site of AChE. A similar binding mode and interaction like donepezil are observed for compound 4a.

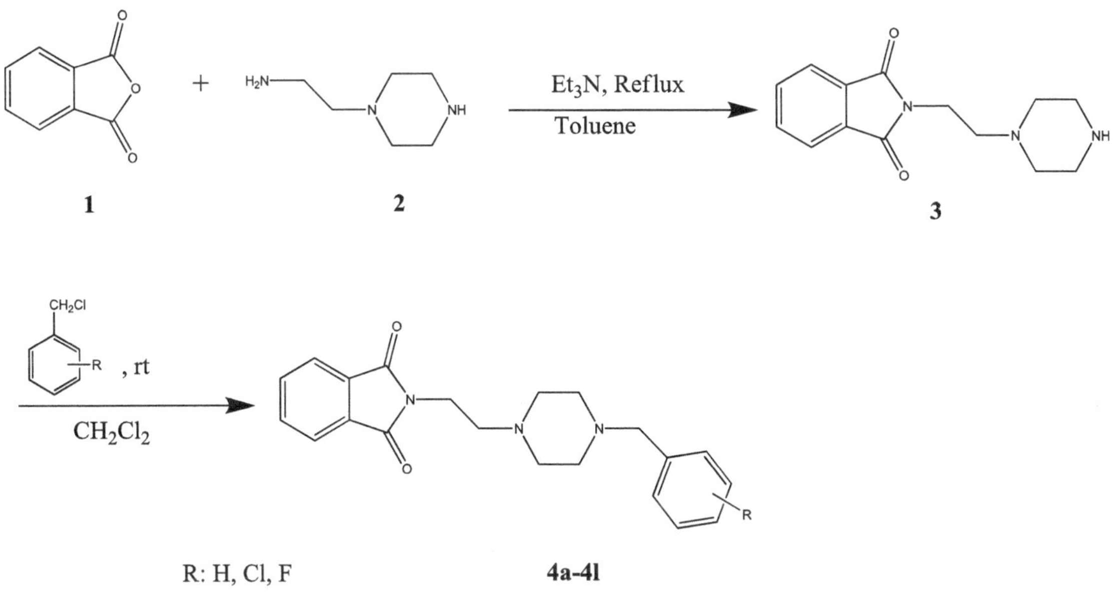

Scheme 1 Synthetic pathway of compounds 4a-4l.

to form the corresponding hydrochloride salt of each derivative. For each compound 2 ml of methanolic solvent was added to the obtained residue and stirred at room temperature for 5–10 minutes. The formed precipitate was filtered, dried and collected.

Different types of substituent consisted of three electron withdrawing substituents (Cl, F, NO_2) and also an electron donating substituent ($-OCH_3$) were synthesized to investigate the electronic effects of various moieties. Furthermore, compound 4l was also synthesized without any group on the phenyl ring to explore the effect of the presence of the substitution on this ring.

Melting points of intermediate and final compounds were obtained using capillary tubes by electrothermal melting point analyzer. A range in melting point was recorded for compounds 3, 4a, 4b, 4f and 4i. In other cases a sharp point was detected and presented in Table 1. ^{1}H NMR, IR and MS spectroscopic methods were applied for characterization and identification of all compounds. Deutrated dimethyl sulfoxide (DMSO-d_6) was used for ^{1}H NMR acquisition and TMS (tetramethyl silane) was applied as internal standard. Infrared spectroscopy was performed for all compounds using KBr disk and outstanding peaks was reported. Molecular ion

Table 1 Properties of synthesized compounds

Compounds	R	Closed formula	MW (g/mol)	mp (°C)	Yield (%)	Appearance
3	-	$C_{14}H_{17}N_3O_2$	259	105-109	61	Yellow
4a	2-Cl	$C_{21}H_{22}ClN_3O_2$	383	105-107	81	Creamy
4b	3-Cl	$C_{21}H_{22}ClN_3O_2$	383	100-103	74	Creamy
4c	4-Cl	$C_{21}H_{22}ClN_3O_2$	383	122	78	Creamy
4d	2-F	$C_{21}H_{22}FN_3O_2$	367	226	96	Yellow
4e	3-F	$C_{21}H_{22}FN_3O_2$	367	225	77	Creamy
4f	4-F	$C_{21}H_{22}FN_3O_2$	367	293-296	77	Yellow
4g	3-OCH_3	$C_{22}H_{25}N_3O_3$	379	259	82	Yellow
4h	4-OCH_3	$C_{22}H_{25}N_3O_3$	379	265	65	Yellow
4i	2-NO_2	$C_{21}H_{22}N_4O_4$	394	118-120	78	Orange
4j	3-NO_2	$C_{21}H_{22}N_4O_4$	394	286	92	Orange
4k	4-NO_2	$C_{21}H_{22}N_4O_4$	394	162	80	Creamy
4l	H	$C_{21}H_{23}N_3O$	349	231	92	Orange

Table 2 Results (IC_{50}, μM) of *in vitro* acetylcholinesterase assay of compounds 4a-4l

Compound	4a	4b	4c	4d	4e	4f	4g	4h	4i	4j	4k	4l	Donepezil
R	2-Cl	3-Cl	4-Cl	2-F	3-F	4-F	3-OCH_3	4-OCH_3	2-NO_2	3-NO_2	4-NO_2	H	-
IC_{50}(μM)	**0.91 ± 0.045**	85 ± 12	26 ± 5	23 ± 7	74 ± 11	42 ± 8	5.5 ± 0.7	72 ± 9	36 ± 5	59 ± 6	40 ± 4	9 ± 2	0.14 ± 0.03

peak of synthesized compounds was recorded in MS spectroscopy. Furthermore, M^{+}+2 was also reported for chlorinated compounds.

Anticholinesterase activity

According to Table 2, all compounds 4a-4l were tested against acetylcholinesterase and related IC_{50} ± SEM were calculated. Compound 4a with *ortho* chlorine substituent on phenyl ring was the most potent one in this series (IC_{50} = 0.91 ± 0.045 μM). *Para* position (compound 4c, IC_{50} = 26 ± 5 μM) was also favorable for anticholinesterase activity but on the other hands *meta* substitution of chlorine (compound 4b, IC_{50} = 85 ± 12 μM) led to the lowest inhibitory effect compared to other position for this moiety. Among compounds 4d-4f with fluorine moiety, compound 4d at position 2(*ortho*) showed the highest inhibitory property toward the acetylcholinesrase. Position 3(*meta*) was the worst position for fluorine and *para* substitution afforded an averaged potency in comparison with other positions. Compound 4g with *meta* substitution of methoxy substituent as electron donating group rendered a high potency derivative with IC_{50} = 5.5 ± 0.7 μM. A similar trend like chlorine and fluorine moieties was also observed for nitro group. Substitution of nitro group as electron withdrawing moiety at position 2(*ortho*) of the phenyl ring in compound 4i afforded the best effect. On the other hands, position 3(*meta*) was the worst position for nitro substituent (compound 4j). Insertion of nitro group at position 4(*para*) in compound 4k led to a moderate affinity for inhibition of acetylcholinesterase compared to positions 2 and 3. Compound 4l without any substituent on the phenyl ring was also one of the most potent inhibitor of acetylcholinesterase in this series. Totally, electron withdrawing moieties such as Cl, F and NO_2 at position 2(*ortho*) of the phenyl ring can enhance the potency of synthesized phthalimide derivatives. Electron donating group like methoxy at position 3 can also increase the enzyme inhibitory effects in these series.

Totally, electron withdrawing substituents are capable to enhance the anticholinestease activity of the phthalimide derivatives that synthesized in this research. Comparison of the different compounds with electron withdrawing moieties showed that *ortho* position is the best position for this type of substituents. Whereas, the *para* position was the worst position for all of the electron withdrawing moieties. Introducing of an electron donating group such as methoxy at *meta* position of the phenyl ring also led to the increasing of the potency. But, this change was not so effective like *ortho* substitution of chlorine atom. Absence of any moiety on the phenyl ring as observed about compound 4l could be an AChE inhibitor with an averaged potency. In fact, this compound exerted potency less than compound 4a with *ortho* chlorine as well as compound 4g with *meta* methoxy substituent.

Molecular modeling

All ligands 4a-4l were docked into the active site of acetylcholinesterase (PDB ID: 1EVE). For performing an accurate docking procedure, the binding site of donepezil was intended as probable binding site for all ligands especially for ligand 4a. Compound 4a as the best inhibitor of AChE *in vitro* was studied *in silico* to reveal the probable binding mode of synthesized compounds perfectly (Figure 3). Superimposed state for this ligand with donepezil was also explored. According to the Figure 4, a similar binding mode and conformation as observed for donepezil, was also seen for this ligand. In fact, the structure of synthesized compounds occupies a similar region like donepezil in the active site of AChE. As seen in Figure 4, phthalimide, piperazine and benzyl rings of compound **4a** adopt a same location like indanone, piperidine and benzyl rings of the donepezil respectively.

Conclusions

A new series of donepezil-like analogs were synthesized based on the phthalimide structure and anticholinesterase activity was assessed using Ellman test. All compounds exhibited a μM range in IC_{50} value (5.5-85 μM) for inhibition of AChE except for compound 4a that exhibited a nM range in IC_{50} value (0.91 μM). *In silico* study of compound 4a by docking method was also confirmed a similar binding mode like donepezil for this ligand.

Competing interests

The authors declare that they have no competing interests.

Acknowledgements

Authors are grateful from the research deputy of Kermanshah University of Medical Sciences for financial support. This work was performed in partial fulfillment of the requirement for PharmD of Mr. Aram Ahmadi.

Author details

[1]Department of Pharmacology, Toxicology and Medical Services, Faculty of Pharmacy, Kermanshah University of Medical Sciences, Kermanshah, Iran. [2]Students Research Committee, Kermanshah University of Medical Sciences, Kermanshah, Iran. [3]Neurobiomedical Research Center, Shahid Sadoughi University of Medical Sciences, Yazd, Iran. [4]Department of Medicinal

Chemistry, Faculty of Pharmacy, Kermanshah University of Medical Sciences, Kermanshah, Iran.

References

1. Sugimoto H, Yamanishi Y, Iimura Y, Kawakami Y: **Donepezil Hydrochloride (E2020) and Other Acetylcholinesterase Inhibitors.** *Curr Med Chem* 2000, **7:**303–339.
2. Mustazza C, Borioni A, Rosaria Del Giudice M, Gatta F, Ferretti R, *et al:* **Synthesis and cholinesterase activity of phenylcarbamates related to Rivastigmine, a therapeutic agent for Alzheimer's disease.** *Eur J Med Chem* 2002, **37:**91–109.
3. Maczurek A, Hager K, Kenklies M, Sharman M, Martins R, Engel J, *et al:* **Lipoic acid as an anti-inflammatory and neuroprotective treatment for Alzheimer's disease.** *Adv Drug Del Rev* 2008, **60:**1463–1470.
4. Scarpini E, Scheltens P, Feldman H: **Treatment of Alzheimer's disease: current status and new perspectives.** *Lancet Neurol* 2003, **2:**539–547.
5. Ucar G, Gokhan N, Yesilada A, Bilgin AA: **1-*N*-Substituted thiocarbamoyl-3 -phenyl-5-thienyl-2-pyrazolines: A novel cholinesterase and selective monoamine oxidase B inhibitors for the treatment of Parkinson's and Alzheimer's diseases.** *Neurosci Lett* 2005, **382:**327–331.
6. Vitorović-Todorović MD, Juranić IO, Mandić LM, Drakulic BJ: **4-Aryl-4-oxo-*N*-phenyl-2-aminylbutyramides as acetyl- and butyrylcholinesterase inhibitors. Preparation, anticholinesterase activity, docking study, and 3D structure–activity relationship based on molecular interaction fields.** *Bioorg Med Chem* 2010, **18:**1181–1193.
7. Araújo JQ, Araújo de Brito M, Bôas Hoelz LV, de Alencastro RB, Castro HC, Rodrigues C, *et al:* **Receptor-dependent (RD) 3D-QSAR approach of a series of benzylpiperidine inhibitors of human acetylcholinesterase (HuAChE).** *Eur J Med Chem* 2011, **46:**39–51.
8. Yu L, Cao R, Yi W, Yan Q, Chen C, Ma L, *et al:* **Synthesis of 4-[(diethylamino) methyl]-phenol derivatives as novel cholinesterase inhibitors with selectivity towards butyrylcholinesterase.** *Bioorg Med Chem Lett* 2010, **20:**3254–3258.
9. Trujillo-Ferrara J, Montoya Cano L, Espinoza-Fonseca M: **Synthesis, Anticholinesterase Activity and Structure-Activity Relationships of *m*-Aminobenzoic Acid Derivatives.** *Bioorg Med Chem Lett* 2003, **13:**1825–1827.
10. Weinstock M, Groner E: **Rational design of a drug for Alzheimer's disease with cholinesterase inhibitory and neuroprotective activity.** *Chem Biol Interact* 2008, **175:**216–221.
11. Liston DR, Nielsen JA, Villalobos A, Chapin D, Jones SB, Hubbard ST, *et al:* **Pharmacology of selective acetylcholinesterase inhibitors: implications for use in Alzheimer's disease.** *Eur J Pharmacol* 2004, **486:**9–17.
12. Racchi M, Mazzucchelli M, Porrello E, Lanni C, Govoni S: **Acetylcholinesterase inhibitors: novel activities of old molecules.** *Pharmacol Res* 2004, **50:**441–451.
13. Zhang J, Zhu D, Sheng R, Wu H, Hu Y, Wang F, *et al:* **BZYX, a novel acetylcholinesterase inhibitor, significantly improved chemicals-induced learning and memory impairments on rodents and protected PC12 cells from apoptosis induced by hydrogen peroxide.** *Eur J Pharmacol* 2009, **613:**1–9.
14. Hassan Khan MT: **Molecular interactions of cholinesterases inhibitors using *in silico* methods: current status and future prospects.** *New Biotechnol* 2009, **5:**331–346.
15. Silman L, Sussman JL: **Acetylcholinesterase: 'classical' and 'non-classical' functions and pharmacology.** *Curr Opin Pharmacol* 2005, **5:**293–302.
16. Kryger G, Silman I, Sussman JL: **Structure of acetylcholinesterase complexed with E2020 (Aricept®): implications for the design of new anti-Alzheimer drugs.** *Structure* 1999, **3:**297–307.
17. Nukoolkarn SV, Saen-oon S, Rungrotmongkol T, Hannongbua S, Ingkaninan K, Suwanborirux K: **Petrosamine, a potent anticholinesterase pyridoacridine alkaloid from a Thai marine sponge Petrosia n. sp.** *Bioorg Med Chem* 2008, **16:**6560–6567.
18. Mukherjee PK, Kumar V, Mal M, Houghton PJ: **Acetylcholinesterase inhibitors from plants.** *Phytomedicine* 2007, **14:**289–300.
19. Razavi SF, Khoobi M, Nadri H, Sakhteman A, Moradi A, Emami S: **Synthesis and evaluation of 4-substituted coumarins as novel acetylcholinesterase inhibitors.** *Eur J Med Chem* 2013, **46:**252–259.
20. Kapková P, Alptüzün V, Frey P, Erciyasb E, Holzgrabe U: **Search for dual function inhibitors for Alzheimer's disease: Synthesis and biological activity of acetylcholinesterase inhibitors of pyridinium-type and their Aβ fibril formation inhibition capacity.** *Bioorg Med Chem* 2006, **14:**472–478.
21. Alonso D, Dorronsoro I, Rubio L, Munoz P, García-Palomero E, Del Monte M, *et al:* **Donepezil-tacrine hybrid related derivatives as new dual binding site inhibitors of AChE.** *Bioorg Med Chem* 2005, **13:**6588–6597.
22. Mary A, Zafiarisoa Renko D, Guillou C, Thal C: **Potent Acetylcholinesterase Inhibitors: Design, Synthesis, and Structure-Activity Relationships of Bis-interacting Ligands in the Galanthamine Series.** *Bioorg Med Chem* 1998, **6:**1835–1850.
23. Zhao Q, Yang G, Mei X, Yuan H, Ning J: **Novel acetylcholinesterase inhibitors: Synthesis and structure-activity relationships of phthalimide alkyloxyphenyl N, N-dimethylcarbamate derivatives.** *Pestic Biochem Phys* 2009, **95:**131–134.
24. Sugimoto H, Iimura Y, Yamanishi Y, Yamatsu K: **Synthesis and Structure-Activity Relationships of Acetylcholinesterase Inhibitors: 1-Benzyl-4-[(5,6-dimethoxy-l-oxoindan-2 yl)methyl]piperidine Hydrochloride and Related Compounds.** *J Med Chem* 1996, **38:**4821–4829.
25. Kaur J, Zhang MQ: **Molecular modelling and QSAR of reversible acetylcholinesterase inhibitors.** *Curr Med Chem* 2000, **7:**273–294.
26. Nadri H, Pirali-Hamedani M, Moradi A, Sakhteman A, Vahidi A, Sheibani V: **5,6-Dimethoxybenzofuran-3-one derivatives: a novel series of dual Acetylcholinesterase/Butyrylcholinesterase inhibitors bearing benzyl pyridinium moiety.** *DARU: J Pharm Sci* 2013, **21:**15. doi:10.1186/2008-2231-21-15.
27. Alipour M, Khoobi M, Foroumadi A, Nadri H, Moradi A, Sakhteman A: **Novel coumarin derivatives bearing *N*-benzyl pyridinium moiety: Potent and dual binding site acetylcholinesterase inhibitors.** *Bioorg Med Chem* 2012, **20:**7214–7222.
28. Ragavendran JV, Sriram D, Patel SK, Reddy IV, Bharathwajan N, Stables J: **Design and synthesis of anticonvulsants from a combined phthalimide-GABA-anilide and hydrazone pharmacophore.** *Eur J Med Chem* 2007, **42:**146–151.
29. Li ZJ, Ren HY, Cui MC, Deuther-Conrad W, Tang RK, Steinbach J, *et al:* **Synthesis and biological evaluation of novel 4-benzylpiperazine ligands for sigma-1 receptor imaging.** *Bioorg Med Chem* 2011, **19:**2911–2917.
30. Nadri H, Pirali-Hamedani M, Shekarchi M, Abdollahi M, Sheibani V, Amanlou M, *et al:* **Design, Synthesis and anticholinesterase activity of a novel series of 1-benzyl-4-((6-alkoxy-3-oxobenzofuran-2(3H)-ylidin) methyl) pyridinum derivatives.** *Bioorg Med Chem* 2010, **18:**6360–6366.
31. ArgusLab 4.0 Mark A: *Thompson Planaria Software LLC.* Seattle, WA. http://www.arguslab.com.
32. Fernandez D, Aviles FX, Vendrell J: *Eur J Med Chem* 2009, **44:**3266–3271.
33. *Brookhaven protein databank.* http://RCSB.org.
34. *Molegro molecular viewer.* http://www.molegro.com.

Immunomodulatory effects of *Ziziphora tenuior* L. extract on the dendritic cells

Abbas Azadmehr[1], Robabeh latifi[2], Sahar Mosalla[2], Reza Hajiaghaee[3] and Mojtaba Shahnazi[2*]

Abstract

Background: *Ziziphora tenuior* L. (Kakuti in Persian) is used in traditional medicine for treatment of gastrointestinal disorders as carminative and analgesic plant. The other usages of this plant are included treatment of diarrhea and nausea. Therefore in the present study we evaluated the immunomodulatory effects of the ethanolic extract of this plant on the dendritic cells (DCs).

Results: *Ziziphora tenuior* L. extract significantly ($p = 0.002$) increased the level of surface expression of CD40 as an important co-stimulatory marker on DCs compared to the control. However this extract did not change CD86 and MHC-II molecules, so it could promote DCs phenotypic maturation. Treatment of DCs with the extract resulted in slightly increased of the production of (IL-12); however, this change was not significant. In addition, the ability of treated DCs to stimulate allogenic T cells proliferation and cytokines secretion was examined in the co-cuture of these cells with T cells in mixed lymphocyte reaction (MLR). *Z. tenuior* L. at the 100 μg/ml concentration inhibited the proliferation of allogenic T cells and also significantly ($P < 0.001$) increased the level of IL-10. Moreover, the extract at 10–100 μg/ml concentration caused slightly increase in IFN-γ production and decreased IL-4 cytokines but these changes were not significant.

Conclusions: These findings indicated that *Z. tenuior* L. extract can modulate immune response by induction of CD40 expression on DCs and cytokine production; whereas it can inhibit T cell stimulating activity of DCs in high concentration. These findings possibly in part explain the traditional use of this plant in treatment of immune-mediated disorders. However future studies are needed.

Keywords: *Ziziphora tenuior* L, Immunomodulation, Dendritic cells, T cell responses, Cytokine

Introduction

Medicinal plants are used to treat immune disorders, such as inflammatory and autoimmune diseases in the worldwide. Previous studies showed that some herbal medicine have immunomodulatory effects [1,2]. *Ziziphora* genus (Lamiacaea) is included of four species namely *Z. tenuior* L., *Z.capitata* L., *Z.clinopodioides* and *Z. Persica Bunge* [3]. *Ziziphora* or Kakuti in Iranian traditional medicine is recognized to dried aerial parts of *Z. tenuior* L. which contains at least 1.2% (volum/weight) of the essential oil [4]. This medicinal plant distributed widely in Iran, Pakistan, Turkmenistan, Afghanistan, Armenia, Anatolia, Syria, Transcaucasia and Central Asia [3]. In traditional medicine, *Ziziphora* is used to treat dysentery, fever, uterus infection and also as analgesic plant [5]. In addition, it is used in the treatment of the gastrointestinal disorder as carminative or treat of vomiting or diarrhea [6,7]. Phytochemical analysis indicated that major components of its essential oil are pulegone, isomenthone, thymol, menthone and piperitone [7-10]. Previous studies showed that these compounds are suggested to be responsible for the mentiond medicinal properties. It has been shown that, *Ziziphora clinopoides* methanolic extract inhibited inflammatory mediators in dextran sodium sulfate induced colitis in mice and also protected acetic acid-induced toxic bowel inflammation through reduction of cellular lipid peroxidation and myeloperoxidase activity [11,12]. On the other hand, Dendritic cells are potential antigen presenting cells for naive T cells and act as a link between the acquired and innate immune systems for the initiation of the protective immune response or the induction of immune tolerance [13]. Maturation status, origin and phenotype are affected on the function of

* Correspondence: shahnazi58@yahoo.com
[2]Parasitology Department, Qazvin University of Medical Sciences, Qazvin, Iran
Full list of author information is available at the end of the article

these cells [14]. The nature of the cytokines produced by DCs in response to various ligands eventually modulates and determines the type of Th cell response. DCs have the exclusive ability to stimulate naive T cells to either Th1 or Th2 cells and also effectively down-regulate T-cell responses through the generation of T regulatory cells [15,16]. It has been demonstrated that immature DCs can effectively present antigen to naive T cells but because of low expression of co-stimulatory molecules such as CD40, CD86 and MHC II they cannot suitably stimulate immune system, finally T cells activation and proliferation are inhibited [14]. In this regards, maturation of DCs converts them to the cells that can stimulate immune system. So, the use of these cells as therapeutic targets by pharmacological compounds such as medicinal plant is a valuable strategy to modulate immune responses. In the present study we have evaluated the immunomodulatory effects of *Z. tenuior* L. extract on the function and maturation of DCs.

Materials and methods

Animals

The male BALB/c and C57BL/6 mice with 6–8 week old were purchased from Razi Institute (Karaj, Iran) and were kept under optimal conditions of hygiene and received standard mouse chow and water *ad libitum*. In this study, all experimental procedures on handling the animals were approved by the ethical committee of Qazvin University of Medical Sciences.

Preparation of DCs from mice spleen

To isolate DCs from spleen, the mice CD11c$^+$ isolation kit (Miltenyi Biotech, Germany), was used as described in previous study [17]. Briefly, the mice spleens were isolated and minced to very small pieces and then suspended in cold (4°C) PBS containing 1.2 mg/ml collagenase D (Roche, Germany).The cell suspension, incubated at 37°C for 40 minutes and was passed through a cell mesh and the collected cells were washed twice. Then, mononuclear cells (MNC) were separated by Nycodenz (Axis-shield, Norway); a material used in density gradient cell separation techniques. According to the manufacturer's protocol, anti-CD11c magnetic beads (Miltenyi Biotech, Germany) were added to the cells and incubated at 4°C for 30 minutes and the non-bonded antibodies were washed out. Using of the minimacs separator (MS) cell columns into the magnetic field (MS separation unit, Miltenyi Biotech, USA) and washed by 1.5 ml EDTA-containing PBS and then passed through the column to absorb the magnetic bead coated DCs and the unwanted cells were washed out using at least 3 washes of 500 µl EDTA-containing PBS. The isolated DCs were collected by disconnecting the column from the magnetic field and injecting 1 ml PBS-EDTA in it under pressure. Purity of the CD11c dendritic cells was determined above 94% using flow cytometry.

Plant material and preparation of the ethanolic extract

Ziziphora tenuior was purchased from herbal market and authenticated by a botanist. Voucher specimens were preserved in the central herbarium of medicinal plants (ACECR). The aerial parts of plant were air-dried at room temperature. This was ground in to powder. The aerial part of plant (50 g) was extracted using percolation method by ethanol (80%) at room temperature. Solvent was completely removed by drying under reduced pressure at 40°C in a rotary evaporator. The samples were stored at 4°C until use (3 g, 6% yield) [18].

Effect of extract on DCs viability

To determine, the effect of cytotoxic concentration of the extract on DCs, 3-(4, 5-dimethylthiazol-2-yl)-2, 5-diphenyltetrazolium bromide (MTT) colorimetric assay was used [15]. Briefly, dendritic cells (10^5 cells/well) were treated with *Z. tenuior* L. extract at 10 to 200 µg/ml concentrations in the cell culture plates for 24 h, and then 10 µl MTT (5 mg/ml, Sigma) was added to each well and cells were incubated for an additional 4 h at 37°C. Dimethyl sulphoxide (DMSO 0.1%) as vehicle and lipopolysaccharides (LPS 1 µg/ml) as DC maturation inducing agent, were used as negative and positive controls, respectively. Finally, the optical density (OD) of each well was measured at 570 with reference at 630 nm on an enzyme-linked immuosorbent assay (ELISA) plate reader and the viability was determined as the follows: (OD of extract-treated cells/OD of DMSO-treated cells) × 100.

Analysis of markers expression of co-stimulatory molecules

In order to evaluate the effect of *Z. tenuior* L. on the expression of co-stimulatory molecules, DCs were treated with the extract for 18 h and analyzed using flow cytometer (FACSCalibur, Beckton Dickinson Biosciences, San Jose, CA). The cells were stained with phycoerithrin (PE)-conjugated anti-CD11c, FITC-conjugated anti-CD86, fluorescence isothiocyanate (FITC)-conjugated anti-CD40, FITC-conjugated anti-MHC II antibody and appropriate conjugated isotypes (Beckton Dickinson (BD) Pharmingen, San Diego, CA). Finally, the percentage of markers expression on extract-treated DCs and DMSO-treated DCs was calculated and the mean florescent intensity (MFI) was analyzed using Win MDI software (Scripps, La Jolla, CA).

Mixed lymphocyte reaction

To determine the proliferative effect of *Z. tenuior* L. extract-treated DCs on T lymphocytes, allogeneic mixed lymphocyte reaction (MLR) assay was used. Briefly, T cells were purified from lymph nodes of C57BL/6 mice using nylon wool. Then, *Z. tenuior* L -treated DCs from BALB/c mice were inactivated with mitomycin C (0.5 mg/ml) for 20 min, and then cells were washed with phosphate buffered saline (PBS) for three times and resuspended in culture medium containing 10% FCS. Mitomycin-treated DCs (10^4 cells/well), as stimulator cells, co-cultured with 10^5 allogenic T cells, as responder cells, in a 96-well culture plate (Nunc, Denmark) in triplicates for 48 h. As negative control, a triplicate wells containing DMSO-treated DCs plus allogenic T cells were used. Finally, T cell proliferation was measured by a 5-Bromo-20-deoxyuridine (BrdU) cell proliferation assay kit (Roche, Germany) according to the manufacturer's instructions. The result was concluded as the follows: (OD of extract-treated culture/OD of DMSO-treated culture) × 100.

Effect of the extract on the cytokines production

In order to evaluate immunomodulatory effect of *Z. tenuior* L. extract on the cytokines production, the enzyme-linked immunosorbent assay (ELISA) method was used. Briefly, the supernatant of extract-treated DCs and MLR cultures were collected and used to measure IFN-γ, IL-4, IL-12 and IL-10 by ELISA kits according to the manufacturer's protocol (eBioscience, USA), respectively.

Statistics analysis

In this study, all data were representative of at least three independent experiments performed in triplicate and presented as mean ± standard deviation (SD). Mann–Whitney test and one-way analysis of variance (ANOVA) were used for the evaluation of statistical differences between the results and p vales less than 0.05 were considered significant.

Results

Viability of DCs after exposure with *Z. tenuior* L. extract

The DCs viability was determined using MTT assay. For this purpose, these cells were treated with different concentrations of the plant extract for 24 h. Our results indicated that this extract at concentration of 10, 50 and 100 μg/ml had no cytotoxic effect on DCs (Figure 1) however the extract at 200 μg/ml had significantly ($P < 0.05$) cytotoxic effect on DCs. Therefore these concentrations (10 to 100 μg/ml) were used as safe dose of *Z. tenuior* L. extract for the next experiments on DCs.

Effect of *Z. tenuior* L. extract on maturation phenotype of DCs

We analyzed the percentage expression and fluorescent intensity of CD86, CD40 and MHC II co-stimulatory molecules on *Z. tenuior* L-treated DCs by flow cytometry. Our results showed that the extract modulate the percentage expression and fluorescent intensity of CD86,

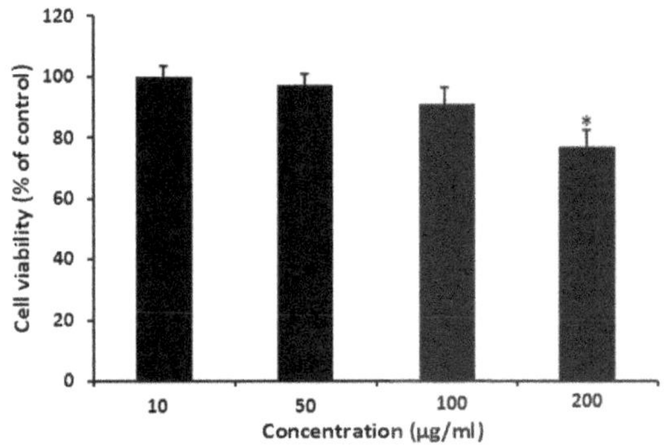

Figure 1 DCs viability after treatment with *Z. tenuior* L. extract. MTT assay was used for determining of DCs viability. These cells were treated with different concentrations of the plant extract for 24 h. DCs treated with DMSO was used as control. The results show mean ± standard deviation of three independent experiments performed in triplicate. The extract at 10 to 100 μg/ml had no significant growth inhibitory effects on DCs. *Significantly ($P < .0.05$) different was between the extract-treated cells and the control cells.

CD40 and MHC II molecules on DCs. As shown in Figure 2, this extract significantly ($P = 0.002$) increased the percentage expression of CD40 molecules at 100 μg/ml compared with negative control. Although, *Z. tenuior* L. Extract increased the percentage expression and fluorescent intensity of CD86 and MHC II on DCs but this effect was not significant comparing with control. These finding showed that *Z. tenuior* L. extract can modulate the maturation phenotype markers on DCs.

Effect of *Z. tenuior* L. extract on allogenic MLR

To determine the effects of the *Z. tenuior* L. extract on allogenic immune response and DCs function, the allogenic T cells from C57BL/6 were co-cultured with DCs isolated from BALB/c mice. For this purpose, the DCs were treated with concentrations of 10 to 100 μg/ml of the extract for 18 h and then cells were co-cultured with allogenic T cells in MLR assay. Finally, the proliferation of T lymphocytes was evaluated using BrdU incorporation assay. As it is shown in Figure 3, the *Z. tenuior* L. extract significantly ($p < 0.05$) decreased the proliferation of T cells at 100 μg/ml. The results indicated that the proliferation of these cells decreased to 76.8 ± 3.4 percent of control when DCs had been treated with 100 μg/ml of the extract concentration.

Effect of *Z. tenuior* L. on the production of cytokines

The concentration of the IL-12 cytokine in the supernatant of the extract-treated DCs was measured. As shown in Figure 4A, treatment of DCs with this extract at 10 to 100 μg/ml resulted in slightly increase of production of IL-12 by these cells comparing with the negative control. However this change was not significant. In

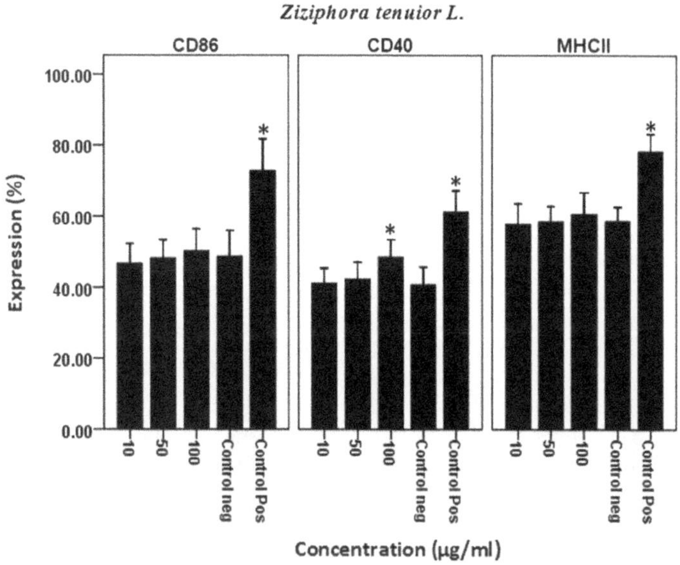

Figure 2 Effect of *Z. tenuior* L. extract on maturation phenotype of DCs. In order to determine the effect of *Z. tenuior* L. extract on maturation phenotype on DCs, these cell were treated with the extract for 18 h and then the expression of CD40, CD86 and MHC II molecules was determined by flow cytomety. DC treated with DMSO as negative control and also lipopolysaccharides (LPS 1 µg/ml) as positive control were considered. The results show mean ± standard deviation of three independent experiments performed in triplicate. *Significantly ($P < 0.05$) different was between the extract-treated cells and the negative control cells.

addition, we measured the effect of the extract on IFN- γ, IL-4 and IL-10 production in MLR. We found that, the extract at 10–100 µg/ml concentrations slightly increased production of IFN-γ and decreased IL-4 cytokines but these changes were not significant (Figure 4B, C). However, as it is shown in Figure 4D, our result indicated that the *Z. tenuior* L. extract at 100 µg/ml concentration significantly ($p < 0.05$) increased IL-10 cytokine production.

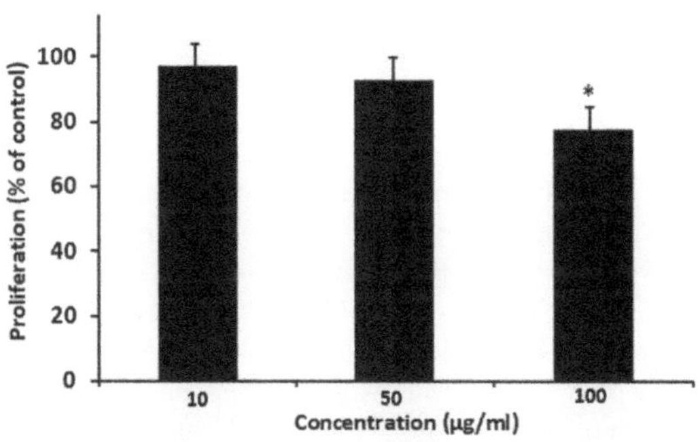

Figure 3 The effect of *Z. tenuior* L. extract on allogenic MLR. In order to find the effects of the *Z. tenuior* L. extract on allogenic immune response, DCs were treated with the extract for 18 h and then co-cultured with allogenic T cells for 48 h. DMSO-treated DCs plus T cells was considered as control. Brdu incorporation assay was used for measuring of cell proliferation. The results show mean ± SD of the cell proliferation in the presence of the extract as compared to the proliferation of controls taken to be 100%. Our results indicated that DCs treated with 100 µg/ml of extract significantly (*$P < 0.05$) have decreased T cells proliferation.

Discussion

In this study, we evaluated the immunomodulatory effects of *Z. tenuior* L. extract on the DCs. Several studies showed that natural agents such as plants can modulate DCs activity [19-21]. Dendritic cells are professional antigen presenting cells for naive T cells and act as a link between the acquired and innate immune systems for the initiation of the protective immune response or the induction of immune tolerance [13]. Therefore, to find out the new DCs immunomodulaters are considered as the important targets for immune response as well as immune regulation. *Ziziphora* is used to treat dysentery, fever, uterus infection and also analgesic plant in traditional medicine [5]. In addition, it is used in the treatment of the gastrointestinal disorder as carminative or treat of vomiting or diarrhea [6,7]. It has been shown that, *Ziziphora clinopoides* methanolic extract inhibited inflammatory mediators in dextran sodium sulfate induced colitis in mice and also protected acetic acid-induced toxic bowel inflammation through reduction of cellular lipid peroxidation and myeloperoxidase activity [11,12].

In the present study, we examined the effect of the *Z. tenuior* L. extract on the phenotypic maturation and function of DCs. The expression of CD86, CD40 and MHC- II molecules are important co-stimulatory and maturation

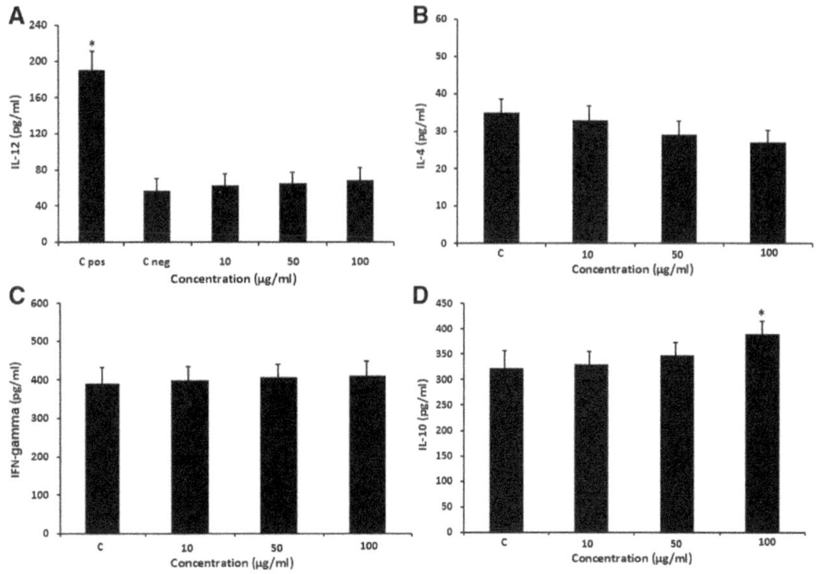

Figure 4 Effect of *Z. tenuior* L. extract on cytokine production. The effect of the *Z. tenuior* L. extract on IL-12 production by DCs after 18 h showed in Figure 4**A**. DMSO treated DCs as control negative (C neg) and LPS as positive control (C pos) were considered. Moreover, the effect of the extract on IFN- γ, IL-4 and IL-10 production in MLR assay showed in Figure 4**B**, **C** and **D**. DMSO-treated DCs plus allogenic T cells as Control considered. *P < 0.05 shows significant difference with the negative control.

markers on DCs and have critical roles in antigen presentation and T cell activation. Our results showed that the extract modulate the percentage expression and fluorescent intensity of CD86, CD40 and MHC II molecules on DCs. Previous studies indicated that some herbal extracts can modulate immune response by immunomodulatory effect on the CD40 expression on the dendritic cells [22,23]. Our results showed that the extract significantly increased the percentage expression of CD40 molecules at 100 μg/ml compared with control negative. Although, *Z. tenuior* L. extract increased the percentage expression and fluorescent intensity of CD86 and MHC II on DCs but this effect was not significant comparing with control. These finding indicated that *Z. tenuior* L. extract can modulate the maturation phenotype markers on DCs.

In addition, we evaluated the immunomodulatory effect of *Z. tenuior* L. extract on the DCs functions by releasing of cytokines and MLR. IL-12 is a cytokine released by DCs which can induce differentiation of T cells to Th1 and cellular immunity, by contrast IL-10 is a Th1 inhibitory cytokine and also, IL-4 and IFN-γ cytokines are landmark of deviation to Th1 or Th2 response [24]. Our results indicated that the treatment of DCs with this extract at 10 to 100 μg/ml concentration increased production of IL-12 comparing with the negative control however this change was not significant. Also, the extract at 10–100 μg/ml concentrations increased production of IFN-γ and decreased IL-4 cytokines but these changes were not significant. However, our result indicated that the *Z. tenuior* L. extract at 100 μg/ml concentration significantly increased IL-10 cytokine production. We assumed that the increased IL-12 production by DCs using 10–100 μg/ml extract concentration along with production of more IFN-γ and less IL-4 by T cells in MLR suggest the ability of *Z. tenuior* L. extract to deviate the cytokine pattern of T cells toward a Th1 response. However, the extract at 100 μg/ml concentration has increased IL-10 secretion in MLR and also reduced the proliferation of T cells in allogenic response, which indicated the inhibitory effect of the extract at higher concentration on the immune response. Moreover, the difference between the effects of the extract at higher concentrations may be attributed to the presence of various constituents in the extract with different mode of actions. So, to confirm Th1/Th2 polarization in co-culture of T cells with *Z. tenuior* L. treated-DCs, study of the T cell signaling activity of DCs and the expression of T bet and GATA-3 as related transcription factors for Th1 and Th2 differentiation is recommended [25]. Future studies are suggested for identifying the main bioactive compound of this plant and other immunomodulatory mechanisms.

Conclusions

Our findings indicated that *Z. tenuior* L. extract can modulate immune response by induction of CD40 expression on DCs and cytokine production; whereas it can inhibit T cell stimulating activity of DCs in high concentration. These findings possibly in part explain the traditional use of this plant in treatment of immune-mediated disorders. However future in vitro and in vivo studies are needed.

Competing interests
The authors declare that they have no competing interests.

Authors' contributions
AA designed and supervised the study and wrote the manuscript. RH provided plant materials. RL and SM carried out the experiments. MSh supervised the study. All authors read and approved the final manuscript.

Acknowledgement
We would like to thank of the Cellular and Molecular Research Center of the Research Vice-Chancellor of Qazvin University of Medical Sciences for financial support and also, the Medicinal Plants Research Center, Institute of Medicinal Plants, (ACECR), Karaj, Iran. This manuscript was a part of thesis for receiving the degree of MSc in medical parasitology in the Qazvin University of Medical Sciences, Qazvin, Iran.

Author details
[1]Immunology Department, Qazvin University of Medical Sciences, Qazvin, Iran. [2]Parasitology Department, Qazvin University of Medical Sciences, Qazvin, Iran. [3]Pharmacognosy and Pharmaceutics department of Medicinal Plants Research Center, Institute of Medicinal Plants, (ACECR), Karaj, Iran.

References

1. Su CA, Xu XY, Liu DY, Wu M, Zeng FQ, Zeng MY, Wei W, Jiang N, Luo X: **Isolation and characterization of exopolysaccharide with immunomodulatory activity from fermentation broth of Morchella conica.** *Daru* 2013, **21**(1):5.
2. Azadmehr A, Hajiaghaee R, Zohal MA, Maliji G: **Protective effects of Scrophularia striata in Ovalbumin-induced mice asthma model.** *Daru* 2013, **21**(1):56.
3. Zohrabi M: *Investigation Botany, Microscopy, Analysis and Indicated Composition of Ziziphora Clinopodioides Subsp.* Tehran: Tehran University; 2000.
4. Davis NC, Newland RC: **The reporting of colorectal cancer: the Australian clinico-pathological staging system.** *Aust N Z J Surg* 1982, **52**(4):395–397.
5. Naeini A, Khosravi AR, Chitsaz M, Shokri H, Kamlnejad M: **Anti-Candida albicans activity of some Iranian plants used in traditional medicine.** *J Med Mycol* 2009, **19**(3):168–172.
6. Naghibi F, Mosaddegh M, Mohammadi Motamed M, Ghorbani A: *Labiatae Family in Folk Medicine in Iran: from Ethnobotany to Pharmacology.* Pharm Res: Iran J; 2010:63–79.
7. Zargari A: *Iranian Medicinal Plants.* Tehran, IR Iran: Tehran university press; 1987.
8. Sezik E, Tümen G, Başer KHC: ***Ziziphora tenuior L.*, a new source of pulegone.** *Flavour Fragrance J* 1991, **6**(1):101–103.
9. Kasumov FY: **Component compositions of the essential oils of some species of the Genus Thymus.** *Chem Nat Comp* 1987, **23**(5):637–638.
10. de Sousa DP, Junior EV, Oliveira FS, de Almeida RN, Nunes XP, Barbosa-Filho JM: **Antinociceptive activity of structural analogues of rotundifolone: structure-activity relationship.** *Z Naturforsch C* 2007, **62**(1–2):39–42.
11. Amini-Shirazi N, Hoseini A, Ranjbar A, Mohammadirad A, Khoshakhlagh P, Yasa N, Abdollahi M: **Inhibition of tumor necrosis factor and nitrosative/oxidative stresses by Ziziphora clinopoides (Kahlioti); a molecular mechanism of protection against dextran sodium sulfate-induced colitis in mice.** *Toxicol Mech Methods* 2009, **19**(2):183–189.
12. Ghafari H, Yasa N, Mohammadirad A, Dehghan G, Zamani MJ, Nikfar S, Khorasani R, Minaie B, Abdollahi M: **Protection by Ziziphora clinopoides of acetic acid-induced toxic bowel inflammation through reduction of cellular lipid peroxidation and myeloperoxidase activity.** *Hum Exp Toxicol* 2006, **25**(6):325–332.
13. Schuurhuis DH, Fu N, Ossendorp F, Melief CJ: **Ins and outs of dendritic cells.** *Int Arch Allergy Immunol* 2006, **140**:53–72.
14. Reis E, Sousa C: **Dendritic cells in a mature age.** *Nat Rev Immunol* 2006, **6**:476–483.
15. Gao Y, Nish SA, Jiang R, Hou L, Licona-Limón P, Weinstein JS, Zhao H, Medzhitov R: **Control of T helper 2 responses by transcription factor IRF4-dependent dendritic cells.** *Immunity* 2013, **17**:722–732.
16. Min WP, Zhou D, Ichim TE, Strejan GH, Xia X, Yang J, Huang X, Garcia B, White D, Dutartre P, Jevnikar AM, Zhong R: **Inhibitory feedback loop between tolerogenic dendritic cells and regulatory T cells in transplant tolerance.** *J Immunol* 2003, **1**:1304–1312.
17. Eftekharian MM, Zarnani AH, Moazzeni SM: **In vivo effects of calcitriol on phenotypic and functional properties of dendritic cells.** *Iran J Immunol* 2010, **7**(2):74–82.
18. Hajiaghaee R, Monsef-Esfahani HR, Khorramizadeh MR, Saadat F, Shahverdi AR, Attar F: **Inhibitory effect of aerial parts of Scrophularia striata on matrix metalloproteinases expression.** *Phytother Res* 2007, **21**(12):1127–1129.
19. Amirghofran Z, Bahmani M, Azadmehr A, Javidnia K, Miri R: **Immunomodulatory activities of various medicinal plant extracts: effects on human lymphocytes apoptosis.** *Immunol Invest* 2009, **38**(2):181–192.
20. Azadmehr A, Afshari A, Baradaran B, Hajiaghaee R, Rezazadeh S, Monsef-Esfahani H: **Suppression of nitric oxide production in activated murine peritoneal macrophages in vitro and ex vivo by Scrophularia striata ethanolic extract.** *J Ethnopharmacol* 2009, **124**(1):166–169.
21. Ghafourian Boroujerdnia M, Azemi ME, Hemmati AA, Taghian A, Azadmehr A: **Immunomodulatory effects of Astragalus gypsicolus hydroalcoholic extract in ovalbumin-induced allergic mice model.** *Iran J Allergy Asthma Immunol* 2011, **10**(4):281–288.
22. Amirghofran Z, Ahmadi H, Karimi MH: **Immunomodulatory activity of the water extract of Thymus vulgaris, Thymus daenensis, and Zataria multiflora on dendritic cells and T cells responses.** *J Immunoassay Immunochem* 2012, **33**(4):388–402.
23. Elluru SR, Duong van Huyen JP, Delignat S, Kazatchkine MD, Friboulet A, Kaveri SV, Bayry J: **Induction of maturation and activation of human dendritic cells: a mechanism underlying the beneficial effect of Viscum album as complimentary therapy in cancer.** *BMC Cancer* 2008, **8**:161.
24. Ho CY, Lau CB, Kim CF, Leung KN, Fung KP, Tse TF, Chan HH, Chow MS: **Differential effect of Coriolus versicolor (Yunzhi) extract on cytokine production by murine lymphocytes in vitro.** *Int Immunopharmacol* 2004, **4**:1549–1557.
25. Kang H, Oh YJ, Choi HY, Ham IH, Bae HS, Kim SH, Ahn KS: **Immunomodulatory effect of Schizonepeta tenuifolia water extract on mouse Th1/Th2 cytokine production in-vivo and in-vitro.** *J Pharm Pharmacol* 2008, **60**:901–907.

Antinociceptive effect of some extracts from *Ajuga chamaecistus* Ging. ssp. *tomentella* (Boiss.) Rech. f. aerial parts

Mahnaz Khanavi[1,2], Araz Mohammad Davoodipoor[1], Seyede Nargess Sadati[2*], Mohammad Reza Shams Ardekani[1,2] and Mohammad Sharifzadeh[3]

Abstract

Background: The genus *Ajuga* is used for the treatment of joint pain, gout, and jaundice in traditional Iranian medicine (TIM). *Ajuga chamaecistus* ssp. *tomentella* is an exclusive subspecies of *Ajuga chamaecistus* in the flora of Iran. The aim of this study was to evaluate antinociceptive properties of some extracts from aerial parts of *A. chamaecistus* ssp. *tomentella*.

Methods: Antinociceptive activities of total water and 80% methanol extracts, hexane, diethyl ether and n-butanolic partition fractions of the methanolic extract were analyzed using the formalin test in mice. Indomethacin (10 mg/kg) and normal saline were employed as positive and negative controls, respectively.

Results: Oral administration of all extracts (200, 400 and 600 mg/kg) 30 min before formalin injection had no effect against the acute phase (0–5 min after formalin injection) of the formalin-induced licking time, but hexane fraction (200 mg/kg) caused a significant effect ($p < 0.001$) on the chronic phase (15–60 min after formalin injection). Total water and diethyl ether extracts at a dose of 400 mg/kg showed a very significant analgesic activity on the chronic phase ($p < 0.001$ and $p < 0.01$, respectively).

Conclusions: The results of this study suggest that the extracts of *A. chamaecistus* ssp. *tomentella* have an analgesic property that supports traditional use of *Ajuga* genus for joint pain and other inflammatory diseases.

Keywords: *Ajuga chamaecistus* ssp. *tomentella*, Antinociceptive effect, Analgesic activity, Formalin test, Mice

Background

Five species of genus *Ajuga* (Lamiaceae) are found in the flora of Iran in which *Ajuga chamaecistus* has been contained several endemic subspecies including *A. chamaecistus* ssp. *tomentella* [1]. Some species which belong to this annual and perennial genus are used as the medicinal plant in the traditional medicine of several countries mostly in Africa, Asia, and China as for wound healing; anthelmintic, antifungal, antifebrile, antitumor, antimicrobial, and diuretic agent, and for the treatment of hypertension, hyperglycemia, joint pain, etc. [2-4]. *Ajuga chamaepitys* (L.) Schreb. which grows in the Middle East and Asia has been used in the treatment of rheumatism, gout, dropsy, jaundice, and sclerosis. *A. decombens* Thunb. that originally grows in East Asia is used for analgesia, inflammation, fever, and joint pain [5]. Moreover in Iranian traditional medicine, the genus *Ajuga* (Kamaphytus) has been used for treatment of joint pain, gout, and jaundice [6].

Also, several biological studies have been performed on many species of this genus which have confirmed their ethno pharmacological properties such as hypoglycemic [7], anti-inflammatory [8], anabolic, analgesic, anti-arthritis, antipyretic, hepatoprotective, antibacterial, antifungal, antioxidant, cardiotonic [5], and antimalarial [9] properties and their application in the treatment of joint diseases [10].

As well, many phytochemical studies on *Ajuga* species have been performed which have led to the isolation of phytoecdysteroids [11,12], neo- clerodanediterpenoids [13],

* Correspondence: n_sadati@sina.tums.ac.ir
[2]Department of Traditional Pharmacy, School of Traditional Iranian Medicine and Traditional Iranian Medicine and Pharmacy Research Center, Tehran University of Medical Sciences, Tehran, Iran
Full list of author information is available at the end of the article

phenylethyl glycosides [3], withanolides [2], iridoids and flavonoids [14], and essential oils [15].

Prior to this study, we have isolated 10 compounds; 20-hydroxyecdysone, cyasterone, ajugalactone, makisterone A, and 24-dehydroprecyasterone (phytoecdysteroids), 8-acetylharpagide (iridoid), *cis-* and *trans-*melilotoside, lavandulifolioside, leonoside B, and martynoside (phenylethanoid glycosides), from diethyl ether and n-butanolic fractions of *Ajuga chamaecistus* ssp. *tomentella.* Cytotoxicity evaluation of some fractions of this plant showed the cytotoxicity of hexane fraction against normal and cancer cell lines. Most of the isolated compounds were inactive in the cytotoxicity assay [16,17].

The aim of this study was to evaluate antinociceptive effects of oral administration of total water and 80% methanolic extracts and partition fractions of hexane, diethyl ether and n- butanol obtained from methanolic extract of aerial parts of *Ajuga chamaecistus* ssp. *tomentella* in an attempt to validate the traditional use of the plants belonging to genus *Ajuga.*

Methods

Plant material

Aerial parts of *Ajuga chamaecistus* Ging. ssp. *tomentella* (Boiss.) Rech. f. were collected from "Sorkhe Hesar", east of Tehran, Iran, in June 2008 and verified by Prof. G. Amin. A voucher specimen (THE-6697) was deposited in the herbarium of the Department of Pharmacognosy, Faculty of Pharmacy, Tehran University of Medical Sciences, Tehran, Iran.

Methanolic extraction

The air-dried and ground aerial parts of *A. chamaecistus* ssp. *tomentella* (250 g) were extracted with methanol 80% (3 × 0.5 L) at room temperature. The solvent was evaporated on a rotary evaporator and in a vacuum oven to give a dark brown extract (45 g). The extract (30 g) was suspended in 80% methanol and partitioned successively between 80% methanol, n-hexane, diethyl ether, and n-butanol. Removal of the solvents with a rotary evaporator resulted in the production of n-hexane, diethyl ether, and n-butanol fractions.

Water extraction

Two hundred and fifty grams of the powdered plant from the aerial parts of *A. chamaecistus* ssp. *tomentella* were extracted with distilled water (3 × 0.5 L) at room temperature. The solvent was removed with a rotary evaporator and freeze drying process to give an extract (30 g).

Administration

The extracts were dissolved in normal saline to achieve the working concentrations. Extracts, standard drug (Indomethacin 10 mg/kg), and normal saline were administered by oral gavage. Three doses of 200, 400 and 600 mg/kg of all extracts were examined.

Animals

Male albino mice weighing 25–30 g were obtained from Pasteur institute and housed in groups of 7 with a 12 h light–dark cycle and constant temperature (22°C). Mice were allowed to acclimatize to the laboratory for 30 min before the experiments began. This study was approved by the ethics committee of the Pharmaceutical Science Research Center of TUMS.

Formalin test in mice

Twenty microliters of formalin (0.5%) was injected subcutaneously according to the previous study [18]. The total time (second) spent on licking in response to the injected paw in the acute phase (0–5 min) and chronic phase (15–60 min) after formalin injection was measured as a pain indicator.

Statistical analysis

Results are expressed as mean ± standard error of mean (S.E.M). Statistical differences between the treatment and control groups were evaluated by one-way ANOVA, followed by Newman–Keuls post hoc test. $p < 0.05$ was considered significant.

Results

In the present study, antinociceptive activity of total water, 80% methanol extracts, and three fractions of methanolic extract from the aerial parts of *Ajuga chamaecistus* ssp. *tomentella* were evaluated in a nociception model in mice. All extracts were administered by a gastrointestinal tube at different doses (200, 400, and 600 mg/kg) 30 min before intraplantar injection of formalin (20 μl, 0.5%). The licking time was 40.29 ± 5.76 for indomethacin (10 mg/kg) in the acute phase. There was no significant difference between indomethacin and all treated extracts (Table 1).

Figure 1 shows the antinociceptive effects of all extracts at different doses on the chronic phase of pain induction. Results demonstrated that hexane fraction (200 mg/kg), diethyl ether fraction and total water extract at a dose of 400 mg/kg significantly ($p < 0.001$) affected the duration of licking in the chronic phase, which was comparable to indomethacin (10 mg/kg). The total methanol extract (600 mg/kg) and n-butanolic (600 mg/kg) fraction also exhibited a reduction on the duration of licking in the chronic phase ($p < 0.01$).

Comparison of the antinociceptive activity of all extracts showed that the maximum inhibitory response was obtained with 200 mg/kg of hexane fraction. According to results, there was no significant difference between the analgesic effect of total water extract and hexane fraction at a dose of 400 mg/kg, diethyl ether fraction (600 mg/kg),

Table 1 Influence of *Ajuga chamaecistus* ssp. *tomentella* extracts on acute phase of formalin- induced pain in mice

Treatment(mg/kg)[b]	Licking time(sec)[a]				
	TW	TM	HEX	DEE	NB
Control	52.14 ± 1.35[C]	52.66 ± 1.47	52.60 ± 1.80	53.00 ± 1.67	52.83 ± 1.38
200	49.00 ± 3.4	53.43 ± 5.35	46.14 ± 2.54	53.86 ± 3.20	48.71 ± 2.02
400	58.86 ± 4.41	59.29 ± 2.41	47.86 ± 3.29	57.43 ± 3.64	46.86 ± 3.46
600	36.00 ± 5.21	59.57 ± 2.04	50.86 ± 3.04	45.71 ± 1.82	47.57 ± 2.44

[a]The amount of time spent licking the injected paw recorded in 0–5 min (acute phase).
[b]Control: Normal saline, TW: Total Water extract, TM: Total Methanol extract, HEX: Hexane fraction, DEE: Diethyl Ether fraction, NB: N-Butanol fraction.
[c]Results are expressed as the mean ± S.E.M (n = 7).

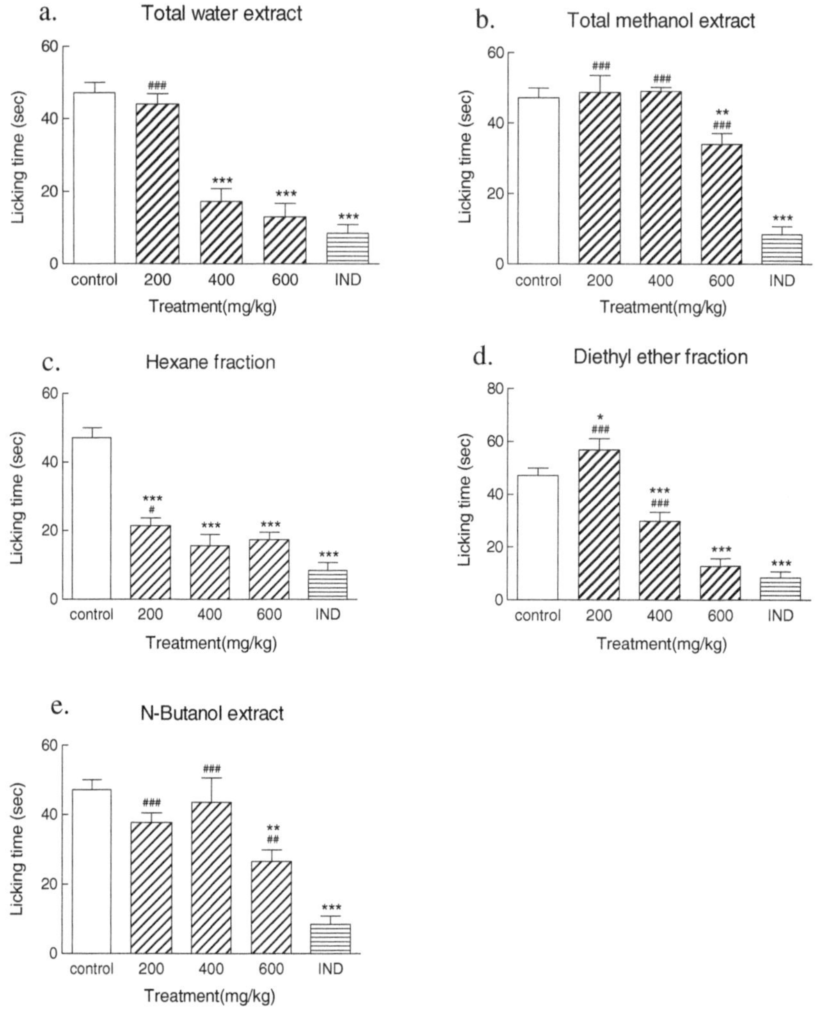

Figure 1 Effects of different extracts of *Ajuga chamaecistus* ssp. *tomentella* on chronic phase of formalin- induced pain. Different doses of all extracts (200, 400, 600 mg/kg), **a)** Total water extract, **b)** Total methanol extract, **c)** Hexane fraction, **d)** Diethyl ether fraction, and **e)** N-Butanol fraction, were administered to mice by oral tube. Control group received normal saline. All extracts of the plant were administered 30 min before formalin injection. Antinociception was recorded 15–60 min (Chronic phase), after formalin injection. Each point is the mean ± S.E.M of at least 7 animals. Control (normal saline), IND (Indomethacin). *$p<0.05$,** $p < 0.01$, ***$p < 0.001$ (as compared with normal saline), #$p<0.05$, ##$p < 0.01$, ###$p < 0.001$ (as compared with Indomethacin).

n-butanol fraction (600 mg/kg), and indomethacin (10 mg/kg) as an NSAID (Figure 2).

Discussion

The formalin test provides a moderate and continuous pain because of tissue injury in the animal, which is a better approach to clinical conditions than more traditional tests of nociception [19]. Subcutaneous injection of formalin induces two distinctive periods of response. The early phase is explained as a direct stimulation of nociceptive neurons, and the late phase occurs secondary to the inflammatory reactions [20,21]. Drugs which affect the central nervous system such as opioids inhibit both phases equally while peripherally acting drugs such as aspirin and indomethacin inhibit the late phase [22]. The early phase of response to the formalin test is insensitive to anti-inflammatory drugs [23]. Inflammation in the late phase is due to the release of chemical mediators, such as serotonin, histamine, bradykinin and prostaglandins and at least to some degree, the sensitization of central nociceptive neurons [24].

The results showed that hexane (200 mg/kg), diethyl ether (400 mg/kg), and n-butanol fractions (600 mg/kg) from the methanolic extract (80%) in addition to total water extract (400 mg/kg) significantly decreased the pain related to the late phase (inflammatory agents) of the formalin test. Since the analgesic properties of effective extracts were observed in late phase like NSAIDs, the antinociceptive activities of the extracts are apparently mediated by interactions with inflammatory mediators especially arachidonic acid metabolites. Recently, [9] reported that 70% ethanol extract of whole plants of *Ajuga bracteosa* showed a significant topical anti-inflammatory activity and a strong in vitro COX-1 and COX-2 inhibitory effect. Among the isolated compounds from this extract, lupulin A (a clerodane diterpenes) exhibited the highest inhibition of COX-1and 6-deoxyharpagide (an iridoid) showed the highest COX-2 inhibition [8]. Cyclooxygenase (COX) catalyzes the biosynthesis of prostaglandin G_2 and H_2 from arachidonic acid. The cyclooxygenase isoforms (COX-1 and COX-2) are the target of the non-steroidal anti-inflammatory drugs (NSAIDs), which provide therapeutic effects in the treatment of pain, fever, and inflammation [25].

Another herb that is used in treatment of pain and arthritis is *Harpagophytum procumbens*, commonly known as

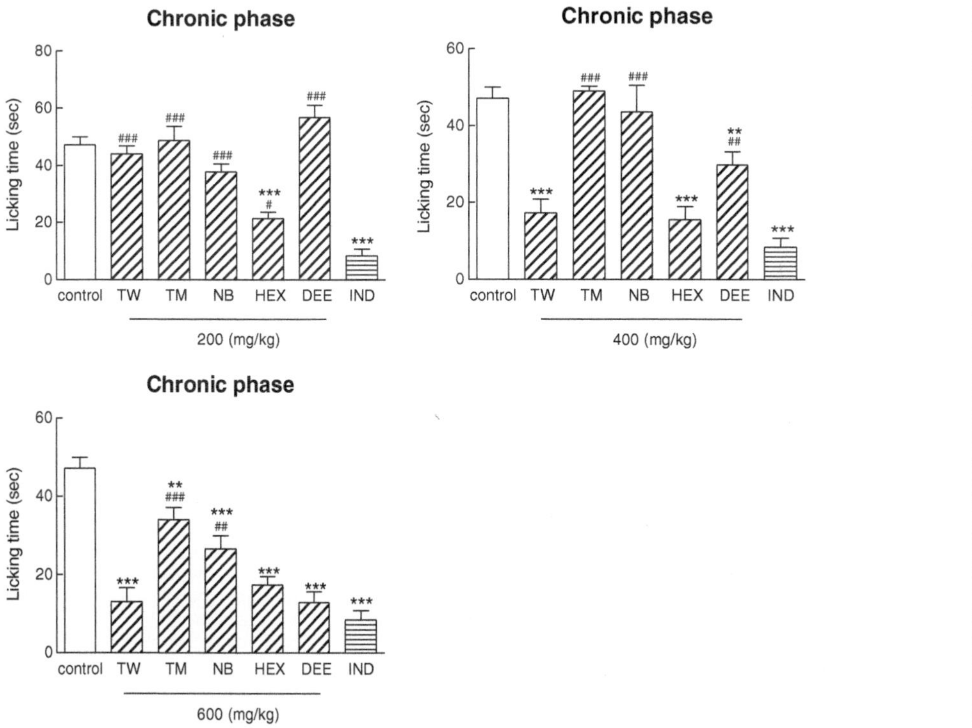

Figure 2 Comparision of different treatments of *Ajuga chamaecistus* ssp. *tomentella* on chronic phase of formalin- induced pain. All samples were administered to mice by oral tube. Control group received normal saline. All extracts of the plant were administered 30 min before formalin injection. Antinociception was recorded 15–60 min (Chronic phase), after formalin injection. Each point is the mean ± S.E.M of at least 7 animals. Control (normal saline), TW (total water), TM (total methanol), NB (n-butanol), HEX (hexane fraction), DEE (diethyl ether fraction). IND (Indomethacin). **p < 0.01, ***p < 0.001 (as compared with normal saline), #p<0.05, ##p < 0.01, ###p < 0.001 (as compared with Indomethacin).

devil's claw. The total water extract of this plant possesses anti-inflammatory and analgesic effects by suppressing cyclooxygenase-2 and inducible nitric oxide synthase expressions. Iridoid glycosides such as harpagoside and harpagide are principal constituent of devil's claw [26,27]. In our previous study, 8-acethyharpagide, an iridoid glycoside, was isolated in a large amount from the diethyl ether fraction [16]. Many studies have exhibited the biological effects of iridoids such as antioxidant, cytotoxic [9], chemoprotective [28], cardiovascular, hypoglycemic and hypolipidemic properties [29]. Li et al. [30] showed that the iridoid glycosides extract of *Lamiophlomis rotate* has a significant antinociceptive effect that was better at the second phase than the first phase of the formalin test [30].

Conclusion

In conclusion, hexane and diethyl ether fractions obtained from the methanolic extract 80%, and total water extract of aerial parts of *Ajuga chamaecistus* ssp. *tomentella* possess significant and promising antinociceptive properties. The mechanism is supposed to be mediated through the inhibition of endogenous mediators release like prostaglandins. According to the previous study, the isolated compound 8-acethylharpagide could be responsible for the antinociceptive effect of the total water extract and diethyl ether fraction. This study confirmed the traditional use of some *Ajuga* plants for the treatment of joint pain and other inflammatory diseases.

Competing interests

The authors declare that they have no competing interests.

Authors' contributions

MK: Participated in introducing the plant and designing the study, AD: carried out the antinociception effect, NS: Participated in extraction of the plant and drafting the manuscript, MRS: Helped to revise the manuscript, MS: Participated in design and interpreting of the data. All authors read and approve the final manuscript.

Acknowledgements

This study was part of a Pharm. D. thesis funded and supported by Tehran University of Medical Sciences (TUMS) (Grant No: 10784-33-02-89). The authors wish to acknowledge the grammatical revision of the manuscript in English carried out by the Consultation Unit, Office of Publications and Scientometrics, Tehran University of Medical Sciences.

Author details

[1]Department of Pharmacognosy and Medicinal Plants Research Center, Faculty of Pharmacy, Tehran University of Medical Sciences, Tehran 14155-6451, Iran. [2]Department of Traditional Pharmacy, School of Traditional Iranian Medicine and Traditional Iranian Medicine and Pharmacy Research Center, Tehran University of Medical Sciences, Tehran, Iran. [3]Department of Pharmacology and Toxicology, Faculty of Pharmacy, Tehran University of Medical Sciences, Tehran, P.O. Box 14155-6451, Iran.

References

1. Mozaffarian V: *A Dictionary of Iranian Plant Names*. Tehran: Farhangmoaser; 2007:21–22.
2. Nawaz HR, Malik A, Khan PM, Ahmed S: **Ajugin E and F: two withanolides from *Ajuga parviflora*.** *Phytochemistry* 1999, **52**:1357–1360.
3. Akbay P, Calis I, Heimann J, Sticher O: **Ionon, iridoid and phenylethanoid glycosides from *Ajuga salicifolia*.** *Z Naturforsch* 2003, **58c**:177–180.
4. Hilaly JE, Israili ZH, Lyoussi B: **Acute and chronic toxicological studies of *Ajuga iva* in experimental animals.** *J Ethnophar* 2004, **91**:43–50.
5. Israili HZ, Lyoussi B: **Ethnopharmacology of the plants of genus *Ajuga*.** *Pak J Pharm Sci* 2009, **22**:425–462.
6. Naghibi F, Mosaddegh M, Mohammadi Motamed S, Ghorbani A: **Labiatae family in folk medicine in Iran: from ethnobotany to pharmacology.** *Iran J Pharm Res* 2005, **2**:63–79.
7. Hilaly JE, Lyoussi B: **Hypoglycemic effect of lyophilized total water extract of *Ajuga iva* in normal and streptozotocin diabetic rats.** *J Ethnophar* 2002, **80**:109–113.
8. Gautam R, Jachak SM, Saklani A: **Anti-inflammatory effect of *Ajuga bracteosa* Wall ex Benth. mediated through cyclooxygenase (COX) inhibition.** *J Ethnophar* 2011, **133**:928–930.
9. Kuria KAM, Coster S, Muriuki G, Masengo W, Kibwage I, Hoogmartens J, Laekeman GM: **Antimalarial activity of *Ajuga remota* Benth (labiatae) and *Caesalpinia volkensii* Harms (Caesalpiniaceae): *in vitro* confirmation of ethnopharmacological use.** *J Ethnophar* 2001, **74**:141–148.
10. Ono Y, Fukaya Y, Imai S, Yamakuni T: **Beneficial effects of *Ajuga decumbens* on osteoprosis and arthritis.** *Biol Pharm Bull* 2008, **31**:1199–1204.
11. Castro A, Coll J, Tandron YA, Pant AK, Mathela C: **Phytoecdysteroids from *Ajuga macrosperma* var. *breviflora* roots.** *J Nat Prod* 2008, **71**:1294–1296.
12. Vanyolos A, Simon A, Toth G, Polgar L, Kele Z, Ilku A, Matyus P, Bathori M: **C-29 Ecdysteroids from *Ajuga reptans*.** *J Nat Prod* 2009, **72**:929–932.
13. Coll J: **NMR shift data of neo-clerodane diterpens from the genus *Ajuga*.** *Phytochem Anal* 2002, **13**:372–380.
14. Manguro LOA, Ogur JA, Okora DM, Wagal SO, Lemen P: **Further flavonol and iridoid glycosides from *Ajuga remota*.** *J Asian Nat Prod Res* 2007, **9**:617–629.
15. Shams Ardekani MR, Khanavi M, Taheri P, Samadi N, Safaripour E, Salimpour F: **The essential oil composition of *Ajuga chamaecistus* Ging. subsp. *tomentella* Rech. f.** *JEOBP* 2010, **13**:45–51.
16. Sadati N, Ostad SN, Karimian Z, Shams Ardekani MR, Akbarzadeh T, Hadjiakhoondi A, Khanavi M: **Phytochemical study and in vitro cytotoxic effect of *Ajuga chamaecistus* ssp. *tomentella*.** *Asian J Chem* 2012, **24**:2871–2874.
17. Sadati N, Jenett-Siems K, Siems K, Shams Ardekani MR, Hadjiakhoondi A, Akbarzadeh T, Ostad SN, Khanavi M: **Major constituents and cytotoxic effects of *Ajuga chamaecistus* subsp. *tomentella*.** *Z Naturforsch* 2012, **67**:275–281.
18. Khanavi M, Sharifzadeh M, Hadjiakhoondi A, Shafiee A: **Phytochemical investigation and anti-inflammatory activity of aerial parts of *Stachys byzanthina* C Koch.** *J Ethnophar* 2005, **97**:463–468.
19. Tjølsen A, Berge O-G, Hunscaar S, Rusland JH, Hole K: **The formalin test: an evaluation of method.** *Pain* 1992, **51**(1):5–17.
20. Dubuisson D, Dennis SG: **The formalin test: a quantitative study of the analgesic effect of morphine, meperidine and brain stem stimulation in rats and cats.** *Pain* 1977, **4**:161–164.
21. Hunskaar S, Berge OG, Hole K: **Dissociation between antinociceptive and anti-inflammatory effects of acetylsalicylic acid and indomethacin in the formalin test.** *Pain* 1986, **25**:125–132.
22. Chen YF, Tsai HY, Wu TS: **Anti-inflammatory and analgesic activity from roots of *Angelica pubescens*.** *Planta Med* 1995, **61**:2–8.
23. Rosland JH, Tjolsen A, Maehle B, Hole K: **The formalin test in mice: effect of formalin concentration.** *Pain* 1990, **42**:235–242.
24. Verma PR, Joharapurkar AA, Chatpalliwar VA, Asnani AJ: **Antinociceptive activity of alcoholic extract of *Hemidesmus indicus* R Br. In mice.** *J Ethnophar* 2005, **102**:298–301.
25. Carol A, Rouzer CA, Marnett LJ: **Cyclooxygenases: structural and functional insights.** *JLR* 2009, **50**:529–534.
26. Jang M-H, Lim S, Han S-M, Park H-J, Shin I, Kim J-W, Kim N-J, Lee J-S, Kim K-A, Kim CJ: ***Harpagophytum procumbens* suppress lipopolysaccharide-stimulated expressions of cyclooxygenase-2 and inducible nitric oxide synthase in fibroblast cell line L929.** *J Pharmacol Sci* 2003, **93**:367–371.
27. Choubey J, Patel A, Verma MK: **Phytotherapy in the treatment of arthritis: a review.** *IJ PSR* 2013, **4**:2853–2865.

28. Konoshima T, Takasaki M, Tokuda H, Nishino H: **Cancer chemoprotective activity of iridoid glycoside, 8-acetylharpagide, from *Ajuga decumbens*.** *Cancer Lett* 2000, **157**:87–92.
29. Bouderbala S, Prost J, Lacaille-Dubois MA, Bouchenak M: **Iridoid extracts from *Ajuga iva* increase the antioxidant enzyme activities in red blood cells of rats fed a cholesterol-rich diet.** *Nut Res* 2010, **30**:358–365.
30. Li M, Shang X, Zhang R, Jia Z, Fan P, Ying Q, Wei L: **Antinociceptive and anti-inflammatory activities of iridoid glycosides extract of *Lamiophlomis rotate* (Benth.) Kudo.** *Fitoter* 2010, **81**:167–172.

Pharmacological evaluation of the semi-purified fractions from the soft coral *Eunicella singularis* and isolation of pure compounds

Monia Deghrigue[1*], Carmen Festa[2], Lotfi Ghribi[3], Maria Valeria D'auria[2], Simona de Marino[2], Hichem Ben Jannet[3], Rafik Ben Said[4] and Abderrahman Bouraoui[1]

Abstract

Background: Gorgonians of the genus *Eunicella* are known for possessing a wide range of pharmacological activities such as antiproliferative and antibacterial effect. The aim of this study was to evaluate the anti-inflammatory and gastroprotective effect of the organic extract and its semi-purified fractions from the white gorgonian *Eunicella singularis* and the isolation and identification of pure compound(s) from the more effective fraction.

Methods: Anti-inflammatory activity was evaluated, using the carrageenan-induced rat paw edema test and in comparison to the reference drug Acetylsalicylate of Lysine. The gastroprotective activity was determined using HCl/EtOH induced gastric ulcers in rats. The purification of compound(s) from the more effective fraction was done by two chromatographic methods (HPLC and MPLC). The structure elucidation was determined by extensive spectroscopic analysis (^1H and ^{13}C NMR, COSY, HMBC, HMQC and NOESY) and by comparison with data reported in the literature.

Results: The evaluation of the anti-inflammatory activity of different fractions from *Eunicella singularis* showed in a dependent dose manner an important anti-inflammatory activity of the ethanol fraction, the percentage of inhibition of edema, 3 h after carrageenan injection was 66.12%, more effective than the reference drug (56.32%). In addition, this ethanolic fraction showed an interesting gastroprotective effect compared to the reference drugs, ranitidine and omeprazol. The percentage of inhibition of gastric ulcer induced by HCl/ethanol in rats was 70.27%. The percentage of the reference drugs (ranitidine and omeprazol) were 65 and 87.53%, respectively. The purification and structure elucidation of compound(s) from this ethanolic fraction were leading to the isolation of five sterols: cholesterol (5α-cholest-5-en-3β-ol) **(1)**; ergosterol (ergosta-5,22-dien-3β-ol) **(2)**; stigmasterol (24-ethylcholesta-5, 22-dien-3b-ol) **(3)**; 5α,8α-epidioxyergosta 6,22-dien-3β-ol **(4)** and 3β-hydroxy-5α,8α-epidioxyergosta-6-ene **(5)**; and one diterpenoid: palmonine D **(6)**.

Conclusion: Based on data presented here, we concluded that diterpenoids and sterols detected in the ethanolic fraction can be responsible for its pharmacological activity.

Keywords: *Eunicella singularis*, Anti-inflammatory activity, Gastroprotective effect, Marine natural product, Diterpenoid, Sterols

* Correspondence: monia.deghrigue@laposte.net
[1]Laboratoire de développement chimique, galénique et pharmacologique des médicaments (LR12ES09). Equipe de Pharmacologie marine, Faculté de pharmacie de Monastir, Université de Monastir, Monastir, Tunisie
Full list of author information is available at the end of the article

Background

Nature has developed an enormous diversity during several billion years of evolution. The Mediterranean Area represents one of the world's major centers of animal diversity; with around 20 gorgonian species, four belong to the genus *Eunicella*: *E. verrucosa*, *E. filiformis*, *E. cavolini* and *E. singularis* [1].

Although natural compounds have been replaced by synthetic chemistry as the main source of new drugs, marine invertebrates remain an unequalled source of biochemical diversity. The studies on gorgonian have great importance in the research of marine resources of active compounds mainly by the pharmaceutical industry or for other uses. In fact, the gorgonians (Anthozoa, Gorgonacea) are known for possessing a wide range of pharmacologic and health promoting properties including antibacterial [2], antiviral [3], antiplasmodial [4], antifouling [5], antiproliferative [6], cytotoxic [7] and insecticidal [8] effects. The gorgonian of the genus *Eunicella* has been demonstrated to contain a wide variety of natural products as steroids and diterpenes [9,10]. These compounds posses anticancer, gastroprotective and anti-inflammatory activities [11]. For many years, our marine pharmacological group in Tunisia has been involved in an accurate research program on gorgonian constituents in order to define both their chemical composition and their biological activities. On the other hand, the use of non-steroidal anti-inflammatory drugs (NSAID) for the treatment of inflammatory diseases is associated with adverse effects as peptic ulcer [12]. Therefore, the research of potent anti-inflammatory drugs from natural sources and with fewer side effects had become necessary. This study has yielded the anti-inflammatory and gastroprotective effects of the organic extract and its semi-purified fractions of the white gorgonian *Eunicella singularis* (Esper, 1791). The structure elucidation of the isolated compounds from the active fraction was done by 1D and 2D NMR experiments and by comparison with literature data.

Methods

General procedures

HPLC was performed using a Waters model 510 pump equipped with Waters Rheodine injector and a differential refractometer, model 401. Medium pressure liquid chromatography (MPLC) was performed on a Buchi apparatus using a silica gel (230–400 mesh) column.

NMR spectra were obtained on Varian Inova 400 and Varian Inova 500 NMR spectrometers (^{1}H at 400 and 500 MHz, ^{13}C at 100 and 125 MHz, respectively) equipped with a Sun hardware, δ (ppm), *J* in hertz, and spectra referred to CD_3Cl_3 (δH=7.27; δC= 70.0) as internal standard. High-resolution ESIMS spectra were performed with a Micromass QTOF Micro mass spectrometer. All reagents were commercially obtained (Aldrich, Fluka) at the highest commercial quality and used without further purification except where noted. All reactions were monitored by TLC on silica gel plates (Macherey–Nagel). Carrageenan (BDH Chemicals Ltd Poole England), Acetylsalicylate of Lysine (ASL) were purchased from Sigma Chemical (Berlin, Germany). Ranitidine was obtained from Medis (Tunis, Tunisia), omeprazole was obtained from AstraZeneca (Monts).

Collection and extraction

E. singularis was collected from the Mediterranean Sea in various areas of the coastal region of Tabarka (Tunisia), in June 2010, at a depth between 20 and 30 m. Identification of specimens was carried out in the National Institute of Marine Sciences and Technologies (Salamboo, Tunisia) where a voucher specimen of *E. singularis* was deposited under the following reference 1132. After maceration of 600 g of the powdered material with methanol and dichloromethane (1:1, v/v) for 48h three times, the organic extract (40 g) was purified, using C18 cartridges (Sep-pack, Supelco), by gradient elution with different organic solvents in the order of decreased polarity: ethanol, acetone and methanol/CH_2Cl_2 (1:1) to give three semi-purified fractions: ethanol (F-EtOH), acetone (F-Ac) and methanol/CH_2Cl_2 (F-MeOH/CH_2Cl_2) fractions. Organic solvents were removed from recuperated fractions using rotating evaporator at 40°C.

Purification, isolation and structure elucidation

F-EtOH (15 g) was fractionated according to the Kupchan partitioning procedure [13] as follow: the ethanolic fraction was dissolved in a mixture of MeOH/H_2O containing 10% H_2O and partitioned against *n*-hexane to give 10.3 g of the crude extract. The water content (% v/v) of the MeOH extract was adjusted to 30% and partitioned against $CHCl_3$ to give 3.9 g of the crude extract. The aqueous phase was concentrated to remove MeOH and then extracted with *n*-BuOH (268 mg of crude extract) (Figure 1). The *n*-hexane extract (5 g) was fractioned by silica gel MPLC using a solvent gradient system from CH_2Cl_2 to MeOH. Fraction eluted with CH_2Cl_2: MeOH 99:1 (307 mg) was purified by HPLC on a Nucleodur 100–5 C18 (5 μm; 10 mm i.d. × 250 mm) with 99% MeOH: H_2O as eluent (flow rate 3mL/min) to give 1.3 mg of 5α-cholest-5-en-3β-ol (**1**) (t_R=55 min) and 2.4 mg of 24-ethylcholesta-5, 22-dien-3β-ol (**3**) (t_R=83min) (Figure 1).

Fraction eluted with CH_2Cl_2:MeOH 95:5 (288 mg) was purified by HPLC on a Nucleodur 100–5 C18 (5 μ, 4.6 mm i.d. × 250 mm) with 95% MeOH:H_2O as eluent (flow rate 1 mL/min) to give 0.1 mg of ergosta-5,22-dien-3β-ol (**2**) (t_R=74 min) (Figure 1).

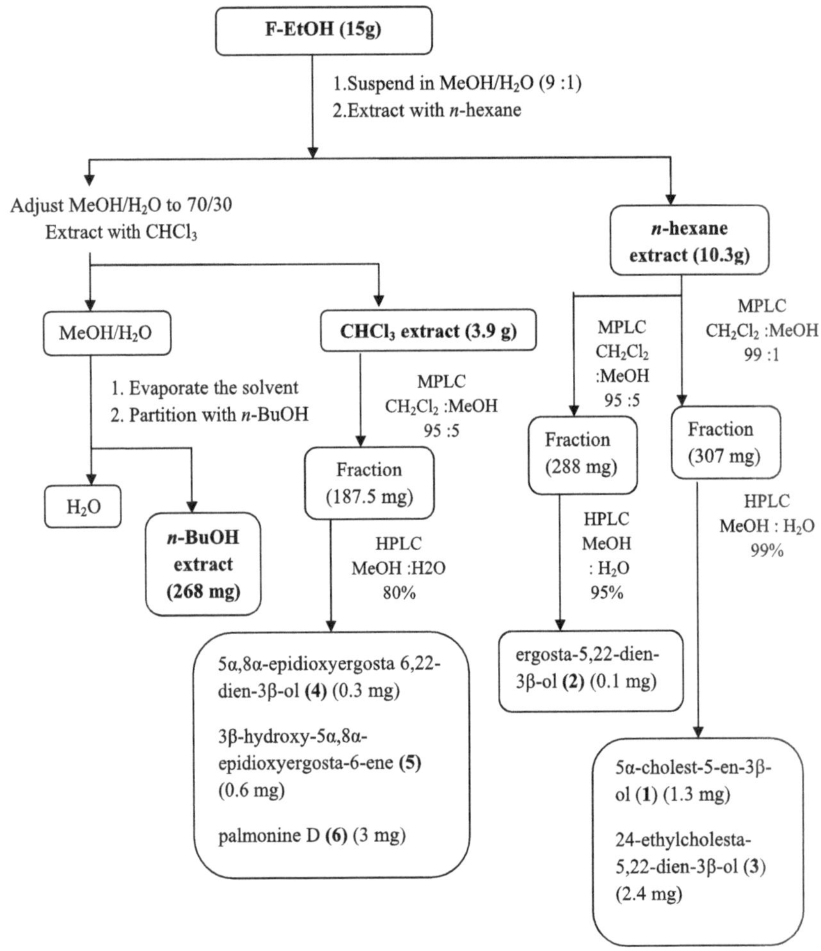

Figure 1 Purification and separation process of the isolation of six compounds from the ethanolic fraction from *E. singularis*.

The $CHCl_3$ extract (3.9 g) was chromatographed by silica gel MPLC using a solvent gradient system from CH_2Cl_2 to CH_2Cl_2: MeOH 1:1.

Fraction eluted with CH_2Cl_2: MeOH 95:5 (187.5 mg) was further purified by HPLC on a Nucleodur 100–5 C18 (5 μ, 4.6 mm i.d. × 250 mm) with 80% MeOH:H_2O as eluent (flow rate 1 mL/min) to give 0.3 mg of 5α,8α-epidioxyergosta 6,22-dien-3β-ol (**4**) (t_R=29 min), and 0.6 mg of 3β-hydroxy-5α,8α-epidioxyergosta-6-ene (**5**) (t_R=2 min) and 3 mg of palmonine D (**6**) (t_R=3 min) (Figure 1).

The purities of compounds were determined to be greater than 95% by HPLC and NMR. Furthermore, HPLC chromatograms and spectroscopic data of each compound were reported (Additional file 1).

Pharmacological evaluation

Animals

Wistar rats of either sex, weighing 150–200 g were obtained from Pasteur Institute (Tunis, Tunisia). Housing conditions and *in vivo* experiments were approved according to the guidelines established by the European Union on Animal Care (CCE Council 86/609).

Carrageenan-Induced Rat Paw Edema

The anti-inflammatory activity of the organic extract and its semi-purified fractions on carrageenan-induced paw edema was determined according to Winter et al. [14]. The animals were divided into eleven groups of six rats each. The control group received an intraperitoneal (i.p.) dose of saline solution (NaCl 9g/L, 2.5 mL/kg), the reference group received Acetylsalicylate of Lysine (ASL) (300 mg/kg, i.p.), and the test groups received the organic extract of *E. singularis* (50, 100 and 200 mg/kg, i.p.) and its semi-purified fractions F-EtOH, F-Ac and F-MeOH/CH_2Cl_2 (25 and 50 mg/kg, i.p.). After 30 min, 0.05mL of a 1% carrageenan suspension was injected into the left hind paw. The paw volume up to the tibiotarsal articulation was measured using a plethysmometer (model

7150, Ugo Basile, Italy). The measures were determined at 0 h (V_0) (before carrageenan injection) and 1, 3 and 5 h later (V_T) (after carrageenan injection). Paw swelling was determined for each rat and the difference between V_T and V_0 was taken as the edema value. The percentages of inhibition were calculated according to the following formula:

$$\% \text{ inhibition} = \left[(V_T - V_0)_{control} - (V_T - V_0)_{treated\ group} / (V_T - V_0)_{control}\right] \times 100$$

Gastric lesions induced by HCl/ethanol

The gastroprotective activity of the organic extract of *E. singularis* and its semi-purified fractions F-EtOH, F-Ac and F-MeOH/CH_2Cl_2 was studied in 150 mM HCl/EtOH induced gastric ulcer [15]. Rats were divided into fifteen groups, fasted for 24 h prior receiving an intraperitoneal doses of vehicle (NaCl 9g/L, 2.5 mL/kg) for the control group, organic extract (50, 100 and 200 mg/kg, i.p.) and its semi-purified fractions F-EtOH, F-Ac and F-MeOH/CH_2Cl_2 (5, 10 and 25 mg/kg, i.p.) for the twelve test groups. Two other groups received ranitidine (60 mg/kg, i.p.) and omeprazole (30 mg/kg, i.p.) as reference drugs. After 30 min, all groups were orally treated with 1mL of 150 mM HCl/EtOH solution for gastric ulcer induction. Animals were killed 1 h after the administration of ulcerogenic agent, their stomachs were excised and opened along the great curvature, washed and stretched on cork plates. The surface was examined for the presence of lesions and the extent of the lesions was measured. The summative length of the lesions along the stomach was recorded (mm) as lesion index.

Statistical analysis

Data are presented as the mean±standard error (s.e.m). Statistical analysis was performed using Student's t-test. The significance of difference was considered to include values of $P<0.05$.

Results and discussion

The current study was carried out to determine the in *vivo* anti-inflammatory and gastroprotective activities of the organic extract of *E. singularis* and its semi-purified fractions. The chemical composition of the more effective fraction was determined by both 1D and 2D NMR experiments.

As shown in Figure 2, 1D and 2D NMR analysis of the ethanolic fraction (F-EtOH) from the gorgonian *E. singularis* resulted in the identification of six compounds.

Compound **1** was isolated as colorless powder. The molecular formula was determined to be $C_{27}H_{46}O$. Analysis of ^1H and ^{13}C NMR data evidenced a Δ^5 dihydroxysteroid structure with a saturated C8 cholestane side chain. Comparison with literature data allowed assigning the 5α-cholest-5-ene-3β-ol (cholesterol) structure [16].

Compound **2** has a molecular formula of $C_{28}H_{46}O$ as determined by HRESIMS. Compound **2** was identified as ergosta-5,22-dien-3β-ol (ergosterol) [17] (Figure 2). This compound was also isolated from the soft coral *Tubastraea coccinea* and *T. tagusensis* [17].

Compound **3** was isolated as colorless powder. The molecular formula was determined to be $C_{28}H_{46}O$. Its identity was determined by 1D and 2D NMR data as 24-ethylcholesta-5,22-dien-3b-ol (stigmasterol) earlier isolated from the halophyte *Salicornia herbacea* [18] and then reported also from the plant *Aglaia eximia* [19].

Compound **4** was isolated as white powder. The molecular formula was determined to be $C_{28}H_{44}O_3$ by HRESIMS data. NMR data disclosed the 5α,8α-epidioxyergosta 6,22-dien-3β-ol structure. This compound was also isolated from the fungus *Sporothrix schenckii* [20] and the fungus *Cryptoporus volvatus* [21].

Compound **5** has a molecular formula of $C_{28}H_{46}O_3$ as determined by HRESIMS. ^1H and ^{13}C NMR indicated that compound **5** is the Δ^{22} derivative of compound **4**. Therefore compound **5** was identified as 3β-hydroxy-5α,8α-epidioxyergosta-6-ene [21].

Compound **6** was isolated as colorless oil. The molecular formula was determined to be $C_{24}H_{36}O_6$ by HRESIMS. The analysis of ^1H NMR spectrum clearly revealed an eunicellin diterpenoid structure. The ^{13}C NMR spectrum revealed 24 carbon signals. ^1H- and ^{13}CNMR assignments were carried out with the aid of the detailed 2D analyses (COSY, HMQC, NOESY, and HMBC) and the resulting NMR evidence revealed **6** to be defined as palmonine D [22]. Three sterols named 5α, 8α-epidioxysterols, pregnanes and 9,11-secosterols were separated from *E. cavolini*, another specie of the genus *Eunicella* [10,11]. The five sterols identified in our study were isolated for the first time from *E. singularis* and were not yet found with another specie from this genus.

Palmonine D is also purified from *E. labiata*, another specie of the genus *Eunicella* [22]. Other researchers reported the isolation of five diterpenoids from the gorgonian *E. labiata*, labiatamide A, labiatamide B, labiatin A, labiatin B and labiatin C [23] but these compounds were not yet separated from *E. singularis*. Massileunicellin A, was obtained from *E. cavolini* [24] but also was not identified from *E.singularis*.

The results reported in Figures 3 and 4 showed the anti-inflammatory effects of organic extract and its semi-purified fractions from *E. singularis* administered intraperitoneally.

E. singularis organic extract presented a dose- related, statistically significant anti-inflammatory activity on carrageenan induced paw edema which was comparable with the reference drug, Acetylsalicylate of Lysine (ASL),

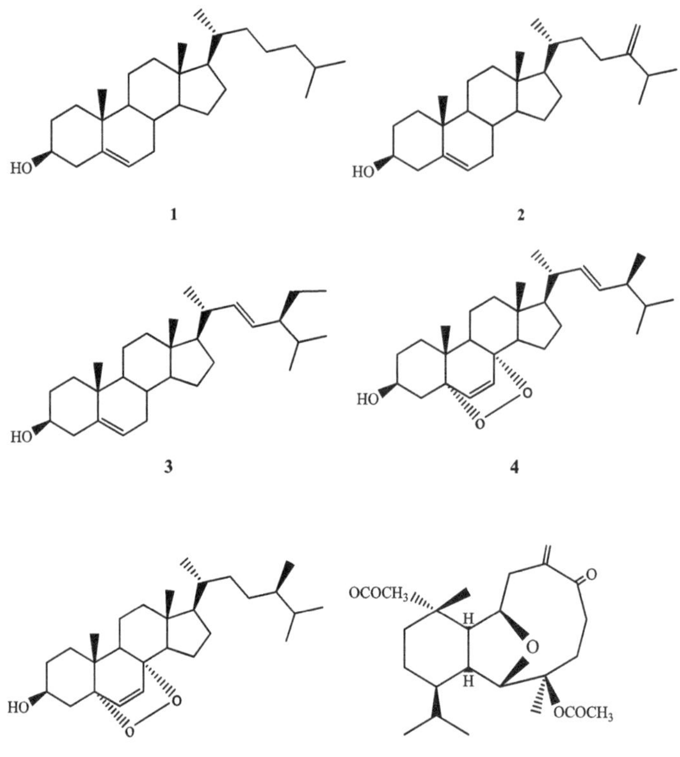

Figure 2 Chemical structures of six compounds isolated from the white gorgonian *E. singularis*. Five sterols **(1-5)**: 5α-cholest-5-en-3β-ol **(1)**; ergosta-5,22-dien-3β-ol **(2)**; 24- ethylcholesta-5,22-dien-3b-ol **(3)**; 5α,8α-epidioxyergosta 6,22-dien-3β-ol **(4)** and 3β-hydroxy- 5α,8α-epidioxyergosta-6-ene **(5)**; and one diterpenoid: palmonine D **(6)**.

a potent inhibitor of cyclooxygenase-2. The percent inhibition of edema at dose levels of 50, 100 and 200 mg/kg were 42.61%, 56.47% and 64.31% (at 3 h), respectively (Table 1). The semi-purified fractions (F-Ac, F-EtOH, F-MeOH/CH_2Cl_2) were assessed for anti-inflammatory effect at 25 and 50 mg/kg. A dose-related anti-inflammatory property was observed for the three fractions with highly significant activity of F-EtOH at dose 50 mg/kg with a percentage of inhibition of 66.12% at 3 h. While F-Ac and F-MeOH/CH_2Cl_2 at a dose of 50 mg/kg reduced

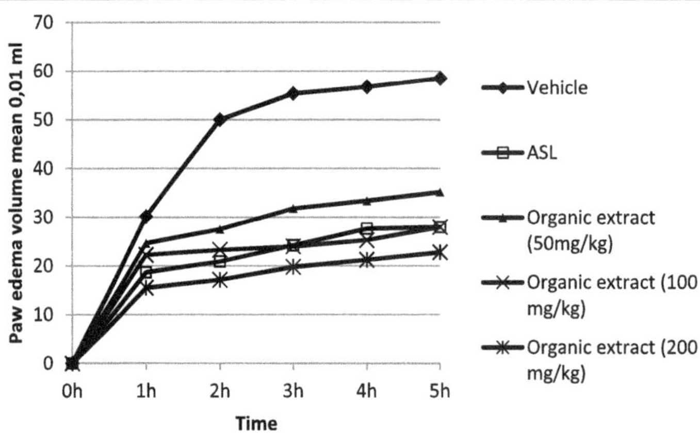

Figure 3 Effect of intraperitoneal administration of the organic extract from *E. singularis* on the carrageenan-induced rat paw edema. Values are mean ± SEM.

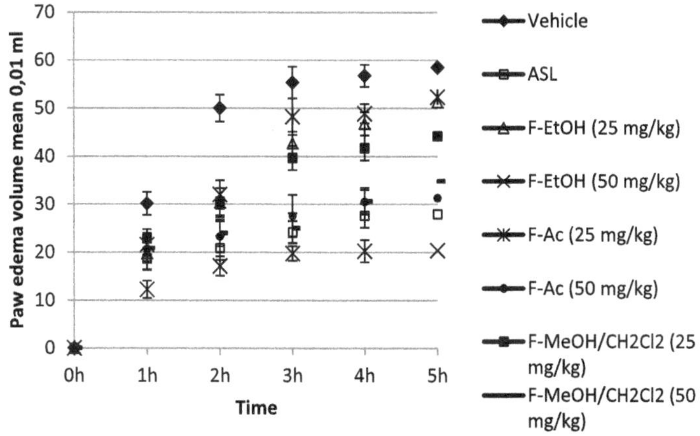

Figure 4 Effect of intraperitoneal administration of semi-purified fractions (F-Ac, F-EtOH and F-MeOH/CH2Cl2 from *E. singularis* on the carrageenan-induced rat paw edema. Values are mean ± SEM.

edema with a percentage of 50.22 and 54.78% (at 3 h), respectively. ASL as a reference standard drug inhibited the edema formation due to carrageenan to an extent of 56.32% (at 3 h) at the dose of 300 mg/kg. The development of edema induced by carrageenan corresponds to the events in the acute phase of inflammation mediated by histamine, bradykinin and prostaglandins produced under an effect of cyclooxygenase-2 (COX-2) [25]. This enzyme is an inducible cyclooxygenase which boosts the inflammatory response by COX-2 mediated prostaglandin E_2 (PGE_2) [26]. Hence, it is probably that the organic extract and its semi-purified fractions from the gorgonian *E. singularis* reduced inflammation by blocking the cyclooxygenase2 (COX-2). Morever, several studies reported that steroids isolated from other species of the genus *Eunicella* have anti-inflammatory activity such as secosteroids [11]. The high anti-inflammatory activity of the fraction F-EtOH can be related with the presence of its main steroid constituents. The chemical analysis of this fraction (F-EtOH) revealed the presence of five sterols: 5α-cholest-5-en-3β-ol (cholesterol) **(1)**; ergosta-5,22-dien-3β-ol (ergosterol) **(2)**; 24-ethylcholesta-5,22-dien-3b-ol (stigmasterol) **(3)**; 5α,8α-epidioxyergosta 6,22-dien-3β-ol **(4)** and 3β-hydroxy-5α,8α-epidioxyergosta-6-ene **(5)**.

The gastroprotective effect of *E. singularis* organic extract and its semi-purified fractions against HCl/EtOH induced gastric damage in rats is shown in (Table 2) and the results are comparable to that of the reference drugs ranitidine, histamine H_2 receptor antagonist, and omeprazole, a proton pump inhibitor [27]. Oral administration of

Table 1 Anti-inflammatory effect of the intraperitoneal administration of *E. singularis* organic extract and its semi-purified fractions (F-EtOH, F-Ac and F-MeOH/CH_2Cl_2) and of reference drug (Acetylsalicylate of Lysine; ASL) in carrageenan-induced rat paw edema test

Treatment	Dose (mg/kg)	Edema (10^{-2}ml) (mean±s. e. m)			Edema inhibition (%)		
		1 h	3 h	5 h	1 h	3 h	5 h
Vehicle	-	30.12±2.38	55.35±3.3	58.5±4.69	-	-	-
Organic extract	50	24.62±2.8	31.76±3.6**	35.14±4.1*	18.26	42.61	39.92
	100	22.22±2.9	23.94±4.1**	27.95±1.5**	32.84	56.47	52.21
	200	15.5±3.2*	19.75±2.4**	22.75±3.6**	48.53	64.31	61.11
F-EtOH	25	19.73±1.6	42.74±2.7	51.26±2.6	34.49	22.78	12.36
	50	12.25±1.5**	18.75±2**	20.37±2.4**	59.32	66.12	65.17
F-Ac	25	21.55±2.6	48.24±2.4	52.33±3.5	28.42	12.84	10.53
	50	20.63±2.4	27.55±3.2**	31.27±2.7*	31.48	50.22	46.54
F-MeOH/CH_2Cl_2	25	22.85±3.2	39.67±2.6	44.2±4.8	24.12	28.32	24.43
	50	20.82±2.4	25.02±2.9**	34.79±3.4*	30.86	54.78	40.52
ASL	300	19.66±3.4	24.17±2.7**	27.95±3.1**	34.71	56.32	52.22

Values are expressed as mean±SEM; n=6 animals. *P<0.01, **P<0.001.

Table 2 Effect of *E. singularis* organic extract and its semi-purified fractions (F-EtOH, F-Ac, F-MeOH/CH_2Cl_2), and of reference drugs (ranitidine and omeprazol) on gastric ulcer induced by HCl/ethanol in rats

Treatment	Dose (mg/kg)	Ulcer index (mm)	Inhibition (%)
Vehicle	-	78.5±3,49	-
Organic extract	50	31.52±2,42**	59.84
	100	24.46±2,48**	68.84
	200	19.49±3,48**	75.16
F-EtOH	5	43.36±1,52*	44.76
	10	37.20±3,05**	52.61
	25	23.33±1**	70.27
F-Ac	25	61.97±0,7	21.05
F-MeOH/CH_2Cl_2	5	66.59±2,33	15.17
	10	58.78±2,82	25.11
	25	29.17±4,04**	62.84
Ranitidine	60	27.47±2.3**	65
Omeprazol	30	9.78±0,81*	87.53

Values are expressed as mean±SEM; n=6 animals. *P<0.01, **P<0.001.

HCl/EtOH produced gastric mucosal damage with severe hemorrhage with lesion index of 78.5 mm in the untreated group. Treatment of rats by organic extract of *E. singularis* produced a significant decrease in gastric hemorrhage and the lesion index was inhibited by 60, 68 and 75% at doses of 50, 100 and 200 mg/kg, respectively. The semi-purified fractions were assessed for gastroprotective activity at 5, 10 and 25 mg/kg. A dose-related gastroprotective effect was observed for the fractions F-EtOH and F-MeOH/CH_2Cl_2 with highly significant activity for the ethanolic fraction (F-EtOH) at 25 mg/kg. The lesion index was inhibited by 44, 52 and 70% at doses of 5, 10 and 25 mg/kg, respectively; while in the ranitidine treated animals (60 mg/kg) the inhibition was 65%. F-Ac failed to protect stomach tissues from mucosal damage. The two classical ulcer drugs ranitidine and omeprazole showed a significant activity with a percentage of inhibition of gastric lesions of 65 and 87%, respectively. Some reports on the gastroprotective effect of diterpenes belonging to different structural skeletons are published [28]. In addition, another studies demonstrated that several terpenes or their derivatives posses gastroprotective activity in different models of induced gastric lesions in animals [29]. This gastroprotective effect seems to be related with an increase of the defensive mechanisms of the stomach, such as prostaglandin synthesis and mucus production [30]. Therefore, the involvement of diterpenoids palmonine D **6** isolated from the active fraction F-EtOH is hypothesized and can be responsible for its high activity.

Furthermore, various phenolic compounds (alkaloids, glycosides, and saponins) detected in *E. singularis* organic extract and fractions [6] may be responsible for its activity. Several studies reported that alkaloids have anti-inflammatory and gastroprotective effects [31]. Also, Glycosides, terpenoids and steroids detected in our samples are known to have anti-inflammatory and gastroprotective properties [10,32] The synergic effect of different compounds of *E. singularis* ethanolic fraction may be responsible for its higher anti-inflammatory and gastroprotective activities. Furthermore, the high free radical scavenging activity of F-EtOH in the DPPH test [6] suggests that the antioxidant activity may be one of the mechanisms of its gastroprotective and anti-inflammatory properties, because both ulcerous and inflammatory processes are related to an increase of free radicals [33].

Conclusion

In conclusion, the obtained results demonstrated that the ethanolic fraction of *E. singularis* had the highest activity in the two tests (anti-inflammatory and gastroprotective). The structure elucidation of compounds isolated from this fraction revealed the presence of five sterols and a eunicellan-based diterpenoid which may be responsible for its activity.

Additional file

Additional file 1: HPLC chromatograms and spectroscopic data of six compounds isolated from the white gorgonian *E. singularis*.

Competing interests
The authors declare that they have no competing interests.

Authors' contributions
AB and HBJ were the supervisors and designed the study. MD carried out pharmacological activities. CF and LG contribute to the chemical study. SDM and MVDA carried out the structure elucidation. RBS made contribution to preparation of organic extract and fractions from *E. singularis*. All authors read and approved the final manuscript.

Author details
[1]Laboratoire de développement chimique, galénique et pharmacologique des médicaments (LR12ES09). Equipe de Pharmacologie marine, Faculté de pharmacie de Monastir, Université de Monastir, Monastir, Tunisie. [2]Department of Pharmacy, University of Naples "Federico II", via D. Montesano 49, I- 80131 Napoli, Italy. [3]Laboratoire de chimie hétérocyclique, produits naturels et réactivité. Equipe de chimie médicinale et produits naturels (LR11ES39), Faculté des sciences de Monastir, Université de Monastir, Monastir, Tunisie. [4]Institut National des Sciences et Technologie de la Mer (INSTM), Salambo, Tunis, Tunisie.

References
1. Gori A, Bramanti L, Lopez-Gonzalez P, Thoma JN, Gili GM, Grinyo J, Uceira V, Rossi S: **Characterization of the zooxanthellate and azooxanthellate morphotypes of the Mediterranean gorgonian *Eunicella singularis*.** *Mar Biol* 2012, **159:**1485-1496.
2. McEnroe FJ, Fenical W: **Structures and synthesis of some new antibacterial sesquiterpenoids from the gorgonian coral *Pseudopterogorgia rigida*.** *Tetrahedron* 1978, **34:**1661-1664.

3. Groweiss A, Look S, Fenical W: **Solenolides, new antiinflammatory and antiviral diterpenoids from a marine octocoral of the genus *Solenopodium*.** *J Org Chem* 1988, **53**:2401-2406.
4. Wei X, Rodriguez AD, Baran P, Raptis RG, Sanchez JA, Ortega-Barria E, Gonzalez J: **Antiplasmodial cembradiene diterpenoids from a Southwestern Caribbean gorgonian octocoral of the genus *Eunicea*.** *Tetrahedron* 2004, **60**:11813-11819.
5. Qi SH, Zhang S, Qian PY, Xiao ZH, Li MY: **Ten new antifouling briarane diterpenoids from the South China Sea gorgonian *Junceella juncea*.** *Tetrahedron* 2006, **62**:9123-9130.
6. Deghrigue M, Dellai A, Bouraoui A: **In vitro antiproliferative and antioxidant activities of the organic extract and its semi-purified fractions from the Mediterranean gorgonian *Eunicella singularis*.** *Int J Pharm Pharm Sci* 2013, **5**:432-439.
7. Sheu JH, Sung PJ, Cheng MC, Liu HY, Fang LS, Duh CY, Chiang MY: **Novel Cytotoxic Diterpenes, Excavatolides A-E, Isolated from the Formosan Gorgonian *Briareum excavatum*.** *J Nat Prod* 1998, **61**:602-608.
8. Grode SH, James TR, Cardellina JH, Onan KD: **Molecular structures of the briantheins, new insecticidal diterpenes from *Briareum polyanthes*.** *J Org Chem* 1983, **48**:5203-5207.
9. Berrue F, Kerr RG: **Diterpenes from gorgonian corals.** *Nat Prod Rep* 2009, **26**:681-710.
10. Ioannou E, Abdel-Razik AF, Alexi X, Vagias C, Alexis MN, Roussis V: **Pregnanes with antiproliferative activity from the gorgonian *Eunicella cavolini*.** *Tetrahedron* 2008, **64**:11797-11801.
11. Ioannou E, Abdel-Razik AF, Alexi X, Vagias C, Alexis MN, Roussis V: **9,11-Secosterols with antiproliferative activity from the gorgonian *Eunicella cavolini*.** *Bioorg Med Chem* 2009, **17**:4537-4541.
12. Hossain H, Al-Mansur A, Akter S, Sara U, Ahmed MR, Jahangir AA: **Evaluation of anti-inflammatory activity and total tannin content from the leaves of *Bacopa monnieri* (Linn.).** *IJPSR* 2014, **5**(4):1246-1252.
13. Kupchan SM, Britton RW, Ziegler MF, Sigel CW: **Bruceantin, a new potent antileukemic simaroubolide from *Brucea antidysenterica*.** *J Org Chem* 1973, **38**:178 179.
14. Winter CA, Risley EA, Nuss GW: **Carrageenan induced edema hind paw of the rat as an easy for anti-inflammatory drugs.** *Proc Soc Exp Biol Med* 1962, **3**:544-547.
15. Mizui T, Doteuchi M: **Effect of polyamines on acidified ethanol-induced gastric lesions in rats.** *Japanese J Pharmacology* 1983, **33**:939-945.
16. Acimovic J, Rozman D: **Steroidal triterpenes of cholesterol synthesis.** *Molecules* 2013, **18**:4002-4017.
17. Lages BG, Fleury BG, Hovell AMC, Rezende CM, Pinto AC, Creed JC: **Proximity to competitors changes secondary metabolites of non-indigenous cup corals, *Tubastraea* spp., in the southwest Atlantic.** *Mar Biol* 2012, **159**:1551-1559.
18. Wang X, Zhang M, Zhao Y, Wang H, Liu T, Xin Z: **Pentadecyl ferulate, a potent antioxidant and antiproliferative agent from the halophyte *Salicornia herbacea*.** *Food Chem* 2013, **141**:2066-2074.
19. Harneti D, Supriadin A, Ulfah M, Safari A, Supratman U, Awang K, Hayashi H: **Cytotoxic constituents from the bark of *Aglaia eximia* (Meliaceae).** *Phytochem Lett* 2014, **8**:28-31.
20. Sgarbi DBG, da Silva AJR, Carlos IZ, Silva CL, Angluster J, Alviano CS: **Isolation of ergosterol peroxide and its reversion to ergosterol in the pathogenic fungus *Sporothrix schenckii*.** *Mycopathologia* 1997, **139**:9-14.
21. Wei-Guang M, Xing-Cong L, De-Zu W, Chong-Ren Y: **Ergosterol peroxides from *Cryptoporus volvatus*.** *Acta Bot Yunnanica* 1994, **16**(2):196-200.
22. Ortega MJ, Zubia E, Salva J: **A new cladiellane diterpenoid from *Eunicella labiata*.** *J Nat Prod* 1997, **60**:485-487.
23. Roussis V, Fenical W, Vagias C, Kornprobst JM, Miralles J: **Labiatamides A, B, and other eunicellan diterpenoids from the Senegalese gorgonian *Eunicella labiata*.** *Tetrahedron* 1996, **52**:2735-2742.
24. Hanson JR: **Diterpenoids.** *Nat Prod Rep* 2001, **18**:88-94.
25. Borgi W, Ghedira K, Chouchane N: **Antiinflammatory and analgesic activities of Zizyphus lotus root barks.** *Fitoterapia* 2007, **78**:16-19.
26. Inoue H, Ohshima H, Kono H, Yamanaka M, Kubota T, Aihara M, Hiroi T, Yago N, Ishida H: **Supressive effects of tranilast on the expression of inducible cyclooxygenase (COX-2) in interleukin-1-β-stimulated fibroblasts.** *Biochem Pharmacol* 1997, **53**:1941-1944.
27. Ishihara M, Ito M: **Influence of aging on gastric ulcer healing activities of cimetidine and omeprazole.** *Eur J Pharmacol* 2002, **444**:209-215.
28. Schmeda-Hirschmann G, Astudillo L, Rodriguez J, Theoduloz C, Yanez T: **Gastroprotective effect of the Mapuche crude drug Araucaria araucana resin and its main constituents.** *J Ethnopharmacol* 2005, **101**:271-276.
29. Farina C, Pinza M, Pifferi G: **Synthesis and anti-ulcer activity of new derivatives of glycyrrhetic, oleanolic and ursolic acids.** *Il Farmaco* 1998, **53**:22-32.
30. Hiruma-Lima CA, Gracioso JS, Toma W, Paula ACB, Almeida ABA, Brasil DD, Muller AH, Souza-Brito AR: **Evaluation of the gastroprotective activity of cordatin, a diterpene isolated from Aparisthmium cordatum (Euphorbiaceae).** *Biol Pharm Bull* 2000, **23**:1465-1469.
31. Moulin M, Coquerel A: *Pharmacologie, connaissance et pratique.* 2èmeth edition. Paris: Masson; 2002:845.
32. Radjasa OK, Vaske YM, Navarro G, Vervoort HC, Tenney K, Linington RG, Crews P: **Highlights of marine invertebrate-derived biosynthetic products: their biomedical potential and possible production by microbial associants.** *Bioorg Med Chem* 2011, **19**:6658-6674.
33. Pedernera AM, Guardia T, Guardia Calderon C, Rotelli AE, de la Rocha NE, Di Genaro S, Pelzer LE: **Anti-ulcerogenic and anti-inflammatory activity of the methanolic extract of *Larrea divaricata* Cav. In rats.** *J Ethnopharmacol* 2006, **105**:415-420.

Potential effects of omega-3 fatty acids on anemia and inflammatory markers in maintenance hemodialysis patients

Afshin Gharekhani[1], Mohammad-Reza Khatami[2], Simin Dashti-Khavidaki[2,3*], Effat Razeghi[2], Alireza Abdollahi[4], Seyed-Saeed Hashemi-Nazari[5] and Mohammad-Ali Mansournia[6]

Abstract

Background: Anemia is a common complication among hemodialysis (HD) patients. Although intravenous iron and erythropoiesis-stimulating agents revolutionized anemia treatment, about 10% of HD patients show suboptimal response to these agents. Systemic inflammation and increased serum hepcidin level may contribute to this hyporesponsiveness. Considering the anti-inflammatory properties of omega-3 fatty acids, this study aimed to evaluate potential role of these fatty acids in improving anemia and inflammation of chronic HD patients.

Methods: In this randomized, placebo-controlled trial, 54 adult patients with HD duration of at least 3 months were randomized to ingest 1800 mg of either omega-3 fatty acids or matching placebo per day for 4 months. Anemia parameters including blood hemoglobin, serum iron, transferrin saturation (TSAT), erythropoietin resistance index, and required dose of intravenous iron and erythropoietin, and serum concentrations of inflammatory/anti-inflammatory markers including interleukin (IL)-6, tumor necrosis factor (TNF)-α, IL-10, C-reactive protein (CRP), hepcidin, ferritin, intact parathyroid hormone (iPTH), and ratios of IL-10 to IL-6 and IL-10 to TNF-α were measured at baseline and after 4 months of the intervention.

Results: 45 subjects (25 in the omega-3 and 20 in the placebo group) completed the study. No significant changes were observed in blood hemoglobin, serum iron, TSAT, and required dose of intravenous iron in either within or between group comparisons. Additionally, erythropoietin resistance index as well as required dose of intravenous erythropoietin showed no significant change in the omega-3 group compared to the placebo group. Although a relative alleviation in inflammatory state appeared in the omega-3 group, the mean differences of inflammatory and anti-inflammatory markers between the two groups did not reach statistically significant level except for IL-10-to-IL-6 ratio and serum ferritin level which showed significant changes in favor of omega-3 treatment ($P < 0.001$ and $P = 0.003$, respectively).

Conclusion: Omega-3 fatty acids relatively improved systemic inflammation of chronic HD patients without any prominent benefits on anemia. However, future well-designed studies on larger number of patients may determine utility of omega-3 fatty acids in HD patients with respect to inflammation and anemia.

Keywords: Anemia, Hemodialysis, Inflammation, Omega-3 fatty acids

* Correspondence: dashtis@sina.tums.ac.ir
[2]Nephrology Research Center, Tehran University of Medical Sciences, Tehran 1417614411, Iran
[3]Faculty of Pharmacy, Tehran University of Medical Sciences, Tehran 1417614411, Iran
Full list of author information is available at the end of the article

Background

Anemia occurs as one of the most common complications of end-stage renal disease (ESRD) in patients undergoing HD [1,2]. It is manifested typically as normocytic and normochromic anemia with normal cellularity of bone marrow [3]. Although erythropoietin (EPO) deficiency is the major reason in the pathogenesis of anemia in ESRD patients, other factors including shortened erythrocyte survival, blood loss, iron and other nutritional deficiencies, hemolysis, oxidative stress, and presence of uremic inhibitors of erythropoiesis seem to play also important roles [4]. Most patients with ESRD and anemia exhibit adequate response to erythropoiesis-stimulating agents (ESA); however, about 10% of the subjects remain hypo- or non-responsive to ESA [2]. Adequate iron supply is necessary to obtain optimal benefit from the ESA therapy. Considering the accelerated erythropoiesis with the initiation of ESA therapy combined with the ongoing uremia- and dialysis-related iron losses, HD patients on ESA are highly predisposed to development of iron-restricted erythropoiesis since the rate of iron release from stores and its delivery to erythroid marrow fail to supply the increased marrow demand. Intravenous (IV) iron supplementation can properly correct limited availability of iron to erythroid marrow and improve hemoglobin concentration [1,5].

On the other hand, dialysis patients have a chronic in flammatory state which may contribute to iron-restricted erythropoiesis via decreasing the mobilization of iron from the reticulo-endothelial system to circulating transferrin, a situation which is associated with the reduced response to ESA therapy and IV iron supplementation [1,3,6]. Several underlying factors have been noted to be responsible for chronic systemic inflammation in HD patients, including the uremic milieu, enhanced infection episodes, greater generation of pro-inflammatory cytokines, widespread atherosclerosis, and the use of bio-incompatible dialysis membrane [3]. Recently, there has been an increasing attention to inflammation in HD patients as a possible cause of disordered iron homeostasis as well as anemia refractory to ESA treatment. Discovery of hepcidin, a 25-amino acid peptide hormone mainly produced in the liver, has dramatically increased our understanding of the molecular basis of iron metabolism over the several past years. It is regarded as the key regulator of iron entry into the systemic circulation [7], and is up-regulated by increased iron stores and inflammation and down-regulated by hypoxia, anemia, and iron deficiency [3,8]. Hepcidin acts by binding to cellular iron exporter ferroportin which is present on the cell membrane of the enterocytes, macrophages and hepatocytes and leads to its internalization and degradation [9]. Thus, the net effect of increased hepcidin synthesis is the reduced absorption of dietary iron and sequestration of iron in hepatocytes and macrophages. It has been reported that dialysis patients have higher serum levels of hepcidin [10-14], probably due to the impaired renal excretion coupled with an enhanced generation secondary to inflammation and iron excess [15]. In addition to limiting iron availability for erythropoiesis, hepcidin may also contribute directly to ESA resistance by an inhibitory impact on erythroid progenitor proliferation and survival [16].

Omega-3 fatty acids have been shown to provide dialysis patients with a host of biochemical and clinical benefits [17]. Nevertheless, it has been shown that dietary fish consumption, as a main source of omega-3 fatty acids, in chronic HD patients was much less than that recommended by American Heart Association, resulting in suboptimal blood levels of omega-3 fatty acids [18]. Similarly, significantly lower concentration of omega-3 fatty acids in erythrocyte membrane phospholipids has been found in HD patients compared with the healthy controls [19], largely due to less consumption of fish or fish-derived products in this patient population [17]. However, the findings of previous studies on anti-inflammatory effects of omega-3 fatty acids supplement in HD patients have been controversial. Some of these studies have indicated positive effects of oral omega-3 supplements on serum systemic inflammatory markers [19-21], while others did not find these effects [22,23]. Furthermore, there is report on positive [19] as well as no effect [24] of oral omega-3 fatty acids on blood hemoglobin level in maintenance HD subjects.

Taking all these data into consideration, our study was aimed to test the hypothesis that administration of omega-3 fatty acids (eicosapentaenoic acid (EPA) and docosahexaenoic acid (DHA)) in maintenance HD patients actually improve systemic inflammation and anemia, and might be useful for reducing serum hepcidin level and consequently required dose of IV iron and EPO.

Methods

Subjects

This is a prospective, randomized, single-blind, placebo-controlled trial on patients in two HD centers in Iran (Imam Khomeini Hospital Complex and Sina Hospital affiliated to Tehran University of Medical Sciences, Tehran, Iran). Adult patients who treated with HD for at least 3 months were selected. Patients with pregnancy, malabsorption syndrome, malignancy, inflammatory or infectious diseases, hypothyroidism, medical or surgical illness in recent 3 months, hemoglobinopathies, asthma, chronic obstructive pulmonary disease, coagulopathies, known psychiatric disorders, lack of tolerance or hypersensitivity to fish products as well as those who were receiving corticosteroid, non-steroidal anti-inflammatory drugs, omega-3 fatty acids in the previous three months, anticoagulants including warfarin, immunomodulator or immunosuppressive were excluded.

Study protocol

The study used a 9-block permuted randomization procedure to allocate subjects randomly into two groups. Each block contained an equal number of omega-3 and control group selections, with the order of the blocks permuted. Random numbers to allocate blocks and randomize group selection were generated using Microsoft Office Excel software. All participants, care providers, and data monitors were blinded to the identity of treatments throughout the study. Patients enrolled into the study were randomized to consume daily dose of either six soft-gel capsules of omega-3 fatty acids (180 mg EPA and 120 mg DHA in each capsule) or matching placebo (containing paraffin oil), provided by Zahravi pharmaceutical company, Tabriz, Iran, for 4 months. Both placebo and omega-3 soft-gel capsules were the same with respect to the size, color, shape, and packaging. All subjects were requested not to alter their habitual diets, drug regimen, and level of physical activity during the study. Adherence to the supplements was assessed by conventional practice of "pill counting", and interviewing with each participant individually thrice weekly. Both omega-3 and placebo capsules were provided free of charge to participants. Furthermore, an attending nephrologist performed a monthly visit for each patient during a routine HD session to encourage adherence to the recommended supplement regimens, and to know adverse effects and tolerability of the supplements. Any changes in the medications as well as patient complaints were recorded during the study period.

At baseline and the end of the study, 10 mL fasting blood were obtained from each patient immediately before HD initiation. The blood samples were centrifuged at 3000 rpm for 10 minutes to separate serum. Serum samples were kept frozen at −70°C for later analysis of serum iron, total iron binding capacity (TIBC), ferritin, hepcidin, iPTH, pro-inflammatory (IL-6, TNF-α, CRP), and anti-inflammatory cytokines (IL-10) concentrations.

The local Ethics Committee of Tehran University of Medical Sciences approved the study protocol, and informed consent was obtained from each patient. The trial was registered in the Iranian Registry of Clinical Trials (registry number: IRCT201202203043N5).

Measurements

Baseline dialysis adequacy (single pool Kt/V urea) was measured for each subject according to pre- and post-dialysis serum urea nitrogen concentrations, ultrafiltration volume, dialysis time, and post-dialysis weight.

Blood hemoglobin concentration was measured using a cell counter (Sysmex K800, Japan); serum CRP level was measured by a turbidimetric method (Autoanalyzer BT3000, Biotechnica, Italy); serum hepcidin, IL-6, IL-10, and TNF-α were measured using ELISA kits (Bioassay Technology laboratory, Shanghai Crystal Day Biotech Co., Ltd., Shanghai, China).

To evaluate the effect of omega-3 fatty acids on iron status and EPO responsiveness, required dose of IV iron and EPO was recorded monthly over the study course. In addition, EPO resistance index (the ratio of weekly EPO dose to hemoglobin concentration per unit of body weight), as well as TSAT (calculated as serum iron × 100/TIBC) were calculated before and after the 4-month intervention period.

Statistical methods

Results were presented as means ± SD or medians (interquartile range). The distribution normality of continuous variables was investigated using quantile normal plot, normal probability plot, and Shapiro-Wilk test. Differences between groups were analyzed using unpaired t-test or two-sample Wilcoxon rank-sum (Mann–Whitney) test, while paired t-test or Wilcoxon matched-pairs signed rank test was used to compare differences within groups. The chi-square test was used to compare differences between categorical variables. Moreover, we estimated the effect of omega-3 supplement on hemoglobin, hepcidin, ferritin, TSAT, iPTH and EPO resistance index using the linear regression model with omega-3 supplement as intervention variable. To adjust for the difference in baseline values and also demographic and clinical characteristics, we also entered these variables in the model. Log-transformation was made in case of TSAT before it was included in regression analysis. Additionally, to normalize the amount of IV EPO and iron required to correct anemia, square root of them was created and then were included in regression analysis. Due to non-normality and heterogeneity of variances of the residual distributions, we used non-parametric bootstrap method with 2000 replications to obtain empirical standard errors and bias-corrected and accelerated (BCa) confidence intervals. In addition, because required dose of IV iron and EPO were recorded four times over the course of the study, to estimate the time trend changes in intervention effect, we also fitted a population-averaged panel-data model by using GEE (generalized estimation equation) with autoregressive one correlation structure to account for within-group correlation structure of individuals. P value of less than 0.05 or confidence interval not including null value was considered as statistically significant. All statistical analyses were carried out using the SPSS version 16.0 (SPSS, Inc., Chicago, IL, USA) and Stata software (StataCorp. 2011. Stata Statistical Software: Release 12. College Station, TX: StataCorp LP).

Results

Figure 1 presents patient randomization and participation procedure in the study. Sixty-four patients were qualified for the study. Of those, 54 patients accepted to

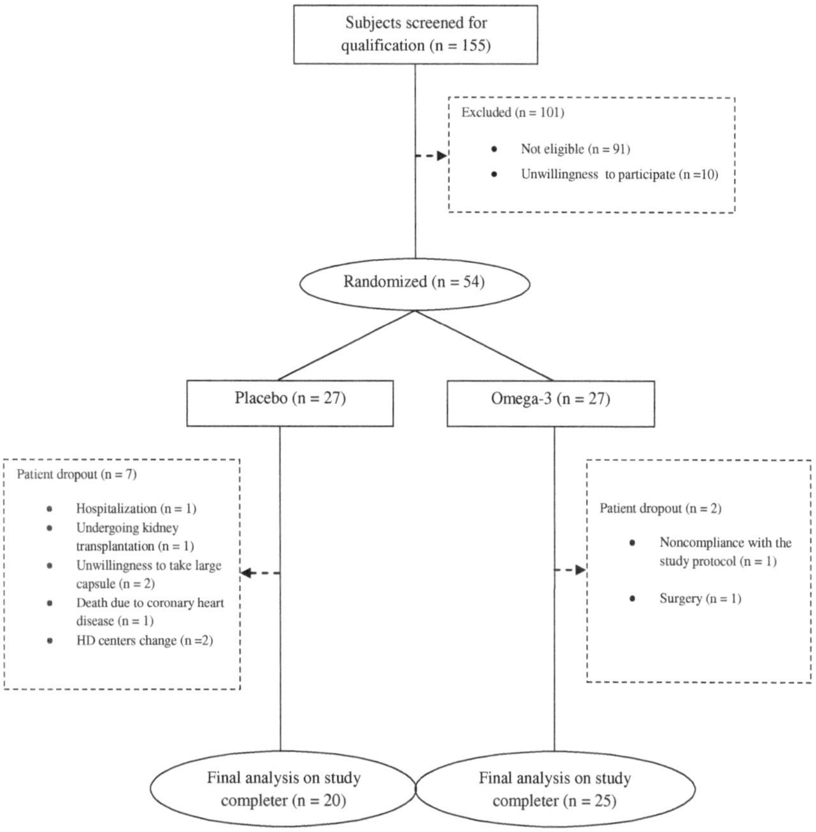

Figure 1 Study's flowchart indicating patient randomization and participation.

participate in the trial. Nine subjects dropped out (7 in the placebo and 2 in the omega-3 group) over the course of the study and thus, 45 (20 placebo and 25 omega-3) completed the study, and their data were used in the final analysis. Table 1 summarizes baseline characteristics of subjects who completed the study. Demographic (gender and age) and clinical (HD duration, dialysis adequacy, and underlying causes of ESRD) data of the patients were comparable between the two study groups at baseline.

Blood hemoglobin levels decreased in both groups during the study period with more decrease in the placebo group. However, the amount of reduction was not significantly different between the two groups ($P = 0.316$). In addition, although serum iron and TSAT showed an

Table 1 Patients' demographic and clinical data at baseline in the placebo and omega-3 group

Characteristics	Placebo (n = 20)	Omega-3 fatty acids (n = 25)	P value
Age (y) (± SD)	57.2 (±15.19)	56.8 (±13.09)	0.925
Sex, n (%)			0.592
Females	8 (40)	12 (48)	
Males	12 (60)	13 (52)	
Hemodialysis duration (mo) (± SD)	72.05 (±60.51)	59.88 (±45.69)	0.450
Dialysis adequacy (Kt/V)	1.27 ± 0.15	1.39 ± 0.22	0.057
Cause of end-stage renal disease, n (%)			0.624
Diabetes	7 (35)	12 (48)	
Hypertension	8 (40)	9 (36)	
Other causes	5 (25)	4 (16)	

Note: Age and hemodialysis duration are expressed as mean ± SD.

increase in the placebo and decrease in the omega-3 group, the magnitude of changes did not reach statistically significance level between the two groups (Table 2). Mean serum TIBC significantly decreased in the omega-3 group at the end of month 4 compared with the placebo group ($P = 0.025$). It is worth noting that before within and between group comparisons were performed on serum hepcidin, four major outlying values were excluded (2 from each group) since they were outside the assay range specified in the package insert of hepcidin kit (> 4000 pg/mL). Thereafter, we observed that serum hepcidin level remained unchanged in the placebo group ($P = 0.756$) at the end of the study compared with baseline, whereas its level increased significantly in the omega-3 group ($P = 0.048$). However, the mean difference of serum hepcidin were comparable between the two groups ($P = 0.145$).

Our results demonstrated that omega-3 treated group had less inflammatory state than placebo group at the end of the study, as reflected in the serum concentrations of IL-6, TNF-α, IL-10, CRP, and anti-inflammatory to pro-inflammatory ratios of IL-10 to TNF-α and IL-10 to IL-6. Although serum levels of iPTH and ferritin, as surrogates of systemic inflammation, increased in both study arms during the study, omega-3 treated subjects experienced much less increase than placebo group. Additionally, comparison of mean differences between the two groups became significant with respect to only serum ferritin level and IL-10 to IL-6 ratio (Table 2).

As shown in Table 3, EPO resistance index showed no significant changes in the omega-3 group compared with the placebo group at the end of the study ($P = 0.086$). At the same time, population-averaged panel-data model did not show any significant change in the required dose of both IV EPO and iron between the two groups in four months of follow-up (Table 4). Of note, omega-3 treatment was weakly and negatively associated with month four IV EPO dose over the course of the study ($P = 0.087$), whereas no such a finding was found regarding the relation between omega-3 treatment and required IV iron dose (Table 4).

Regression analysis with bootstrap method illustrated that among anemia parameters studied in this study, omega-3 treatment was a significant predictor of only serum ferritin level after adjustment for patients' baseline demographic and clinical characteristics (Table 5).

Discussion

Anemia occurs as a common complication in patients with chronic kidney disease and associated with a poor quality of life and bothersome symptoms including fatigue, headache, dyspnea, and light-headedness [25]. Notably, it contributes to the high prevalence of left ventricular hypertrophy in chronic kidney disease patients, even prior to the onset of dialysis, which has been associated with cardiovascular mortality [26]. Thus, careful detection and treatment of anemia is of clinical importance in dialysis patients.

We aimed to investigate the potential benefits of omega-3 fatty acids as adjunct to IV iron and EPO treatment in correction of anemia in maintenance HD patients. Our study showed that administration of omega-3 fatty acids for 4 months caused no change in blood hemoglobin level. This finding was in line with that of Kooshki *et al.*'s study, in that they showed no significant change in blood hemoglobin level following a 10-week supplementation of HD patients with 2080 mg omega-3 fatty acids per day [24]. Additionally, Donnelly *et al.* illustrated that daily ingestion of 3.6 g omega-3 fatty acids by HD patients for 4 weeks produced no significant change in blood hemoglobin concentration [27]. Conversely, Perunicic-Pekovic *et al.* indicated that daily supplementation of HD patients with 2.4 g omega-3 fatty acids for 8 weeks caused a significant increase in blood hemoglobin concentration [19]. The observed discrepancies may in part be related to the diversity in study design, duration and dosage of omega-3 supplementation, varied dietary intake, and baseline blood hemoglobin concentration of the patients.

Supplemental use of omega-3 fatty acids for 4 months also failed to increase TSAT as representative of available serum iron for erythropoiesis. Although we found no similar study in available literature regarding the effect of omega-3 fatty acids on available serum iron to be compared with our results, it seems that inability of omega-3 supplement to improve TSAT might be related to lower dosage of omega-3 supplement (1800 mg per day), relatively favorable TSAT at baseline, or uncontrolled dietary intake of iron.

Moreover, serum TIBC showed a significant reduction in the omega-3 group compared to the placebo group over the course of the study. This finding was in contrast to that of Kalantar-Zadeh *et al.*'s study, in which they observed a significant increase in serum TIBC in hypoalbuminemic HD patients who consumed a nutritional oral supplement containing 1680 mg omega-3 fatty acids [28]. Although the supplement was used during each HD session for 4 weeks, the complex composition of the supplement makes it impossible to distinguish the potential positive effect of omega-3 fatty acids on serum TIBC from other constituents. In addition, Szklarek-Kubicka *et al.* found no marked effects of intradialytic intravenous administration of omega-3 emulsion (containing 2g EPA and 2g DHA) on serum transferrin after 11 consecutive HD sessions [29]. Because dietary protein intake can influence serum transferrin concentration, as a correlate of TIBC, uncontrolled patients' diet in our study might have led to this controversial result. Altogether, considering no significant change in TSAT along with relative attenuated inflammatory state in the omega-3 group, conflicting result

Table 2 Effects of 4 months omega-3 vs. placebo supplementation on hematological and inflammatory parameters

	Placebo (n = 20)				Omega-3 (n = 25)				
	Baseline	Month-4	Diff	P	Baseline	Month-4	Diff	P	P overall
Hgb (g/dL)									
Mean ± SD	11.14 ± 1.62	10.17 ± 1.62	**−0.97 ± 2**	0.055	11.14 ± 2.27	10.86 ± 1.30	**−0.28 ± 2.21**	0.567	**0.316**
Median (IQR)	10.90 (10.10, 12.30)	10.40 (9.02, 11.20)			11.10 (9.45, 12.15)	10.70 (10, 11.45)			
Serum iron (μg/dL)									
Mean ± SD	86.11 ± 37.52	87 ± 43.44	**0.89 ± 49.23**		117.45 ± 117.65	71.85 ± 48.05	**−45.60 ± 115.34**		
Median (IQR)	80 (54.25, 109.50)	66 (53, 132.75)		0.647	66 (48.25, 113.25)	52.50 (45.50, 96)		0.296	**0.781**
TIBC (μg/dL)									
Mean ± SD	281 ± 78.09	264 ± 95.29	**−17 ± 125.98**		318.81 ± 75.26	224.60 ± 52.23	**−94.21 ± 77.28**	0.000	**0.025**
Median (IQR)	252.50 (234.50, 297.50)	232 (200, 283.25)		0.446	310 (255, 383)	210 (182, 272)			
TSAT%									
Mean ± SD	33.36 ± 16.99	38.56 ± 26.20	**5.20 ± 28.06**		35.15 ± 29.12	32.77 ± 22.19	**−2.37 ± 30.49**		
Median (IQR)	30.41 (19.70, 45.80)	29.19 (18.62, 53.28)		0.711	23.67 (14.08, 42.29)	25.68 (17.65, 42.26)		0.575	**1.000**
Ferritin (ng/mL)									
Mean ± SD	345.91 ± 168.90	1236 ± 885.85	**890.05 ± 862.71**		839.63 ± 719.81	1005.10 ± 1185.70	**165.45 ± 886.59**		
Median (IQR)	445.50 (187, 467.50)	1033 (750, 1767)		0.000	596.50 (213.25, 1225.80)	739.50 (126, 1267.50)		0.681	**0.000**
Hepcidin (pg/mL)									
Mean ± SD	584.81 ± 654.45	557.25 ± 401.96	**−27.56 ± 650.83**		579.74 ± 340.81	729.48 ± 661.81	**149.74 ± 574.87**		
Median (IQR)	358.50 (306.50, 546.50)	377 (334.50, 812.25)		0.756	392 (318, 983)	443 (335, 856)		0.048	**0.145**
IL-6 (ng/L)									
Mean ± SD	103.54 ± 145.18	106.48 ± 136.51	**2.94 ± 206.17**		144.38 ± 167.66	136.85 ± 183.56	**−7.53 ± 126.01**		
Median (IQR)	44.90 (40.22, 87.32)	52.85 (40.55, 98.62)		0.695	56.30 (46.90, 151.45)	50 (29.20, 123.50)		0.034	**0.115**
TNF-α (ng/L)									
Mean ± SD	80.93 ± 64.89	77.43 ± 59.82	**−3.50 ± 49.21**		122.09 ± 171.69	116.57 ± 172.32	**−5.52 ± 46.92**		
Median (IQR)	48.05 (42.42, 95.57)	48.05 (44.17, 99.22)		0.616	67 (44.30, 127.20)	58.60 (44.55, 112.80)		0.346	**0.971**
IL-10 (pg/mL)									
Mean ± SD	111.76 ± 67.39	107.24 ± 63.01	**−4.51 ± 90.79**		123.94 ± 71.91	132.06 ± 94.81	**8.11 ± 57.63**		
Median (IQR)	78.05 (72.80, 119.08)	83 (68.20, 128.30)		0.446	91.80 (71.80, 154.10)	87.70 (69.90, 149.60)		0.798	**0.445**
IL-10 / IL-6									
Mean ± SD	1.57 ± 0.42	1.39 ± 0.35	**−0.18 ± 0.53**		1.32 ± 0.55	1.96 ± 1.19	**0.64 ± 1.14**		
Median (IQR)	1.74 (1.56, 1.79)	1.48 (1.27, 1.66)		0.078	1.48 (0.97, 1.56)	1.59 (1.05, 2.77)		0.013	**0.003**

Table 2 Effects of 4 months omega-3 vs. placebo supplementation on hematological and inflammatory parameters *(Continued)*

IL-10 / TNF-α									
Mean ± SD	1.85 ± 1.19	1.69 ± 0.95	**−0.16 ± 1.17**		1.35 ± 0.29	1.44 ± 0.28	**0.09 ± 0.25**		**0.399**
Median (IQR)	1.62 (1.26, 2.07)	1.49 (0.91, 2.08)		0.349	1.39 (1.20, 1.58)	1.50 (1.27, 1.64)		0.139	
CRP (mg/L)									
Mean ± SD	7.73 ± 4.89	12.69 ± 14.02	**4.96 ± 12.59**		9.24 ± 8.79	8 ± 6.78	**−1.24 ± 5.68**		
Median (IQR)	6.19 (4.79, 8.93)	6.26 (3.55, 18.81)		0.246	6.23 (4.87, 10.26)	5.91 (3.25, 10.72)		0.414	**0.143**
iPTH (pg/mL)									
Mean ± SD	271.18 ± 233.60	654.57 ± 1082.30	**383.39 ± 927.49**		333.42 ± 567.22	348.07 ± 723	**14.65 ± 235.88**		
Median (IQR)	180 (95, 507.50)	224 (110.40, 980.50)		0.006	118 (91.35, 316)	167 (97.15, 286)		0.455	**0.17**

Notes: Data are mean ± SD and median (IQR). P values for each group were derived from paired t-test or Wilcoxon signed ranks test between baseline versus month-4 comparison (within group comparison). Overall P values were derived using independent t-test or Mann–Whitney U test, comparing mean differences of parameters between omega-3 and placebo group (between group comparisons of mean differences) (bold faces).

Abbreviations and definitions: IQR, Interquartile range; IL, Interleukin; TNF-α, Tumor necrosis factor alpha; CRP, C-reactive protein; iPTH, Intact parathyroid hormone; Hgb, Hemoglobin; TSAT, Transferrin saturation; TIBC, Total iron binding capacity; Diff, Mean difference of month-4 minus baseline.

Table 3 Mean dose of IV iron and EPO and calculated EPO resistance index in two groups

Groups	Baseline	Month 2	Month 3	Month 4	Difference	P value
IV iron (mg/week)						
Omega-3	65.22 ± 91.93	49 ± 63.11	37 ± 61.29	37.30 ± 76.78	**−27.91 ± 128.96**	**0.554**
Placebo	54.17 ± 44.76	36.84 ± 34.73	56.94 ± 71.13	23.61 ± 33.73	**−30.56 ± 64.49**	
IV EPO (unit/week)						
Omega-3	8695.70 ± 8059	9960 ± 7236.90	8640 ± 7846.80	8956.50 ± 8019.70	**260.87 ± 4013.81**	**0.086**
Placebo	6888.90 ± 4861.40	9052.60 ± 4440.60	8333.30 ± 4186.80	9666.70 ± 5005.80	**2777.78 ± 5493.91**	
EPO resistance index (unit/week per Hgb per weight)						
Omega-3	14.64 ± 15.12	-	-	15.03 ± 13.40	**0.39 ± 7.82**	**0.086**
Placebo	11.17 ± 8.72	-	-	17.26 ± 12.02	**6.09 ± 11.89**	

Notes: All values are mean ± SD. Difference indicates mean difference of month-4 minus baseline. P values were derived using independent t-test or Mann–Whitney U test, comparing mean differences of parameters between two groups (bold faces). P value < 0.05 was considered as statistically significant.
Abbreviations: *Hgb* Hemoglobin, *IV* Intravenous, *EPO* Erythropoietin.

of our study remains to be elucidated in more controlled studies.

In the present work, serum ferritin level increased in both groups during the study period with much more retarded increase in the omega-3 group. In contrast, Rasic-Milutinovic *et al.* showed that daily administration of 2.4 g omega-3 fatty acids for 8 weeks significantly lowered serum ferritin level in maintenance HD patients [21]. Huang *et al.* failed to demonstrate an association between plasma omega-3 fatty acids concentration and systemic inflammation in dialysis patients [30]. We used a moderate dose of 1800 mg omega-3 supplement per day for 4 months, which may be insufficient to replace membrane phospholipids' fatty acids beside plasma free fatty acids to exert prominent anti-inflammatory effects. However, omega-3 supplement in our study was a significant and independent predictor of reduction in serum ferritin. Given the unchanged TSAT in both arms of this study, it is conceivable that changes in serum ferritin, as an acute phase protein, was more reflective of systemic inflammation rather than iron stores. This concept was further supported when serum ferritin increased more restrictedly in omega-3 treated patients who experienced slight alleviation in systemic inflammation (Table 2).

The mean difference of required IV EPO dose in the omega-3 group was lower than that in the placebo group (Table 3). Consistently, population-averaged panel-data model revealed that omega-3 supplement was a weakly predictor of reduced IV EPO dose in month four of intervention. Therefore, more pronounced reduction in IV EPO dose might likely appear with omega-3 supplementation if the study period was expanded. In contrast, Kooshki *et al.* found no significant changes in mean dose of IV EPO in either omega-3 (2080 mg/day) or placebo group during their 10-week study period [24]. In our study, EPO resistance index indicated no significant improvement in omega-3 treated subjects compared with the placebo group during the study period. In contrast to this finding, Himmelfarb *et al.* demonstrated that daily administration of gamma-tocopherol-enriched mixture of DHA (containing 924 mg gamma-tocopherol and 1200 mg DHA) for 8 weeks caused a significant reduction in the serum IL-6 and erythropoietic index (weekly EPO dose divided by hematocrit) in maintenance HD patients [31]. In

Table 4 Population-averaged panel-data model by using GEE for evaluating the effects of omega-3 supplement on required dose of IV iron and EPO during the study, with time being considered as a possible interacting factor

	Independent variables			
Dependent variable	**Omega-3†**	**Baseline value**	**Time**	**Time*Omega-3**
Post-IV EPO dose	β = −15.57 95%CI (−32.93 , 2.93) P = 0.087	β = 0.48 95%CI (0.27 , 0.68) P = 0.000	β = 1.71 95%CI (−3.24 , 6.36) P = 0.493	β = −7.04 95%CI (−17.52 , 2.29) P = 0.150
Post-IV iron dose	β = −0.42 95%CI (−3.13 , 2.59) P = 0.771	β = 0.18 95%CI (−0.03 , 0.45) P = 0.166	β = −0.73 95%CI (−1.94 , 0.66) P = 0.279	β = 0.18 95%CI (−1.67 , 2.21) P = 0.856

Notes: Square root of intravenous erythropoietin and iron were included in regression analysis.
Abbreviations: *EPO* Erythropoietin, *IV* Intravenous, *Post-* Post-intervention, *TSAT* Transferrin saturation, *CI* Bias-corrected confidence interval.
†The coefficient indicates predictive value of omega-3 treatment on the difference in square root of outcome variables measured at the end of the study between omega-3 and placebo groups.
P value < 0.05 or 95%CI not including null value was considered as statistically significant.

Table 5 Effects of omega-3 supplement on anemia parameters and iPTH in multiple linear regression model

Independent variable		Dependent variable†					
		Post-Hemoglobin	Post-Hepcidin	Post-Ferritin	Post-TSAT^Ψ	Post-EPO resistance index	Post-iPTH
Omega-3 supplement	Coefficient (β)	0.683	67.979	−922.484	−0.273	−5.404	−414.247
	Bootstrap standard error	0.547	147.169	282.992	0.218	3.899	213.935
	P value	0.212	0.644	**0.001***	0.211	0.166	0.053
	95% CI	(−0.361, 1.776)	(−203.593, 362.789)	(−1533.274, -412.422)	(−0.671, 0.193)	(−12.844, 2.466)	(**−1150.008, -129.641**)*

Abbreviations: *EPO* Erythropoietin, *Post-* Post-intervention, *TSAT* Transferrin saturation, *iPTH* Intact parathyroid hormone, *CI* Bias-corrected and accelerated confidence interval.
†All analyses were adjusted for age, gender, hemodialysis duration, and baseline values of Kt/V and outcome variables.
ΨBoth baseline and post-intervention TSAT were included in regression analysis in logarithmic scale.
*P value < 0.05 or 95%CI (with bootstrap method) not including null value was considered as statistically significant.

spite of the contributory role of inflammation in the EPO resistance [32-34], relative attenuated inflammation by omega-3 supplement in our study was not sufficient to cause favorable changes in EPO resistance.

Unexpectedly, required dose of IV iron decreased in both groups through the study period with no significant difference between the mean differences of the two groups (Table 3). Additionally, population-averaged panel-data model showed no role of omega-3 supplement over time in the prediction of post-treatment IV iron dose. Unfortunately, we were not able to interpret such a finding using available data.

In our study, although omega-3 treated patients experienced significant increase in the ratio of IL-10 to IL-6 and marked favorable changes in the serum ferritin level compared to the placebo group, other serum inflammatory markers including IL-6, TNF-α, CRP, IL-10, iPTH and IL-10-to-TNF-α ratio also desirably changed in this group. Inability of omega-3 supplement to provide marked anti-inflammatory effects in this study may be due to limited statistical power, small dosage of omega-3 fatty acids supplement, shorter observation period, or all of these. It should be mentioned that results of the majority of the studies evaluating the effects of omega-3 fatty acids on inflammatory markers in HD patients are inconclusive, largely due to diversity in study design, supplement dosage, and study length. Saifullah *et al.* showed that daily administration of 1.3 g omega-3 fatty acids for 12 weeks induced a significant reduction in serum CRP levels of HD patients [20]. In addition, Perunicic-Pekovic *et al.* demonstrated significant decline in serum IL-6 and TNF-α levels of HD subjects following daily consumption of 2.4 g of omega-3 fatty acids for 2 months [19]. Bowden *et al.* treated maintenance HD patients with 1560 mg omega-3 fatty acids per day for 6 months, and found a significant decrease in serum CRP level [35]. In contrast, a recent study by Kooshki *et al.* failed to demonstrate any effects of omega-3 fatty acids (2080 mg per day for 10 weeks) on serum CRP, TNF-α, and IL-6 concentration in HD patients [36]. In agreement with our results, Hassan *et al.* found insignificant decrease in the serum concentrations of CRP, TNF-α, and IL-6 after 8 weeks of oral omega-3 supplementation (3.4 g EPA and DHA per day) in peritoneal dialysis patients [37]. Also our results were in line with those of Poulia *et al.*'s study, that daily ingestion of 1680 mg omega-3 fatty acids for 4 weeks caused an insignificant decline in serum CRP concentrations in chronic HD subjects [38].

Additionally, omega-3 supplement was a significant predictor of reduced serum iPTH level in our study (Table 5). None of the participants ingested cinacalcet to control hyperparathyroidism, and the number of subjects receiving calcitriol was comparable between the two study arms. Thus, significant association of omega-3 supplementation with reduced serum iPTH levels might largely be related to partial decline in systemic inflammation following 4 months of omega-3 administration.

In addition, serum hepcidin level showed no significant change in the omega-3 group compared with the placebo group. There are conflicting reports with respect to the relation between inflammation markers and serum hepcidin. Some studies have detected a positive association [39,40], while others have not [15,41,42]. Our study showed a relative improvement in systemic inflammation by omega-3 treatment, whereas serum hepcidin level showed a significant increase in this group. Also TSAT, as an important regulator of hepcidin synthesis [43], had no significant changes within and between the two groups during the study period. Actually, we found no similar study in available literature regarding the effect of omega-3 supplement on serum hepcidin to compare our result. However, some reasons could be provided for the observed discrepancy. First, dosage of omega-3 fatty acids used in our study might not be sufficient to exert pronounced suppression on systemic inflammatory markers in general, and serum hepcidin in particular. Second, considering normal value of inflammation markers in healthy individuals [44,45], our study subjects had no overt sever inflammation at baseline or at the end of the study, that this state might partly weaken the anti-inflammatory effect of omega-3 fatty acids on hepcidin production. Third, elevated serum hepcidin may not be necessarily needed to maintain a mild iron deficiency and anemia of inflammation because other inflammatory mediators have a similar effect, and normal serum hepcidin level is also able to sufficiently restrict iron supply and prevent the correction of the established anemia [41]. Finally, interrelations among the response to EPO, serum iron status, iron therapy, and serum hepcidin increase the complexity of interpretations in this area. For instance, some iron parameters are representative of both iron stores and inflammation (i.e. ferritin) or have a mixed inflammatory and nutritional significance (i.e. transferrin) [46,47].

Our study may be criticized for some limitations, as follows: low statistical power to detect meaningful differences between the groups due to the small sample size and short observation period, monitoring of patient compliance with "pill counting" practice instead of in vivo measurement of omega-3 fatty acids, lack of interim analysis on all outcome variables to identify a potential trend over time and reduce variance of estimates of treatment effects, distortion of subject blindness in the placebo arm due to "Fishy" smells of omega-3 soft-gel capsules, and lack of careful assessment of patients' dietary intake. Despite the above-mentioned limitations, our trial had several strengths including placebo-controlled design, relatively longer duration of the study compared with previous ones, relatively comprehensive assessment of anemia and inflammation markers, absent serious adverse effects causing patient withdrawal, and enhanced patient adherence via more frequent interviews compared with previous studies.

In summary, the present study showed a mild attenuation in systemic inflammation of chronic HD patients by omega-3 fatty acids supplement. Although omega-3 supplement failed to improve anemia, its positive, though slight, effects on serum inflammation markers including ferritin were encouraging. Considering elevated serum hepcidin in the presence of unchanged TSAT and weakened inflammation in the omega-3 group, it can be speculated that other impressive factor(s) not controlled in our study might contribute to these contradictory results. Therefore, there is a need for further well-designed studies to precisely determine utility of omega-3 fatty acids in HD patients with respect to inflammation and anemia.

Competing interests
The authors declare that they have no competing interest.

Authors' contribution
AG: made substantial contributions to study design, acquisition and interpretation of data and drafting the manuscript and revising it. MRK: have been involved in drafting the manuscript and revising it critically for important intellectual content. SDK: have made substantial contributions to conception and design of the study, have been involved in drafting the manuscript or revising it critically for important intellectual content, and final approval of the manuscript. ER: made substantial contributions to data acquisition. AA: made substantial contributions to data acquisition. SSHN: made substantial contributions to data analysis. MAM: made substantial contributions to data analysis. All authors read and approved the final manuscript.

Acknowledgements
This study has been supported by Tehran University of Medical Sciences (grant No: 17020). The Authors thank Zahravi Pharmaceutical Co., Tehran, Iran for providing placebo free of charge and Dr Amir Hekmat for his kind coordinating between researchers' team and the pharmaceutical company. The authors also appreciate valuable helps of hemodialysis nursery teams of Imam-Khomeini Hospital complex and Sina Hospital, especially Mrs. Abdpoor.

Author details
[1]Resident of Clinical Pharmacy, Faculty of Pharmacy, Tehran University of Medical Sciences, Tehran 1417614411, Iran. [2]Nephrology Research Center, Tehran University of Medical Sciences, Tehran 1417614411, Iran. [3]Faculty of Pharmacy, Tehran University of Medical Sciences, Tehran 1417614411, Iran. [4]Vali-e-Asr Hospital, Tehran University of Medical Sciences, Tehran 1417614411, Iran. [5]Department of Epidemiology, School of Public Health, Shahid Beheshti University of Medical Sciences, Tehran 1417614411, Iran. [6]Department of Epidemiology and Biostatistics, School of Public Health, Tehran University of Medical Sciences, Tehran 1417614411, Iran.

References
1. Tessitore N, Girelli D, Campostrini N, Bedogna V, Solero GP, Castagna A, Melilli E, Mantovani W, Matteis GD, Olivieri O, *et al*: **Hepcidin is not useful as a biomarker for iron needs in haemodialysis patients on maintenance erythropoiesis-stimulating agents.** *Nephrol Dial Transplant* 2010, **25:**3996–4002.
2. Swinkels DW, Wetzels JFM: **Hepcidin: a new tool in the management of anaemia in patients with chronic kidney disease?** *Nephrol Dial Transplant* 2008, **23:**2450–2453.
3. Malyszko J, Malyszko JS, Mysliwiec M: **Hyporesponsiveness to erythropoietin therapy in hemodialyzed patients: potential role of prohepcidin, hepcidin, and inflammation.** *Ren Fail* 2009, **31:**544–548.
4. Malyszko J, Mysliwiec: **Hepcidin in anemia and inflammation in chronic kidney disease.** *Kidney Blood Press Res* 2007, **30:**15–30.
5. Macdougall IC, Tucker B, Thompson J, Tomson CR, Baker LR, Raine AE: **A randomized controlled study of iron supplementation in patients treated with erythropoietin.** *Kidney Int* 1996, **50:**1694–1699.
6. Barany P, Divino Filho JC, Bergstrom J: **High C-reactive protein is a strong predictor of resistance to erythropoietin in hemodialysis patients.** *Am J Kidney Dis* 1997, **29:**565–568.
7. Ganz T: **Molecular control of iron transport.** *J Am Soc Nephrol* 2007, **18:**394–400.
8. Nicolas G, Viatte L, Bennoun M, Beaumont C, Kahn A, Vaulont S: **Hepcidin, a new iron regulatory peptide.** *Blood Cells Mol Dis* 2002, **29:**327–335.
9. Putten KVD, Jie KE, Broek DVD, Kraaijenhagen RJ, Laarakkers C, Swinkels DW, Braam B, Gaillard CA: **Hepcidin-25 is a marker of the response rather than resistance to exogenous erythropoietin in chronic kidney disease/ chronic heart failure patients.** *Eur J Heart Fail* 2010, **12:**943–950.
10. Zaritsky J, Young B, Gales B, Wang H, Rastogi A, Westerman M, Nemeth E, Ganz T, Salusky IB: **Reduction of serum hepcidin by hemodialysis in pediatric and adult patients.** *Clin J Am Soc Nephrol* 2010, **5:**1010–1014.
11. Tomosugi N, Kawabata H, Wakatabe R, Higuchi M, Yamaya H, Umehara H, Ishikawa I: **Detection of serum hepcidin in renal failure and inflammation by using ProteinChip system.** *Blood* 2006, **108:**1381–1387.
12. Zaritsky J, Young B, Wang H, Westerman M, Olbina G, Nemeth E, Ganz T, Rivera S, Nissenson AR, Salusky IB: **Hepcidin-a potential novel biomarker for iron status in chronic kidney disease.** *Clin J Am Soc Nephrol* 2009, **4:**1051–1056.
13. Valenti L, Girelli D, Valenti GF, Castagna A, Como G, Campostrini N, Rametta R, Dongiovanni P, Messa P, Fargion S: **HEF mutations modulate the effect of iron on serum hepcidin-25 in chronic hemodialysis patients.** *Clin J Am Soc Nephrol* 2009, **4:**1331–1337.
14. Peters HPE, Laarakkers CMM, Swinkels DW, Wetzels JFM: **Serum hepcidin-25 levels in patients with chronic kidney disease are independent of glomerular filtration rate.** *Nephrol Dial Transplant* 2010, **25:**848–853.

15. Weiss G, Theurl I, Eder S, Koppelstaetter C, Kurz K, Sonnweber T, Kobold U, Mayer G: **Serum hepcidin concentration in chronic haemodialysis patients: associations and effects of dialysis, iron and erythropoietin therapy.** *Eur J Clin Invest* 2009, **39**:883–890.
16. Dallalio G, Law E, Means RT Jr: **Hepcidin inhibits in vitro erythroid colony formation at reduced erythropoietin concentrations.** *Blood* 2006, **107**:2702–2704.
17. Friedman A, Moe S: **Review of the effects of omega-3 supplementation in dialysis patients.** *Clin J Am Soc Nephrol* 2006, **1**:182–192.
18. Friedman AN, Moe SM, Perkins SM, Li Y, Watkins BA: **Fish consumption and omega-3 fatty acid status and determinants in long-term hemodialysis.** *Am J Kidney Dis* 2006, **47**:1064–1071.
19. Perunicic-Pekovic GB, Rasic ZR, Pljesa SI, Sobajic SS, Djuricic I, Maletic R, Ristic-Medic DK: **Effect of n-3 fatty acids on nutritional status and inflammatory markers in haemodialysis patients.** *Nephrology* 2007, **12**:331–336.
20. Saifullah A, Watkins BA, Saha C, Li Y, Moe SM, Friedman AN: **Oral fish oil supplementation raises blood omega-3 levels and lowers C-reactive protein in haemodialysis patients-a pilot study.** *Nephrol Dial Transplant* 2007, **22**:3561–3567.
21. Rasic-Milutinovic Z, Perunicic G, Pljesa S, Gluvic Z, Sobajic S, Djuric I, Ristic D: **Effects of n-3 PUFAs supplementation on insulin resistance and inflammatory biomarkers in hemodialysis patients.** *Ren Fail* 2007, **29**:321–329.
22. Fiedler R, Mall M, Wand C, Osten B: **Short-term administration of omega-3 fatty acids in hemodialysis patients with balanced lipid metabolism.** *J Ren Nutr* 2005, **15**:253–256.
23. Madsen T, Schmidt EB, Christensen JH: **The effect of n-3 fatty acids on C-reactive protein levels in patients with chronic renal failure.** *J Ren Nutr* 2007, **17**:258–263.
24. Kooshki A, Taleban FA, Tabibi H, Hedayati M: **Effects of omega-3 fatty acids on serum lipids, lipoprotein (a), and hematologic factors in hemodialysis patients.** *Ren Fail* 2011, **33**:892–898.
25. Guidi GC, Santonastaso CL: **Advancements in anemias related to chronic conditions.** *Clin Chem Lab Med* 2010, **48**:1217–1226.
26. Levin A: **Anemia and left ventricular hypertrophy in chronic kidney disease populations: a review of the current state of knowledge.** *Kidney Int Suppl* 2002, **80**:35–38.
27. Donnelly SM, Ali MA, Churchill DN: **Effect of n-3 fatty acids from fish oil on hemostasis, blood pressure, and lipid profile of dialysis patients.** *J Am Soc Nephrol* 1992, **2**:1634–1639.
28. Kalantar-Zadeh K, Braglia A, Chow J, Kwon O, Kuwae N, Colman S, Cockram DB, Kopple JD: **An anti-inflammatory and antioxidant nutritional supplement for hypoalbuminemic hemodialysis patients: a pilot/feasibility study.** *J Ren Nutr* 2005, **15**:318–331.
29. Szklarek-Kubicka M, Fijałkowska-Morawska J, Zaremba-Drobnik D, Uciński A, Czekalski S, Nowicki M: **Effect of intradialytic intravenous administration of ω-3 fatty acids on nutritional status and inflammatory response in hemodialysis patients: a pilot study.** *J Ren Nutr* 2009, **19**:487–493.
30. Huang X, Stenvinkel P, Qureshi AR, Risérus U, Cederholm T, Bárány P, Heimbürger O, Lindholm B, Carrero JJ: **Essential polyunsaturated fatty acids, inflammation and mortality in dialysis patients.** *Nephrol Dial Transplant* 2012, **27**:3615–3620.
31. Himmelfarb J, Phinney S, Ikizler TA, Kane J, McMonagle E, Miller G: **Gamma-tocopherol and docosahexaenoic acid decrease inflammation in dialysis patients.** *J Ren Nutr* 2007, **17**:296–304.
32. Eleftheriadis T, Kartsios C, Liakopoulos V, Antoniadi G, Ditsa M, Papadopoulos C, Anifandis G, Skirta A, Markala D, Stefanidis I: **Does hepcidin affect erythropoiesis in hemodialysis patients?** *Acta Haematol* 2006, **116**:238–244.
33. Malyszko J, Malyszko JS, Pawlak K, Drozdowska-Rams L, Brzosko S, Mysliwiec M: **Hepcidin is linked to anemia and inflammation in peritoneal dialysis patients.** *Perit Dial Int* 2008, **28**:418–421.
34. Ashby DR, Gale DP, Busbridge M, Murphy KG, Duncan ND, Cairns TD, Taube DH, Bloom SR, Tam FW, Chapman RS, *et al*: **Plasma hepcidin levels are elevated but responsive to erythropoietin therapy in renal disease.** *Kidney Int* 2009, **75**:976–981.
35. Bowden RG, Jitomir J, Wilson RL, Gentile M: **Effects of omega-3 fatty acid supplementation on lipid levels in endstage renal disease patients.** *J Ren Nutr* 2009, **19**:259–266.
36. Kooshki A, Taleban FA, Tabibi H, Hedayati M: **Effects of marine omega-3 fatty acids on serum systemic and vascular inflammation markers and oxidative stress in hemodialysis patients.** *Ann Nutr Metab* 2011, **58**:197–202.
37. Hassan KS, Hassan SK, Hijazi EG, Khazim KO: **Effects of omega-3 on lipid profile and inflammation markers in peritoneal dialysis patients.** *Ren Fail* 2010, **32**:1031–1035.
38. Poulia KA, Panagiotakos DB, Tourlede E, Rezou A, Stamatiadis D, Boletis J, Zampelas A: **Omega-3 fatty acids supplementation does not affect serum lipids in chronic hemodialysis patients.** *J Ren Nutr* 2011, **21**:479–484.
39. Nemeth E, Valore EV, Territo M, Schiller G, Lichtenstein A, Ganz T: **Hepcidin, a putative mediator of anemia of inflammation, is a type II acute-phase protein.** *Blood* 2003, **101**:2461–2463.
40. Kuragano T, Shimonaka Y, Kida A, Furuta M, Nanami M, Otaki Y, Hasuike Y, Nonoguchi H, Nakanishi T: **Determinants of hepcidin in patients on maintenance hemodialysis: role of inflammation.** *Am J Nephrol* 2010, **31**:534–540.
41. Ferrucci L, Semba RD, Guralnik JM, Ershler WB, Bandinelli S, Patel KV, Sun K, Woodman RC, Andrews NC, Cotter RJ, *et al*: **Proinflammatory state, hepcidin, and anemia in older persons.** *Blood* 2010, **115**:3810–3816.
42. Kato A, Tsuji T, Luo J, Sakao Y, Yasuda H, Hishida A: **Association of prohepcidin and hepcidin-25 with erythropoietin response and ferritin in hemodialysis patients.** *Am J Nephrol* 2008, **28**:115–121.
43. Price EA, Schrier SL: **Unexplained aspects of anemia of inflammation.** *Adv Hematol* 2010, **2010**:1–5.
44. Ravishankaran P, Karunanithi R: **Clinical significance of preoperative serum interleukin-6 and C-reactive protein level in breast cancer patients.** *World J Surg Oncol* 2011, **9**:1–6.
45. Rose WE, Eickhoff JC, Shukla SK, Pantrangi M, Rooijakkers S, Cosgrove SE, Nizet V, Sakoulas G: **Elevated serum interleukin-10 at time of hospital admission is predictive of mortality in patients with *Staphylococcus aureus* bacteremia.** *J Infect Dis* 2012, **206**:1604–1611.
46. Locatelli F, Andrulli S, Memoli B, Maffei C, Del Vecchio L, Aterini S, De Simone W, Mandalari A, Brunori G, Amato M, *et al*: **Nutritional-inflammation status and resistance to erythropoietin therapy in haemodialysis patients.** *Nephrol Dial Transplant* 2006, **21**:991–998.
47. Eleftheriadis T, Liakopoulos V, Antoniadi G, Kartsios C, Stefanidis I: **The role of hepcidin in iron homeostasis and anemia in hemodialysis patients.** *Semin Dial* 2009, **22**:70–77.

11

Comparative amino acid decomposition analysis of potent type I p38α inhibitors

Ahmad Ebadi[1,2], Nima Razzaghi-Asl[1,2], Mehdi Khoshneviszadeh[1] and Ramin Miri[1,2*]

Abstract

Background and purpose of the study: p38α is a member of mitogen-activated protein kinases (MAPK) considered as a prominent target in development of anti-inflammatory agents. Any abnormality in the phosphorylation process leads to the different human diseases such as cancer, diabetes and inflammatory diseases. Several small molecule p38α inhibitors have been developed up to now. In this regard, structural elucidation of p38 inhibitors needs to be done enabling us in rational lead development strategies.

Methods: Various interactions of three potent inhibitors with p38α active site have been evaluated in terms of binding energies and bond lengths via density function theory and MD simulations.

Results: Our comparative study showed that both *ab initio* and MD simulation led to the relatively similar results in pharmacophore discrimination of p38α inhibitors.

Conclusion: The results of the present study may find their usefulness in pharmacophore based modification of p38α inhibitors.

Keywords: p38α, Anti-inflammatory, Amino acid decomposition analysis, DFT, Molecular dynamic

Introduction

In the process of drug discovery, lead generation is a key bottleneck. The costly experimental testing of so many compounds leads to a real challenge in high throughput screening (HTS) method and makes it critical to perform virtual screening techniques to reduce the size of chemical collection richen in active compounds [1]. Computer based prescreening of chemical databases has found its key role in lead identification and is known as *in silico* drug design. Generally speaking, *in silico* drug design falls into four categories that are related to each other depending on the structural information on targets and their ligand. These methods are structure-based design, ligand-based design, combinatorial chemistry-based design and de novo design [2].

De novo design techniques are used in the case of known receptor structure and unknown ligand structure. One of the most efficient and rational methods to afford this challenge is fragment based drug design [3,4]. In fragment based drug design, binding of small molecule fragments ($MW < 300$, No. H-donors < 3, No. H-acceptors < 3, $ClogP < 3$) [5] to specific domain of active site is evaluated. Based on the binding energies, best fragments are selected and bridged together with appropriate linker(s) to generate new scaffolds. The reverse process, *i.e.* fragmentation of ligands to constructing fragments, can be used for modification of known ligands. By fragmentation, the chemical diversity of fragment database decreases and the chance of achievement to new lead compound increases. In this process, assessment of interaction between fragments and receptor is the rate limiting step. Estimating the contribution of individual amino acid-ligand interaction energies in total binding energy, *i.e.* Amino acid Decomposition Analysis (ADA) [6-8], would be a very useful trend in fragment development. ADA is based on receptor structure and could be applied to different types of scaffolds. The power of ADA in predicting the effect of individual residues on ligand-receptor interactions can be used as supporting information in drug design. In this regard, estimation of the optimum binding geometry could assist in choosing the best fragment(s) leading to the improved ligand potency profiles.

* Correspondence: mirir@sums.ac.ir
[1]Medicinal and Natural Products Chemistry Research Center, Shiraz University of Medical Sciences, PO Box 3288-71345, Shiraz, Iran
[2]Department of Medicinal Chemistry, School of Pharmacy, Shiraz University of Medical Sciences, PO Box 1583-71345, Shiraz, Iran

The phosphorylation of proteins by protein kinases, the largest family of signaling proteins, regulates cell life. More than 500 protein kinases are encoded by the human genome and it is no surprise that any abnormality in the phosphorylation process would lead to the different human diseases such as cancer, diabetes and inflammatory diseases. Different types of these regulating enzymes are introduced as therapeutic target. The active site conservation between protein kinases makes it a real challenge to design selective agents [9-12]. Therefore evaluation of structural features of these protein kinases and the role of fragments to achieve selectivity may be regarded as an important topic.

p38 belongs to the family of mitogen-activated protein kinases (MAPK). p38 MAPKs are generally divided to various isoforms including α, β, γ and δ types [13,14]. p38α and p38β are vital biological targets in inflammatory pathways [15]. MAP kinase kinase3 and 6 (MKK3, 6) are activated by inflammatory factors such as IL-1, TNFα and cell stress [16-18]. MKK3 and 6 are upstream kinases that phosphorylate the tyrosine and threonine residues in p38α and hence activate it [19]. The activated p38α stimulates the IL-1, TNFα and COX-2, enhances the transcription of inflammatory genes, and also has been found to stabilize the inflammatory response protein mRNAs [20,21].

Considering the important role in inflammatory pathways, p38 can be regarded as an attractive target to design and develop anti-inflammatory agents. Indeed, p38α is a distinguished target in development of anti-inflammatory agents. Different classes of p38α inhibitors have been developed up to now and their pharmacophore were evaluated in detail [22-27]. In the present contribution, we used MD simulations and *ab initio* method to evaluate pharmacophore model of three potent type I p38α inhibitors comprehensively. The results of both MD and *ab initio* methods were reported and compared with each other. Three different inhibitors, diarylimidazole [28], dihydroquinazolinone [29] and 2-arylpyridazin-3-one [30] scaffolds were selected for our study (Figure 1). These inhibitors are direct ATP-binding site inhibitors with sub-micromolar to nanomolar activity. **SB203580** inhibits p38α and β with almost similar potency. This compound is ~10 times selective towards p38α/β compared to p38γ/δ [31].

In the case of **SB203580**, crystallographic studies (PDB code 1A9u, resolution: 2.50 Å) demonstrated that pyridyl nitrogen formed a hydrogen bond with Met109 (Figure 2). Moreover; 4-fluorophenyl ring occupied the hydrophobic pocket adjacent to the Met109. These two types of interactions have been observed in most of the ATP-binding inhibitors [32]. Nitrogen atom of imidazole ring interacts with Lys53 via hydrogen bond and electrostatic forces. Electrostatic forces are long range interactions between ligand and receptor and have determinant effect on ultimate ligand-receptor complex stability.

For dihydroquinazolinone (PDB code: 1M7Q, resolution: 2.40 Å) and 2-arylpyridazin-3-one (PDB code: 2I0H, resolution: 2.00) scaffolds, the same pattern of binding in the p38α active site have been reported (Figure 2) [29,30]. Both of these inhibitors have a carbonyl moiety that interacts with Met109 and Gly110 backbone NH via hydrogen bonds. 2,4-diflourophenyl and 2-chloro-4-flouropheny moieties in dihydroquinazolinone and 2-arylpyridazin-3-one inhibitors occupied the hydrophobic pocket in the proximity of Met109. Dihydroquinazolinone scaffold has an additional hydrogen bond with His107 and 2-arylpyridazin-3-one has more hydrophobic interactions when compared with dihydroquinazolinone.

In this project we used *ab initio* method and MD simulations to pharmacophore modeling of these three potent inhibitors via ADA strategy. B3LYP functional [33] and BP86 functional [34] together supplemented with triple-ζ basis set (TZV) [35] were used with the aim of:

- Evaluation of ligand-p38α stability via molecular dynamic simulations
- ADA through MD simulations and *ab initio* method to detect hot spots in p38α active site
- Comparative evaluation of MD and *ab initio* results

Materials and methods

Preparation of data set

X-ray crystallographic structures of p38α with its cognate ligands were obtained from Brook Haven Protein databank (www.rcsb.org). The Swiss PDB Viewer program (http://www.expasy.org/spdbv) [36] was used to rebuilt and add missed atoms of Lys15 and Arg173 in 1M7Q and 2I0H PDB structures. The crystallographic *holo* structures were used as a starting point for MD simulations. The force field parameters of ligands were obtained using PRODRG, an automated topology generation tool web server [37]. The electrostatic potential (ESP) derived charges of ligands were all recalculated according to Breneman and Wiberg [38] by using B3LYP/TZV(2d,2p) method and were adjusted in topology file.

The evaluated amino acid residues were selected on the basis of information from schematic 2D representations of ligand-receptor interactions produced by LIGPLOT program [39].

In *ab initio* studies, all amino acids were considered in their real electrostatic state. Each residue under study was truncated at the C-terminal and N-terminal. N-terminal was acetylated and C-terminal was methyl amidated to mimic the original electron density profile. All conformational and configurational features were the same as the X-ray structure. Molecular images were produced using VMD program [40].

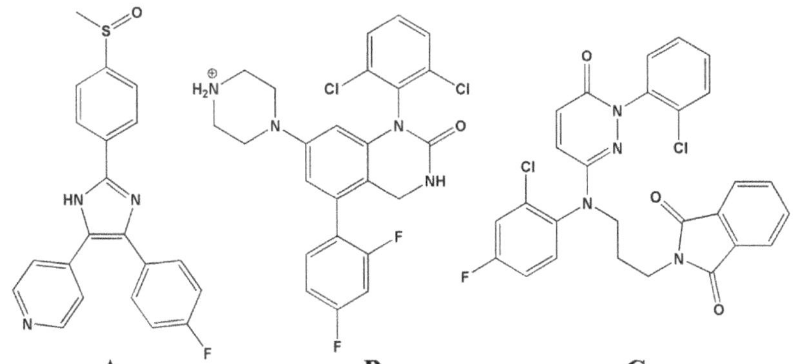

Figure 1 Structure of diarylimidazole (SB203580) IC_{50}: 4.8 nM (A), dihydroquinazolinone IC_{50}: 2.6 nM (B) and 2-arylpyridazin-3-one IC_{50}: 5 nM (C) p38α type I inhibitors.

Molecular dynamics simulations

Molecular dynamics simulations were carried out using GROMACS 4 package with the standard GROMOS96 force field [41]. In each case, the p38-ligand complex was solvated in a cubic box with the dimension of 95 × 95 × 95 (all in Å). Explicit simple point charge model (SPC216) was used to represent water molecules [42]. Na^+ atoms were added to neutralize the total charge of the systems. Short-range interactions were evaluated using a twin-rang cutoff with van der Waals and electrostatic interactions truncated at 12 and 10 Å, respectively. Particle mesh Ewald (PME) method was used to evaluate long-range electrostatic interactions. The protein-ligand complex and waters along with ions were coupled in a temperature bath at 300K, separately ($\tau_T = 0.1$ ps). Berendsen barostat ($\tau_P = 1$ ps) was used to maintain pressure in 1.0 atm [43,44]. Linear constraint solver (LINCS) was applied to constrain all bonds [45].

In the first step, energy minimization was performed using steepest descent integrator realized in GROMACS package. After energy minimization, 100 ps NVT and NPT ensembles were used to equilibrate system. During NVT and NPT ensembles a harmonic position restrain (1000 kJ mol^{-1} nm^{-1}) was applied to all the heavy atoms of the p38α and ligand. Following equilibration step, production of MD simulation was conducted for 20 ns without any constrains. Finally, analysis programs included in GROMACS package were used to evaluate trajectories.

Ab initio method

All calculations were performed on a structure that obtained by averaging over last 10 ns of MD simulations. Heavy atom-hydrogen bonds were optimized by using heavy atom fixing approximation (constrained optimizations). Constrained optimization was used to prevent irrational movement of the side chains. Otherwise the position of ligand and relevant residue could be changed drastically. Neese and Bykov evaluated optimization errors of this type [46]. According to their evaluation, obtained results are reliable. BP86 functional together in association with triple-ζ basis set (TZV) was used in optimization process. Resolution-of-identity (RI) approximation [47] together with fitting auxiliary basis set TZV/J [48] was applied for all atoms.

Energy calculations were done using B3LYP (Becke-Lee-Yang-Parr) functional in association with triple-ζ basis set (TZV) on optimized structures. For these calculations, chain-of-spheres (RIJCOSX) approximation [49] was invoked. Two set of first polarization functions were applied on hydrogen and non-hydrogen atoms [TZV(2d,2p)]. To consider long-range dielectric effect of protein in our calculation, COSMO model [50] with a dielectric constant of 4.8 was applied [51]. All calculations were done using the ORCA quantum chemistry package [52].

Ligand-residue binding energies (ΔE_b) were calculated using the previously introduced equation [53]. Counterpoise correction [54] was used to take into account basis set superposition error (BSSE). In the case of **SB203580**, Potential Energy Surface (PES) scan were performed in the direction of hydrogen bond with Met109 in forty steps considering 0.05Å step sizes. The PES calculations were performed by the same method and basis set as mentioned above.

Results and discussion

MD simulations

Crystallographic structure of p38α with its cognate ligands enabled us to perform MD simulations and evaluate the role of individual amino acids in total binding energy. This structure was used as starting conformation for our simulations. In the first step, we performed a 20 ns MD simulation to reach a stable trajectory.

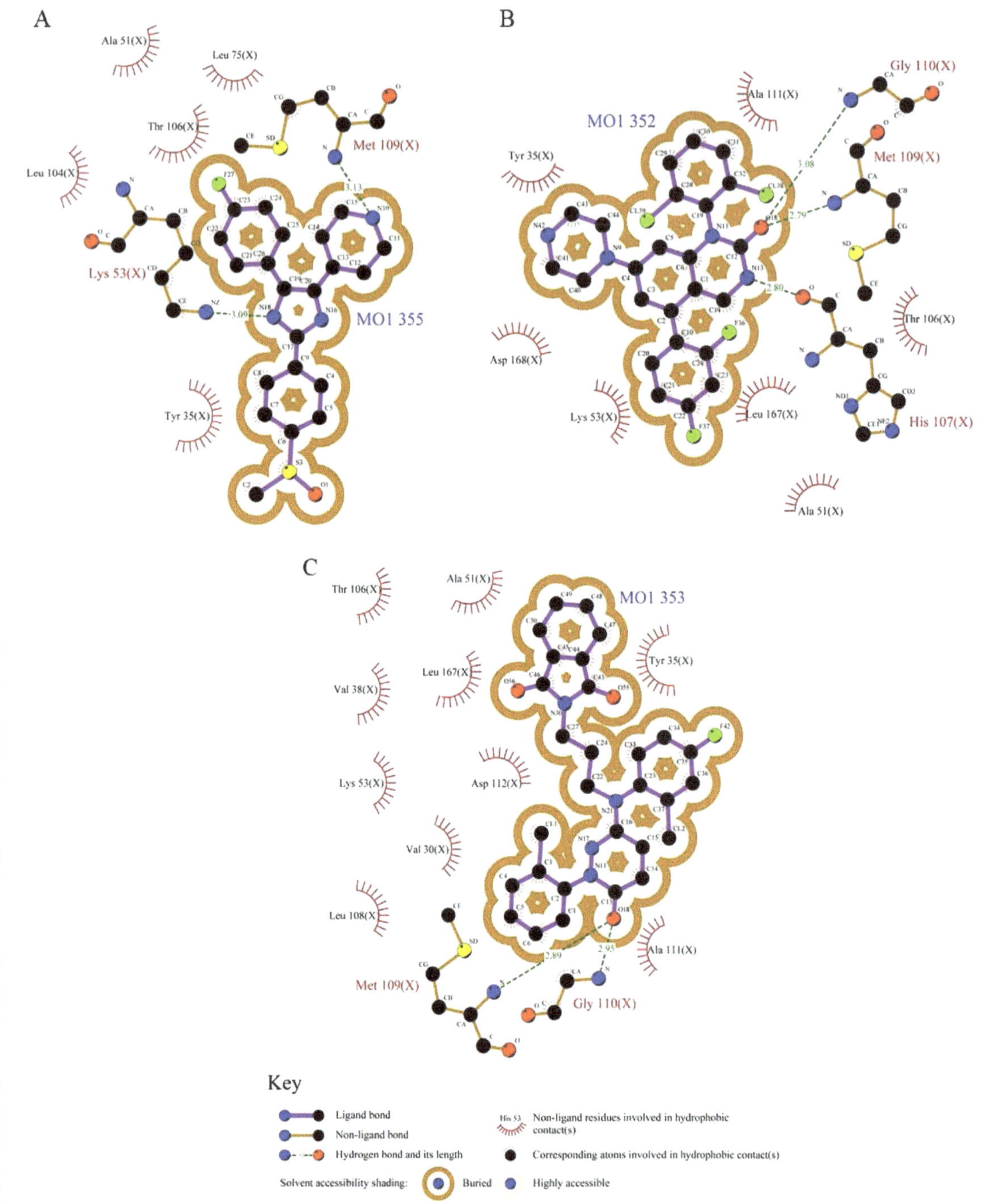

Figure 2 **2D schematic representation of interactions between SB203580 (A), dihydroquinazolinone (B) and 2-arylpyridazin-3-one (C) scaffolds and p38α active site generated by LIGPLOT.**

The stabilities of trajectories were confirmed by assessment of total energy, temperature and RMSD (Figures 3 and 4).

The Average temperature during 20 ns MD simulation at 300.0K was found to be 300K (±1.32, 1.34 and 1.33 respectively) for these systems (Figure 3). These results

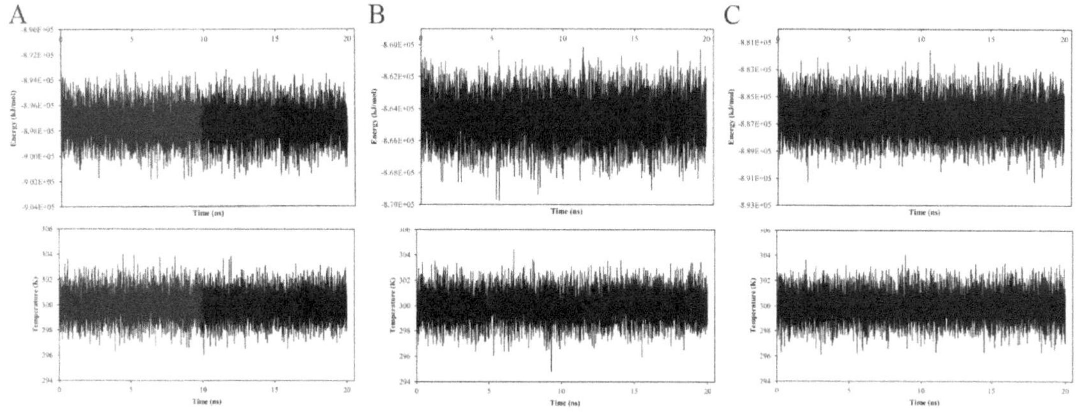

Figure 3 Total energy and temperature variations during 20 ns MD simulation; SB203580 (A), dihydroquinazolinone (B) and 2-arylpyridazin-3-one (C).

represented that the obtained equilibriums and energy conservations for the studied systems were desirable.

The RMSDs of ligands in the active site of p38α with respect to their initial structures were used to evaluate the stabilities of these three complexes.

In the case of **SB203580** (Figure 4A), RMSD rose up to 1.13 Å at the beginning of MD simulations and fluctuated around this value (± 0.15) for the rest of simulation. This distribution pattern demonstrated us that ligand achieved to the equilibrium state just after 1 ns distinguished by the RMSD profile. For dihydroquinazolinone scaffold (1M7Q), RMSD increased to 0.71 Å and leveled off to nearly 3 ns (Figure 4B). At this point of simulation, RMSD rose up again to 1 Å and leveled off (± 0.13). In the case of 2-arylpyridazin-3-one scaffold, RMSD increased to 0.76 Å and fluctuated around (± 0.16) over the course of MD simulation time (Figure 4C). These data showed that evaluated ligands reached to an equilibrium state after preliminary fluctuations.

During MD simulations the average of 1.2 H-bond(s) could be detected between **SB203580** and p38α active site residues (Figure 5A). The variation of donor-acceptor

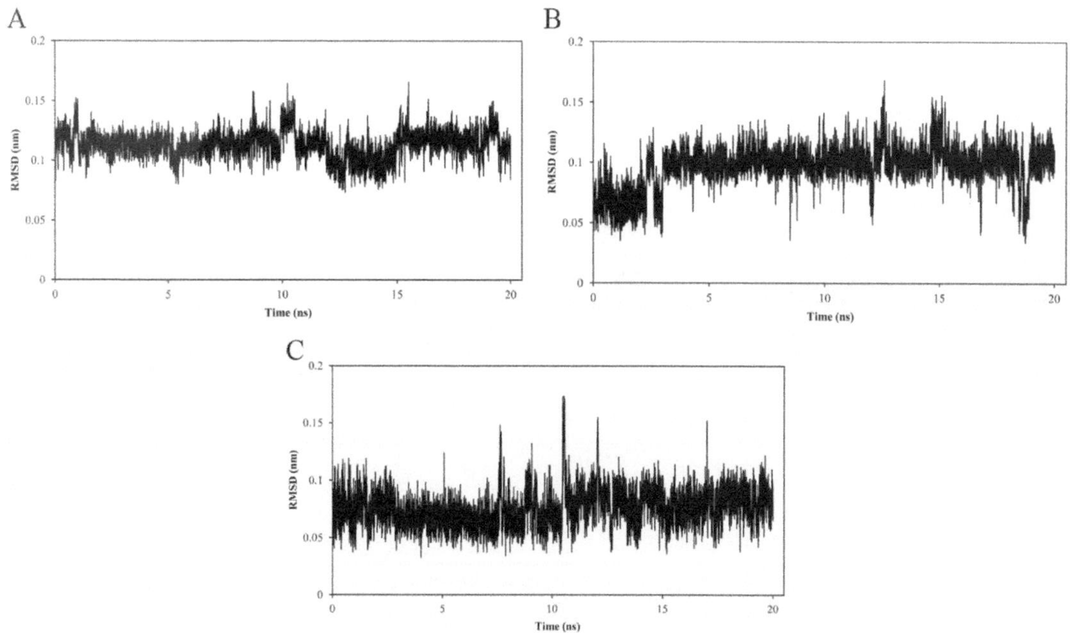

Figure 4 RMSD of ligand atoms; SB203580 (A), dihydroquinazolinone (B) and 2-arylpyridazin-3-one (C).

distance during MD simulation could be used to evaluate the forming and breaking of H-bonds. Over the whole process, the donor-acceptor distances less than 3.5 Å demonstrated hydrogen bond formation. As can be seen in Figure 5A, pyridine nitrogen-Met109 NH distance remained less than 3 Å for the whole simulation time (green). This fact could convince us in considering a permanent H-bond between these two moieties. But hydrogen bond between imidazole nitrogen and quaternary amine hydrogen of Lys53 was significantly less detectable. This hydrogen bond was formed and broken frequently during MD simulations (Figure 5A blue).

In the case of dihydroquinazolinone scaffold, an average of 1.5 H-bond(s) with p38α active site residues (Figure 5B) could be detected. Results showed that H-bond between Met109 NH and ligand O18 atoms (green) existed during whole MD simulation period. The distance between His107 O and ligand HN13 atoms remained less than 3.5 Å during MD simulation (blue). According to obtained results, these two hydrogen bonds are permanent during 20 ns MD simulations. The Gly110 NH-ligand O18 distance (red) fluctuated between 5 ns and 20 ns. However the averaged distance remained higher than 0.35 Å for 98.8% of the simulation period (Temporary H-bond, Table 1).

2-arylpyridazin-3-one scaffold formed an average of 1.2 H-bond(s) with Met109 and Gly110 during MD simulation (Figure 5C). In this case, the distance between Met109 NH and ligand O18 atoms was almost under 0.35 Å in the whole period (green). But the distance between Gly110 NH and ligand O18 atoms was higher than 0.35 Å in 49.5% of simulation period (blue). These outcomes showed that Met109-ligand and Gly110-ligand H-bonds were of permanent and temporary types, respectively.

On the basis of results (Table 1), it might be concluded that hydrogen bond between ligand and Met109 is the key structural point in binding to the receptor. This interaction is the common structural feature of all type I p38α inhibitors. More detailed analysis of H-bonds between p38α active site residues and evaluated ligands is summarized in Table 1.

After obtaining an equilibrium system, ADA was carried out as follow: participation of each amino acid in total binding energy was computed by evaluation of Lennard-Jones (LJ) and coulombic interaction energies between each amino acid and ligands via performing an additional 1 ns MD simulation in each case. The results of ADA are shown in Figure 6 and Table 2. Negative energy shifts showed that the residue made favorable contribution to ligand-receptor interactions.

LIGPLOT program [39] was used to detect residues that interact with ligand in each case. Based on the obtained data, same binding pattern to p38α active site could be detected in all the scaffolds. Interaction energies with hinge region residues (Met109, Gly110, and Ala111) are significant and in each case at least, there is one interaction with these amino acids. Residues constructing hydrophobic pocket in the proximity of Met109 were almost involved in interactions with ligand.

In **SB203580**, Lys53 was found to be the most significant residue in ligand-receptor interactions (ΔE: -5.77 kcal/mol). Nitrogen atom of an imidazole ring participated in H-bond with quaternary amine hydrogen of Lys53. In fact electrostatic forces between these groups made it a favorable interaction. Lys53 had maximum coulombic and LJ interaction energies in these series (−1.64 and −4.13 kcal/mol, respectively). Electrostatic interactions are important forces in primary approach of ligand and receptor to each other. These types of interactions are of long-range type

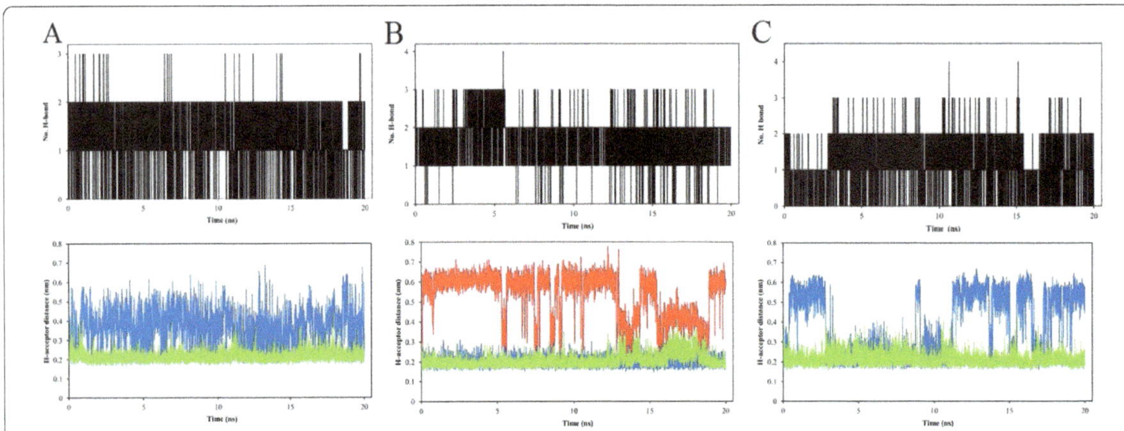

Figure 5 Number and distance of H-bonds between ligands and p38α active site residues; SB203580 (A), dihydroquinazolinone (B) and 2-arylpyridazin-3-one (C).

Table 1 Hydrogen bond analysis between evaluated ligands and p38α residues

System	Donor	Acceptor[1]	H-bond distance[2] (Å)	H-bond angle[3] (degree)	Occupancy (%)
1A9U	Met109 NH	Ligand N10	2.14 (± 0.24)	14.2 (± 8.78)	99.8
	Lys53 HZ	Ligand N18	3.66 (± 0.85)	58.5 (± 23.7)	39.7
1M7Q	Met109 NH	Ligand O18	2.06 (± 0.32)	14.4 (± 11.4)	99.8
	Gly110 NH	Ligand O18	5.30 (± 1.15)	55.1 (± 29.0)	11.2
	Ligand HN13	His107 O	1.98 (± 0.20)	14.4 (± 8.10)	100
2I0H	Met109 NH	Ligand O18	2.09 (± 0.28)	23.9 (± 14.8)	99.8
	Gly110 NH	Ligand O18	3.81 (± 1.58)	38.2 (± 28.5)	50.5

[1]Atom numbers are according to Figure 2.
[2]The average H-bond distance with standard deviation in parentheses.
[3]The average H-bond angle with standard deviation in parentheses.

and determinative in the final ligand-receptor complex stability. According to the obtained results, imidazole ring (interacting with Lys53) is a very important moiety in diarylimidazole based p38α inhibitors.

Met109 backbone hydrogen formed a hydrogen bond with pyridine nitrogen (ΔE: -4.61 kcal/mol). Hydrogen bond with hinge region residue (Met109) is the key feature of ATP binding site (type I) inhibitors and could be observed in all type I inhibitors. Accumulated negative charge on pyridine ring of **SB203580** formed a favorable interaction (hydrogen bond and electrostatic forces) with Met109.

Ala51, Leu75, Leu104 and Thr106 contributed to important hydrophobic contacts in the hydrophobic pocket (ΔE: -2.76, -0.87, -2.83 and −2.34 kcal/mol, respectively). These hydrophobic interactions had minimum coulombic interaction energies (Table 2). Due to the reported pharmacophore models of diverse classes of p38 MAPK [22], interactions with Met109 and this hydrophobic pocket are the chemical features designated for type I p38α inhibitors. Tyr35 participated in π-π stacking interaction with *para*-methylsulfinyl phenyl ring of **SB203580** (ΔE: -3.59 kcal/mol).

In the case of dihydroquinazolinone scaffold (1M7Q), His107 (−4.28 kcal/mol), Met109 (−4.24 kcal/mol), Gly110 (−4.72 kcal/mol) and Asp168 (−4.86 kcal/mol) residues had maximum binding energies. His107, Met109 and

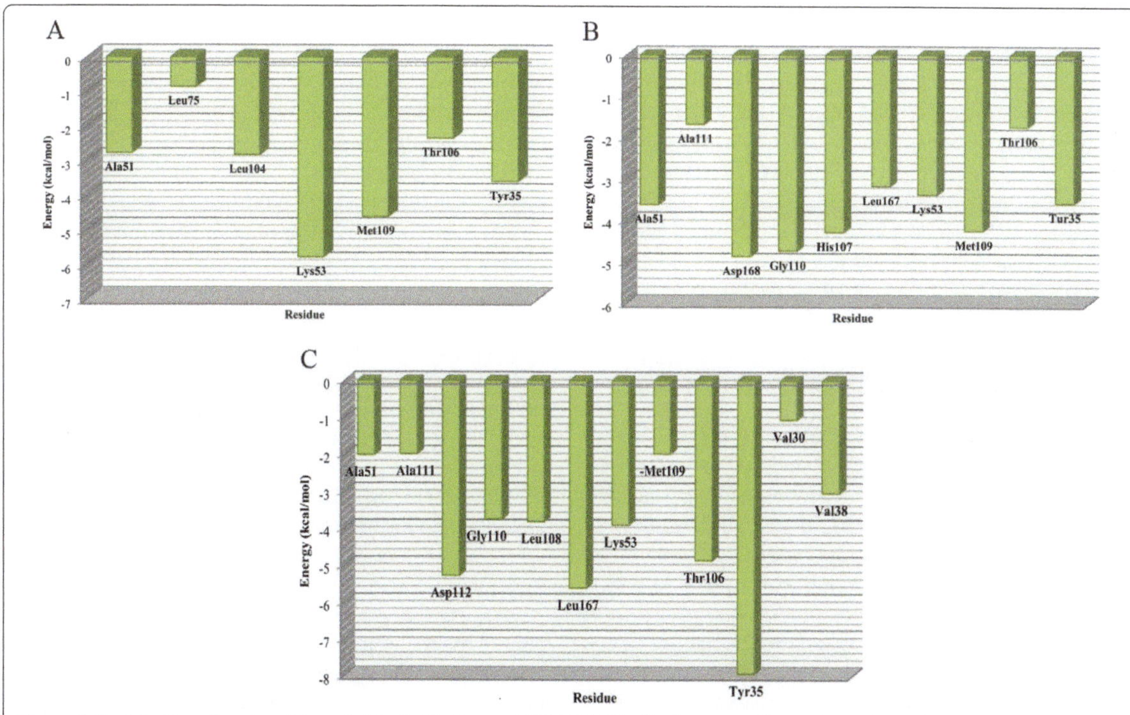

Figure 6 Contribution of each residue of p38α in binding to SB203580 (A), dihydroquinazolinone (B) and 2-arylpyridazin-3-one (C) scaffolds (calculated by MD simulations).

Table 2 LJ and coulombic interaction energies (kcal/mol) between p38α active site residues and evaluated ligands

1A9U			1M7Q			2IOH		
Residue	Coul	LJ	Residue	Coul	LJ	Residue	Coul	LJ
Ala51	−0.23	−2.53	Ala51	−0.39	−3.21	Ala51	−0.05	−1.95
Leu75	0.00	−0.87	Ala111	0.11	−1.79	Ala111	0.08	−2.06
Leu104	−0.48	−2.35	Asp168	−3.56	−1.30	Asp112	−1.61	−3.66
Lys53	−1.64	−4.13	Gly110	−2.09	−2.63	Gly110	−1.31	−2.44
Met109	−2.87	−1.74	His107	−3.56	−0.72	Leu108	−0.32	−3.49
Thr106	0.10	−2.44	Leu167	0.00	−3.15	Leu167	0.01	−5.62
Tyr35	0.11	−3.70	Lys53	0.69	−4.04	Lys53	0.21	−4.11
			Met109	−2.23	−2.01	Met109	−0.58	−1.39
			Thr106	0.12	−1.85	Thr106	−1.48	−3.37
			Tyr35	−1.15	−2.41	Tyr35	−0.07	−7.86
						Val30	0.01	−1.06
						Val38	0.00	−3.04

Gly110 interact via hydrogen binding and Asp168 interact via electrostatic interactions (maximum coulombic interaction −3.56 kcal/mol). Lys53 had minimum coulombic interaction energy (0.69 kcal/mol) due to nearness of Lys53 quaternary amine to positive N42 atom in this ligand.

2-arylpyridazin-3-one scaffold (2IOH) had maximum biding energy with Tyr35. Our model indicated that Isoindoline-1,3-dione ring interacted with Tyr35 via π-π stacking. This interaction was associated with maximum LJ interaction energy (−7.86 kcal/mol). Met109 (−1.97 kcal/mol) and Gly110 (−3.75 kcal/mol) backbone NHs interacted with ligand O18 atom via H-bond. This ligand had more hydrophobic interactions in comparison with previous ones. LJ and coulombic interaction energies in each case were summarized in Table 2.

By using ADA we could model the binding mode of three different p38α inhibitors. Obtained results were in good agreement with evaluated pharmacophore models in the literature [22].

Ab initio evaluation

In this part we used *ab initio* method to evaluate contribution of individual amino acid-ligand interaction energies in total binding energy and compare obtaining results with MD simulations.

The constrained optimization process was done using BP86/TZV method on a structure which was obtained by averaging over last 10 ns MD simulations. All *ab initio* studies were done on achieved optimized structure.

Various interaction energies between studied p38α inhibitors and selected residues in the active site were obtained independently. The relevant data are shown in Figure 7.

Interactions between imidazole nitrogen and quaternary amine of Lys53 in **SB203580** had the most considerable interaction energy (−4.66 kcal/mol) (Figure 7A). This strong interaction occurred as a result of electrostatic forces between positive nitrogen (cationic Lys53, atomic partial charge: +0.51) and partially negative imidazole N1 atom (atomic partial charge: -0.62). This ionic dipole interaction had determinant participation in total ligand-receptor binding energy.

Another important interaction could be recorded between Met109 and pyridine nitrogen (−2.30 kcal/mol). Interestingly, residues participated in hydrophobic interactions exhibited repulsive interaction with evaluated inhibitor. In the case of Tyr35, the repulsive interaction may be interpreted on the basis of inappropriate orientation of ligand *para*-methylsulfinyl phenyl ring versus Tyr35 phenyl ring. It should be noted, p38α inhibitors lacking this moiety might not have any significant effect on ligand potency [28].

Asp168 carboxylic moiety interacts via electrostatic forces with quaternary amine in dihydroquinazolinone ligand. This major interaction had prominent binding energy in this series of residues. Hydrogen bond between Met109 backbone NH and ligand O18 atom had binding energy equal to −8.78 kcal/mol. Negative binding energies could be detected between His107 backbone NH and HN18 (−6.34 kcal/mol), Gly110 backbone NH and ligand O18 atom (−4.16 kcal/mol) but like the other ones all hydrophobic interactions had positive contribution in binding energy. Proximity of Lys53 and ligand quaternary amines made this interaction inefficient.

In the case of 2-arylpyridazin-3-one scaffold, Cation-π interaction could be detected between Lys53 and 4-flouro-2-methilphenyl moiety. This interaction had maximum binding energy. Hydrogen binding could be

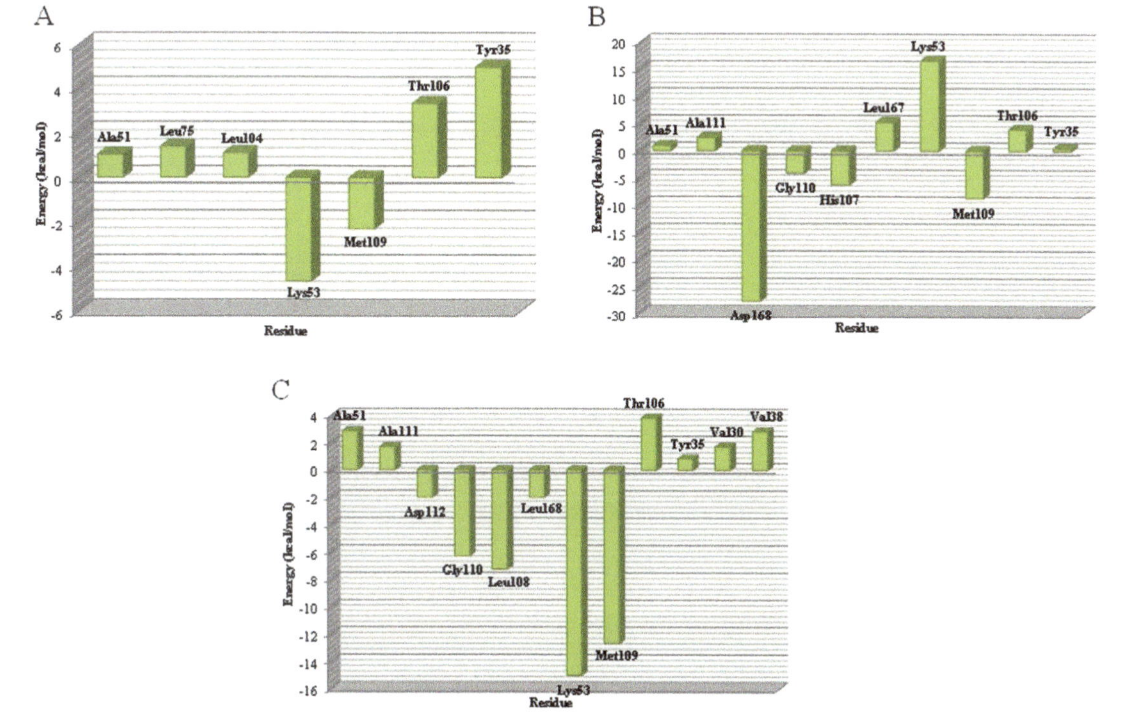

Figure 7 Contribution of each residue of p38α in binding to SB203580 (A), dihydroquinazolinone (B) and 2-arylpyridazin-3-one (C) scaffolds (calculated by *ab initio*).

detected between Met109 and Gly110 backbones NH and ligand O18 atom (−12.66 and −6.27 kcal/mol, respectively).

Owing to the important role of hydrogen bond with Met109 in type I inhibitors, we decided to optimize the geometric position of the involving functional group in the **SB203580** ligand. For this purpose, hydrogen bond distance between Met109 backbone hydrogen and pyridyl nitrogen in **SB203580** was scanned in the original direction. The maximum interaction energy was found in the 2.25 Å bond length (data was not shown). The optimum distance between pyridine nitrogen and Met109 backbone hydrogen after 20 ns MD simulation was calculated to be 2.14 Å. These findings interestingly showed that *ab initio* method and MD simulations converged to the same results. Moreover, it was demonstrated that crystallographic structures may not be appropriate starting points for *ab initio* calculations in all cases.

Comparison of the two methods

MD simulations and *ab initio* methods were used to calculate the involvement of each amino acid in total binding energy. The results of applied methods were compared to reveal the accuracy and efficiency levels. Our calculations revealed that MD simulations and *ab initio* based studies led to the similar trends in estimation of amino acid-ligand binding energies. In both methods residues responsible for major interactions in the p38α active site could be recognized with adaptable level of reproducibility (Figures 6 and 7).

For p38α active site, *ab initio* method resulted in more repulsive hydrophobic and more attractive electrostatic interactions when compared to MD simulations (Figure 8). This effect seemed to be probably related to the solvent effect and also interactions among adjacent residues. Moreover B3LYP method tended to produce more polarized wave function in electrostatic interactions [55] leading to false positive values.

For instance in p38α, Lys53 interacted with Asp168 and this electrostatic interaction decreased the attractive interaction between Lys53 and **SB203580** in MD simulations. But in *ab initio* study, just the interaction between Lys53 (truncated at N-terminal and C-terminal) and ligand was considered. Similar binding patterns for nearly all residues could be detected while in the case of charge-assisted interactions (Lys53, Asp168), significant deviations were seen (Figure 8). However, relatively similar

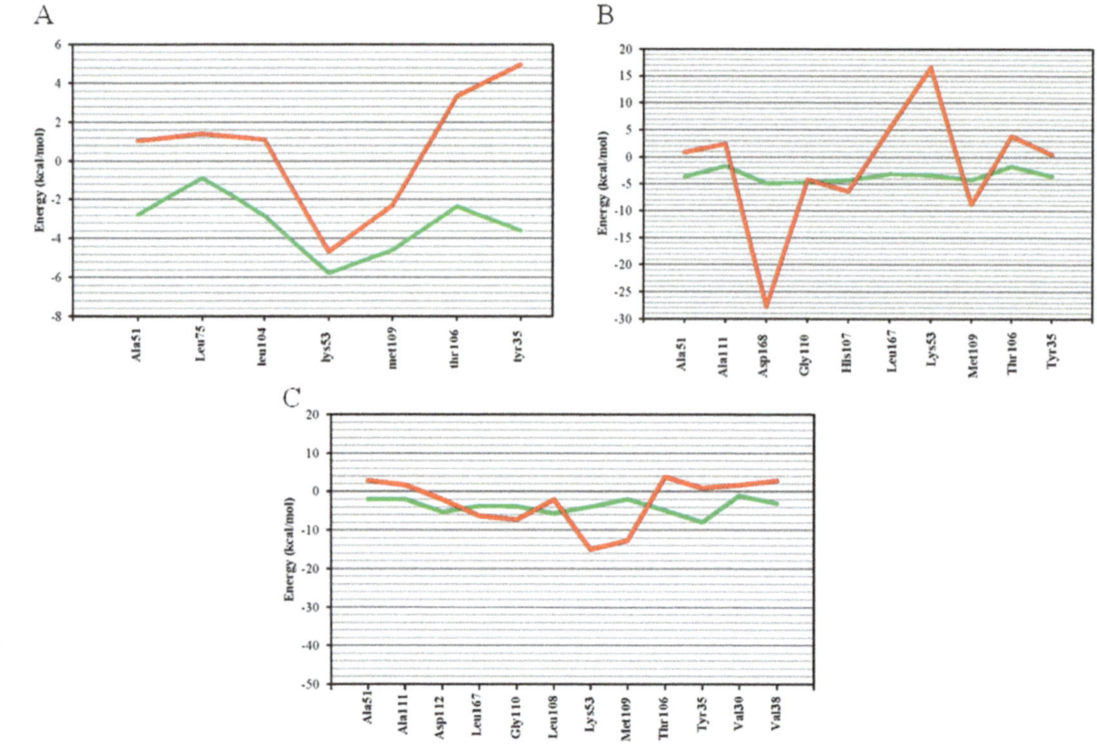

Figure 8 Comparative results of MD simulations (green) and *ab initio* studies (red) in SB203580 (A), dihydroquinazolinone (B) and 2-arylpyridazin-3-one (C) scaffolds.

binding energies were estimated for Lys53 in **SB203580**. Two rationales might be envisaged for this different trend:

- Solvent effects were attended in MD simulations while *ab initio* studies were performed in vacuum
- In SB203580, Lys53 interacted with partially negative imidazole sp^2 nitrogen atom
- Probable repulsive forces between dihydroquinazolinone piperazinium and Lys53 quaternary amine
- 2-arylpyridazin-3-one scaffold contributed in cation-π interaction with Lys53

Conclusion

We applied totally 60 ns MD simulations and *ab initio* method to evaluate and compare the accuracy of these methods in predicting pharmacophore models of three different p38α MAPK inhibitors. Both methodologies were able to unravel key interactions with different p38α inhibitors. One advantageous feature of DFT-based calculations is their relatively adaptable outputs regarding significantly shorter processing times due to the incorporated approximations. Results indicated that LJ interactions contributed significantly to binding of **SB203580**, dihydroquinazolinone and 2-arylpyridazin-3-one scaffolds despite the important role of electrostatic interactions in initial approach of ligands to the receptor. We used enzyme structure that was obtained by averaging over last 10 ns of MD simulations for our *ab initio* studies. This technique led to the results indicating that crystallographic primary structures may be used with care in such calculations. Further investigations would be required to rule out widespread structure activity relationships of p38α inhibitory activity. Finally the results of the present study may find their usefulness in pharmacophore based modification of p38α inhibitors.

Competing interests

The authors declare that they have no competing interests.

Authors' contributions

AE: Molecular Dynamics, NR-A: ab Initio, MK: ab Initio, RM: Molecular Dynamic, ab Initio, All authors read and approved the final manuscript.

Acknowledgements

Financial supports of this project by research council of Shiraz University of Medical Sciences are acknowledged.

References

1. Leach AR, Hann MM: **The in silico world of virtual libraries.** *Drug Discov Today* 2000, **5**:326–336.
2. Foye WO, Lemke TL, Williams DA: *Foye's principles of medicinal chemistry.* Lippincott Williams & Wilkins; 2007.
3. Warr WA: **Fragment-based drug discovery.** *J Comput Aided Mol Des* 2009, **23**:453–458.
4. Erlanson DA, McDowell RS, O'Brien T: **Fragment-based drug discovery.** *J Med Chem* 2004, **47**:3463–3482.
5. Congreve M, Carr R, Murray C, Jhoti H: **A'rule of three'for fragment-based lead discovery?** *Drug Discov Today* 2003, **8**:876.
6. Hensen C, Hermann JC, Nam K, Ma S, Gao J, Höltje HD: **A combined QM/MM approach to protein-ligand interactions: polarization effects of the HIV-1 protease on selected high affinity inhibitors.** *J Med Chem* 2004, **47**:6673–6680.
7. Thangapandian S, John S, Lee KW: **Molecular Dynamics Simulation Study Explaining Inhibitor Selectivity in Different Class of Histone Deacetylases.** *J Biomol Struct Dyn* 2012, **29**:677–698.
8. de Brito MA, Rodrigues CR, Cirino JJV, Araújo JQ, Honório T, Cabral LM, de Alencastro RB, Castro HC, Albuquerque MG: **Residue-Ligand Interaction Energy (ReLIE) on a Receptor-Dependent 3D-QSAR Analysis of S-and NH-DABOs as Non-Nucleoside Reverse Transcriptase Inhibitors.** *Molecules* 2012, **17**:7666–7694.
9. Noble MEM, Endicott JA, Johnson LN: **Protein kinase inhibitors: insights into drug design from structure.** *Science Signalling* 1800, **2004**:303.
10. Weinmann H, Metternich R: **Editorial: drug discovery process for kinease inhibitors.** *ChemBioChem* 2005, **6**:455–459.
11. Davies SP, Reddy H, Caivano M, Cohen P: **Specificity and mechanism of action of some commonly used protein kinase inhibitors.** *Biochem J* 2000, **351**:95.
12. Bain J, McLauchlan H, Elliott M, Cohen P: **The specificities of protein kinase inhibitors: an update.** *Biochem J* 2003, **371**:199.
13. Saklatvala J: **The p38 MAP kinase pathway as a therapeutic target in inflammatory disease.** *Curr Opinin Pharmacol* 2004, **4**:372–377.
14. Chen Z, Gibson TB, Robinson F, Silvestro L, Pearson G, Xu B, Wright A, Vanderbilt C, Cobb MH: **MAP kinases.** *Chem Rev* 2001, **101**:2449–2476.
15. Hale KKTD, Rihanek M, Manthey CL: **Differential expression and activation of p38 mitogen-activated protein kinase alpha, beta, gamma, and delta in inflammatory cell lineages.** *J Immunol* 1999, **162**:4246–4252.
16. Han J, Lee JD, Jiang Y, Li Z, Feng L, Ulevitch RJ: **Characterization of the structure and function of a novel MAP kinase kinase (MKK6).** *J Biol Chem* 1996, **271**:2886–2891.
17. Derijard B, Raingeaud J, Barrett T, Wu IH, Han J, Ulevitch RJ, Davis RJ: **Independent human MAP-kinase signal transduction pathways defined by MEK and MKK isoforms.** *Science* 1995, **267**:682–685.
18. Schieven GL: **The p38 kinase plays a central role in inflammation.** *Curr Top Med Chem* 2009, **9**:1038–1048.
19. Enslen H, Raingeaud J, Davis RJ: **Selective activation of p38 mitogen-activated protein (MAP) kinase isoforms by the MAP kinase kinases MKK3 and MKK6.** *J Biol Chem* 1998, **273**:1741–1748.
20. Kracht M, Saklatvala J: **Transcriptional and post-transcriptional control of gene expression in inflammation.** *Cytokine* 2002, **20**:91–106.
21. Clark AR, Dean JLE, Saklatvala J: **Post-transcriptional regulation of gene expression by mitogen-activated protein kinase p38.** *FEBS Lett* 2003, **546**:37–44.
22. Sarma R, Sinha S, Ravikumar M, Kishore Kumar M, Mahmood S: **Pharmacophore modeling of diverse classes of p38 MAP kinase inhibitors.** *Eur J Med Chem* 2008, **43**:2870–2876.
23. Wrobleski ST, Doweyko AM: **Structural comparison of p38 inhibitor-protein complexes: a review of recent p38 inhibitors having unique binding interactions.** *Curr Top Med Chem* 2005, **5**:1005–1016.
24. Karcher SC, Laufer SA: **Successful structure-based design of recent p38 MAP kinase inhibitors.** *Curr Top Med Chem* 2009, **9**:655–676.
25. Pettus LH, Wurz RP: **Small molecule p38 MAP kinase inhibitors for the treatment of inflammatory diseases: novel structures and developments during 2006–2008.** *Curr Top Med Chem* 2008, **8**:1452–1467.
26. Hynes J, Leftheris K: **Small molecule p38 inhibitors: novel structural features and advances from 2002–2005.** *Curr Top Med Chem* 2005, **5**:967–985.
27. Bolos J: **Structure-activity relationships of p38 mitogen-activated protein kinase inhibitors.** *Mini Rev Med Chem* 2005, **5**:857–868.
28. Wang Z, Canagarajah BJ, Boehm JC, Kassis S, Cobb MH, Young PR, Abdel-Meguid S, Adams JL, Goldsmith EJ: **Structural basis of inhibitor selectivity in MAP kinases.** *Structure* 1998, **6**:1117–1128.
29. Stelmach JE, Liu L, Patel SB, Pivnichny JV, Scapin G, Singh S, Hop CECA, Wang Z, Strauss JR, Cameron PM: **Design and synthesis of potent, orally bioavailable dihydroquinazolinone inhibitors of p38 MAP kinase.** *Bioorg Med Chem Lett* 2003, **13**:277–280.
30. Natarajan SR, Heller ST, Nam K, Singh SB, Scapin G, Patel S, Thompson JE, Fitzgerald CE, O'Keefe SJ: **p38 MAP kinase inhibitors. Part 6: 2-Arylpyridazin-3-ones as templates for inhibitor design.** *Bioorg Med Chem Lett* 2006, **16**:5809–5813.
31. Bain J, Plater L, Elliott M, Shpiro N, Hastie CJ, Mclauchlan H, Klevernic I, Arthur JSC, Alessi DR, Cohen P: **The selectivity of protein kinase inhibitors: a further update.** *Biochem J* 2007, **408**:297.
32. Wagner G, Laufer S: **Small molecular anti cytokine agents.** *Med Res Rev* 2006, **26**:1–62.
33. Becke AD: **A new mixing of Hartree–Fock and local density-functional theories.** *J Chem Phys* 1993, **98**:1372.
34. Becke AD: **Density functional calculations of molecular bond energies.** *J Chem Phys* 1986, **84**:4524.
35. The TurboMole basis sets can be obtained from: [ftp.chemie.uni--karlsruhe.de/pub in the directories basen jac].
36. Guex N, Peitsch MC: **SWISS-MODEL and the Swiss-Pdb Viewer: an environment for comparative protein modeling.** *Electrophoresis* 1997, **18**:2714–2723.
37. Aalten DMF, Bywater R, Findlay J, Hendlich M, Hooft R, Vriend G: **PRODRG, a program for generating molecular topologies and unique molecular descriptors from coordinates of small molecules.** *J Comput Aided Mol Des* 1996, **10**:255–262.
38. Breneman CM, Wiberg KB: **Determining atom-centered monopoles from molecular electrostatic potentials. The need for high sampling density in formamide conformational analysis.** *J Comput Chem* 1990, **11**:361–373.
39. Wallace AC, Laskowski RA, Thornton JM: **Ligplot—a program to generate schematic diagrams of protein ligand interactions.** *Protein Eng* 1995, **8**:127–134.
40. Humphrey W, Dalke A, Schulten K: **VMD: visual molecular dynamics.** *J Mol Graphics* 1996, **14**:33.
41. Van Der Spoel D, Lindahl E, Hess B, Groenhof G, Mark AE, Berendsen HJC: **GROMACS: fast, flexible, and free.** *J Comput Chem* 2005, **26**:1701–1718.
42. Rivail L, Chipot C, Maigret B, Bestel I, Sicsic S, Tarek M: **Large-scale molecular dynamics of a G protein-coupled receptor, the human 5-HT < sub > 4</sub > serotonin receptor, in a lipid bilayer.** *J Mol Struct (THEOCHEM)* 2007, **817**:19–26.
43. Bussi G, Donadio D, Parrinello M: **Canonical sampling through velocity-rescaling.** *arXiv preprint arXiv:08034060* 2008.
44. Berendsen HJC, Postma JPM, van Gunsteren WF, DiNola A, Haak J: **Molecular dynamics with coupling to an external bath.** *J Chem Phys* 1984, **81**:3684–3690.
45. Hess B, Bekker H, Berendsen HJC, Fraaije JGEM: **LINCS: a linear constraint solver for molecular simulations.** *J Comput Chem* 1997, **18**:1463–1472.
46. Bykov D, Neese F: **Substrate binding and activation in the active site of cytochrome c nitrite reductase: a density functional study.** *J Biol Inorg Chem* 2011, **16**:417–430.
47. Neese F: **An improvement of the resolution of the identity approximation for the formation of the Coulomb matrix.** *J Comput Chem* 2003, **24**:1740–1747.
48. Eichkorn K, Treutler O, Öhm H, Häser M, Ahlrichs R: **Auxiliary basis sets to approximate Coulomb potentials.** *Chem Phys Lett* 1995, **240**:283–290.
49. Neese F, Wennmohs F, Hansen A, Becker U: **Efficient, approximate and parallel Hartree–Fock and hybrid DFT calculations. A 'chain-of-spheres' algorithm for the Hartree–Fock exchange.** *Chem Phys* 2009, **356**:98–109.
50. Klamt A, Schüürmann G: **COSMO: a new approach to dielectric screening in solvents with explicit expressions for the screening energy and its gradient.** *J Chem Soc Perkin Trans 2* 1993, **5**:799–805.
51. Bykov D, Neese F: **Reductive activation of the heme iron-nitrosyl intermediate in the reaction mechanism of cytochrome c nitrite reductase: a theoretical study.** *J Biol Inorg Chem* 2012, **17**:1–20.
52. Neese F: *ORCA – an ab initio, Density Functional and Semiempirical program package, Version 2.8.0.* University of Bonn; 2011.

53. Razzaghi-Asl N, Ebadi A, Edraki N, Shahabipour S, Miri R: ***Ab initio* modeling of a potent isophthalamide-based BACE-1 inhibitor: amino acid decomposition analysis.** *Med Chem Res* 2013, **22**:3259–3269.
54. Boys S, Bernardi F: **The calculation of small molecular interactions by the differences of separate total energies. Some procedures with reduced errors.** *Mol Phys* 1970, **19**:553–566.
55. Cramer CJ: *Essentials of computational chemistry: theories and models.* Wiley; 2005.

12

Tacrolimus ameliorates functional disturbances and oxidative stress in isoproterenol-induced myocardial infarction

Arash Khorrami[1,2], Mojtaba Hammami[2], Mehraveh Garjani[2], Nasrin Maleki-Dizaji[1] and Alireza Garjani[1*]

Abstract

Background: The inflammatory responses play a major role in the pathogenesis of acute myocardial infarction (MI). Early inhibition of inflammation may improve post MI cardiac function. The aim of this study was to investigate the effects of tacrolimus on cardiac function, hemodynamic parameters as well as histopathologic and electrocardiographic changes in isoproterenol-induced myocardial infarction.

Methods: Male Wistar rats were randomly divided into six groups of control, isoproterenol alone, tacrolimus alone, and isoproterenol plus tacrolimus (0.5, 1 and 2 mg/kg). Isoproterenol (100 mg/kg) was injected subcutaneously for two consecutive days to induce myocardial infarction, and simultaneously tacrolimus was administered orally twice a day for three days.

Results and conclusions: Administration of isoproterenol resulted in myocardial edema and necrosis as well as a marked reduction in the left ventricular systolic pressure (LVSP), left ventricular contractility ($LVdP/dt_{max}$) and relaxation ($LVdP/dt_{min}$) along with a severe elevation in left ventricular end-diastolic pressure (LVEDP). Isoproterenol also elevated the ST-segment and suppressed the R-amplitude and R-R interval on ECG. It was found that all doses of tacrolimus could amend the ECG pattern and ameliorated the isoproterenol induced disturbances in cardiac function. Acute and short term treatment with tacrolimus at dose of 2 mg/kg significantly ($P < 0.001$) improved $LVdP/dt_{max}$ from 2712 ± 82 in myocardial infarcted rats to 4592 ± 149 mmHg/sec. Similarly, tacrolimus lowered LVEDP from 17.6 ± 0.68 in MI group to the value of 5.6 ± 0.22 mmHg ($P < 0.001$). Furthermore, tacrolimus was found to reduce malondialdehyde concentration in serum and myocardium by 50-70% ($P < 0.001$).
The results of this study showed that acute treatment with tacrolimus, coincided with the occurrence of myocardial infarction, strongly protected the myocardium against the isoproterenol-induced myocardial infarction; where this might be due to the anti-inflammatory properties of tacrolimus.

Keywords: Tacrolimus, Myocardial infarction, Isoproterenol, Electrocardiography

Background

Cardiovascular disease (CVD), predominantly myocardial infarction, is the leading cause of death worldwide [1,2]. Reductions in the myocardial blood flow due to the coronary artery occlusion can considerably compromise the energy metabolism. Coronary artery occlusion, only as short as 5 minutes, can lead to oxidative stress and then functional abnormalities of the myocardium that persist up to 24–48 hours after reperfusion [3-5].

The existing therapeutic approaches are designed to reduce the myocardial necrosis and also amendment of cardiac function after a myocardial infarction. Several studies have shown that consecutive vigorous inflammatory and immune reactions increases the generation of cytokines and oxidative stress, recruits inflammatory and T cells, and initiates the complement cascade [6,7]. The inflammatory responses induced by myocardial ischemia play a major role in the pathogenesis of acute myocardial infarction (AMI). In addition, recent studies have demonstrated that myocardial necrosis and subsequent oxidative stress trigger a cytokine cascade initiated by Tumor Necrosis Factor (TNF)-α. These inflammatory responses

* Correspondence: garjania2002@yahoo.com
[1]Department of Pharmacology and Toxicology, Faculty of Pharmacy, Tabriz University of Medical Sciences, Tabriz, Iran
Full list of author information is available at the end of the article

are found to exacerbate myocardial injury and remodeling after AMI [1,6,8], which lead to a progressive and irreversible myocardial damage. One of the principal interventions that exist for AMI is early inhibition of the inflammatory cycle and thus achieves a better recovery of the myocardium.

Tacrolimus (FK506) is a macrolide produced by the bacteria *Streptomyces tsukubaensis*. It is an immunosuppressant mainly used in organ transplantation in order to reduce the risk of graft rejection. Activation of T cells by allogenic antigens in transplanted tissue increases intracellular calcium concentration that contributes to the calcium-calmodulin complex formation. Calcium-calmodulin complex, in turn, activates calcineurin, a crucial phosphatase for T cell signaling [9,10]. Tacrolimus binding to the FK506 binding protein (FKBP), a respective cytoplasmic receptor, inactivates calcineurin, thereby the inflammatory response. FKBP is present in most tissues, including the myocardium. In addition to the anti-inflammatory effects of FK506-FKBP complex, it plays a critical role in modulating myocardial calcium homeostasis and rhythm regulation by stabilizing Ryanodine receptors [7,11]. The complex of FK506-FKBP inhibits the phosphatase activity of calcineurin and the calcium-dependent inflammatory responses. Moreover, some experimental studies have revealed that tacrolimus can effectively inhibit MAPK and PI3K-Akt signaling pathways in various inflammatory diseases [7].

Isoproterenol (ISO) is a synthetic beta-adernoceptor agonist and its subcutaneous injection induces irreversible cellular damage and ultimately myocardial infarction in rats. The acute hemodynamic and electrocardiographic changes in isoproterenol induced myocardial infarction resemble closely to those occurring in patients with myocardial infarction [12]. Therefore, the rat model of isoproterenol induced myocardial infarction offers a reliable non-invasive technique for studying the effects of various potentially cardioprotective agents [13].

The aim of the present study was to investigate the potential cardioprotective effects of tacrolimus on acute heart remodeling, hemodynamic, electrocardiographic, and biochemical changes in isoproterenol-induced myocardial infarction in rats.

Materials and methods

Animals

Male albino Wistar rats weighing between 260 and 280 g were used in the present study. The animals were housed in standard polypropylene cages (six per cage) under a 12/12 h light/dark cycle at a constant temperature of 20 ± 1.8°C and ambient humidity of 50 ± 10%. The rats were given food and water freely. This study was performed in accordance with the Guide for the Care and Use of Laboratory Animals of Tabriz University of Medical Sciences, Tabriz-Iran (National Institutes of Health publication No 85–23, revised 1985).

Induction of acute myocardial infarction

Isoproterenol (Sigma Co; USA) was dissolved in normal saline and injected subcutaneously to rats (100 mg/kg) for two consecutive days at an interval of 24 hours to induce acute myocardial infarction. Animals were sacrificed 48 hours after the first injection of isoproterenol [13].

Experimental protocol

The animals were randomly divided into six groups consisting of six rats each. Rats in group1 (normal control) received a subcutaneous injection of normal saline (0.5 ml) and were left untreated for the entire experimental period. Rats in group 2 (sham) were received an oral administration of tacrolimus (2 mg/kg; twice daily) for two consecutive days and were subcutaneously injected with normal saline. To induce myocardial infarction, rats in group 3 (MI control; ISO) were subcutaneously (SC) injected with isoproterenol (100 mg/kg) dissolved in normal saline as a vehicle (0.5 ml) for two consecutive days at an interval of 24 h. Rats in groups 4 to 6 were orally treated with tacrolimus at 0.5, 1 and 2 mg/kg twice daily. The treatment was started immediately prior to induction of MI (SC injection of isoproterenol) for the ensuing 2 days.

Hemodynamic measurements

About 24 to 48 hours after the last administration of drug, the animals were anesthetized by the intraperitoneal injection of a mixture of ketamine (50 mg/kg), xylazine (30 mg/kg), and acepromazine (20 mg/kg). When rats did not respond to noxious stimuli, a standard limb lead (II) observed constantly during the experimental period and any changes in ECG pattern were documented. To observe the hemodynamic parameters, a ventral midline skin incision was made from the lower mandible posteriorly to the sternum (~3 cm) and the left common carotid artery was isolated. The artery was temporary occluded toward the heart using a dieffenbach serrefines clamp (Elcon; Germany). Vannas micro iris scissors (Medi Plus; USA) was used to make a tiny incision on the carotid artery. A polyethylene cannula (Protex; OD 0.98 mm, ID 0.58 mm), coupled to a pressure transducer (Powerlab system; AD Instruments, Australia), was inserted into the artery for the recording systemic arterial blood pressure. The mean arterial blood pressure was calculated from the systolic and diastolic blood pressure traces. To assess the cardiac left ventricular function, a Mikro-Tip® catheter transducer (Millar Instruments, INC) was inserted to the lumen of the left ventricle. This helped to measure the left ventricular systolic pressure (LVSP), left ventricular end-diastolic pressure (LVEDP), maximum and minimum rates of developed left ventricular pressure ($LVdP/dt_{max}$ and $LVdP/dt_{min}$

respectively) and the rate of pressure change at a fixed left ventricular pressure (LVdP/dt/P). All the parameters were continuously recorded using a Powerlab system (AD Instruments, Australia) [14].

Tissue weights

Subsequent to hemodynamic measurements, the animals were euthanized, the hearts were removed, weighed, and histological examinations were done. The wet heart weight to body weight ratio was calculated to assess the degree of myocardial weight gain.

Determination of lipid peroxidation in serum and myocardium

Malondialdehyde (MDA), a thiobarbiturate reactive substance, was measured as a marker for oxidative stress in serum and myocardial homogenates using a method prescribed by Satoh [15]. To prepare the homogenates, another set of experiment (n = 6) including all groups was repeated and 500 mg of heart tissues from apex were homogenized in a ratio of 1:10 in 0.15% KCl by means of a homogenizer. Consequently the homogenates were centrifuged at 4 000 rpm at 4°C for 10 min. Then 3 mL of phosphoric acid and 1 mL of TBA 0.67% were added to 250 μL of supernatant of each homogenate to analyze the MDA level in tissue samples. After addition of 3 mL of n-Butanol to each sample, they heated in a water bath for 40 min and the absorbance of MDA was measured spectrophotometrically. The lipid peroxidation level expressed as nanomole MDA production per gram myocardium and nonomole per milliliter serum.

Histopathological examination

The hearts were fixed in 10% buffered formalin. The heart tissues were embedded in paraffin, sectioned at 5 μm, and stained with hematoxylin and eosin (H&E) for histologic evaluation and observed microscopically. Myocardial necrosis and edematous were evaluated in each of the four quadrants of the left ventricular cross section in each heart in the zone lying within 1.5 mm of the ventricular endocardium, using a morphometric point-counting procedure [16]. Two persons graded the histopathological changes as 1, 2, 3, and 4 for low, moderate (focal myocyte damage or small multifocal degeneration with slight degree of inflammation), high (extensive myofibrillar degeneration and/or diffuse inflammatory process), and intensive (necrosis with diffuse inflammatory process) pathological changes, respectively.

Measurements of serum TNF-α level by ELISA

The serum level of TNF-α was determined using an enzyme-linked immunosorbent assay (ELISA) (Rat TNF-α, IBL, Hamburg, Germany) according to the manufacture's instruction. Briefly, the samples were homogenized or mixed in an ice-cold solution containing 50 mM Tris–HCl, 150 mM NaCl, 5 mM Sodium Pyrophosphate (NaPPi), 50 mM NaF, 1 mM EDTA, 1 mM.

dithiothreitol (DTT), 0.1%SDS (w/v), 1% TXT-100 (v/v), and protease inhibitor cocktail (Roche, Mannheim, Germany). The samples were then centrifuged twice at 10,000 (rpm) for 10 min at 4°C. The resulting supernatants were used for assay. The concentration of the cytokines was expressed as pg/ml of serum.

Statistics

Data were presented as mean ± SEM. One-way ANOVA was used to make comparisons between the groups. If the ANOVA analysis indicated significant differences, Student–Newman–Keuls post test was employed to compare the mean values between the treatment groups and the control. Differences between the groups were considered significant if $P < 0.05$.

Results

Effects of tacrolimus on electrocardiogram

The Lead II electrocardiograms obtained from animals were shown in Figure 1. The rats were received tacrolimus alone (sham) showed normal patterns of ECG, while the rats treated with isoproterenol alone (MI group) demonstrated significant changes in ECG pattern. The changes included a marked elevation of ST segment from 95 ± 5.2 μv in control group to 194 ± 14.2 μv in ISO-treated group ($P < 0.001$), and a reduction in R wave amplitude from 448 ± 27 μv in control group to 267 ± 15 μv in ISO-treated group ($P < 0.001$) which both are indicative of myocardial infarction (Figure 2). Oral treatment with tacrolimus at doses of 0.5, 1 and 2 mg/kg significantly suppressed the isoproterenol-induced ST-segment elevation from 194 ± 14.2 μv in ISO-treated group to 169 ± 12.7, 113 ± 8.4 and 121 ± 11 μv in tacrolimus-treated groups, respectively.

Furthermore, treatment with all doses of tacrolimus resulted in a significant increase in the R-amplitude ($P < 0.001$) as compared to the rats treated with isoproterenol alone (Figure 2).

Effects of tacrolimus on hemodynamic responses

The mean arterial pressure (MAP) was significantly decreased from 79.5 ± 1.78 mmHg in control group to 37 ± 1 mmHg in isoproterenol-treated group ($P < 0.001$; Table 1). There was a significant increase in the mean arterial pressure to the value of 52 ± 1.12, 79 ± 1.86 and 78.2 ± 2 mmHg, respectively, after administration of 0.5, 1 and 2 mg/kg tacrolimus.

The intraventricular pressure was measured to determine the degree of left ventricular response to isoproterenol. Isoproterenol reduced the LVSP from 112.8 ± 2.71 mmHg in the control group to 72.8 ± 1.38 mmHg ($P < 0.001$).

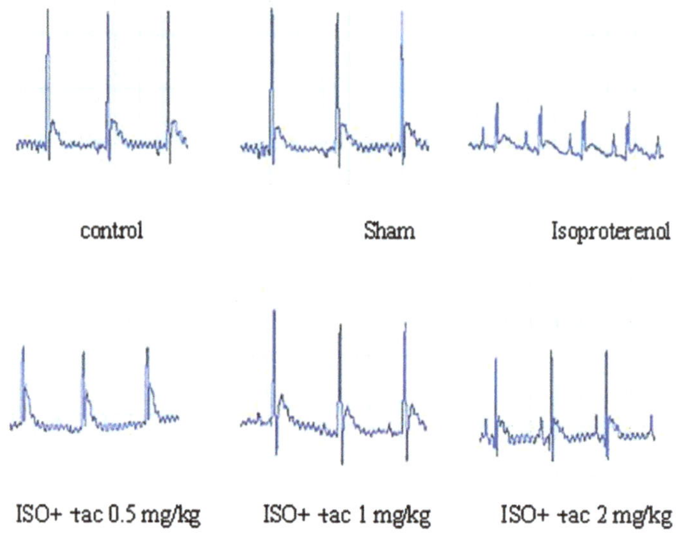

Figure 1 Effect of tacrolimus on electrocardiographic patterns and changes (recorded from limb lead II) in normal control, tacrolimus alone treated group (Sham), isoproterenol alone injected (ISO), and rats treated with tacrolimus (Tac: 0.5, 1, 2 mg/kg).

Tacrolimus was found to increase the LVSP toward the normal value in a dose-dependent manner.

Furthermore, isoproterenol treatment leads to almost a three-fold elevation in LVEDP, which was indicative of left ventricular dysfunction. All three doses of tacrolimus remarkably ($P < 0.01$) improved the left ventricular function by lowering LVEDP from 17.6 ± 0.68 mmHg in isoproterenol-treated rats to 10.2 ± 0.45, 6 ± 0.24 and 5.6 ± 0.22, respectively (Table 1).

Compared with the control group, the rats with left ventricular dysfunction (MI group) demonstrated a reduction in the value of left ventricular maximal and minimal rates of pressure (LV dP/dt_{max}; LV dP/dt_{min}; $P < 0.01$; Figure 3) as well as a lower rate of pressure change at a fixed ventricular pressure (LV dP/dt/P; $P < 0.05$; Table 1). The mentioned indices of myocardial contractility, along with LVSP, were considerably improved by administration of all three doses of tacrolimus (Figure 3). In this regard, tacrolimus at doses of 0.5, 1 and 2 mg/kg significantly increased LV dP/dt_{Max} to 3702 ± 308 ($P < 0.05$), 4484 ± 318 ($P < 0.001$) and 4592 ± 333 mmHg/s ($P < 0.001$), respectively, from 2712 ± 181 mmHg/s in isoproterenol alone treated group. Tacrolimus had a similar effect on LV dP/dt_{Min}.

Effects of tacrolimus on the heart weight to body weight ratio

The heart weight to body weight ratio (mg/kg) was determined to evaluate the amount of heart weight gain developed by the injection of isoproterenol (Figure 4). Isoproterenol injection significantly increased the ratio from 2.58 ± 0.22 in control group to 3.94 ± 0.14 ($P < 0.01$). Acute treatment with 1 mg/kg of tacrolimus resulted in a substantial ($P < 0.01$) reduction in the heart to body weight ratio in comparison to the isoproterenol alone treated rats.

Effects of tacrolimus on lipid peroxidation

To determine the lipid peroxidation, MDA levels were measured in serum and myocardial homogenates. Both serum and heart MDA levels were considerably increased ($P < 0.001$) in isoproterenol alone treated rats in comparison with normal control group (Table 2). However, treatment with tacrolimus significantly suppressed the rise of MDA levels of serum and myocardium ($P < 0.001$; Table 2).

Histopathological examination of the cardiac tissue

In the control group, myocardial fibers were arranged regularly with clear striations, without any damage or necrosis in the tissue (Figure 5). Histopathological sections of the isoproterenol alone treated hearts displayed extensive hypertrophy, necrosis and increased edematous inter muscular space. Scoring the necrosis showed that all three doses of tacrolimus significantly prevented inflammatory responses. Tacrolimus at doses of 0.5, 1 and 2 mg/kg reduced isoproterenol-induced edema and necrosis by 28% ($P < 0.05$), 35% ($P < 0.01$) and 24% ($P < 0.05$), respectively (Figure 6).

Effects of tacrolimus on the level of TNF-α in serum after myocardial infarction

In the present study, the effects of tacrolimus on the concentration of TNF-α in serum of rats with isoproterenol

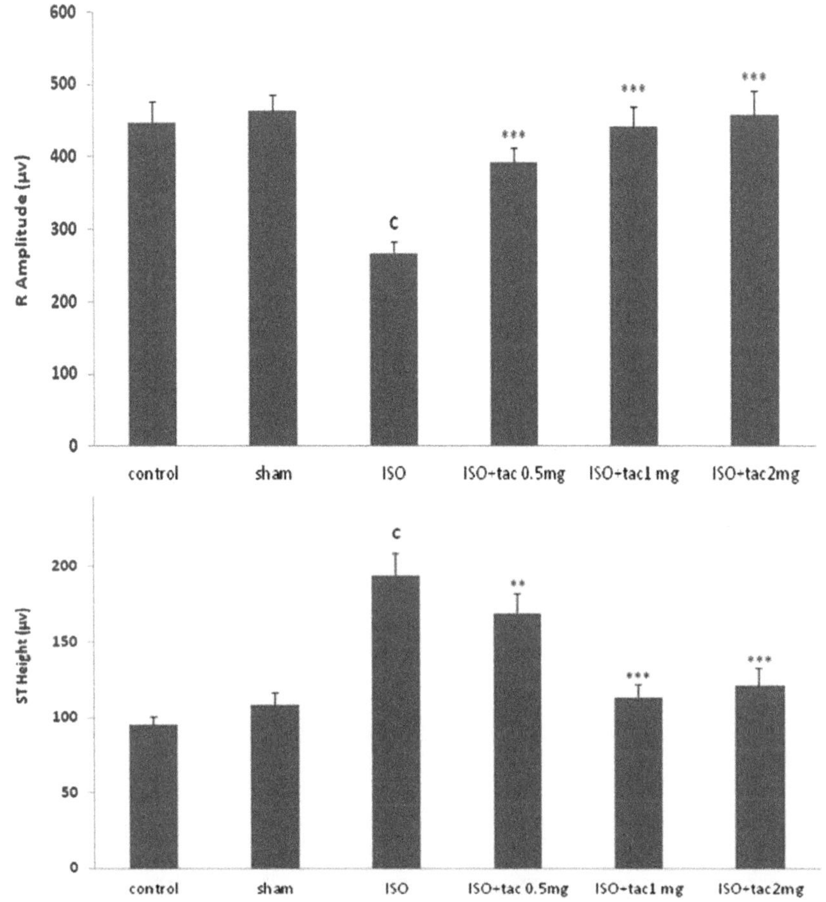

Figure 2 Effects of oral administration of tacrolimus (tac) on ST segment and R-amplitude (recorded from limb lead II). $^{c}P < 0.001$ compared to normal controls. $^{**}P < 0.01$ and $^{***}P < 0.001$ as compared to the ISO-treated group. Data are reported as mean ± SEM (n = 6).

induced MI were also investigated in order to determine whether inflammatory condition in myocardium are associated with the level of pro-inflammatory cytokines. It was found that the level of TNF-α was profoundly increased in the isoproterenol group in comparison to the control group (P < 0.001) in serum (Figure 7). It was observed that tacrolimus alone (100 mg/kg/12 h) in the sham group had no effect on the level of TNF-α in serum. The increased level of TNF-α by isoproterenol was markedly decreased by treatment with tacrolimus serum. The maximal effect

Table 1 Effects of short term oral administration of tacrolimus (tac) on hemodynamic parameters in normal and isoproterenol (ISO) induced myocardial infarction rats

Groups	MAP ± SEM (mmHg)	HR ± SEM (bpm)	LVSP ± SEM (mmHg)	LVEDP ± SEM (mmHg)	LVdp/dt/p ± SEM (1/sec)
Control	79.5 ± 1.78	197.8 ± 3.05	112.8 ± 2.71	6.3 ± 0.21	85.2 ± 1.49
Sham	80.4 ± 2.52	216.4 ± 6.21	117.6 ± 4.03	5.4 ± 0.36	85.6 ± 1.52
ISO	37 ± 1.05^{c}	290 ± 7.9^{c}	72.8 ± 1.389^{c}	17.6 ± 0.68^{c}	53.4 ± 1.07^{a}
ISO + tac 0.5 mg	52 ± 1.12*	247 ± 7.35*	83.4 ± 1.57	10.2 ± 0.45***	65 ± 1.96*
ISO + tac 1 mg	79.8 ± 1.86***	200.2 ± 4.84***	120.6 ± 3.76***	6 ± 0.24***	86.6 ± 2.07***
ISO + tac 2 mg	78.2 ± 2.06***	212.8 ± 5.43***	117.8 ± 3.24***	5.6 ± 0.22***	83.4 ± 1.95***

$^{a}P < 0.05$, $^{c}P < 0.001$ compared to normal control group. $^{*}P < 0.05$ and $^{***}P < 0.001$ as compared to the ISO-treated group. Mean arterial pressure (MAP), heart rate (HR), left ventricular systolic pressure (LVSP), left ventricular end diastolic pressure (LVEDP), left ventricular pressure changes at a fixed pressure (LV dP/dt/P). Data are shown as mean ± SEM (n = 6).

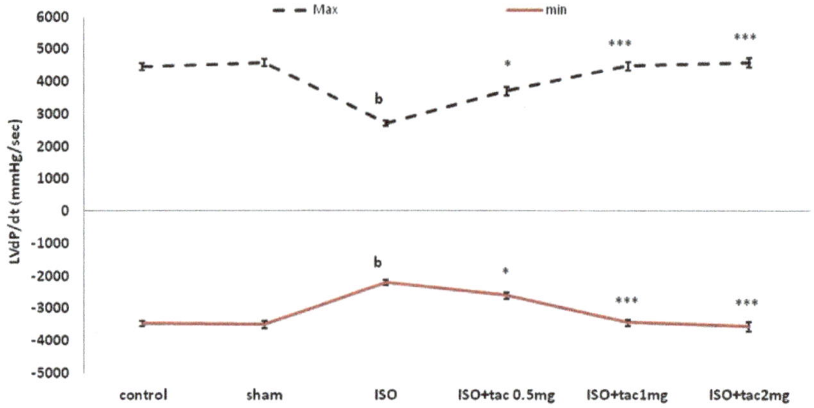

Figure 3 The effect of oral administration of tacrolimus (tac) on the minimum and maximum left ventricular pressure ($LVdP/dt_{Max}$, $LVdP/dt_{Min}$). $^{c}P < 0.001$ as compared to the normal control group, $^{*}P < 0.05$ and $^{***}P < 0.001$ as compared to the ISO-treated group. Data are reported as mean ± SEM (n = 6).

was seen by 1 mg/kg of tacrolimus, where the concentration of TNF-α was significantly reduced from 410 ± 22 pg/mL of serum to 160 ± 14 pg/mL (P < 0.001) (Figure 7).

Discussion

Electrocardiogram (ECG) is considered the most important clinical tool for the diagnosis of many types of myocardial infarction, especially for detection of ST segment elevation myocardial infarction (STEMI). Subcutaneous injection of isoproterenol (100 mg/kg) for two consecutive days caused ST- segment elevation and R-amplitude depression. The elevated ST-segment implies the loss of cell membrane function and the consequent potential difference between the ischemic and non-ischemic regions and the depressed R-amplitude might be due to the isoproterenol-induced myocardial edema [14]. Tacrolimus administration significantly amended the ECG pattern, indicating its protective effects on cell membrane function and electrical discharges.

Isoproterenol injection was followed by a significant decrease in arterial pressure indices, including ventricular contractility ($LVdP/dt_{max}$) and relaxation ($LVdP/dt_{min}$), as well as an increase in the left ventricular end-diastolic pressure (LVEDP). These disturbances were compatible with the hemodynamic changes occurring in the acute myocardial infarction.

The principal goal of post-MI therapy is to preserve the contractility of the heart ($LVdP/dt_{max}$ and $LVdP/dt_{min}$) and to decrease the elevated LVEDP. Lower values of LVEDP result in improved blood flow to the subendocardial tissue, which is greatly susceptible to ischemic necrosis.

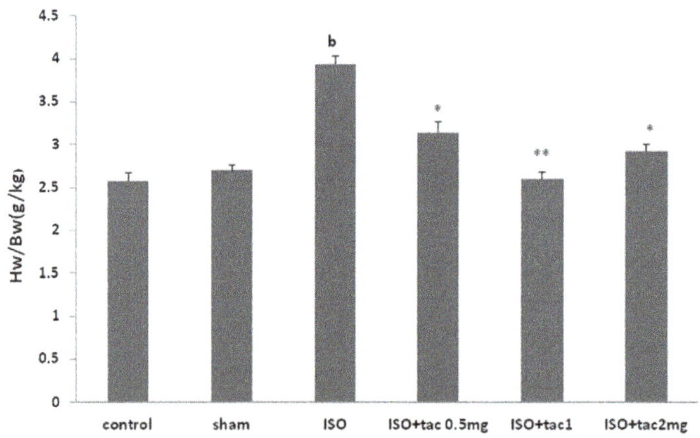

Figure 4 Effects of isoproterenol (ISO) injection as well as tacrolimus (tac) on heart weight (HW) to body weight (BW) ratio as an index of tissue edemathose in different groups. $^{b}P < 0.01$ compared to respective group in healthy animals, $^{*}P < 0.05$ and $^{**}P < 0.01$ as compared to isoproterenol (ISO) treated group. Data are reported as mean ± SEM (n = 6).

Table 2 The effects of acute treatment with tacrolimus (tac) on malondialdehyde (MDA) levels in the serum and heart tissue of control and rats with myocardial infarction

Groups (n = 6)	MDA (nmol/mL serum)	MDA (nmol/g tissue)
Control	5.4 ± 0.48	2.7 ± 0.08
sham	4.9 ± 0.3	2.4 ± 0.09
Isoproterenol (Iso)	13.7 ± 0.2[a]	5.78 ± 0.17[c]
Iso + tac (0.5 mg/kg)	7.8 ± 1.7***	4.54 ± 0.12**
Iso + tac (1 mg/kg)	7.2 ± 0.6***	2.9 ± 0.06***
Iso + tac (2 mg/kg)	4.2 ± 0.5***	2.5 ± 0.09***

[a]P < 0.001, [c]P < 0.01 from respective control value; *P < 0.05, **P < 0.01 and ***P < 0.001 as compared with ISO-treated group. Data are expressed as mean ± SEM (n = 6).

The results of the present study clearly demonstrated the beneficial effects of acute treatment with tacrolimus, administered concurrently with the induction of myocardial infarction, on various parameters of cardiac function. Tacrolimus was found to effectively raise the arterial blood pressure and myocardial contractility, along with decreasing the left ventricular end diastolic pressure.

Tacrolimus had more significant protective effects on the left ventricular function at the low dose of 1 mg/kg compared with the dose of 2 mg/kg. This might be due to the paradoxical effects of the high dose of tacrolimus on inflammatory process and on intracellular calcium homestasis. Tacrolimus binds to FKBP and suppresses inflammatory responses. On the other hand, since FKBP plays a critical role in modulating myocardial calcium homeostasis by stabilizing ryanodine receptors, the binding may disturbs the calcium homeostasis and therefore, reverse the protective effects of the drug [7,11]. It seems

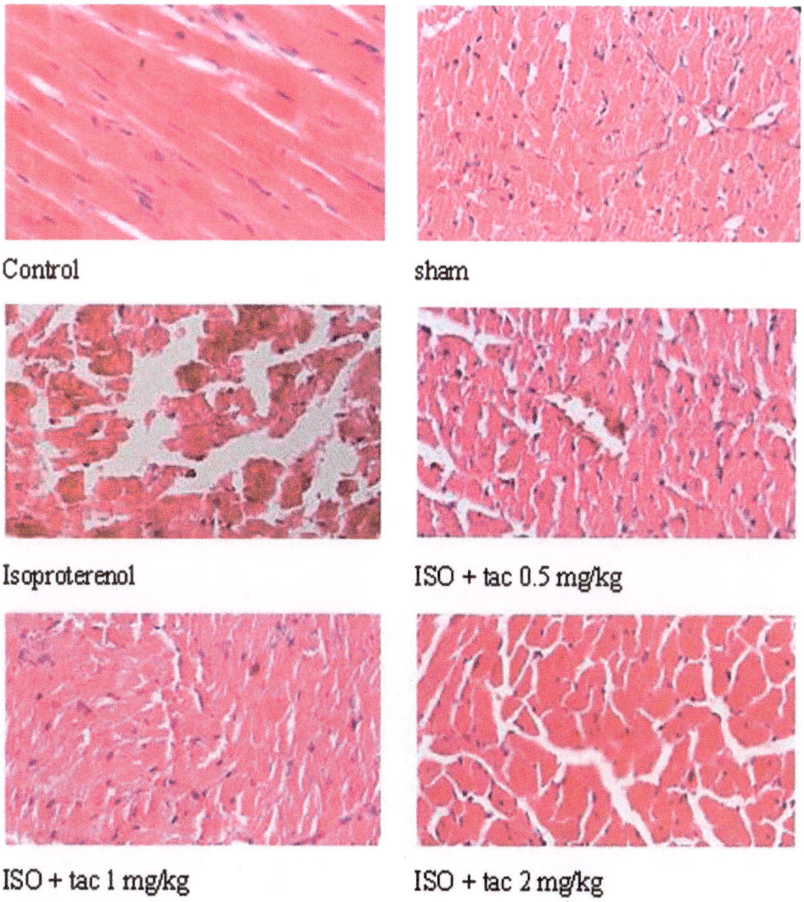

Figure 5 Photomicrographs of sections of rat cardiac apexes. Heart tissue of a rat treated with isoproterenol (ISO) showed intensive cardiomyocyte necrosis and increased edematous intramuscular space. Acute treatment with tacrolimus (tac) demonstrated a marked improvement. H&E (40' magnification).

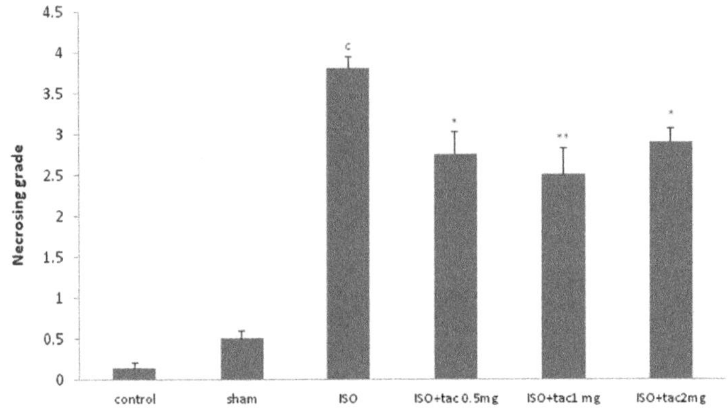

Figure 6 Grading of histopathological changes in the rat's cardiac apex tissues. Grades 1, 2, 3, and 4 showed low, moderate, high and intensive pathological changes, respectively. $^{c}P < 0.001$ compared to respective group in healthy animals, $^{*}P < 0.05$ and $^{**}P < 0.01$ as compared to isoproterenol treated group. Data are reported as mean ± SEM (n = 6).

that the high dose of the drug reduces remodeling by suppressing inflammatory responses and meanwhile, it inhibits the stabilizing effects of FKBP on ryanodine receptors by binding to it [17].

The importance of oxidative stress is implicated in the pathology of myocardial infarction. There is appreciable evidence validating the direct toxic effects of free radicals on heart tissue [18]. In fact, one of the mechanisms of isoproterenol-induced myocardial infarction is to generate highly cytotoxic free radicals, as superoxide. Malondialdehyde, a product of the oxidative degradation of unsaturated fatty acids, is a biomarker of oxidative stress, and the concentration increases in response to the free radical production in myocardial infarction, and decreases by antioxidant systems [19,20]. The results of the present study suggest that tacrolimus possesses an in vivo antioxidant activity. Tacrolimus administration substantially reduced peroxylipid levels by 50 - 70% in isoproterenol-induced myocardial infarction. This reduction may relate to blunted polymorphonuclear leukocyte accumulation [21]. Tacrolimus treatment ameliorates oxidative stress augmentation which plays a pivotal role in the myocardial infarction pathology.

Histopathological examination of infarcted myocardial tissue elucidated extensive hypertrophy, subendocardial necrosis, and edema. All three doses of tacrolimus considerably attenuated the edema and necrosis in the isoproterenol-treated heart.

The heart to body weight ratio was significantly increased following isoproterenol injection. The heart weight gain might be due to water absorption and increase in protein content of muscular cells. Cardiac hypertrophy is due to increased cardiac performance. Treatment with all doses of tacrolimus markedly reduced the heart to body weight ratio. However, the drug was very effective at the low dose of 1 mg/kg.

Conclusions

Limited data are available on the cardioprotective effects of tacrolimus. However, our study finds that administration of tacrolimus, simultaneous to the myocardial infarction incidence, has a remarkable protective potential

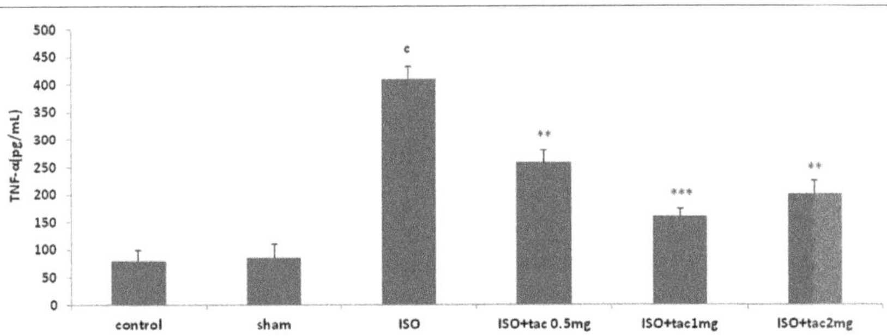

Figure 7 The effect of acute and short term treatment with tacrolimus (tac) at the doses of 0.5, 1 and 2 mg/kg/12 h on TNFα concentration in serum. $^{c}P < 0.001$ from respective control value; $^{**}P < 0.01$ and $^{***}P < 0.001$ as compared with isoproterenol (ISO) injected group. Data are reported as mean ± SEM (n = 6).

against damages caused by isoproterenol-induced myocardial infarction. The cardioprotective effects of acute treatment with tacrolimus are confirmed by amending electrocardiographic pattern, improvement of hemodynamic and left ventricular functions, and less histopathological damage following isoproterenol-induced myocardial infarction. It is proposed that tacrolimus exerts this cardioprotective effects through its anti-inflammatory and antioxidant properties. Although this study has provided a possible new therapeutic tool for myocardial infarction, more studies are required to elucidate the precise mechanism of tacrolimus in reversing the pathogenesis of myocardial infarction.

Competing interests
The authors declare that they have no competing interests.

Authors' contribution
MH Carried out animals grouping and handling and the biochemical experiments. AK Carried out the hemodynamic experiments. MG Accompanied Mojtaba Hammami in MI induction and helped in preparing manuscript. NM Histopathological works and interpretations. AG Supervising and directing the project carried out the data analysis and interpretations and prepared the manuscript. All authors read and approved the final manuscript.

Acknowledgments
The present study was supported by a grant from the Research Vice Chancellors of Tabriz University of Medical Sciences; Tabriz, Iran. This article is based on a thesis submitted for PharmD degree (No: 5/4/3419) in Faculty of Pharmacy, Tabriz University of Medical Sciences, Tabriz, Iran.

Author details
[1]Department of Pharmacology and Toxicology, Faculty of Pharmacy, Tabriz University of Medical Sciences, Tabriz, Iran. [2]Student Research Committee, Tabriz University of Medical Sciences, Tabriz, Iran.

References
1. Xie N, Zhang W, Li J, Liang H, Zhou H, Duan W, Xu X, Yu S, Zhang H, Yi D: **α-linolenic acid intake attenuates myocardial ischemia/reperfusion injury through anti-inflammatory and anti-oxidative stress effects in diabetic but not normal rats.** *Arch Med Res* 2011, **42**:171–181.
2. Colditz GA, Rimm EB, Giovannucci E, Stampfer MJ, Rosner B, Willett WC: **A prospective study of parental history off myocardial infarction and coronary artery disease in men.** *Am J Cardiol* 1991, **67**:933–938.
3. Neumar RW, Browns CG, Robitaille P-ML, Altschul RA: **Myocardial high energy phosphate metabolism during ventricular fibrillation with total circulatory arrest.** *Resuscitation* 1990, **19**:199–226.
4. Ivan Hall R, Amos Moffitt E: **The effects of anaesthetics on coronary artery blood flow and myocardial metabolism: a review of studies in animals and man.** *Baillières Clin Anaesthesiol* 1989, **3**:27–46.
5. Bodi V, Sanchis J, Morales JM, Marrachelli VG, Nunez J, Forteza MJ, Chaustre F, Gomez C, Mainar L, Minana G, Rumiz E, Husser O, Noguera I, Diaz A, Moratal D, Carratala A, Bosch X, Llacer A, Chorro FJ, Viña JR, Monleon D: **Metabolomic profile of human myocardial ischemia by nuclear magnetic resonance spectroscopy of peripheral blood serum: a translational study based on transient coronary occlusion models.** *J Am Coll Cardiol* 2012, **59**:1629–1641.
6. Maekawa N, Wada H, Kanda T, Niwa T, Yamada Y, Saito K, Fujiwara H, Sekikawa K, Seishima M: **Improved myocardial ischemia/reperfusion injury in mice lacking tumor necrosis factor-α.** *J Am Coll Cardiol* 2002, **39**:1229–1235.
7. Yang CH, Sheu JJ, Tsai TH, Chua S, Chang LT, Chang HW, Lee FY, Chen YL, Chung SY, Sun CK, Leu S, Yen CH, Yip HK: **Effect of tacrolimus on myocardial infarction is associated with inflammation, ROS, MAP kinase and Akt pathways in mini-pigs.** *J Atheroscler Thromb* 2013, **20**:9–22.
8. Mazzone A, Cusa C, Mazzucchelli I, Vezzoli M, Ottini E, Pacifici R, Zuccaro P, Falcone C: **Increased production of inflammatory cytokines in patients with silent myocardial ischemia.** *J Am Coll Cardiol* 2001, **38**:1895–1901.
9. Van Rossum H, Romijn F, Smit N, de Fijter J, Van Pelt J: **Everolimus and sirolimus antagonize tacrolimus based calcineurin inhibition via competition for FK-binding protein 12.** *Biochem Pharmacol* 2009, **77**:1206–1212.
10. Chua S, Leu S, Sheu JJ, Lin YC, Chang LT, Kao YH, Yen CH, Tsai TH, Chen YL, Chang HW, Sun CK, Yip HK: **Intra-coronary administration of tacrolimus markedly attenuates infarct size and preserves heart function in porcine myocardial infarction.** *J Inflamm* 2012, **9**:21–33.
11. Su Z, Sugishita K, Li F, Ritter M, Barry W: **Effects of FK506 on [Ca2+]i differ in mouse and rabbit ventricular myocytes.** *J Pharmacol Exp Ther* 2003, **304**:334–341.
12. Yousefi K, Soraya H, Fathiazad F, Khorrami A, Hamedeyazdan S, Maleki-Dizaji N, Garjani A: **Cardioprotective effect of methanolic extract of Marrubium vulgare L. on isoproterenol-induced acute myocardial infarction in rats.** *Indian J Exp Biol* 2013, **51**:653–660.
13. Fathiazad F, Matlobi A, Khorrami A, Hamedeyazdan S, Soraya H, Hammami M, Maleki-Dizaji N, Garjani A: **Phytochemical screening and evaluation of cardioprotective activity of ethanolic extract of Ocimum basilicum L. (basil) against isoproterenol induced myocardial infarction in rats.** *DARU J Pharm Sci* 2012, **20**:87–97.
14. Garjani A, Andalib S, Biabani S, Soraya H, Doustar Y, Garjani A, Maleki-Dizaji N: **Combined atorvastatin and coenzyme Q10 improve the left ventricular function in isoproterenol-induced heart failure in rat.** *Eur J Pharmacol* 2011, **666**:135–141.
15. Satoh K: **Serum lipid peroxide in cerebrovascular disorders determined by a new colorimetric method.** *Clinica Chimica Acta* 1978, **90**:37–43.
16. Benjamin IJ, Jalil JE, Tan LB, Cho K, Weber KT, Clark WA: **Isoproterenol-induced myocardial fibrosis in relation to myocyte necrosis.** *Circ Res* 1989, **65**:657–670.
17. Shawn D, St. P, Adyr AM, David CM: **Effects of tacrolimus on ischemia-reperfusion injury.** *Liver Transpl* 2003, **9**:105–116.
18. Rona G: **Catecholamine cardiotoxicity.** *J Mol Cell Cardiol* 1985, **7**:291–306.
19. Radovanovic S, Savic-Radojevic A, Pljesa-Ercegovac M, Djukic T, Suvakov S, Krotin M, Simic DV, Matic M, Radojicic Z, Pekmezovic T, Simic T: **Markers of oxidative damage and antioxidant enzyme activities as predictors of morbidity and mortality in patients with chronic heart failure.** *J Card Fail* 2012, **18**:493–501.
20. Ho E, Karimi Galougahi K, Liu C-C, Bhindi R, Figtree GA: **Biological markers of oxidative stress: applications to cardiovascular research and practice.** *Redox Biol* 2013, **1**:483–491.
21. Squadrito F, Altavilla D, Squadrito G, Saitta A, Deodato B, Arlotta M, Minutoli L, Quartarone C, Ferlito M, Caputi AP: **Tacrolimus limits polymorphonuclear leucocyte accumulation and protects against myocardial ischaemia–reperfusion injury.** *J Mol Cell Cardiol* 2000, **32**:429–440.

13

Formulation of inhalable lipid-based salbutamol sulfate microparticles by spray drying technique

Zahra Daman[1], Kambiz Gilani[1,2*], Abdolhossein Rouholamini Najafabadi[1], Hamid Reza Eftekhari[1] and Mohammad Ali Barghi[3]

Abstract

Background: The aim of this work was to develop dry powder inhaler (DPI) formulations of salbutamol sulfate (SS) by the aid of solid lipid microparticles (SLmPs), composed of biocompatible phospholipids or cholesterol.

Methods: The SLmPs were prepared by using two different solvent systems (ethanol and water-ethanol) and lipid carriers (dipalmitoylphosphatidylcholine (DPPC) and cholesterol) with/without L-leucine in the spray drying process. The spray-dried microparticles were physically-mixed with coarse lactose monohydrate in order to make our final DPI formulations and were investigated in terms of physical characteristics as well as in vitro drug release profile and aerosolization behavior.

Results: We observed significant differences in the sizes, morphologies, and in vitro pulmonary depositions between the formulations. In particular, the SS-containing SLmPs prepared with water-ethanol (30:70 v/v) solution of DPPC and L-leucine which had then been blended with coarse lactose (1:9 w/w) exhibited the highest emitted dose (87.9%) and fine particle fraction (42.7%) among the formulations. In vitro drug release study indicated that despite of having a significant initial burst release for both cholesterol and DPPC-based microparticles, the remained drug released more slowly than the pure drug.

Conclusion: This study demonstrated the potential of using lipid carriers as well as L-leucine in DPI formulations of SS to improve its aerosolization behavior and retard the release profile of the drug.

Keywords: Dry powder inhalation, Spray drying, Salbutamol sulfate, Solid lipid microparticles, Particle engineering, L-leucine

Background

Local administration of drugs to the lungs presents several advantages, especially, in patients with specific pulmonary diseases, such as asthma, pulmonary infections or lung cancer. The advantages include reduction in systemic side effects, elevated drug concentration at the site of action, and reduction in amount of drug administered to the patient compared to traditional routs [1-3]. In this regard, the area of particle engineering is becoming increasingly attractive for the development of more efficient inhaled therapeutics.

One of the attractive applications of particle engineering is to develop a sustained release (SR) formulation by using suitable carriers, a kind of formulation that has not been marketed yet, despite active research conducted on this subject. A SR formulation will provide the active drug over an extended duration of time, and therefore may improve therapy by enhancing the compliance of the patients. In such formulations, it is expected that the overall amount of drug and the side effects will be reduced [4-6]. However, the efforts for finding suitable, non-toxic excipients, which can produce a desired drug release profile and improve the respirable fraction of the inhaled particles to maximize drug deposition into smaller airways are continuous and extensive.

One approach to SR delivery to the respiratory tract utilizes liposomal formulations. Liposomes are promising vehicles for pulmonary drug delivery owing to their

* Correspondence: gilani@tums.ac.ir
[1]Aerosol Research Laboratory, Department of Pharmaceutics, School of Pharmacy, Tehran University of Medical Sciences, Tehran, Iran
[2]Medicinal Plants Research Center, Tehran University of Medical Sciences, Tehran, Iran
Full list of author information is available at the end of the article

capacity to increase drug retention time and reduce the toxicity of drugs after administration [7,8]. Several factors such as the composition of lipids and the size of liposomes can affect the performance of the system [9-11]. Many studies have shown the applicability of liposomes in lung delivery of a large variety of drugs such as cytotoxic agents, anti-asthma drugs, antimicrobial agents, and drugs for systemic action like insulin and other proteins [4,10]. However, there are some disadvantages about liposomal vehicles that limits their application as commercial formulations such as high production cost and instability during storage even at low temperatures [12], and nebulization [13,14] that can cause premature release of the entrapped drug. The latter problem has been reported even about the dry powder formulations prepared by jet milling micronization of lyophilized liposomes, which deleteriously affected their integrity [15].

Another approach for development of an inhalable SR formulation is to produce solid lipid microparticles (SLmPs). It has been suggested that SLmPs offer high tolerability in the pulmonary tract, as they are mainly made of biocompatible and biodegradable materials [16,17]. Moreover, they possess several other advantages compared to traditional vehicles such as polymeric drug carriers, micelles or liposomes, including more physiochemical stability, incorporation of both lipophilic and hydrophilic drugs, low large-scale production cost and having no significant biotoxicity [16-19]. Phospholipids and cholesterol have been previously used in inhalation formulations as solid lipid carriers or fillers to improve drug targeting to the lung. The prepared SLmPs presented spherical shapes, reduced agglomeration tendency and high fine particle fraction (FPF) [17,20].

Spray drying is an attractive solidification technique in the field of respiratory drug delivery, with respect to its relative simplicity, availability of large-scale equipment, capability to produce homogenous particle size distribution, and ability to control various parameters that optimize the particulate product characteristics such as size, size distribution, shape, morphology and density [21-23]. Therefore, it can be used as a suitable technology to produce dry powder inhaler (DPI) products, which possess several advantages over pressurized metered dose inhalers (pMDI), such as being breath-activated and having no requirement of any propellant [24].

Thus, the aim of this study was to design SLmPs using cholesterol or dipalmitoylphosphatidylcholine (DPPC) by spray drying method. The idea was emerged from the potential ability of these excipients to entrap both water-soluble and water-insoluble drugs, as well as providing a prolonged local drug release [6,16]. Moreover, the safety issue of these SLmPs over other vehicles was a key consideration in our design process, since they are mainly made from endogenous materials [25,26]. For this purpose, we chose to work with SS, a short acting beta2-adrenoceptor stimulant with plasma half-life of 4–6 hours, which requires frequent dosing for daily management of asthma. A SR preparation of this agent is desirable approach to improve therapy of asthma, especially in non-compliant patients and also for covering the nocturnal decline of the drug [27], when administered at the bed time.

Aside from SR properties, an effective DPI formulation should offer optimum particle characteristics to achieve high FPF and reduce the central deposition in pulmonary airways. In other words, a suitable DPI formulation should have the ability to reach deep lung regions and disperse adequately within the airflow of the patient. Indeed, decreasing of both particle size and density can be achieved by spray drying technique in order to generate particles with satisfactory respirable fraction [23]. However, the dispersibility of the particles is another factor that has to be taken into consideration. The particle aggregation associated with cohesive forces between them can be regulated using excipients such as coarse crystalline lactose, which is currently serving as the drug carrier and also the bulking agent in most available DPI products [23]. Usually, drug particles and such excipients are combined in a physical blending process during which the microparticles are attached to the surface of the carrier. Therefore, our final DPI formulations consisted of physically-mixed SLmPs with large coarse lactose carrier particles. To aid dispersibility, it has been also proven that co-spray drying of simple amino acids, especially the hydrophobic ones such as L-leucine, can improve dispersion of the powder and may enhance the fraction of respirable particles [28]. Thus, we used this amino acid in our spray drying process to evaluate its effects on the aerodynamic performance of the resultant DPI formulation.

In the present study, the obtained SLmPs were further characterized for their physical properties, in vitro aerosolization behavior, and their potential of being a SR delivery system.

Methods

Materials

SS was supplied as micronized powder from Darupakhsh (Iran). Cholesterol was purchased from Merck (Germany), and the phospholipid, DPPC, was supplied from Lipoid (Germany). Inhalation grade lactose (Pharmatose 325 M) with D50% of about 60 μm was obtained from DMV Internationals (The Netherlands). Other chemical reagents and solvents including the HPLC grade ones were purchased from either Merck or Sigma. L-Leucine was also supplied from Merck (Germany).

Preparation of the lipid-based microparticles

The SLmPs were prepared, at laboratory scale, by spray drying method using a Büchi Minispray dryer B-191-a from Büchi Laboratory-Technique (Switzerland). In this study, we decided to improve the drying efficiency of the lipid excipients by using a jacketed cyclone with cold-water circulation, to cool down the cyclone separator wall and thus decrease the lipid particles' adhesion and agglomeration.

Two different types of formulations were spray dried for the preparation of SLmPs. The first type was prepared by dispersing the SS microparticles within an ethanol solution of the hydrophobic excipients, cholesterol or DPPC. The suspensions were sonicated for 10 min before spray drying to ensure the adequate dispersion of the drug. The second type of formulations was obtained from spray drying of water-ethanol (30:70 v/v) solution of the drug and the lipid materials. Details are shown in Table 1.

The spray drying conditions were as following: Solid content, 5% w/v; Nozzle size, 0.5 mm; Inlet temperature, 80/100°C (depending on the solvent system); Outlet temperature, 54/65°C (depending on the inlet temperature); Spraying air flow rate, 800 L/h; Feed rate, 0.2 g/min; Cold water circulation in the jacketed cyclone, 0°C.

Furthermore, as shown in Table 1, L-leucine was co-spray dried at the amount of 10% w/w with respect to the solid content with water-ethanol solution of DPPC and SS. Finally, all the obtained formulations were physically blended with inhalation grade lactose monohydrate (Pharmatose® 325 M) at a ratio of 1:9 w/w in a Turbula mixer from Dorsa Novin (Iran) for 60 min at a low speed (46 rpm).

Determination of SS content

Quantification of CIP was conducted by HPLC using a mobile phase consisting of water, methanol and phosphate buffer (pH 2.8) in the ratio of 60:20:20 at a flow rate of 1 mL/min. The phosphate buffer was prepared by dissolving 2.625 g ammonium phosphate in 50 mL purified deionized water, adding 2.8 mL of phosphoric acid (85%) and diluting to 100 mL with purified deionized water. The HPLC system consisted of a pump (Waters 600E, Millipore, USA), a C18 Tracer Excel column (15 × 0.46 cm, 5 μm, Spain) and a UV detector (Waters 486, USA) at 276 nm. Bamethan sulfate (to final concentration of 10 μg/mL) was added as the internal standard to each sample just before analysis. From the relative area under the peak, linearity (R2 = 0.999) was achieved using standard aqueous solutions of SS between 0.5 and 50 μg/mL.

For all the prepared DPI formulations, the content uniformity was evaluated by taking 10 random samples, each weighing 10 mg powder which were subjected to lipid extraction by adding 1.5 mL chloroform to each one and centrifugation at 37565 × g for 20 min. The recovered drug was diluted with mobile phase before being subjected to HPLC analysis. Mixtures with relative standard deviation values of less than 10%, as recommended by The United States Pharmacopeia, were considered to be satisfactorily mixed.

Particle size measurement

The size distribution of the microparticles was determined by laser diffraction method using Malvern Mastersizer X (UK) after the formulations had been dispersed in appropriate medium (saturated solution of SS in water) and sonicated for 2 min. The geometrical diameter was expressed as volume median diameter (D50%). Also the Span values of formulations were defined as $\frac{D90\%-D10\%}{D50\%}$, which represents the breadth of the particle distribution. Each measurement was repeated in triplicate.

Scanning electron microscopy

Particle morphology was observed by scanning electron microscopy (SEM) using Philips XL30 equipment (The Netherlands). The samples were coated with gold under relative vacuum by means of Bal-Tec/SCDOOS sputter coater (Switzerland) and were examined under an accelerating voltage of 25 kv.

Determination of true density

The density was assessed with Quantachrome helium pycnometer (USA). The basis of this method is on putting the sample of known mass into a cell of known volume. Briefly, when helium penetrates into the cell at a vacuum, it occupies the entire volume of the cell, so the actual volume of the sample can be determined since the volume

Table 1 Composition of different spray-dried formulations

Formulation number	Drug conc. (%)*	Excipients	Solvent system	Inlet temperature (°C)
1	12.5	cholesterol	Ethanol	80
2	25	cholesterol	Ethanol	80
3	37.5	cholesterol	Ethanol	80
4	37.5	DPPC	Ethanol	80
5	37.5	cholesterol	Water/Ethanol	100
6	37.5	DPPC	Water/Ethanol	100
7	37.5	DPPC + Leucine	Water/Ethanol	100

*Percentage of the total solid content (w/w).

of the cell is known. So, the actual densities of the samples were accurately calculated. Each sample was analyzed thrice.

Aerosol performance of SLmPs

The in vitro pulmonary deposition of the powders was determined by Twin Stage Impinger (TSI) glass apparatus from Copley Scientific (UK). A dry powder formulation device, Novartis Cyclohaler® (Switzerland), was filled with a hard gelatin capsule loaded with 10 mg of each formulation. On the other hand, the mobile phase was introduced to stage 1 (7 mL) and stage 2 (30 mL) of the TSI. Once the assembly had been checked to be tight and vertical, the Cyclohaler® had been inserted to the rubber mouthpiece attached to the throat part of the impinger. The test was operated at 60 L/min for 4 s. The flow rate was achieved using a rotary vein pump from Copley Scientific (UK). After the operation, the impinger components had been washed into separate volumetrics (25 mL for the throat and stage 1, and 50 mL for the device and stage 2) with the same solution. Their contents were assayed for SS, after the lipid had been extracted with certain ratio of chloroform.

Fine particle dose (FPD) was considered as the amount of drug deposited in stage 2 (dae < 6.4 μm). The emitted dose (ED) was determined as a percent of total powder exiting the capsule and the device. The FPF was calculated as the percent of the ratio of FPD to the total amount of drug emitted per capsule.

Determination of drug release from SLmPs

Since the volume of surface liquid in the respiratory tract is relatively low, the conventional European Pharmacopeia methods cannot be used for exact evaluation of dissolution behavior of inhaled drugs due to their large volumes of dissolution media (900–1000 mL) [29]. Hence we used a dispersion method to measure in vitro release of the drug from SLmPs. Briefly, 10 mg of each formulation was suspended individually in 10 mL phosphate buffered saline (PBS, PH = 7.4) in test tubes and incubated in a shaker (Grant instruments, Cambridge, England) at 37°C on 50 rpm. At certain time intervals of 0.25, 0.5, 1, 2, 4, 8, and 12 hours, three tubes were picked and individually assayed for SS after being filtered. The mean value of the tree tubes for each time interval was calculated, and plotted as cumulative amount of SS released over 12 hours.

Statistical analysis

Data for all measurements were considered as the mean ± standard deviation (SD) of at least three separate experiments. One-way analysis of variance (ANOVA) test was used for statistical comparison of the results while $p < 0.05$ was considered significant in all cases.

Results and discussion

Different powder compositions were formulated using the spray drying technique, with the aim of studying the influence of lipid composition and the solvent type on the physiochemical properties and the aerosolization behavior of the powders. Table 1 gives an overview of all the prepared powder formulations. It should be mentioned that the content uniformity test was conducted for both spray-dried formulations and the physical blends, using a conventional invasive sampling method. The active drug content was quantified by HPLC, and ranged between 95 ± 2% and 103 ± 3% for different formulations.

Evaluation of physiochemical properties of aerosol particles

The particle size characteristics of the formulations are summarized in Table 2. The results showed that for the same lipid and solvent composition of the formulations (cholesterol in ethanol), the percentage of SS in the suspensions used for spray drying had no significant effect on the size of resultant SLmPs ($p > 0.05$). Additionally, the D50% of the spray dried formulations obtained from ethanol suspension of the drug were shown to be dependent

Table 2 Particle size measurement obtained by laser diffraction method (mean ± SD)

Formulation number	Drug conc. (%)*	Excipients	Solvent system	Inlet temp. (°C)	D50%	Span
1	12.5	cholesterol	Ethanol	80	3.23 ± 0.48	3.19
2	25	cholesterol	Ethanol	80	5.04 ± 0.66	1.75
3	37.5	cholesterol	Ethanol	80	4.16 ± 0.32	1.66
4	37.5	DPPC	Ethanol	80	1.42 ± 0.15	0.87
5	37.5	cholesterol	Water-Ethanol	100	7.32 ± 0.28	2.26
6	37.5	DPPC	Water-Ethanol	100	4.02 ± 0.18	2.54
7	37.5	DPPC + Leucine	Water-Ethanol	100	4.04 ± 0.25	2.23
C_1	100	-	Ethanol	80	3.70 ± 0.13	2.47
C_2	100	-	Water-Ethanol	100	5.83 ± 0.21	1.82

*Percentage of the total solid content (w/w).

on the type of lipid component, which was much smaller for DPPC-based microparticles than cholesterol ($p < 0.05$). Changing the solvent from ethanol to water-ethanol (30:70 v/v) resulted in an increase in D50% values of both DPPC and cholesterol-based particles ($p < 0.05$). It seems that the enhancement in the inlet temperature of spray drying process has contributed to the particle size enlargement, as it was previously proven that adding in tempe rature will lead to increase in the diameter of particles [30,31]. Furthermore, the laser diffraction particle size analysis showed that co-spray drying of L-leucine with DPPC and SS did not significantly change the particle size distribution with respect to the counterpart sample without L-leucine ($p > 0.05$).

Scanning electron microphotographs of the SLmPs are shown in Figure 1. As shown in Figure 1a-c, changing the solvent in the feed solution did not seriously change the spherical shape of cholesterol-based SLmPs which is typically obtained via spray drying technique [32]. Processing of the drug and DPPC in ethanol produced particles similar to that of cholesterol-based samples (Figure 1d). However, as it is indicated in Figure 1e, applying a mixed solution of water-ethanol (30:70 v/v) in formulations consisted of DPPC resulted in production of wrinkled particles which used to be mostly spherical when pure ethanol was applied as the solvent. It is supposed that the solubility saturation of the formulation components upon former evaporation of the more volatile solvent (ethanol) leads to formation of a primary solid shell which then collapses as the core's water content evaporates [33]. In this case, the surface-active DPPC could have contributed to the formation of this primary solid shell during particle formation stage. Incorporation of L-leucine within this formulation led the spherical shape back to the particles, as it is clearly shown in Figure 1f. It seems that the more tendency of L-leucine to water than ethanol and its subsequent localization in the core of the primary particles inhibited the shell to completely collapse after water evaporation. Figure 2 shows the attachment of SLmPs obtained from water-ethanol (30:70 v/v) solution of DPPC and SS to the large lactose surface. In fact, physical blending of the formulations with lactose monohydrate as the coarse carrier promoted the adhesion of SLmPs onto its surface. This process was expected to aid the deaggregation and dispersion of particles within the respiratory flow [34].

The true density values of the spray dried samples obtained by helium pycnometry are shown in Table 3. SS powders, which were spray dried from both kinds of the solvent systems, were used as controls. The results suggested that utilizing the lipid components along with the drug could result in reduction of the true density of the spray-dried powders. Actually, particle's aerodynamic diameter (d_a) is a function of particle's geometric diameter (d), density (ρ) and morphology (χ, shape factor) according to the following equation:

$$d_a = d\sqrt{(\rho/\chi)}$$

In other words, particles with low density have smaller aerodynamic diameter than their geometric diameter. Thus, it can be of great value to reduce the density and affect the aerodynamic diameter of the particles by changing a DPI formulation composition. In this regard, Scalia et al. had previously reported the true density values of lower than 1 g cm^{-3} for the lipid microparticles obtained by melt emulsification technique [35].

Aerosol performance of the SLmPs

Table 4 shows the ED (%), FPD (μg) and FPF (%) values of the spray dried SLmPs (formulations number 1 to 7) along with the same powders mixed with lactose carrier in the ratio of 1:9 w/w (formulations number 8 to 12). The aerodynamic characteristics were measured using a TSI at the flow rate of 60 L/min after aerosolization by

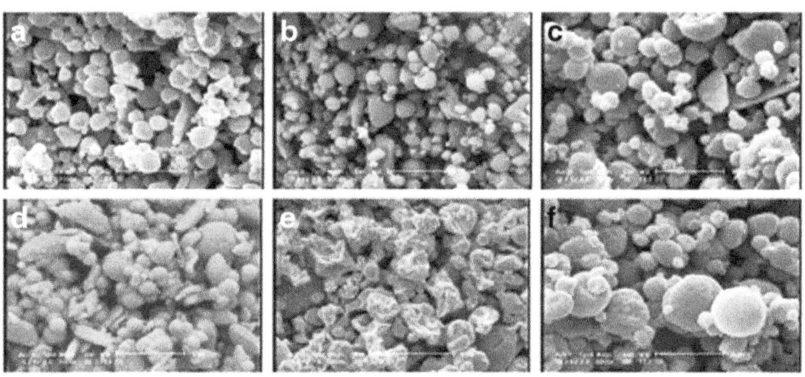

Figure 1 Scanning electron micrographs of SLmPs containing salbutamol sulfate in different formulations: a) F2, b) F3, c) F5, d) F4, e) F6, f) F7.

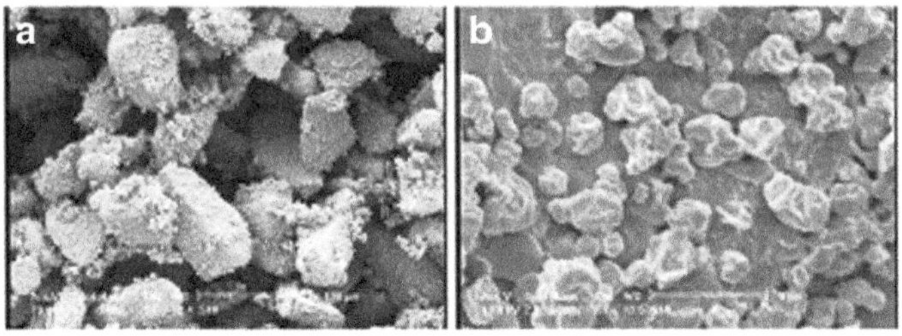

Figure 2 Scanning electron micrographs of SLmPs blended with lactose. a) magnification ×240, **b)** more magnification (×5000) representing SLmPs deposited on the surface of lactose carriers.

Cyclohaler®. It should be noted that SS recoveries from the inhaler and the different parts of the TSI ranged between 90.1-95.2% of the total loaded drug.

It seems that the type of solvent system and lipid excipients had a direct effect on aerosolization properties of the powders. Among the formulations prepared by cholesterol and ethanol, increasing the drug content from 12.5% to 25% did not make a significant change on FPF values ($P > 0.05$), but the initial drug content of 37.5% (Formulation No. 3) appeared to have higher FPF (%) than the others ($P < 0.05$). However, changing the type of cholesterol solvent to 30:70 v/v water-ethanol (Formulation No. 5) resulted in FPF reduction which seems to be due to particle size enlargement of the resultant SLmPs [36,37]. The difference between FPF values associated with the type of solvent was more noticeable when DPPC was used as the lipid excipient. The consequence of changing the solvent from pure ethanol to 30:70 v/v water-ethanol was a noticeable increase in FPF values from 4.1% to 22.5% for DPPC-based formulations ($P < 0.05$). The latter results are not in accordance with the particle size determinations obtained by laser diffraction, since the formulation prepared by the aid of ethanol solution of DPPC had smaller size than that of water-ethanol solution of it. In this case, the particle aggregation of very small particles (D50% =1.42 μm) made up of DPPC as the lipid excipient and ethanol as the solvent, seemed to be the main cause of owning the lowest FPF value. In addition, wrinkled particles usually improve the respirable fraction of a DPI formulation by decreasing the interparticulate cohesion forces as well as enhancing the powder dispersibility [38].

The incorporation of L-leucine to the formulation number 6 which was prepared from 30:70 v/v water-ethanol solution of DPPC and SS resulted in insignificant FPF improvement ($P > 0.05$). As mentioned earlier, both kinds of formulations (F6 and F7) had almost similar particle average diameters, but different shapes. Although L-leucine plays a role of anti-adherent amino acid that can improve the deagglomeration of SLmPs [29], it seems that the corrugated particles made from spray-dried SS and DPPC could compensate the absence of L-leucine and act as favorably as the spherical particles of F7 in the in vitro pulmonary deposition test.

Moreover, simple blending of micron-sized SLmPs with coarse lactose monohydrate terminated in noticeable FPF elevation, compared to the FPF values of uncombined SLmPs. It seems that the absorption of the SLmPs to the surface of lactose, and the subsequent improvement in the dispersibility and deaggregation of them within the airflow resulted in elevated drug deposition in stage 2 of the TSI [24,34]. Finally, we found that co spray-dried DPPC/L-leucine, which had then been blended with coarse lactose (in the ratio of 1:9 w/w), was the most appropriate formulation for SS in term of aerosol performance.

In vitro drug release study

The release profiles of SS from SLmPs are reported in Figure 3. It should be noted that release of pure micronized SS was rapid as nearly all the amount of the drug was

Table 3 True density values obtained by the helium pycnometer

Drug conc. (%)*	Excipients	Solvent system	Inlet temp. (°C)	Density (g/cm^3)
37.5	Cholesterol	Ethanol	80	1.11 ± 0.09
37.5	Cholesterol	Water/Ethanol	100	1.15 ± 0.10
37.5	DPPC	Ethanol	80	1.15 ± 0.08
37.5	DPPC	Water/Ethanol	100	1.18 ± 0.07
100	-	Ethanol	80	1.33 ± 0.11
100	-	Water/Ethanol	100	1.41 ± o.12

*Percentage of the total solid content (w/w).

Table 4 Fine particle dose (FPD), emitted dose (ED) and fine particle fraction (FPF) of salbutamol sulfate after aerosolization from different formulations (mean ± SD)

Formulation number	Lipid excipients	Solvent system**	Inlet temp.(°C)	Blending excipient**	FPF(%)	FPD(μg)	ED(%)
1	Cholesterol	E	80	-	16.7 ± 0.8	165 ± 4.4	79.2 ± 2.1
2	Cholesterol	E	80	-	16.5 ± 1.2	305 ± 5.7	74.1 ± 2.5
3	Cholesterol	E	80	-	21.1 ± 0.9	575 ± 7.3	74.8 ± 1.8
4	DPPC	E	80	-	4.1 ± 0.3	138 ± 3.2	89.3 ± 1.6
5	Cholesterol	W/E	100	-	12.1 ± 0.7	310 ± 4.8	69.1 ± 2.1
6	DPPC	W/E	100	-	22.5 ± 1.3	686 ± 7.5	81.1 ± 2.3
7	DPPC + leucine	W/E	100	-	23.7 ± 1.1	712 ± 6.9	80.2 ± 1.9
8	Cholesterol	E	80	Lac.	24.1 ± 1.4	75 ± 3.1	82.6 ± 2.5
9	Cholesterol	W/E	100	Lac.	20.3 ± 0.8	61 ± 3.5	80.1 ± 2.2
10	DPPC	E	80	Lac.	16.6 ± 0.9	50 ± 2.8	80.1 ± 1.6
11	DPPC	W/E	100	Lac.	33.7 ± 1.5	108 ± 3.7	85.3 ± 2.7
12	DPPC + leucine	W/E	100	Lac.	42.7 ± 1.7	141 ± 4.1	87.9 ± 2.3
C_1^*	-	E	80	Lac.	17.6 ± 1.0	146 ± 2.8	83.4 ± 1.9
C_2^*	-	W/E	100	Lac.	14.4 ± 0.8	116 ± 2.2	81.1 ± 2.1

*C_1 and C_2 are control formulations of 5% (w/v) salbutamol sulfate in spray drying solution.
**E stands for Ethanol, W for Water, and Lac for lactose.

released in less than 30 min, which is in accordance with other studies [35]. In this study, generating inhalable microspheres from SS, cholesterol and ethanol provided a SR profile of the drug. In this regard, several other studies had shown the usefulness of SLmPs in developing SR formulations [7,17,18]. As shown in Figure 3, the release profile of SS from SLmPs produced from cholesterol and ethanol exhibited a burst release of approximately 50%, followed by a sustained SS release pattern over 12 hours, whilst in cholesterol-based SLmPs obtained from water-ethanol solution of SS, no SR profile was observed. This observation can be explained by the fact that the drug has a hydrophilic and ionized nature and does not dissolve in ethanol, so upon application of water and ethanol as the mixed solvent system, the drug mainly partitions into the water phase during the particle formation stage in spray drying chamber, and thus accumulates on the surface of the particle as the water evaporates. However, when the ethanol suspension of the drug is used, it is more likely for SS to be entrapped within the core of SLmPs as it does not dissolve in ethanol and thus does not migrate to lipid surface of the generating microparticles. In contrast, DPPC-based microparticles from ethanol suspension of SS did not show any SR profile, while changing the feed solvent from ethanol to water-ethanol (30:70 v/v) improved the drug entrapment within these DPPC-based SLmPs and exhibited a SR profile over 12 hours with a burst release of nearly 35%. In fact, besides the effect of the solvent, the affinity between the drug and lipid material is another efficient factor, which determines the retention capacity of SLmPs [17]. Herein, DPPC tends to place at the surface of the particles while the drug mostly remains within the aqueous core of the primary particles in the drying chamber before all the water content is subjected to evaporation. Thus, it is possible for DPPC to serve as a SS-retarding carrier in the mentioned inhalable formulation.

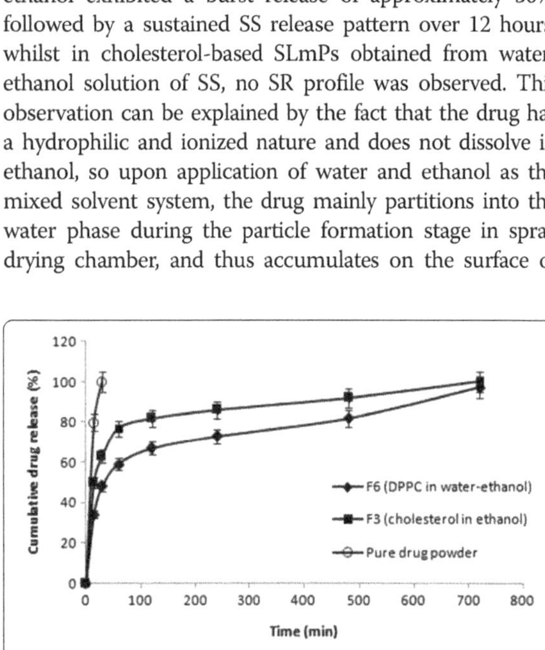

Figure 3 ***In vitro*** **release profile of salbutamol sulfate from different formulations.**

It worth mentioning that, this kind of SR pattern should be justified according to the dissolution rate of the pure drug powder as well as its specific pulmonary delivery rout. In this regard, it can be an acceptable SR pattern for SS DPI formulation since the lung retention time of microparticles is dependent on the generation number of the airway where the inhaled particles are deposited, and our SLmPs showed high FPF indicating that they have the potential to sufficiently penetrate deep into the lungs and avoid mucociliary clearance in the conducting airways. So the prolonged duration of the effect of SS can be expected by the aid of these SLmPs.

Conclusions

The type of lipid, presence of L-leucine in the feed solution, and the solvent system from which the SS-containing SLmPs were spray dried were the factors, which greatly affected the particle morphologies and aerosolization properties. We also observed substantial effects that physical mixing of spray-dried microparticles with coarse carrier can have on the aerosol performance. Among different DPI formulations, powders spray dried from water-ethanol solution of the drug, DPPC and L-leucine which were also physically blended with coarse lactose exhibited the best aerosolization properties. Despite having noticeable burst release during the first hour of the study, some SS-containing SLmPs showed significant release retardation compared the pure drug. The present study suggests that DPPC and L-leucine can be interesting additives for further developments of SS inhalable powder formulations.

Competing interests

The authors declare that they have no competing interests.

Authors' contributions

ZD: Carried out the preparation and characterization of the DPI formulations and drafted the manuscript. KM: Supervisor andparticipated in drafting the manuscript. ARN: Supervisor. HRF: participated in analysis of the drug. MAB: participated in characterization of the powders. All authors read and approved the final manuscript.

Acknowledgements

This study was funded and supported by Tehran University ofMedical Sciences (TUMS); grant no. 87-03-33-7715.

Author details

[1]Aerosol Research Laboratory, Department of Pharmaceutics, School of Pharmacy, Tehran University of Medical Sciences, Tehran, Iran. [2]Medicinal Plants Research Center, Tehran University of Medical Sciences, Tehran, Iran. [3]XRD Research Laboratory, School of Sciences, Tehran University, Tehran, Iran.

References

1. Courrier H, Butz N, Vandamme TF: **Pulmonary drug delivery systems: recent developments and prospects.** *Crit Rev Ther Drug Carrier Syst* 2002, **19**:no. 4–no. 5.
2. Groneberg D, Witt C, Wagner U, Chung K, Fischer A: **Fundamentals of pulmonary drug delivery.** *Resp Med* 2003, **97**:382–387.
3. Labiris N, Dolovich M: **Pulmonary drug delivery. Part I: physiological factors affecting therapeutic effectiveness of aerosolized medications.** *Brit J Clin Pharmacol* 2003, **56**:588–599.
4. Zeng XM, Martin GP, Marriott C: **The controlled delivery of drugs to the lung.** *Int J Pharm* 1995, **124**:149–164.
5. Hardy JG, Chadwick TS: **Sustained release drug delivery to the lungs.** *Clin Pharmacokin* 2000, **39**:1–4.
6. Cook RO, Pannu RK, Kellaway IW: **Novel sustained release microspheres for pulmonary drug delivery.** *J Control Rel* 2005, **104**:79–90.
7. Schreier H, Gonzalez-Rothi RJ, Stecenko AA: **Pulmonary delivery of liposomes.** *J Control Rel* 1993, **24**:209–223.
8. Lu D, Hickey AJ: **Liposomal dry powders as aerosols for pulmonary delivery of proteins.** *AAPS PharmSciTech* 2005, **6**:E641–E648.
9. Abra R, Mihalko PJ, Schreier H: **The effect of lipid composition upon the encapsulation and in vitro leakage of metaproterenol sulfate from 0.2 μm diameter, extruded, multilamellar liposomes.** *J Control Rel* 1990, **14**:71–78.
10. Parthasarathy R, Gilbert B, Mehta K: **Aerosol delivery of liposomal all-trans-retinoic acid to the lungs.** *Cancer Chemother Pharmacol* 1999, **43**:277–283.
11. Pilcer G, Amighi K: **Formulation strategy and use of excipients in pulmonary drug delivery.** *Int J Pharm* 2010, **392**:1–19.
12. Taylor KM, Fan SJ: **Liposomes for drug delivery to the respiratory tract.** *Drug Dev Ind Pharm* 1993, **19**:123–142.
13. Kellaway IW, Farr SJ: **Liposomes as drug delivery systems to the lung.** *Adv Drug Deliv Rev* 1990, **5**:149–161.
14. Niven RW, Schreier H: **Nebulization of liposomes. I. Effects of lipid composition.** *Pharm Res* 1990, **7**:1127–1133.
15. Desai TR, Hancock RE, Finlay WH: **Delivery of liposomes in dry powder form: aerodynamic dispersion properties.** *Eur J Pharm Sci* 2003, **20**:459–467.
16. Jaspart S, Bertholet P, Piel G, Dogné J-M, Delattre L, Evrard B: **Solid lipid microparticles as a sustained release system for pulmonary drug delivery.** *Eur J Pharm Biopharm* 2007, **65**:47–56.
17. Sebti T, Amighi K: **Preparation and in vitro evaluation of lipidic carriers and fillers for inhalation.** *Eur J of Pharm Biopharm* 2006, **63**:51–58.
18. Müller RH, Mäder K, Gohla S: **Solid lipid nanoparticles (SLN) for controlled drug delivery–a review of the state of the art.** *Eur J Pharm Biopharm* 2000, **50**:161–177.
19. Trotta M, Cavalli R, Carlotti M, Battaglia L, Debernardi F: **Solid lipid micro-particles carrying insulin formed by solvent-in-water emulsion–diffusion technique.** *Int J Pharm* 2005, **288**:281–288.
20. Pilcer G, Sebti T, Amighi K: **Formulation and characterization of lipid-coated tobramycin particles for dry powder inhalation.** *Pharm Res* 2006, **23**:931–940.
21. Masters K: *Spray drying handbook.* 5th edition. New York: Longman; 1991.
22. Steckel H, Brandes HG: **A novel spray-drying technique to produce low density particles for pulmonary delivery.** *Int J Pharm* 2004, **278**:187–195.
23. Chow AH, Tong HH, Chattopadhyay P, Shekunov BY: **Particle engineering for pulmonary drug delivery.** *Pharm Res* 2007, **24**:411–437.
24. Son Y-J, McConville JT: **Advancements in dry powder delivery to the lung.** *Drug Dev Ind Pharm* 2008, **34**:948–959.
25. Sanna V, Kirschvink N, Gustin P, Gavini E, Roland I, Delattre L, Evrard B: **Preparation and in vivo toxicity study of solid lipid microparticles as carrier for pulmonary administration.** *AAPS PharmSciTech* 2004, **5**:17–23.
26. Nassimi M, Schleh C, Lauenstein H, Hussein R, Hoymann H, Koch W, Pohlmann G, Krug N, Sewald K, Rittinghausen S: **A toxicological evaluation of inhaled solid lipid nanoparticles used as a potential drug delivery system for the lung.** *Eur J Pharm Biopharm* 2010, **75**:107–116.
27. Smolensky M, D'alonzo G, Kunkel G, Barnes P: **Day-night patterns in bronchial patency and dyspnea: basis for once-daily and unequally divided twice-daily theophylline dosing schedules.** *Chronobiol Int* 1987, **4**:303–317.
28. Chew NY, Shekunov BY, Tong HH, Chow AH, Savage C, Wu J, Chan HK: **Effect of amino acids on the dispersion of disodium cromoglycate powders.** *J Pharm Sci* 2005, **94**:2289–2300.
29. Salama RO, Traini D, Chan H-K, Young PM: **Preparation and characterisation of controlled release co-spray dried drug–polymer microparticles for inhalation 2: Evaluation of in vitro release profiling methodologies for controlled release respiratory aerosols.** *Eur J Pharm Biopharm* 2008, **70**:145–152.
30. Al-Asheh S, Jumah R, Banat F, Hammad S: **The use of experimental factorial design for analysing the effect of spray dryer operating variables on the production of tomato powder.** *Food Bioprod Process* 2003, **81**:81–88.
31. Ståhl K, Claesson M, Lilliehorn P, Lindén H, Bäckström K: **The effect of process variables on the degradation and physical properties of spray dried insulin intended for inhalation.** *Int J Pharm* 2002, **233**:227–237.
32. Vehring R: **Pharmaceutical particle engineering via spray drying.** *Pharm Res* 2008, **25**:999–1022.
33. Lechuga-Ballesteros D, Charan C, Stults CL, Stevenson CL, Miller DP, Vehring R, Tep V, Kuo MC: **Trileucine improves aerosol performance and stability of spray-dried powders for inhalation.** *J Pharm Sci* 2008, **97**:287–302.
34. Srichana T, Brain A, Marriott C, Martin GP: **A study of drug-carrier interactions in dry powder inhaler formulations using the Andersen cascade impactor, X-ray microanalysis and time of flight aerosol beam spectrometry (TOFABS).** *Chem Pharm Bull* 2000, **48**:167–174.
35. Scalia S, Salama R, Young P, Traini D: **Preparation and in vitro evaluation of salbutamol-loaded lipid microparticles for sustained release pulmonary therapy.** *J Microencap* 2012, **29**:225–233.

36. Yu J, Chien YW: **Pulmonary drug delivery: physiologic and mechanistic aspects.** *Crit Rev Ther Drug Carrier Syst* 1997, **14**:395–453.
37. Bosquillon C, Lombry C, Preat V, Vanbever R: **Comparison of particle sizing techniques in the case of inhalation dry powders.** *J Pharm Sci* 2001, **90**:2032–2041.
38. Zeng XM, Martin GP, Marriott C: *Particulate Interactions in Dry Powder Formulation for Inhalation.* London: Taylor & Francis; 2000.

14

Surface modification of PLGA nanoparticles via human serum albumin conjugation for controlled delivery of docetaxel

Saeed Manoochehri[1], Behrad Darvishi[1], Golnaz Kamalinia[2], Mohsen Amini[3], Mahdieh Fallah[4], Seyed Naser Ostad[5], Fatemeh Atyabi[1,2] and Rassoul Dinarvand[1,2*]

Abstract

Background: Poly lactic-co-glycolic acid (PLGA) based nanoparticles are considered to be a promising drug carrier in tumor targeting but suffer from the high level of opsonization by reticuloendothelial system due to their hydrophobic structure. As a result surface modification of these nanoparticles has been widely studied as an essential step in their development. Among various surface modifications, human serum albumin (HSA) possesses advantages including small size, hydrophilic surface and accumulation in leaky vasculature of tumors through passive targeting and a probable active transport into tumor tissues.

Methods: PLGA nanoparticles of docetaxel were prepared by emulsification evaporation method and were surface conjugated with human serum albumin. Fourier transform infrared spectrum was used to confirm the conjugation reaction where nuclear magnetic resonance was utilized for conjugation ratio determination. In addition, transmission electron microscopy showed two different contrast media in conjugated nanoparticles. Furthermore, cytotoxicity of free docetaxel, unconjugated and conjugated PLGA nanoparticles was studied in HepG2 cells.

Results: Size, zeta potential and drug loading of PLGA nanoparticles were about 199 nm, −11.07 mV, and 4%, respectively where size, zeta potential and drug loading of conjugated nanoparticles were found to be 204 nm, −5.6 mV and 3.6% respectively. Conjugated nanoparticles represented a three-phasic release pattern with a 20% burst effect for docetaxel on the first day. Cytotoxicity experiment showed that the IC50 of HSA conjugated PLGA nanoparticles (5.4 μg) was significantly lower than both free docetaxel (20.2 μg) and unconjugated PLGA nanoparticles (6.2 μg).

Conclusion: In conclusion surface modification of PLGA nanoparticles through HSA conjugation results in more cytotoxicity against tumor cell lines compared with free docetaxel and unconjugated PLGA nanoparticles. Albumin conjugated PLGA nanoparticles may represent a promising drug delivery system in cancer therapy.

Keywords: PLGA nanoparticles, Surface modification, Human serum albumin, Emulsion evaporation, Tumor targeting, Docetaxel

* Correspondence: dinarvand@tums.ac.ir
[1]Department of Pharmaceutics, Faculty of Pharmacy, Tehran University of Medical Sciences, Tehran 1417614411, Iran
[2]Nanotechnology Research Centre, Tehran University of Medical Sciences, Tehran, Iran
Full list of author information is available at the end of the article

Background

Polymeric nanoparticles are considered as one of the most promising carrier systems for cytotoxic drug delivery and have received a great deal of attention during the recent years. Poly lactic-co-glycolic acid (PLGA) based nanoparticulate system is one of the most successful and interesting colloidal systems. PLGA nanoparticles (NPs) protect the therapeutic agents and increase their stability and can be used for controlled delivery of therapeutics with improved pharmacokinetic and pharmacodynamic profile. Furthermore, PLGA is approved by United States Food and Drug Administration (FDA) and European Medicine Agency (EMA) for various drug delivery formulations. However, PLGA NPs, suffer from a significant limitation due to their high level of opsonization by reticuloendothelial system (RES) [1]. To address this negative aspect, several methods and procedures have been utilized for surface modification of PLGA NPs in order to produce PLGA based nanoparticulate systems which are not readily recognized by RES. This goal has been achieved by PLGA NPs surface coating with more hydrophilic agents to cover their hydrophobic surface and provide stealth nanoparticles. Various agents have been used for this purpose including polyethylene glycol (PEG), poloxamers and chitosan molecules to neutralize or reduce the negative zeta potential of PLGA NPs and reduce their phagocytosis by RES [2]. However, surface modified PLGA NPs have been found to highly localize in liver tissue due to the rigidity of the PLGA core which has triggered many research studies to improve surface modification methods for achieving better outcomes [3,4].

Among various available agents, human serum albumin (HSA) seems to be a promising molecule for surface modification of PLGA NPs. HSA is known to be the most abundant native protein in human body which has various advantages including ready availability, biodegradability, and low toxicity and immunogenicity [5]. HSA has received special interest in drug delivery studies due to its ability for passive targeting through enhanced permeation and retention (EPR) effect which is related to both "enhanced permeation" of macromolecules through the fenestrated structure of tumor vasculature in addition to an "enhanced retention" which is considered to be related to the lack of effective lymphatic drainage in tumor tissues [6]. Furthermore it has been postulated that active targeting of HSA coated nanoparticles occurs through special albumin receptors on tumor cell membranes [7].

Surface modification of PLGA NPs by grafting protein molecules has been previously reported and various proteins including transferrin and wheat germ agglutinin have been coated on the surface of PLGA NPs through covalent conjugation. The created stealth NPs have successfully increased the cellular uptake of PLGA NPs and have resulted in a greater antiproliferative activity and better cytotoxicity in vitro. In addition in vivo experiments have confirmed a higher tumor accumulation for the above surface coated NPs [8-10]. HSA coating by non-covalent interactions have also been studied where protein molecules only saturate the nanoparticles surface and no covalent linking occurs [11].

Herein, docetaxel (DTX), a cytostatic agent with very low water solubility was encapsulated in PLGA NPs produced by a modified emulsification evaporation method and was subjected to surface modification by HSA molecules through a carbodiimide conjugation reaction. Surface modification created a stealth core shell structure and was used to reduce the negative charge on PLGA NPs along with an increase in drug efficiency through passive targeting. These newly developed fully biodegradable HSA coated PLGA NPs can increase DTX water solubility and will eliminate the need for Tween 80 utilization in DTX formulations which has been taken responsible for many of DTX injections side effects including hypersensitivity reactions [12]. The nanoparticles were further evaluated for their cytotoxic effect in HepG2 cell line. The present evidences suggest that HSA stealth PLGA NPs may represent a promising nanoparticulate drug delivery system for DTX and other anticancer agents.

Methods

Materials

PLGA (50:50, 504H, MW = 48 kDa) was purchased from Boehringer-Ingelheim (Ingelheim, Germany). HSA, 1-ethyl-3-(3-dimethylaminopropyl) carbodiimide (EDC), N–hydroxysuccinimide (NHS) and 3-(4,5-dimethyathiazol-2-yl)-2,5-diphenyltetrazoliumbromide (MTT) were purchased from Sigma-Aldrich (St. Louis, MO, USA). Dulbecco's modified eagle's medium (DMEM), fetal bovine serum (FBS) and penicillin and streptomycin antibiotic mixture were obtained from Life technologies (grand Island, NY, USA).Polyvinyl alcohol (PVA) was obtained from Acros (Geel, Belgium). 2-(N-morpholinoethansulfonicacid) (MES) was purchased from Fluka (St. Louis, MO, USA). DTX was from Cipla (Mumbai, India). All other solvents and reagents unless otherwise stated were from Merck (Darmstadt, Germany).

Preparation of PLGA nanoparticles

PLGA NPs were fabricated using a modified emulsification/ evaporation method [12]. Briefly, PVA (0.5% w/w) was dissolved in deionized water providing the aqueous phase where MES buffer (50 mmol) was used for pH adjustment (pH = 5). In organic phase, PLGA and docetaxel were dissolved in mixtures with various ratios of acetone and dichloromethane and the resulting organic phase was slowly added to the aqueous phase using an ultrasonic probe (Misonix, USA) equipped with a microtip (power: 11 watt, time: 5 min). During sonication, the whole system was placed in an ice bath to prevent any loss of the oil phase due to evaporation and the mixture was magnetically stirred overnight. The experiment was conducted with 10% and 20% organic phase to water phase ratio to evaluate the effect of oil: water ratio on the formed nanoparticles characteristics. Purification of nanoparticles was achieved by three times centrifugation with a high speed centrifuge (21,000 g for 30 minutes) at 10°C (Sigma 3 K30, Ostrode, Germany) to remove any extra PVA from the NPs surface. The isolated NPs were then lyophilized into a fine cake.

Surface modification of PLGA NPs by HSA conjugation

PLGA NPs were conjugated with HSA through a carbodiimide coupling reaction. For this purpose, PLGA carboxylic functional groups were first activated through exposure with 15 mg EDC and 12 mg NHS for 5 h right after their preparation in a medium consisting of MES buffer (pH = 5, 50 mmol). The activated NPs were then purified by three times centrifugation (21,000 g for 30 minutes) at 10°C to remove any remnants of PVA, EDC and NHS.

The activated PLGA nanoparticles were then exposed to HSA solution in 40 ml phosphate buffered saline (PBS, pH = 7.4) with an equimolar concentration in a dropwise manner and under constant stirring. The conjugated NPs were then isolated by a centrifugation step (15,000 g for 30 minutes) at 10°C and the supernatant was removed. Conjugated NPs were then subjected to the lyophilization process for long term storage.

Determination of HSA conjugated PLGA NPs molecular structure

For determining the number of free carboxylic moieties in activated PLGA NPs and further calculation of the activation ratio a Bruker 500 MHz ^{1}H-NMR system (Bruker, Germany) was used and the resulting nuclear magnetic resonance (NMR) spectrum was utilized to characterize the substitution degree of activated PLGA.

Fourier transform infrared (FT-IR) spectroscopy was used to characterize the molecular structure of PLGA NPs conjugated with HSA and to confirm the structural changes occurred after HSA conjugation. Lyophilized samples were placed on KBr disks and their FT-IR spectra were recorded by a Nicolet (Magna IR-550, USA) spectrophotometer.

NPs characterization and morphology evaluation

PLGA and PLGA NPs conjugated with HSA were fully characterized and their size, poly dispersity index (PDI) and zeta potential were determined by dynamic light scattering (DLS) (Malvern Zetasizer, ZS, Malvern, UK).

To evaluate the particles morphology, PLGA NPs were coated with gold under vacuum conditions and their morphology was evaluated by scanning electron microscopy (SEM) (FE-SEM, S4160, Hitachi, Japan).

Furthermore, transmission electron microscope (TEM) (Zeiss EM10C, Carl Zeiss AG, Oberkochen, Germany) was used to evaluate the surface morphology of PLGA NPs conjugated with HSA.

Differential scanning calorimetry (DSC) was performed for PLGA NPs conjugated with HSA in addition to a physical mixture of PLGA, HSA and DTX with a Mettler DSC 823 unit (Mettler Toledo, Switzerland) and a Julabo thermocryostate model FT100Y (Julabo labortechnik, Germany) where Indium was utilized for instrument calibration. The scanning took place between 20 to 200°C with a thermal scan rate of 10°C per minute.

Determination of DTX concentration, drug loading and entrapment efficiency in nanoparticles

The extent of DTX loading in PLGA and PLGA NPs conjugated with HSA was investigated by a previously published method [13]. Briefly, a small amount of PLGA NPs (2 mg) was dispersed in 2 ml acetonitrile resulting in PLGA and DTX dissolution in acetonitrile medium. In the next step methanol was added to the above mixture and resulted in PLGA precipitation. This solution only contained DTX and was injected to high pressure liquid chromatography (HPLC) (Knauer apparatus model K-1001 Wellchrome (Berlin, Germany) equipped with a PDA K-2700 ultraviolet Detector (Knauer, Berlin, Germany). A C18 column (internal diameter: 0.46 cm, length: 25 cm, pore size: 5 μm, ODS 3-MZ, Germany) was used as stationary phase and acetonitrile: water mixture (65: 35) was used as the mobile phase. The analysis was performed in 230 nm wavelength at 25°C and DTX concentration was evaluated accordingly. Furthermore, "drug loading" which is calculated as the ratio between DTX (expressed as μg) and the PLGA NPs (expressed as mg) in addition to "entrapment efficiency" or the percent of drug loaded in PLGA nanoparticles to the initial amount of DTX were determined.

DTX release from PLGA nanoparticles

Dialysis technique was used to evaluate drug release from PLGA NPs [14]. A dialysis tube (molecular weight cut-off: 8 kDa) containing 2 mg of nanoparticles suspended in 5 ml PBS (pH = 7.4) was dipped in a medium consisting of 20 ml PBS (pH =7.4) containing 0.1% Tween 80 and was continuously stirred on a shaker incubator for over 14 days at 37°C. At selected time intervals, 15 mL of the medium was removed and the medium was replenished with freshly prepared PBS. The aliquots were then exposed to dichloromethane for liquid-liquid extraction of DTX. The extraction procedure was repeated three times and the extracted organic phase was evaporated and the remnants were dissolved in 200 μl acetonitrile and were subjected to

HPLC analysis. Drug release data were expressed as the percentage of the cumulative amount of drug release.

In vitro cytotoxicity of DTX encapsulated NPs

HepG2 (Human hepatocellular carcinoma) cells were obtained from Pasteur Institute of Iran (Tehran, Iran) and were cultivated and maintained in DMEM growth media supplemented with 10% FBS and 1% penicillin streptomycin antibiotic mixture. The cells were incubated at 37°C in a humidified atmosphere with 5% CO_2 and the culture media was exchanged every other day. Cells were seeded in 96 wells with a density of 1×10^4 cells per well and were incubated for 24 h to allow cellular attachment. Cells were then treated with different concentrations of free DTX, PLGA NPs and PLGA NPs conjugated with HSA for 96 hand were then exposed to 20 μL of MTT reagent (5 mg/mL per well) for an additional 4 h. The culture media was then discarded and 200 μL dimethylsulfoxide was added to each well to dissolve the formed formazan crystals. Optical density was then measured at 570 nm with a 660 nm background using a microplate reader (Anthos 2020; Anthos Labtec Instruments, Wals, Austria). Each experiment was performed in triplicate and cellular viability was expressed as the percentage of viable cells to control. IC50 was calculated from the cell viability data as the drug concentration in which cell growth was inhibited by 50%. Furthermore similar MTT assays were performed with drug free PLGA NPs and conjugated PLGA NPs with HSA to assess any intrinsic carrier toxicity.

Results and Discussion

PLGA nanoparticles preparation and characterization

PLGA nanoparticles were prepared by a modified emulsification evaporation method (Figure 1). In this method the organic phase solution containing DTX and PLGA provides the oil phase (O) and PVA aqueous solution serves as the water phase (W) in an O/W emulsion. Physical sonication induction reduces the size of nano droplets in this emulsion. The particulate characteristics of prepared PLGA NPs in addition to their drug loading and entrapment efficiency are shown in Table 1. As it is observed PLGA NPs had an average size of 180 to 221 nm and were monodispersed as confirmed by their PDI amounts which was less than or equal to 0.23. Nanoparticles drug loading was achieved by drug incorporation into PLGA NPs during the production process and a maximum 5.35% drug loading with about 48% entrapment efficiency was achieved. The formed NPs carried a negatively charged zeta potential of about -11mv.

Size is the most important and effective parameter in determining the cellular uptake and biological functions of colloidal systems where a reduced size will usually result in significantly better uptake of nanoparticles by tumor cells [15]. It has been demonstrated that emulsion fabrication is the most critical step during the preparation of nanoparticles where the size of emulsion droplets is directly relevant to the final nanoparticles size [16,17]. Various factors may affect the size of PLGA NPs including the stabilizer type and the oil phase solvent mixture composition.

The oil phase solvent mixture here was composed of various ratios of dichloromethane and acetone. As shown in Figure 2A, nanoparticles size decreased as a result of reducing the acetone to dichloromethane ratio in the oil phase mixture where the smallest size was achieved by a 40:60 (acetone: dichloromethane) ratio. This may be due to a decrease in the interfacial tension between the oil phase and aqueous phase with increasing the portion of acetone in the oil phase mixture. It has been reported that

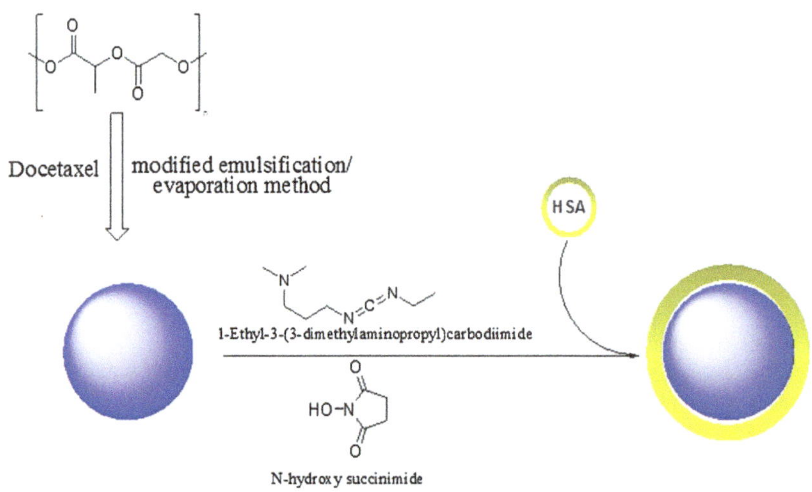

Figure 1 PLGA and conjugated PLGA nanoparticles with HSA formation process.

Table 1 PLGA nanoparticles and PLGA nanoparticles conjugated with HSA characteristics (DCM: dichloromethane, O: oil phase, W: water phase, HSA: human serum albumin, PLGA: Poly (lactic-co-glycolic acid), PDI: polydispersity index and EE: entrapment efficiency)

Sample	Acetone: DCM	O:W ratio (%)	HSA:PLGA	Size (nm)	PDI	Zeta potential (mv)	E.E (%)	Loading (μg/mg)
1	2.5:97.5	20	-	221 ± 25	0.23 ± 0.02	−13.48 ± 1.8	18.5 ± 2.1	2.06 ± 0.18
2	10:90	20	-	195 ± 19	0.15 ± 0.01	−11.71 ± 2.1	25.2 ± 1.8	2.8 ± 0.41
3	20:80	20	-	188 ± 28	0.14 ± 0.01	−15.32 ± 2.3	9.3 ± 1.6	1.0 ± 0.2
4	40:60	20	-	180 ± 29	0.20 ± 0.02	−11.13 ± 1.9	6.2 ± 1.1	0.7 ± 0.05
5	5:95	10	-	204 ± 20	0.15 ± 0.02	−11.52 ± 1.5	13.5 ± 1.1	1.5 ± 0.1
6	10:90	10	-	199 ± 22	0.17 ± 0.01	−11.07 ± 1.8	48.2 ± 2.3	5.35 ± 0.33
7	20:80	10	-	189 ± 19	0.18 ± 0.02	−9.83 ± 1.3	9.46 ± 1.4	1.05 ± 0.07
8	30:70	10	-	186 ± 22	0.16 ± 0.01	−11.08 ± 1.4	2.8 ± 0.7	0.3 ± 0.03
9	40:60	10	-	180 ± 21	0.20 ± 0.02	−11.02 ± 1.7	7.6 ± 1.5	0.85 ± 0.1
10	10:90	10	50:50	204 ± 15	0.14 ± 0.01	−5.6 ± 0.21	33.7 ± 2.6	3.62 ± 0.42
11	10:90	10	75:25	221 ± 24	0.17 ± 0.01	−5.45 ± 0.24	34.2 ± 2.1	3.53 ± 0.37

during the emulsification process the two organic and aqueous phases are not in equilibrium and the acetone concentration is not homogenous at the interface of oil and water phases. Acetone diffuses through the higher viscosity oil phase resulting in an acetone concentration gradient which creates some perturbation and turbulence in the interface of the two phases. This perturbation further results in a larger interface area between the oil droplets and aqueous medium and creates extremely fine nano droplets which result in the formation of small sized nanoparticles. The interfacial tension decrease between the oil and water phases due to the presence of acetone in the organic solvent mixture in addition to acetone passive diffusion from nano droplets and the subsequent spontaneous mixing will result in PLGA NPs formation with a much smaller size [17].

Besides the size of NPs, loading and entrapment efficiency are also affected by acetone to dichloromethane ratio. As it is observed in Figure 2B, loading is decreased with increasing the acetone: dichloromethane ratio from 10:90 to 40:60. In addition entrapment efficiency shows the same trend and a decrease in this parameter is observed with increasing acetone to dichloromethane ratio. DTX has poor water solubility and favors the organic phase during oil in water emulsion preparation. This higher drug affinity to the oil core results in a higher drug loading and better entrapment efficiency [18]. However when acetone to dichloromethane ratio is very low, both loading and entrapment efficiency are significantly decreased which may be related to the high DTX solubility in acetone solutions [19]. On the other hand when acetone to dichloromethane ratio is increased, some of the drug molecules dissolved in the oil core may disperse out along with acetone. This results in some sort of drug leak and will decrease the drug loading [17].

In addition to the oil phase composition, the ratio of oil to water is another factor which may impact the evaporation phase and nanoparticles formation process. Decreasing the

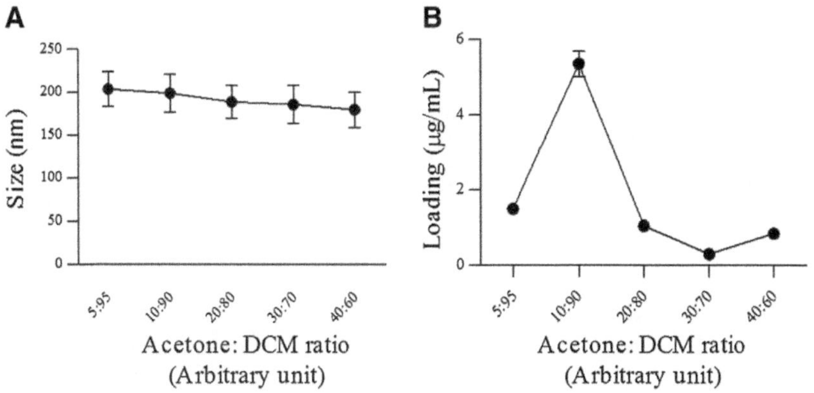

Figure 2 The effect of acetone to dichloromethane ratio on PLGA nanoparticles size (A) and drug loading (B).

oil to water ratio from 20% to 10% has mildly increased the nanoparticles size along with a slight increase in their entrapment efficiency and drug loading (Table 1). It has been postulated that when the aqueous phase volume is increased in relation to oil phase, the droplets external energy which is the cause of droplets breakage is distributed in a higher volume and a lower droplet breakage and an elevated particle size will be achieved [20,21].

Nanoparticles stabilization and protection of the droplets is another important step in the emulsification process which is achieved by addition of surfactant molecules. These surfactants prevent drops coalescence and result in a better size. In this study 0.5% PVA was used as a stabilizer to create a cover between organic and aqueous phases interface and provide effective stabilization [22,23].

PLGA NPs size and morphology was further evaluated by SEM microscopy which showed roughly spherical particles (Figure 3). It is noteworthy that NPs showed a larger size when evaluated by DLS compared to SEM images which may be due to the swelling of particles when dispersed in the aqueous medium [16].

Characterization of PLGA nanoparticles conjugated with HSA

HSA was conjugated to carboxylic functional groups on PLGA structure through a carbodiimide meditated coupling reaction Figure 1). FT-IR spectra of PLGA, HSA, their physical mixture and PLGA NPs conjugated with HSA are shown in Figure 4. As it can be seen, free PLGA ester and acid bonds absorption peaks can be observed in 1760 (cm^{-1}) and 1713 (cm^{-1}). In free HSA the amide bond stretch region was observed in 1650 (cm^{-1}). When HSA conjugated PLGA nanoparticles spectrum was evaluated, 1760 (cm^{-1}), 1713 (cm^{-1}) and 1650 (cm^{-1}) absorption peaks were observed which confirms the presence of both PLGA and HSA structures in the conjugated NPs.

Activated PLGA NPs structure was further evaluated by its ^{1}H NMR spectra to predict the ratio of covalently conjugated carboxylic functional groups on PLGA NPs. For this purpose area under the curve of NHS peak at 2.0 ppm was compared with area under the curve of PLGA peaks at 5.4, 4.9 and 1.5 ppm in activated PLGA NMR spectra. It was found that about 30% of PLGA carboxylic acid moieties were involved in PLGA activation reaction where about 70% of carboxylic functional groups remained free. This suggests a 30% conjugation ratio between PLGA and HSA.

To further evaluate HSA conjugated PLGA nanoparticles, size and zeta potential of these particles were evaluated and were compared with unconjugated PLGA NPs (Table 1). As it is observed, the size of PLGA NPs conjugated with HSA was slightly increased in comparison to PLGA NPs.

Zeta potential which is another important nanoparticle characteristic and can influence particle stability and cell adhesion was also measured in PLGA NPs conjugated with HSA [24]. As shown in Table 1, the zeta potential of PLGA NPs conjugated with HSA showed a negative zeta potential, which was smaller than that of PLGA NPs (-11.07 ± 1.8 mV vs. -5.6 ± 0.21 mV). This decrease in negative zeta potential is probably due to the involvement of carboxylic functional groups on PLGA NPs in amide bond formation with amino moieties on lysine amino acids in HSA primary structure [25].

Entrapment efficiency and loading of PLGA NPs and PLGA NPs conjugated with HSA are shown in Table 1. As it is shown, the entrapment efficiency and drug loading in PLGA NPs conjugated with HSA were slightly less than PLGA NPs.

PLGA NPs morphology was evaluated by TEM imaging (Figure 5). As it is observed PLGA NPs were almost spherical with a size of about 200 nm where HSA conjugated NPs showed a slightly larger size. PLGA NPs were uniform but a notable outer layer was observed in

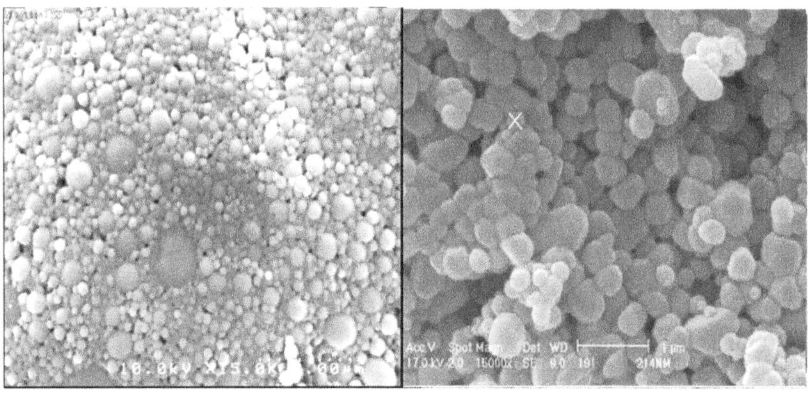

Figure 3 Poly (lactic-co-glycolic acid) (PLGA) nanoparticles morphology acquired by scanning electron microscopy with 15,000 times magnification.

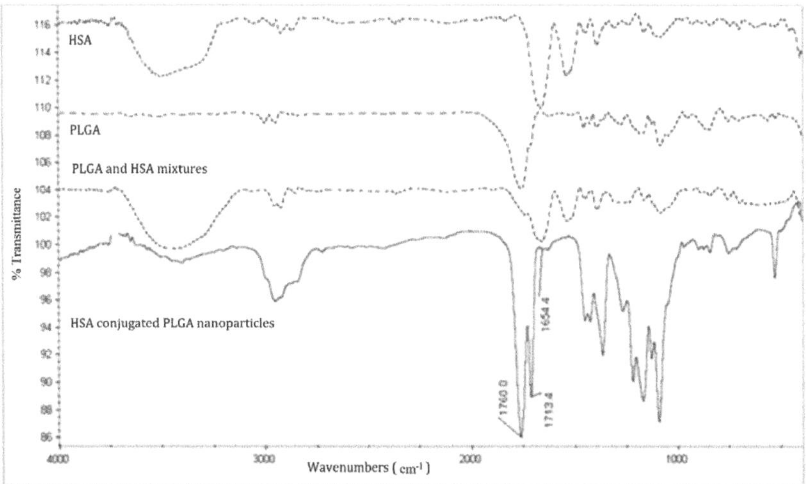

Figure 4 FT-IR spectrum of HSA, PLGA, their physical mixture and PLGA NPs conjugated with HSA (PLGA major absorption peaks are observed in 1760 (cm^{-1}) and 1713 (cm^{-1}) where HSA major absorption peak comes in 1650 (cm^{-1})).

conjugated NPs. It seems that HSA, have formed a mushroom structure on NPs surface which is in accordance with the predicted core-shell structure and may be able to prevent PLGA NPs opsonization more effectively [26].

Drug polymer mixtures may exist in various forms and structures for example amorphous or crystalline drug in combination with an amorphous or crystalline polymer [27]. DSC was utilized here to examine the thermal transitions in PLGA NPs and PLGA NPs conjugated with HSA.

Figure 6 shows DSC thermograms of PLGA, DTX, HSA, PLGA NPs and PLGA NPs conjugated with HSA in addition to a physical mixture of PLGA, DTX and HSA. As it can be seen, PLGA has an endothermic glassy transition temperature around 50°C. Glassy transition endothermic process for HSA conjugated NPs was observed at about 60°C. In the physical mixture thermogram a peak is observed in 160°C which stands for DTX melting point peak in its crystalline form. This peak is not observed in PLGA NPs and PLGA NPs conjugated with HSA which suggests an absence of crystallinity and an amorphous structure for DTX molecules in these NPs [28,29].

DTX release pattern from PLGA and HSA conjugated PLGA NPs

Various factors may affect drug release behavior from PLGA NPs including the polymer type and composition and drug-polymer interactions. In vitro drug release pattern from PLGA and PLGA NPs conjugated with HSA is shown as the cumulative percentage of release in Figure 7. DTX release from PLGA NPs followed a bi-phasic pattern. As shown in Figure 7, a burst release occurs within 10 h when roughly 40% of the drug was released from the

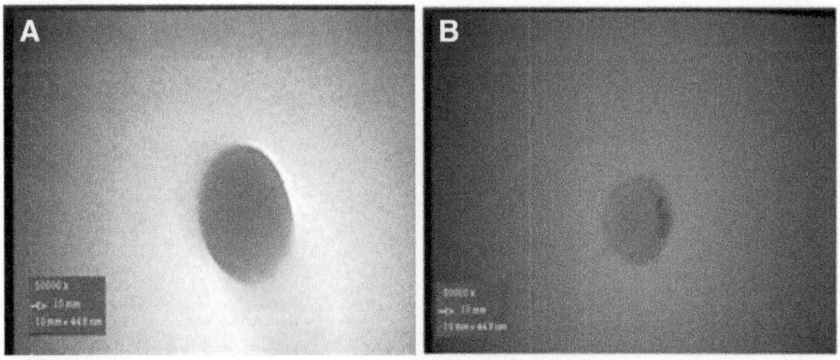

Figure 5 Appearance of A) PLGA nanoparticle and B) PLGA nanoparticle conjugated with HSA acquired by transmission electron microscopy with 50,000 times magnification (Conjugation has occurred in the surface of PLGA nanoparticles where phase contrast is clearly observe).

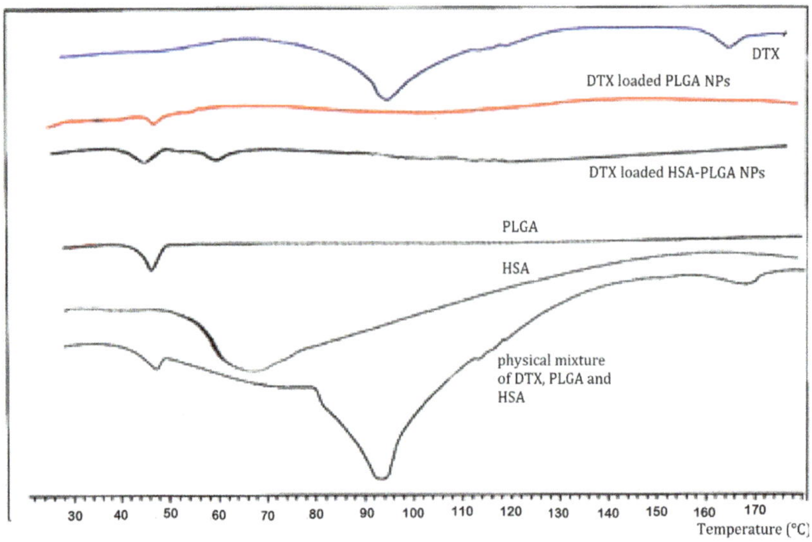

Figure 6 DSC thermograms of PLGA, HSA, DTX and DTX loaded in PLGA NP conjugated with HSA (Peaks of PLGA, HSA, and DTX was observed at 48°C, 60°C and 160°C. In DTX encapsulated HSA-PLGA nanoparticles, PLGA peak was observed at 48°C, HSA peak was observed at 60°C and no peak was observed at 160°C indicating the amorphous structure of DTX in this nanoparticulate formulation).

nanoparticles. The rest of DTX was released with a slower rate within 12 days. This initial burst release may be related to the portion of DTX molecules which are adsorbed on nanoparticle's surface and the diffusion controlled drug dissolution of drug molecules at nanoparticles and medium interface [30]. In addition the release of DTX molecules which are encapsulated near the surface of PLGA NPs may also contribute in this initial burst release. The slower second phase is related to the entrapped DTX inside the polymeric NPs.

The release profile of DTX from PLGA NPs conjugated with HSA exhibited a three-phasic pattern (Figure 7). 20% initial burst release occurred at the first day and in the next 8 days 75% of DTX was released. The rest of the drug was eventually released within 4 days. Comparing the release pattern of these two nanoparticles demonstrated that the release rate of DTX from conjugated NPs was slower and followed a three phasic pattern including an initial burst phase, a second release phase and a much slower final drug release phase.

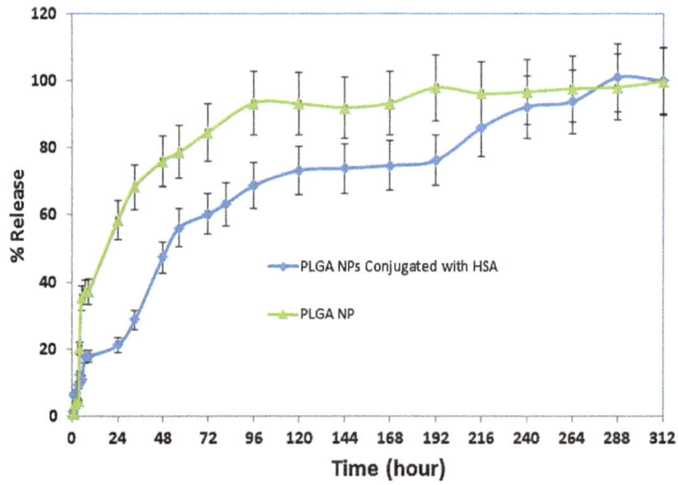

Figure 7 DTX release pattern from PLGA NPs and PLGA NPs conjugated with HSA in PBS medium (pH = 7.4). In PLGA NPs, 40% burst release of DTX occurred in the first 10 hours. The drug was then released slowly within 12 days (green line); In PLGA NPs conjugated with HSA, 20% burst release of DTX occurred within 24 hours and the overall release rate was much slower compared to PLGA NPs (blue line).

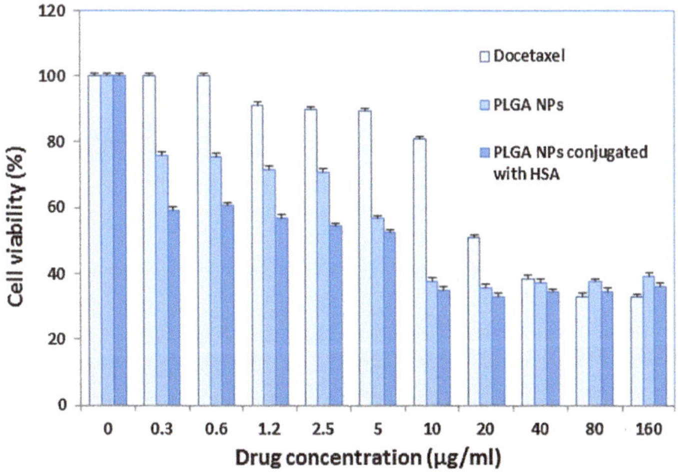

Figure 8 Cell viability in HepG2 cell line in exposure to free DTX, DTX encapsulated PLGA NPs and DTX encapsulated HSA-PLG NPs with various concentrations against Hep-G2 assessed by MTT assay (n = 3).

The graph shows that surface treatment with HSA molecules has resulted in a reduced initial burst where only 20% of drug is released during the first 24 h from HSA conjugated NPs in comparison to around 60% in unconjugated NPs. This lower burst effect is probably due to a decrease in the amount of drug which is adsorbed on the surface of conjugated NPs [9].

In vitro cytotoxicity assay

To assess the cellular cytotoxicity of PLGA NPs and PLGA NPs conjugated with HSA, HepG2 cell line was used. HepG2 cell line has been recognized as a suitable model for cytotoxicity evaluating studies [31]. Following 72 h of exposure to both unconjugated and conjugated NPs, cell viability was assessed by MTT assay and IC50 values of free DTX and its formulations were estimated from the results as presented in Figure 8. The IC50 of free DTX, PLGA NPs and PLGA NPs conjugated with HSA were 20.2 ± 0.28, 6.2 ± 0.23 and 5.4 ± 0.21 μg respectively after 72 h incubation with the cell line ($n = 3$). These results may be explained by drug release pattern of various PLGA particulate formulations and their degradation profiles. When DTX is encapsulated in PLGA or PLGA NPs conjugated with HSA a higher DTX concentration may be delivered to the intracellular space which may be the result of the small size of nanoparticles and the passive targeting of macromolecules due to EPR effect. As a result a better efficacy and a lower IC50 is observed for HSA conjugated with PLGA NPs [32].

It should be mentioned that in PLGA NPs conjugated with HSA, the outer layer, HSA, creates a stealth surface which reduces NPs interaction (both interactions between NPs and interaction between cells and NPs) [33].

It is noteworthy that no cellular cytotoxic effect was observed when drug free PLGA NPs and drug free PLGA NPs conjugated with HSA were exposed to HepG2 cell line which confirms these carriers safety.

Conclusions

In this study surface modified PLGA NPs with HSA were developed to prepare a novel drug delivery particulate system which may preferentially target tumor tissues through passive targeting. Specific features of HSA such as its biocompatibility and accumulation in inflamed and tumor tissues make it a good candidate for surface functionalization of carriers. Herein, PLGA NPs conjugated with HSA were developed and fully characterized. The newly developed NPs had an acceptable size and zeta potential and showed promising results in cell culture investigation where a lower IC50 was observed for the conjugated nanoparticles in comparison with free DTX and unconjugated PLGA NPs. It seems that surface modification of PLGA NPs with human serum albumin may represent a promising approach for nanoparticulate delivery system for cytostatic agent delivery.

Competing interests

The authors declare that they have no competing interests.

Authors' contributions

SM conceived the study, carried out the experiments and drafted the manuscript. BD helped with the characterization of the nanoparticles, GK reviewed and revised the manuscript. MA supervised the synthesis and characterization of copolymers, MF assisted in preparation of the manuscript, SNO supervised the MTT assay and cell culture study, FA co-supervised the study, RD designed, coordinated and supervised the study and is the corresponding author of the manuscript. All authors read and approved the final manuscript.

Acknowledgements
This paper is the outcome of a PhD thesis of the first author and was financially supported by Nanotechnology Research Centre, Faculty of Pharmacy, Tehran University of Medical Sciences.

Author details
[1]Department of Pharmaceutics, Faculty of Pharmacy, Tehran University of Medical Sciences, Tehran 1417614411, Iran. [2]Nanotechnology Research Centre, Tehran University of Medical Sciences, Tehran, Iran. [3]Department of Medicinal Chemistry, Faculty of Pharmacy, Tehran University of Medical Sciences, Tehran, Iran. [4]Arash Hospital, Faculty of Medicine, Tehran University of Medical Sciences, Tehran, Iran. [5]Department of Toxicology and Pharmacology, Faculty of Pharmacy, Tehran University of Medical Sciences, Tehran, Iran.

References

1. Dinarvand R, Sepehri N, Manoochehri S, Rouhani H, Atyabi F: **Polylactide-co-glycolide nanoparticles for controlled delivery of anticancer agents.** *Int J Nanomedicine* 2011, **6**:877.
2. Danhier F, Ansorena E, Silva JM, Coco R, Le Breton A, Préat V: **PLGA-based nanoparticles: an overview of biomedical applications.** *J Control Release* 2012, **161**:505–522.
3. Chung YI, Kim JC, Kim YH, Tae G, Lee SY, Kim K, Kwon IC: **The effect of surface functionalization of PLGA nanoparticles by heparin-or chitosan-conjugated Pluronic on tumor targeting.** *J Control Release* 2010, **143**:374–382.
4. Park J, Mattessich T, Jay SM, Agawu A, Saltzman WM, Fahmy TM: **Enhancement of surface ligand display on PLGA nanoparticles with amphiphilic ligand conjugates.** *J Control Release* 2011, **156**:109–115.
5. Kratz F: **Albumin as a drug carrier: design of prodrugs, drug conjugates and nanoparticles.** *J Control Release* 2008, **132**:171–183.
6. Maeda H, Wu J, Sawa T, Matsumura Y, Hori K: **Tumor vascular permeability and the EPR effect in macromolecular therapeutics: a review.** *J Control Release* 2000, **65**:271–284.
7. Taheri A, Atyabi F, Nouri FS, Ahadi F, Derakhshan MA, Amini M, Ghahremani MH, Ostad SN, Mansoori P, Dinarvand R: **Nanoparticles of conjugated methotrexate-human serum albumin: preparation and cytotoxicity evaluations.** *J Nanomaterials* 2011, **2011**:5.
8. Sahoo SK, Labhasetwar V: **Enhanced antiproliferative activity of transferrin-conjugated paclitaxel-loaded nanoparticles is mediated via sustained intracellular drug retention.** *Mol Pharm* 2005, **2**:373–383.
9. Shah N, Chaudhari K, Dantuluri P, Murthy R, Das S: **Paclitaxel-loaded PLGA nanoparticles surface modified with transferrin and Pluronic® P85, an in vitro cell line and in vivo biodistribution studies on rat model.** *J Drug Target* 2009, **17**:533–542.
10. Mo Y, Lim LY: **Paclitaxel-loaded PLGA nanoparticles: potentiation of anticancer activity by surface conjugation with wheat germ agglutinin.** *J Control Release* 2005, **108**:244–262.
11. Bazile D, Ropert C, Huve P, Verrecchia T, Mariard M, Frydman A, Veillard M, Spenlehauer G: **Body distribution of fully biodegradable [^{14}C]-poly (lactic acid) nanoparticles coated with albumin after parenteral administration to rats.** *Biomaterials* 1992, **13**:1093–1102.
12. Esmaeili F, Dinarvand R, Ghahremani MH, Ostad SN, Esmaily H, Atyabi F: **Cellular cytotoxicity and in-vivo biodistribution of docetaxel poly (lactide-co-glycolide) nanoparticles.** *Anticancer Drugs* 2010, **21**:43.
13. Esmaeili F, Hosseini-Nasr M, Rad-Malekshahi M, Samadi N, Atyabi F, Dinarvand R: **Preparation and antibacterial activity evaluation of rifampicin-loaded poly lactide-co-glycolide nanoparticles.** *Nanomedicine* 2007, **3**:161–167.
14. D'Souza SS, DeLuca PP: **Development of a dialysis in vitro release method for biodegradable microspheres.** *AAPS PharmSciTech* 2005, **6**:E323–E328.
15. He C, Hu Y, Yin L, Tang C, Yin C: **Effects of particle size and surface charge on cellular uptake and biodistribution of polymeric nanoparticles.** *Biomaterials* 2010, **31**:3657–3666.
16. Manchanda R, Fernandez-Fernandez A, Nagesetti A, McGoron AJ: **Preparation and characterization of a polymeric (PLGA) nanoparticulate drug delivery system with simultaneous incorporation of chemotherapeutic and thermo-optical agents.** *Colloids Surf B Biointerfaces* 2010, **75**:260–267.
17. Niwa T, Takeuchi H, Hino T, Kunou N, Kawashima Y: **Preparations of biodegradable nanospheres of water-soluble and insoluble drugs with D, L-lactide/glycolide copolymer by a novel spontaneous emulsification solvent diffusion method, and the drug release behavior.** *J Control Release* 1993, **25**:89–98.
18. Feng L, Wu H, Ma P, Mumper RJ, Benhabbour SR: **Development and optimization of oil-filled lipid nanoparticles containing docetaxel conjugates designed to control the drug release rate in vitro and in vivo.** *Int J Nanomedicine* 2011, **6**:2545.
19. Zaske L, Perrin MA, Leveiller F: **Docetaxel: solid state characterization by X-ray powder diffraction and thermogravimetry.** *Le Journal de Physique IV* 2001, **11**:Pr20-221–Pr210-226.
20. Budhian A, Siegel SJ, Winey KI: **Haloperidol-loaded PLGA nanoparticles: systematic study of particle size and drug content.** *Int J Pharm* 2007, **336**:367–375.
21. Song X, Zhao Y, Wu W, Bi Y, Cai Z, Chen Q, Li Y, Hou S: **PLGA nanoparticles simultaneously loaded with vincristine sulfate and verapamil hydrochloride: systematic study of particle size and drug entrapment efficiency.** *Int J Pharm* 2008, **350**:320–329.
22. Mainardes RM, Evangelista RC: **PLGA nanoparticles containing praziquantel: effect of formulation variables on size distribution.** *Int J Pharm* 2005, **290**:137–144.
23. Quintanar-Guerrero D, Fessi H, Allemann E, Doelker E: **Influence of stabilizing agents and preparative variables on the formation of poly (D, L-lactic acid) nanoparticles by an emulsification-diffusion technique.** *Int J Pharm* 1996, **143**:133–141.
24. Chen H, Yang W, Liu L, Gao F, Yang X, Jiang Q, Zhang Q, Wang Y: **Surface modification of mitoxantrone-loaded PLGA nanospheres with chitosan.** *Colloids Surf B Biointerfaces* 2009, **73**:212–218.
25. Misra R, Sahoo SK: **Intracellular trafficking of nuclear localization signal conjugated nanoparticles for cancer therapy.** *Eur J Pharm Sci* 2010, **39**:152–163.
26. Hu Y, Xie J, Tong YW, Wang CH: **Effect of PEG conformation and particle size on the cellular uptake efficiency of nanoparticles with the HepG2 cells.** *J Control Release* 2007, **118**:7–17.
27. Esmaeili F, Ghahremani MH, Esmaeili B, Khoshayand MR, Atyabi F, Dinarvand R: **PLGA nanoparticles of different surface properties: preparation and evaluation of their body distribution.** *Int J Pharm* 2008, **349**:249–255.
28. Musumeci T, Ventura CA, Giannone I, Ruozi B, Montenegro L, Pignatello R, Puglisi G: **PLA/PLGA nanoparticles for sustained release of docetaxel.** *Int J Pharm* 2006, **325**:172–179.
29. Yallapu MM, Gupta BK, Jaggi M, Chauhan SC: **Fabrication of curcumin encapsulated PLGA nanoparticles for improved therapeutic effects in metastatic cancer cells.** *J Colloid Interface Sci* 2010, **351**:19–29.
30. Magenheim B, Levy M, Benita S: **A new in vitro technique for the evaluation of drug release profile from colloidal carriers-ultrafiltration technique at low pressure.** *Int J Pharm* 1993, **94**:115–123.
31. Yoo HS, Oh JE, Lee KH, Park TG: **Biodegradable nanoparticles containing doxorubicin-PLGA conjugate for sustained release.** *Pharm Res* 1999, **16**:1114–1118.
32. Senthilkumar M, Mishra P, Jain NK: **Long circulating PEGylated poly (D, L-lactide-co-glycolide) nanoparticulate delivery of Docetaxel to solid tumors.** *J Drug Target* 2008, **16**:424–435.
33. Panyam J, Labhasetwar V: **Dynamics of endocytosis and exocytosis of poly (D, L-lactide-co-glycolide) nanoparticles in vascular smooth muscle cells.** *Pharm Res* 2003, **20**:212–220.

15

Toxicity of nanomaterials; an undermined issue

Mehdi Mogharabi[1,2], Mohammad Abdollahi[2] and Mohammad Ali Faramarzi[1,2*]

Abstract

Nanomaterials are employed in extensive variety of commercial products such as electronic components, cosmetics, food, sports equipment, biomedical applications, and medicine. With the increasing utilization of engineered nanomaterials, the potential exposure of human to nanoparticles is rapidly increasing. Nowadays when new nanomaterials with new applications are introduced, mostly good and positive effects are mentioned whereas possible hazards arising from nanosize of the compounds are undermined. Toxicology studies of nanomaterials demonstrate some adverse effects in some human organs such as central nerve system, immune system, and lung. There is lack of complete information about human toxicity and environmental waste of nanomaterials. We aimed to highlight current toxicological concerns of potentially useful nanomaterials which are now used in pharmaceutical and biomedical sciences.

Keywords: Adverse health effects, Drug delivery, Nanomaterials, Nanomedicine, Toxicity

Nanotechnology possesses a progressively sophisticated ability to manipulate matter at the nanoscale, making new materials, products, and devices that demonstrate new and unique behavior. Despite this explosive growth, the potential safety risks associated with consumer products containing nanoscale materials are still being learned. Exposure to products containing nanomaterials may cause effects which differ from those observed with conventionally scaled materials. Nowadays when new nanomaterials with new applications are introduced, mostly good and positive effects are mentioned whereas possible hazards arising from nanosize of the compounds are undermined. In addition to the chance of direct exposure to nanocompounds if used in human as a medicine, there are concerns on exposure during product manufacturing or through waste sources. Development of nanomaterials with numerous industrial applications such as electronic components, medical devices, tires, food and beverage, pharmaceuticals, and cosmetics has increased the chance of accumulation in the environment and consequent entering into food chain and human body (Figure 1) [1,2]. As an example, Australian government surprisingly reported that 30% of zinc sunscreens and 70% of titanium sunscreens are now formulated with nanosized ingredients (http://www.tga.gov.au/; accessed June 17, 2014). Also, several new products containing nanoparticles are being launched by food industries with the understanding to improve appearance, efficiency, and packaging of foods [3]. For instance, ZnO and MgO nanoparticles due to their antibacterial activities are used as the additive to polymer matrix of food packing [4]. On the other hand, there has been progressive interest in the pharmaceutical companies to use nanomaterials with the aim to better drug delivery. In this way, some drugs have got approval for use in human such as Doxil® known as one of several nanoparticle formulations of doxorubicin or Abraxane® that is an albumin-based nanoparticle formulation of paclitaxel used to treat different kinds of cancers and acquired immunodeficiency syndrome. Poly ethylene glycol (PEG)-linked proteins also represent an important group of therapeutic macromolecules that have been widely investigated within the context of nanoparticles. Covalent attachment of PEG to proteins has been demonstrated to prolong their circulation due to the size of molecule and reduced kidney clearance. Oncospar®, Pegasys®, and Neulasta® are approved by FDA as PEGylated protein for acute lymphoblastic leukemia, hepatitis C, and neutropenia, respectively. Macugen® (Pegaptanib) is an approved nanoscaled formulation of aptamer applied as an antagonist to vascular endothelial growth factor that lessens growth of the vessels located within the eye (Table 1) [5]. Besides the

* Correspondence: faramarz@tums.ac.ir
[1]Department of Pharmaceutical Biotechnology, Faculty of Pharmacy & Biotechnology Research Center, Tehran University of Medical Sciences, Tehran 1417614411, Iran
[2]Department of Toxicology and Pharmacology, Faculty of Pharmacy and Pharmaceutical Sciences Research Center, Tehran University of Medical Sciences, Tehran 1417614411, Iran

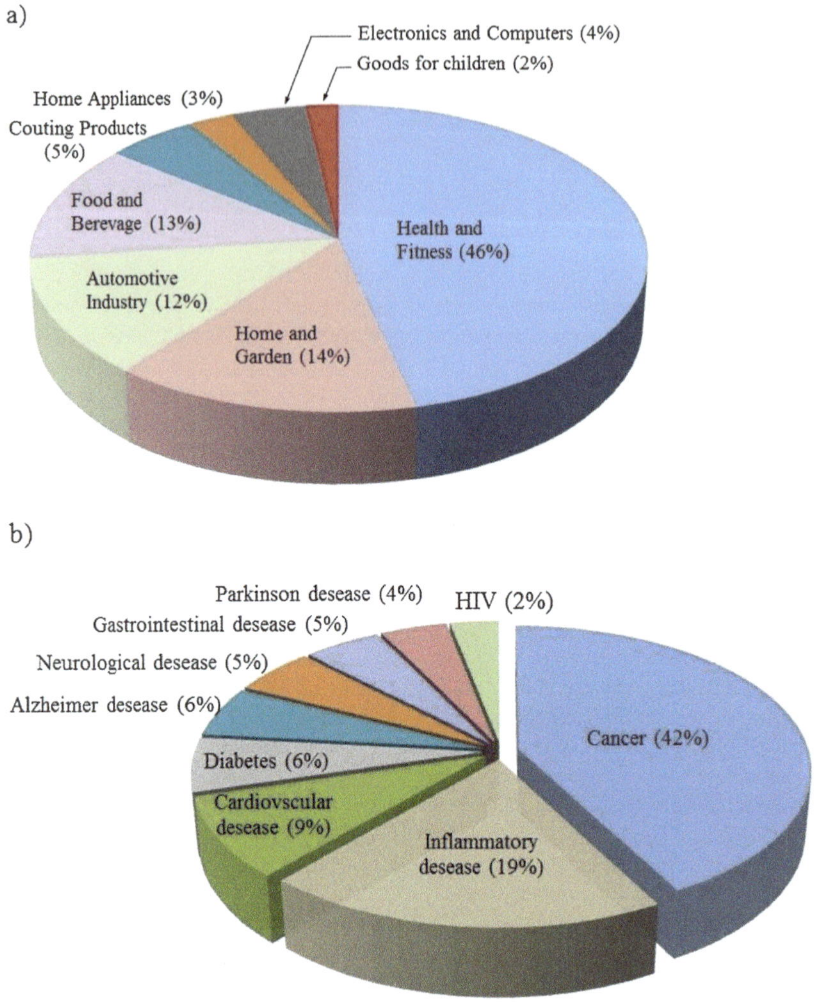

Figure 1 **Percent of various consumer products containing nanomaterials (a), percentage of articles published in scientific journals addressing the application of nanoparticles in various diseases (b), based on data obtained from Consumer Products Inventory [http://www.nanotechproject.org/] and Scopus (accessed June 17, 2014).**

Table 1 Some of clinically available nanoparticle containing drugs

Trade name	Nanomaterial	Company	Application
Abraxane	Albumin	Abraxis Oncology	Cancer treatment
Basulin	Polyglutamate polymer dotted with insulin	Advanced Magnetics	Type I diabetes
Biovant	Nanosized calcium phosphate	BioSante Pharmaceuticals	Vaccine component
Combidex	Iron oxide nanoparticles	Advanced Magnetics	Tumor imaging
Doxil	PEGylated liposome	Orthobiotech	Cancer treatment
Oncospar	PEGylated asparaginase	Medac GmbH	Leukemia treatment
Opaxio™	Polyglutamic acid	Cell Therapeutics, Inc.	Cancer treatment

growth in applications of nanomaterials in various aspects of human life, concerns on potential adverse human health effects of nanoparticles are escalating. Intravenous and subcutaneous injections of nanomaterial-based carriers delivers exogenous nanoparticles into the body with the aim to better distribution whereas broader spread may cause toxicity and undesirable interaction with biological macromolecules. Injected nanomaterials smaller than 100 nm are efficiently transported via interstitial flow to the draining lymphatics and lymph nodes. Meanwhile, they can reach most of organs dependent on the size of particle and surface characteristics. Besides injection, other routs of exposure like dermal, inhalation, and ingestion are also common. The penetration to skin by use of cosmetics with nanoparticles is the most relevant dermal route of exposure in human. Studies show that metallic nanoparticles smaller than 10 nm are able to penetrate the epidermal layers [1,6]. Larese et al. [7] demonstrated the permeation of silver nanoparticles through the stratum corneum of damaged skin in an in vitro diffusion cell system. Nanoparticles possess the ability to induce lung inflammation by not only stimulating pulmonary epithelial cells to generate proinflammatory cytokines, but also via causing endothelial cells to produce leukocyte adhesion molecules and circulating leukocytes [8]. Non-surprisingly destructive effects of metal containing nanomaterials on the brain vasculature have grown the toxicity concerns. For instance, it has been demonstrated that silver nanoparticles disrupt blood brain barrier and cause neuronal degeneration [9]. A major challenge in drug delivery is to improve selective targeting and safe strategies but major caution should be made in especial group of patients like pregnant women, infants, and aged people. Giving examples about pregnant group, studies have shown that nanoparticles can easily cross the placental barrier and induce pregnancy complications [10] that is a serious matter. A toxicology study carried out on pregnant mice investigated the effect of fullerene solubilized with poly (vinylpyrrolidone) in water when injected intraperitoneally to pregnant mice at varying concentrations. The results demonstrated that fullerene nanoparticles were traced in the embryos and at higher doses caused significant toxicity and death [11]. In addition, titanium oxide nanoparticles, which are widely used in consumer products, possess the ability to transfer from pregnant mice to their offspring affecting the central nerve and genital systems [12].

Using nanoparticles in medicine and drug delivery is growing rapidly while there are still non-resolved concerns about their risk of toxicity. It should not be forgotten that every material with smaller size can cross the cell membrane easier than materials with normal size. As a matter of fact, most of information about kinetics of materials come from tests of materials in the normal size and non-surprisingly there is a lack of data about kinetics of nanosized materials that has a major role in toxicity [13,14]. Graphene is a good example of a new nanomaterial that has raised new toxicological concerns [2]. Concerns on the use of nanomaterials also back to their waste in the environment. At the moment there is lack of information about pattern of accumulation of nanomaterials waste and their possible entrance into food chain. Here the facility of in-silico toxicology should come into help [15]. Therefore, scientists need a databank of biological effects, toxicity, biokinetics, as well as structure and molecular size of nanomaterials to be able to predict their toxicity. In other words, current need is to estimate different physical and chemical properties of the nanomaterials relevant to toxicity, environmental fate, and transport.

Competing interests
The authors declare that they have no competing interests.

Authors' contributions
Authors contributed equally to the paper. Authors read and approved the final manuscript.

References

1. Faramarzi MA, Sadighi A: **Insights into biogenic and chemical production of inorganic nanomaterials and nanostructures.** *Adv Colloid Interface Sci* 2013, **189–190:**1–20.
2. Mogharabi M, Abdollahi M, Faramarzi MA: **Safety concerns to application of graphene compounds in pharmacy and medicine.** *Daru* 2014, **22:**23.
3. Sharifi S, Behzadi S, Laurent S, Forrest ML, Stroeve P, Mahmoudi M: **Toxicity of nanomaterials.** *Chem Soc Rev* 2012, **41:**2323–2343.
4. Cushen M, Kerry J, Morris M, Cruz-Romero M, Cummins E: **Nanotechnologies in the food industry recent developments, risks and regulation.** *Food Sci Technol* 2012, **24:**30–46.
5. Heidel JD, Davis ME: **Clinical developments in nanotechnology for cancer therapy.** *Pharm Res* 2011, **28:**187–199.
6. Baroli B, Ennas MG, Loffredo F, Isola M, Pinna R, Lopez-Quintela MA: **Penetration of metallic nanoparticles in human full-thickness skin.** *J Investig Dermatol* 2007, **127:**1701–1712.
7. Larese FF, D'Agostin F, Crosera M, Adami G, Renzi N, Bovenzi M, Maina G: **Human skin penetration of silver nanoparticles through intact and damaged skin.** *Toxicology* 2009, **255:**33–37.
8. Nel A, Xia T, Mädler L, Li N: **Toxic potential of materials at the nanolevel.** *Science* 2006, **311:**622–627.
9. Sharma HS, Sharma A: **Nanoparticles aggravate heat stress induced cognitive deficits, blood–brain barrier disruption, edema formation and brain pathology.** *Prog Brain Res* 2007, **162:**245–273.
10. Wick P, Malek A, Manser P, Meili D, Maeder-Althaus X, Diener L, Diener P-A, Zisch A, Krug HF, von Mandach U: **Barrier capacity of human placenta for nanosized materials.** *Environ Health Perspect* 2010, **18:**432–436.
11. Tsuchiya T, Oguri I, Yamakoshi YN, Miyata N: **Novel harmful effects of [60] fullerene on mouse embryos in vitro and in vivo.** *FEBS Lett* 1996, **393:**139–145.
12. Takeda K, Suzuki KI, Ishihara A, Kubo-Irie M, Fujimoto R, Tabata M, Oshio S, Nihei Y, Ihara T, Sugamata M: **Nanoparticles transferred from pregnant mice to their offspring can damage the genital and cranial nerve systems.** *J Health Sci* 2009, **55:**95–102.

13. Mostafalou S, Mohammadi H, Ramazani A, Abdollahi M: **Different biokinetics of nanomedicines linking to their toxicity; an overview.** *Daru* 2013, **21**:14.
14. Pourmand A, Abdollahi M: **Current opinion on nanotoxicology.** *Daru* 2012, **20**:95.
15. Saeidnia S, Manayi A, Abdollahi M: **The pros and cons of the in-silico phannaco-toxicology in drug discovery and development.** *Int J Pharmacol* 2013, **9**:176–181.

Discovery of new angiotensin converting enzyme (ACE) inhibitors from medicinal plants to treat hypertension using an *in vitro* assay

Niusha Sharifi[1], Effat Souri[1], Seyed Ali Ziai[2], Gholamreza Amin[3] and Massoud Amanlou[1,4*]

Abstract

Background and purpose of the study: Angiotensin converting enzyme (ACE) inhibitors plays a critical role in treating hypertension. The purpose of the present investigation was to evaluate ACE inhibition activity of 50 Iranian medicinal plants using an *in vitro* assay.

Methods: The ACE activity was evaluated by determining the hydrolysis rate of substrate, hippuryl-L-histidyl-L-leucine (HHL), using reverse phase high performance liquid chromatography (RP-HPLC). Total phenolic content and antioxidant activity were determined by Folin-Ciocalteu colorimetric method and DPPH radical scavenging assay respectively.

Results: Six extracts revealed > 50% ACE inhibition activity at 330 μg/ml concentration. They were *Berberis integerrima* Bunge. (Berberidaceae) (88.2 ± 1.7%), *Crataegus microphylla* C. Koch (Rosaceae) (80.9 ± 1.3%), *Nymphaea alba* L. (Nymphaeaceae) (66.3 ± 1.2%), *Onopordon acanthium* L. (Asteraceae) (80.2 ± 2.0%), *Quercus infectoria* G. Olivier. (Fagaceae) (93.9 ± 2.5%) and *Rubus* sp. (Rosaceae) (51.3 ± 1.0%). *Q. infectoria* possessed the highest total phenolic content with 7410 ± 101 mg gallic acid/100 g dry plant. Antioxidant activity of *Q. infectoria* (IC_{50} value 1.7 ± 0.03 μg/ml) was more than that of BHT (IC_{50} value of 10.3 ± 0.15 μg/ml) and Trolox (IC_{50} value of 3.2 ± 0.06 μg/ml) as the positive controls.

Conclusions: In this study, we introduced six medicinal plants with ACE inhibition activity. Despite the high ACE inhibition and antioxidant activity of *Q. infectoria*, due to its tannin content (tannins interfere in ACE activity), another plant, *O. acanthium*, which also had high ACE inhibition and antioxidant activity, but contained no tannin, could be utilized in further studies for isolation of active compounds.

Keywords: Angiotensin converting enzyme, Screening, Medicinal plants, Total phenolic content, Antioxidant activity

Introduction

In 2000, 26.4% of the world's population suffered hypertension and it is predicted that this rate would increase by 60% in 2025 [1]. Since the proportion of hypertensive people will increase rapidly, new therapeutic approaches for management of hypertension are essential. High blood pressure is a silent killer, causing several serious diseases such as heart failure, kidney failure and stroke. There are a number of choices for the treatment of hypertension. Some treatments include diuretics, β-blockers, calcium channel blockers and angiotensin II receptor blockers, the most common of which is angiotensin converting enzyme inhibitors.

Angiotensin converting enzyme, EC 3.4.15.1, is a zinc metallopeptidase that converts the angiotensin I (inactive decapeptide) to angiotensin II (a potent vasoconstrictor), and bradykinin (a hypotensive peptide) to inactive components [2]. High ACE activity leads to increased concentration of angiotensin II and hypertension. Therefore, development of agents that inhibit the conversion of angiotensin I to angiotensin II, and bradykinin to inactive components began as a therapeutic strategy to treat hypertension. ACE inhibitors such as captopril and lisinopril play key roles in treating hypertension and maintaining the electrolyte balance [3]. They are commonly used as they are safe and well tolerated with few side effects.

* Correspondence: amanlou@tums.ac.ir
[1]Department of Medicinal Chemistry, Faculty of Pharmacy, Tehran University of Medical Sciences, Tehran, Iran
[4]Medicinal Plants Research Center, Faculty of Pharmacy, Tehran University of Medical Sciences, Tehran, Iran
Full list of author information is available at the end of the article

Tannins are plant polyphenolic compounds that precipitate proteins and interfere in the functions of many macromolecules including ACE. Therefore, plants with ≥ 50% ACE inhibition activity would be further tested for the presence of tannins in order to eliminate false positives [4].

Furthermore, reactive oxygen species (ROS) play a significant role in cardiovascular diseases such as hypertension and congestive heart failure. In hypertensive patients, angiotensin II increases chronically and nicotinamide adenine dinucleotide phosphate (NADPH) oxidase is activated, which causes a rise in ROS. As a result, it is more beneficial for an antihypertensive drug to have antioxidant effect [5]. Phenolic compounds have antioxidant activity and are effective agents to prevent oxidative stress.

Natural products could be important sources of ACE inhibitors such as captopril, a synthetic antihypertensive drug, which is developed by changing and optimizing the structure of the venom of the Brazilian viper. Active substances derived from medicinal plants can also be a source of new ACE inhibitors. Moreover, some plants contain a great amount of phenolic compounds, so consequently, they have antioxidant activity.

In this study, some medicinal plants that are used to manage different diseases were screened to discover possible new ACE inhibition activity using an *in vitro* ACE inhibition assay. Among the plants tested, the most active ones were examined for total phenolic content and antioxidant activity.

Material and methods

Chemicals

Angiotensin converting enzyme (ACE) from rabbit lung, hippuryl-L-histidyl-L-leucine (HHL), 4-(2-hydroxyethyl)-1-piperazineethanesulfonic acid (HEPES) buffer, hippuric acid (HA) and captopril were purchased from Sigma-Aldrich Co. (England). HCl, KH_2PO_4, methanol (HPLC grade), 2,2-diphenyl-1-picrylhydrazyl (DPPH), Folin-Ciocalteu reagent, Na_2CO_3, gallic acid, butylated hydroxyl toluene (BHT), 6-hydroxy-2,5,7,8-tetramethylchroman-2-carboxylic acid (Trolox), $FeCl_3$, NaCl, NaOH and dimethyl sulfoxide (DMSO) were purchased from Merck Co. (Germany). Ultrapure water was applied to prepare all of the aqueous solutions.

Apparatus

Enzymatic incubation was performed in a thermomixer eppendorf comfort (Germany). HPLC analysis was carried out by a Knauer liquid chromatograph, with an ODS Eurospher column (250 × 4.6 mm, 100–5; C18), protected by a C18 precolumn (Perfectsil Target, ODS-3 (5 μm)) and a 20 μl injection loop. A smartline Photodiode Array (PDA) detector 2850 (Knauer, Germany) was used to detect analytes, and a Chromgate software version 3.3, was used for data processing. A Cecil UV/Vis spectrophotometer (series 9000) was utilized to measure the absorbances.

Plant materials

Some of the studied plants (41 plants) were purchased from a local herbal store located in Tehran, Iran (June 2011). *Rubus* sp. was collected from north of Iran, Mazandaran province (June 2012), and 8 other plants were collected from Herburatum of Faculty of Pharmacy, Tehran University of Medical Sciences (June 2011). All of the mentioned plants were identified by Prof. G. Amin. Voucher specimens of the collected plants were deposited in the Herbarium of Tehran University of Medical Sciences.

Preparation of crude extracts

Dried plant materials (1 g) were extracted with 20 ml methanol:water (80:20, v/v) at room temperature for 24 h and then over 2 h in an ultrasonic bath [6]. The extracts were filtered and concentrated under reduced pressure, using a rotary evaporator at room temperature and then they were lyophilized.

ACE inhibition assay

In this study, the assay method is based on the hydrolysis of the substrate HHL by ACE, and measuring the amount of HA using RP-HPLC [6-9]. HEPES buffer solution used in this assay was prepared by dissolving 50 mM HEPES and 300 mM NaCl in 1000 ml water and adjusting the solution to pH 8.3 by 1 M NaOH solution. The substrate solution (9 mM) was prepared by dissolving HHL (19.74 mg) in 5 ml of HEPES buffer. Herbal extract (1 mg) was dissolved in 1 ml of solvent containing buffer/DMSO (90:10, v/v) to provide 330 μg/ml concentration (a comparable scale all over the world) [10].

First, ACE solution (25 μl) (80 mU/ml) was added to 25 μl of inhibitor solution (or solvent as negative control). After 3 min preincubation at 37°C, 25 μl substrate solution was added and the mixture was incubated at 37°C for 30 min with shaking at 300 rpm in an Eppendorf thermomixer. After 30 min, the reaction was stopped by addition of 50 μl of 1 M HCl and then the reaction mixture was subjected to RP-HPLC. The mobile phase was an isocratic system consisting of a mixture of 10 mM KH_2PO_4 (adjusted to pH 3 with H_3PO_4) and methanol (50:50, v/v). The flow rate was 1 ml/min and the injection volume was 20 μl. Analytes were detected by a PDA detector at the wavelength of 228 nm.

ACE inhibition measurement

ACE inhibition calculation was based on the ratio of the area under curve (AUC) of HA peak in an inhibitor

Table 1 Angiotensin converting enzyme (ACE) inhibition activity of the 50 studied plants*

Scientific name and plant family	Common name in Persian	Part used	Collection site	Medicinal use	Voucher No	Inhibition%
Abrus precatorius L. (Leguminosae)	Cheshm- e Khorus	Seed	LHS[a]	Tonic, astringent	PMP - 725[b]	−13.1
Alcea sp. (Malvaceae)	Khatmi	Flower	LHS	Diuretic, demulcent, disinfectant	PMP - 503	−27.3
Allium cepa L. (Alliaceae)	Tokhm- e pyaz	Seed	LHS	Anti-typhoid fever	PMP - 726	21.2
Amaranthus lividus L. (Amaranthaceae)	Tokhm- e tajkhorus	Seed	LHS	Treatment of anemia	PMP - 723	−13.9
Amomum subulatum Roxb. (Zingiberaceae)	Hel- e bad	Fruit	LHS	Stomach tonic, carminative	PMP - 634	−11.6
Arnebia euchroma (Royle) I. M. Johnst. (Boraginaceae)	Havachobe	Root	LHS	Disinfectant	PMP - 211	−8.1
Artemisia sp. (Asteraceae)	Afsantin	Herb	H[a]	Stomach tonic, increasing the appetite	83004	−8.5
Berberis integerrima Bunge. (Berberidaceae)	Zereshk- e abi	Fruit	LHS	Tonic, laxative, refrigerant, antiseptic	PMP - 619	88.2 ± 1.7[c]
Biebersteinia sp. (Geraniaceae)	Chelledaghi	Root	LHS	Anti-rheumatic	PMP - 215	22.7
Cerasus avium (L.) Moench (Rosaceae)	Dom- e gilas	Tail	LHS	Cardiac tonic, diuretic	PMP - 309	28.4
Chelidonium majus L. (Papaveraceae)	Mamiran	Root	LHS	Anti-diarrhea, anti-liver disease	PMP - 314	0.0
Cichorium intybus L. (Compositae)	Kasni	Root	LHS	Diuretic, analgesic, anti-fever	PMP - 213	13.2
Colchicum sp. (Colchicaceae)	Suranjan	Rhizome	LHS	Anti-pain in gout	PMP - 214	19.6
Commiphora sp. (Burseraceae)	Moql	Resin	LHS	Anti-rheumatic	PMP - 812	20.8
Cordia myxa L. (Boraginaceae)	Sepestan	Fruit	LHS	Mucilage, anti-chest complaints	PMP - 730	−15.9
Crataegus microphylla C. Koch (Rosaceae)	Sorkhevalik	Leaf	LHS	Cardiac tonic, diuretic, hypotensive	PMP - 306	80.9 ± 1.3
Cucurbita pepo L. (Cucurbitaceae)	Tokhm- e kadu	Seed	LHS	Anti-fever, anti-gastrointestinal parasites	PMP - 729	−31.5
Cynodon dactylon (L.) Pers. (Gramineae)	Margh	Rhizome	LHS	Diuretic	PMP - 312	9.6
Datura stramonium L. (Solanaceae)	Tature	Leaf	LHS	Anti-asthma	PMP - 728	22.3
Dorema ammoniacum Don. (Umbelliferae)	Vasha	Resin	LHS	Anti-gastrointestinal parasites	PMP - 815	14.2
Echinacea purpurea (L.) Moench (Asteraceae)	Sarkhargol	Aerial part	H	Anti-inflammatory, immune-stimulant	84159	−50.4
Echinops sp. (Compositae)	Shekartighal	Resin	LHS	Demulcent, anti-cough, anti-fever	PMP - 817	2.1
Elettaria cardamomum (L.) Maton (Zingiberaceae)	Hel- e sabz	Fruit	LHS	Spice, stomach tonic, carminative	PMP - 630	−25.7
Entada rheedii Spreng. (Leguminosae)	Qorc- e kamar	Seed	LHS	Ointment for backache	PMP - 724	17.3
Eugenia caryophyllata Thunb. (Myrtaceae)	Mikhak	Flower	LHS	Anti-dental pain, disinfectant	PMP - 504	−34.4
Ferula asssa-foetida L. (Umbelliferae)	Anqoze	Resin	LHS	Anti-gastrointestinal parasites	PMP - 816	−40.3
Ferula gumosa Boiss. (Umbelliferae)	Barije	Resin	LHS	Stomach tonic	PMP - 814	−36.7
Foeniculum vulgare Mill. (Umbelliferae)	Razyane	Seed	LHS	Tonic, diuretic, carminative	PMP - 632	−9.2

Table 1 Angiotensin converting enzyme (ACE) inhibition activity of the 50 studied plants* *(Continued)*

Heracleum persicum Desf. (Umbelliferae)	Golpar	Fruit	LHS	Spice, disinfectant, carminative	PMP - 631	4.7
Iris sp. (Iridaceae)	Rishe- e irisa	Root	LHS	Diuretic, cathartic	PMP - 212	0.0
Lepidium sativum L. (Cruciferae)	Tokhm- e shahi	Seed	LHS	Tonic	PMP - 722	−2.2
Malva sylvestris L. (Malvaceae)	Panirak	Flower	H	Mucilage, anti-cough	84450	21.7
Matricaria inodora L. (Asteraceae)	Babuneh	Flower	H	Carminative, febrifuge	83452	−7.5
Nymphaea alba L. (Nymphaeaceae)	Gol- e nilufar	Flower	LHS	Diuretic, sedative	PMP - 501	66.3 ± 1.2
Onopordon acanthium L. (Asteraceae)	Khajebashi	Seed	LHS	Hypotensive, diuretic, cardiac tonic	PMP - 714	80.2 ± 2.0
Passiflora caerulea L. (Passifloraceae)	Gol- e saati	Flower	H	Spinal depressant, respiratory stimulant	84568	−33.2
Plantago ovata Phil. (Plantaginaceae)	Esfarze	Seed	LHS	Laxative, anti-hemorrhoids	PMP - 731	−24.2
Quercus infectoria G.Olivier. (Fagaceae)	Jaft	Bark	LHS	Anti-diarrhea, astringent, antibacterial	PMP - 621	93.9 ± 2.5
Rosmarinus officinalis L. (Lamiaceae)	Rosaemary	Leaf	H	Spice, herb, carminative, GI irritant	83636	0.0
Rubus sp. (Rosaceae)	Tameshk	Leaf	N[a]	Hypotensive, anti-diarrhea	PMP - 404	51.3 ± 1.0
Salvia macrosiphon Boiss. (Labiatae)	Tokhm- e marv	Seed	LHS	Demulcent, anti-cough	PMP - 721	−11.7
Saponaria officinalis L. (Caryophyllaceae)	Gol- e sabooni	Flower	H	Expectorant, laxative	84680	−33.6
Satureja hortensis L. (Labiatae)	Tokhm- e marze	Seed	LHS	Anti-muscle pain, anti-rheumatic	PMP - 732	34.4
Tanacetum Balsamita L. (Compositae)	Shahesparam	Leaf	LHS	Stomach tonic, anti-nausea	PMP - 405	−15.2
Terminalia chebula Retz. (Combretaceae)	Halil- e zard	Fruit	LHS	Stomach tonic, anti-diarrhea	PMP - 633	17.9
Terminalia chebula Retz. (Combretaceae)	Halil- e siah	Fruit	LHS	Cathartic	PMP - 629	15.2
Teucrium polium L. (Labiatae)	Maryam nokhodi	Aerial part	LHS	Cold treatment, anti-fever	PMP - 313	2.1
Vitex agnus-castus L. (Verbenaceae)	Panj anghosht	Flower	H	Anti-androgen, carminative	84802	31.4
Zataria multiflora Boiss. (Labiatae)	Avishan- e shirazi	Leaf	LHS	Cold treatment, carminative	PMP - 310	24.8
Zea mays L. (Gramineae)	Kakol- e zhorrat	Herb	LHS	Diuretic, urethra antiseptic	PMP - 311	−35.7

*All medicinal plants were collected in June 2011 except *Rubus* sp. which is collected in June 2012.
[a]LHS, Local Herbal Store; H, Herburatum of Tehran University of Medical Sciences (http://pharmacy.tums.ac.ir); N, North of Iran (Mazandaran province).
[b]PMP, Popular Medicinal Plant.
[c]Values are means ± SD of three measurements for 6 active plants.

sample to that of negative control sample as it is expressed by equation 1:

$$\text{ACE inhibition } (\%) = [1\text{-}(\text{AUC}_{\text{inhibitor}}/\text{AUC}_{\text{control}})] \times 100 \quad (1)$$

$\text{AUC}_{\text{inhibitor}}$: AUC of the HA peak with inhibitor

$\text{AUC}_{\text{control}}$: AUC of the HA peak of control sample without inhibitor

Gelatin salt block test (eliminating false positive results)

In order to detect tannins, extracts with ≥ 50% ACE inhibition activity were tested under gelatin salt block test. Active extracts (200 mg) were dissolved in 4 ml water (50°C) and allowed to reach room temperature. To remove non-tannin compounds, a few drops of an aqueous 10% NaCl solution was added to the extracts. After filtration, the filtrate (1 ml) was added to four test tubes. Tube 1 contained 4–5 drops of 1% gelatin solution. Tube 2 contained 4–5 drops of 1% gelatin + 10% NaCl solution. Tube 3 contained 3–4 drops of 10% ferric chloride solution, and tube 4, was a control sample containing no reagent. Tube 1 and 2 were observed for the formation of precipitate, while tube 3 was observed for color [4].

The presence of greenish-blue or greenish-black color following the addition of ferric chloride indicates the presence of condensed tannins, and bluish-black color accounts for the presence of pyrogallol type tannins (assuming that precipitation is the result of gelatin salt block test). The presence of greenish-black or bluish-black color after the addition of ferric chloride with negative gelatin salt block test indicated no tannins in that extract.

Total phenolic content (TP)

Folin-Ciocalteu colorimetric method [11] was used to determine the total phenolic content of extracts. First, Folin-Ciocalteu reagent (0.5 ml) was added to 0.5 ml of methanol extract solution (100 mg/ml). Then Na_2CO_3 (0.5 ml) (100 mg/ml) was added to the mixture. The absorbance was measured at 760 nm, after 60 min incubation at room temperature. Calibration curve of gallic acid in different concentrations (1, 10, 100, 500 and 1000 μg/ml) was prepared using the same method. Total phenolic content of each extract was calculated from calibration curve of gallic acid and reported as mg of gallic acid equivalent in 100 g dry of plant [12].

DPPH radical scavenging activity

The DPPH radical scavenging activity assay is a method for determining the ability of extracts to trap free radicals [13]. First, DPPH methanol solution (2.0 ml) (0.16 mM) was added to 2.0 ml of extract methanol solutions in different concentrations. Next the same sample was prepared with 2.0 ml methanol replacing extract methanol solution as control. After that the mixtures were vortexed for 1 min and left at room temperature for 30 min. Later the absorbance (Abs) were read at 517 nm. For calculating radical scavenging activity (RSA), the equation 2 was used:

$$\text{RSA}\ (\%) = [1 - (\text{Abs}_{\text{extract}}/\text{Abs}_{\text{control}})] \times 100 \quad (2)$$

$\text{Abs}_{\text{extract}}$: Absorbance of the extract sample
$\text{Abs}_{\text{control}}$: Absorbance of the control sample

Radical scavenging activity of extracts was compared with those of BHT and Trolox as the positive controls.

Table 2 The active medicinal plants with more than 50% ACE inhibition activity at 330 μg/ml concentration

Scientific name	Percent of inhibition[a]
B. integerrima	88.2 ± 1.7
C. microphylla	80.9 ± 1.3
N. alba	66.3 ± 1.2
O. acanthium	80.2 ± 2.0
Q. infectoria	93.9 ± 2.5
Rubus sp.	51.3 ± 1.0

[a]Values are means ± SD of three measurements.

Table 3 Results of gelatin salt block test in order to detect tannin in extracts

Scientific name	1% Gelatin	1% gelatin + 10% NaCl	Ferric chloride
B. integerrima	NP[a]	NP	Green/black
C. microphylla	NP	NP	Green/black
N. alba	NP	NP	Blue/black
O. acanthium	NP	NP	Green/black
Q. infectoria	P[b]	P	Green/black
Rubus sp.	NP	NP	Blue/black

[a]NP, no precipitate; [b]P, precipitate.

Establishing the sensitivity of the ACE assay system

The half maximal inhibitory concentration (IC_{50}) value of captopril was determined from concentration - response curve by nonlinear regression, using GraphPad Prism software version 5, and it was compared with the value in the literature. The IC_{50} value for captopril determined in this study was 25 ± 2.6 nM, which was close to the value (23 nM) in the literature [14].

Results

ACE inhibition activity

Table 1 illustrates scientific names, plant families, common names in Persian, parts used, collection sites, collection times, medicinal uses, voucher numbers and ACE inhibition activities of herbal extracts. Of a total of fifty herbal extracts, six extracts have shown inhibition activity more than 50% at 330 μg/ml concentration (Table 2). They were *B. integerrima* (88.2 ± 1.7%), *C. microphylla* (80.9 ± 1.3%), *N. alba* (66.3 ± 1.2%), *O. acanthium* (80.2 ± 2.0%), *Q. infectoria* (93.9 ± 2.5%) and *Rubus* sp. (51.3 ± 1.0%).

Tannin test

Out of six active extracts investigated in this study, only the extract of *Q. infectoria* produced a positive gelatin salt block test (Table 3). The presence of greenish-black

Table 4 Total phenolic content and antioxidant activity of active extracts

Scientific name	Tp[a] (mg gallic acid/100 g dry plant)	IC_{50}[b](μg/ml)
B. integerrima	2250 ± 37	15.3 ± 0.20
C. microphylla	2000 ± 29	13.1 ± 0.20
N. alba	3860 ± 36	10.2 ± 0.15
O. acanthium	2740 ± 26	7.0 ± 0.09
Q. infectoria	7410 ± 101	1.7 ± 0.03
Rubus sp.	3870 ± 26	11.3 ± 0.22
BHT	–	10.3 ± 0.15
Trolox	–	3.2 ± 0.06

[a]Tp, Total phenolic content.
[b]IC_{50}, radical scavenging activity in DPPH assay.
Values are means ± SD of three independent measurements.

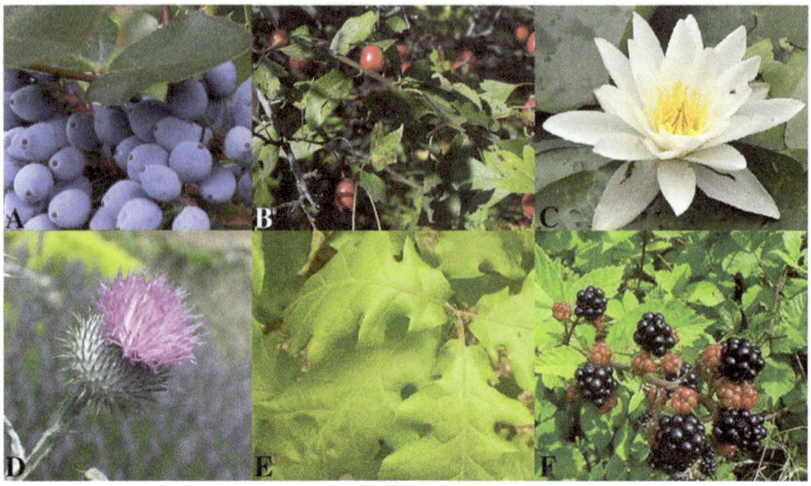

Figure 1 The picture of active medicinal plants with more than 50% angiotensin converting enzyme inhibitory activity. A) *B. integerrima* **B)** *C. microphylla* **C)** *N. alba* **D)** *O. acanthium* **E)** *Q. infectoria* **F)** *Rubus* sp [26-31].

or bluish-black color after the addition of ferric chloride with negative gelatin salt block test indicated no tannins in other extracts.

Total phenolic content and radical scavenging activity

Oxidative stress plays a critical role in cardiovascular disease [15]. Phenolic compounds are responsible for antioxidant activity due to their ability for scavenging free radicals. Therefore, total phenolic content and radical scavenging activities of these six medicinal plants were determined (Table 4). Most of these six extracts had a large phenolic content. In DPPH radical scavenging assay, IC_{50} values of six plant extracts were determined and compared with those of BHT and Trolox as the positive controls (Table 4). *Q. infectoria* possessed more antioxidant activity (IC_{50} value of 1.7 ± 0.03 μg/ml), compared to that of BHT (IC_{50} value of 10.3 ± 0.15 μg/ml) and Trolox (IC_{50} value of 3.2 ± 0.06 μg/ml).

Discussion

Hypertension, a worldwide illness, is a major factor in cardiovascular diseases that affects a large population of adults. One of the most effective medications for the treatment of hypertension is angiotensin converting enzyme inhibitors. Meanwhile, medicinal plants have been used for treating illnesses. Therefore, they can be important resources to develop new drug candidates [16].

As illustrated in Table 1 six extracts showed inhibition activity more than 50%, nineteen extracts showed inhibition activity less than 50% and 25 of them showed no inhibition activity at 330 μg/ml concentration. Among these active medicinal plants, three ones (*C. microphylla*,

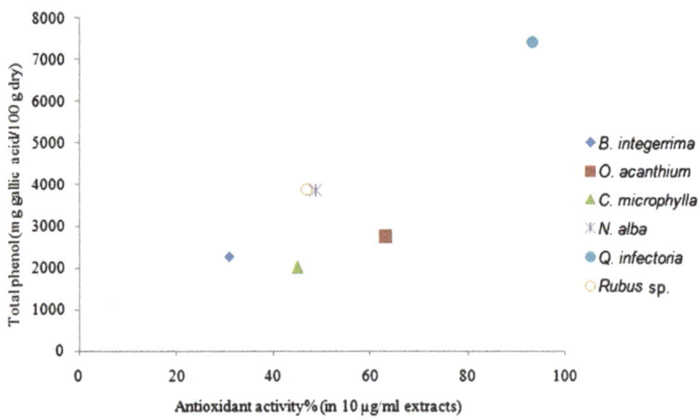

Figure 2 The correlation between total phenolic content and DPPH radical scavenging activity for six plant extracts.

O. acanthium and *Rubus* sp.) are utilized for the treatment of hypertension in traditional medicine and this research revealed that the mechanism of action of the three mentioned plants in treatment of hypertension could be done through ACE inhibition.

In addition, Antihypertensive activity is reported in traditional medicine for similar species of the above mentioned plants including *Crataegus oxyacantha* [17], *Onopordon leptolepis* and *Onopordon carmanicum* [18].

Flavonoids [19], flavanols [20], flavonols [21], anthocyanins [22], isoflavones [23], flavones [24] and other phenolic compounds have proved to be effective in decreasing the ACE activity. Therefore, the above mentioned secondary metabolites could be responsible for ACE inhibition activity in these 6 active extracts.

On the other hand, such ACE inhibitors with antioxidant activity might be useful to treat other diseases which are caused as a result of a rise in ROS production [25].

The highest ACE inhibition activity (93.9 ± 2.5%) was observed at 330 μg/ml concentration in *Q. infectoria*. It is clear that tannins are phenolic natural products that interfere in enzymatic activity. Consequently, we checked for its presence in our active extracts (extracts with ≥ 50% ACE inhibition activity). Unfortunately, greenish-black color after the addition of ferric chloride with positive gelatin salt block test indicated the presence of condensed tannins in *Q. infectoria* extract. Therefore, in spite of high ACE inhibition and antioxidant activity, it is not the plant of choice for further studies to isolate the active compounds.

Among other active medicinal plants, three ones including *B. integerrima, C. microphylla* and *O. acanthium* possessed > 80% ACE inhibition activity. Out of the three mentioned plants, *O. acanthium* possessed more antioxidant activity (IC_{50} value of 7 ± 0.09 μg/ml), compared to that of *B. integerrima* (IC_{50} value of 15.3 ± 0.2 μg/ml) and *C. microphylla* (IC_{50} value of 13.1 ± 0.2 μg/ml). Therefore, because of high ACE inhibition and antioxidant activity, *O. acanthium* is a valuable medicinal plant for isolation of active compounds.

Furthermore, *N. alba* and *Rubus* sp. are moderate ACE inhibitors and after the above three mentioned plants, are valuable plants for isolation of active compounds in further studies.

Conclusions

Medicinal plants presented in Table 2 are potential sources for developing new ACE inhibitors (Figure 1) [26-31]. There was a linear relationship between total phenolic content and radical scavenging activity with equation formula, y = 83.53 × - 823.4; R^2 = 0.714 (Figure 2). As shown in Tables 2, 3 and 4, in spite of possessing the highest ACE inhibition and antioxidant activity, *Q. infectoria* had tannin content. On the other hand, *O. acanthium*, which also had high ACE inhibition and antioxidant activity containing no tannin, and could be used in further studies for isolation of active compounds.

Competing interests

The authors have no conflict of interests to declare.

Authors' contributions

NS: Performed the experimental work including plant extraction, biological tests, data interpretation, and manuscript preparation. ES: Was responsible for HPLC analysis. SAZ: Was involved in designing the experiments. GHA: Identified all plants. MA: Was responsible for the study registration, financial and administrative support, and also gave final approval of the version to be published. All authors read and approved the final manuscript.

Acknowledgment

The financial support of the Research Council of the Tehran University of Medical Sciences is gratefully acknowledged.

Author details

[1]Department of Medicinal Chemistry, Faculty of Pharmacy, Tehran University of Medical Sciences, Tehran, Iran. [2]Department of Pharmacology, Faculty of Medicine, Shahid Beheshti University of Medical Sciences, Tehran, Iran. [3]Department of Pharmacognosy, Faculty of Pharmacy, Tehran University of Medical Sciences, Tehran, Iran. [4]Medicinal Plants Research Center, Faculty of Pharmacy, Tehran University of Medical Sciences, Tehran, Iran.

References

1. Kearney PM, Whelton M, Reynolds K, Muntner P, Whelton PK, He J: **Global burden of hypertension: analysis of worldwide data.** *Lancet* 2005, **365:**217–223.
2. Skeggs SLT, Kahn JR, Shumway NP: **The preparation and function of the angiotensin I converting enzyme.** *J Exp Med* 1956, **103:**295–299.
3. Carretero OA, Oparil S: **Essential hypertension.Part I: definition and etiology.** *Circulation* 2000, **101:**329–335.
4. Duncan AC, Jager AK, Staden JV: **Screening of Zulu medicinal plants for angiotensin converting enzyme (ACE) inhibitors.** *J Ethnopharmacol* 1999, **68:**63–70.
5. Griendling KK, Candace A, Minieri CA, Ollerenshaw JD, Alexander RW: **Angiotensin II stimulates NADH and NADPH oxidase activity in cultured vascular smooth muscle cells.** *Circ Res* 1994, **74:**1141–1148.
6. Kouchmeshky A, Jameie SB, Amin G, Ziai SA: **Investigation of angiotensin-converting enzyme inhibitory effects of medicinal plants used in traditional Persian medicine for treatment of hypertension, screening study.** *Thrita Stud J Med Sci* 2012, **1:**13–23.
7. Horiuchi M, Fujimura K, Terashima T, Iso T: **Method for determination of angiotensin converting enzyme activity in blood and tissue by high performance liquid chromatography.** *J Chromatogr* 1982, **233:**123–130.
8. Mehanna AS, Dowling M: **Liquid chromatographic determination of hippuric acid for the evaluation of ethacrynic acid as angiotensin converting enzyme inhibitor.** *J Pharm Biomed Anal* 1999, **19:**967–973.
9. Schnaith E, Beyrau R, Buckner B, Klein RM, Rick W: **Optimized determination of angiotensin I converting enzyme activity with hippuril-L-histidyl-L-leucine as substrate.** *Clin Chim Acta* 1994, **227:**145–158.
10. Tundis R, Loizzo MR, Statti GA, Deguin B, Amissah R, Houghton PJ, *et al*: **Chemical composition of and inhibition of angiotensin-converting enzyme by Senecio samnitum huet.** *Pharm Biol* 2005, **43:**605–608.
11. Singleton VL, Orthofer R, Lamuela-Raventos RM: **Analysis of total phenols and other oxidation substrates and antioxidants by means of Folin-Ciocalteu reagent.** *Methods Enzymol* 1999, **299:**152–178.
12. Lachman J, Hamouz K, Orsak M, Pivec V: **Potato tubers as a significant source of antioxidant human nutrition.** *Rostl Vyr* 2000, **46:**231–236.
13. Yen GC, Chen HY: **Antioxidant activity of various tea extracts in relation to their antimutagenicity.** *J Agric Food Chem* 1995, **43:**27–37.
14. Ondetti MA: **Structural relationships of angiotensin converting enzyme inhibitors to pharmacologic activity.** *Circulation* 1988, **77:**74–78.
15. Dhalla NS, Temsah RM, Netticadan T: **Role of oxidative stress in cardiovascular diseases.** *J Hypertens* 2000, **18:**655–673.

16. Lipp FJ: **The efficacy, history, and politics of medicinal plants.** *Altern Ther Health Med* 1996, **2:**36–41.
17. Lacaille-Dubois MA, Franck U, Wagner H: **Search for potential Angiotensin Converting Enzyme (ACE)-inhibitors from plants.** *Phytomedicine* 2001, **8:**47–52.
18. Esmaeili A, Saremnia B: **Preparation of extract-loaded nanocapsules from Onopordon leptolepis DC.** *Ind Crop Prod* 2012, **37:**259–263.
19. Ojeda D, Jiménez-Ferrer E, Zamilpa A, Herrera-Arellano A, Tortoriello J, Alvarez L: **Inhibition of angiotensin converting enzyme (ACE) activity by the anthocyanins delphinidin- and cyanidin-3-O-sambubiosides from Hibiscus sabdariffa.** *J Ethnopharmacol* 2010, **127:**7–10.
20. Ottaviani JI, Actis-Goretta L, Villordo JJ, Fraga CG: **Procyanidin structure defines the extent and specificity of angiotensin I converting enzyme inhibition.** *Biochimie* 2006, **88:**359–365.
21. Oh H, Kang DG, Kwon JW, Kwon TO, Lee SY, Lee DB, *et al*: **Isolation of angiotensin converting enzyme (ACE) inhibitory flavonoids from Sedum sarmentosum.** *Biol Pharm Bull* 2004, **27:**2035–2037.
22. Kwon EK, Lee DY, Lee H, Kim DO, Baek NI, Kim YE, *et al*: **Flavonoids from the buds of Rosa damascena inhibit the activity of 3-hydroxy-3-methylglutaryl-coenzyme a reductase and angiotensin I-converting enzyme.** *J Agric Food Chem* 2010, **58:**882–886.
23. Montenegro MF, Pessa LR, Tanus-Santos JE: **Isoflavone genistein inhibits the angiotensin converting enzyme and alters the vascular responses to angiotensin I and bradykinin.** *Eur J Pharmacol* 2009, **607:**173–177.
24. Loizzo MR, Said A, Tundis R, Rashed K, Statti GA, Hufner A, *et al*: **Inhibition of angiotensin converting enzyme (ACE) by flavonoids isolated from Ailanthus excels (Roxb) (Simaroubaceae).** *Phytother Res* 2007, **21:**32–36.
25. Hasani-Ranjbar S, Larijani B, Abdollahi M: **A systematic review of the potential herbal sources of future drugs effective in oxidant-related diseases.** *Inflamm Allergy Drug Targets* 2009, **8:**2–10.
26. *Berberis integerrima.* http://www.plantsystematics.org/imgs/kcn2/r/Berberidaceae_Berberis_sp_1445.html. webcite (accessed September 6, 2013).
27. *Crategus microphylla.* http://www.plantarium.ru/page/image/id/155248.html. webcite (accessed September 6, 2013).
28. Wikipedia contributors: *Nymphaea alba.* Wikipedia, The Free Encyclopedia. http://en.wikipedia.org/wiki/Nymphaea_alba. webcite (accessed September 6, 2013).
29. Wikipedia contributors: *Ononpordum acanthium.* Wikipedia, The Free Encyclopedia. http://en.wikipedia.org/wiki/Onopordum_acanthium. webcite (accessed September 6, 2013).
30. *Quercus infectoria.* http://www.biolib.cz/en/taxonimage/id77341 webcite (Pavel Bursik). (accessed September 6, 2013).
31. Wikipedia contributors: *Rubus sp..* Wikipedia, The Free Encyclopedia. http://en.wikipedia.org/wiki/Rubus webcite (accessed September 6, 2013).

Computational investigation of inhibitory mechanism of flavonoids as bovine serum albumin anti-glycation agents

Anahita Johari[1,2], Ali Akbar Moosavi-Movahedi[2] and Massoud Amanlou[1*]

Abstract

Background: Glycation of serum albumin and its consequence products were considered as an important factor in drug distribution and diabetic complications, therefore finding the glycation inhibitors and their inhibitory mechanisms became a valuable field of study. In this work, bovine serum albumin (BSA) became a subject as a model protein for analyzing the inhibitory mechanism of flavonoids, known as natural BSA glycation inhibitors in the early stage of glycation.

Methods: Firstly, for theoretical study, the three-dimensional model of BSA structure was generated by homology modeling and refined through molecular dynamic simulation. Secondly, several validation methods (statistical assessment methods and also neural network methods) by simultaneous docking study were employed for insurance about accuracy of our simulation. Then docking studies were performed for visualizing the relation between flavonoids' binding sites and BSA glycation sites besides, the correlation analyzes between calculated binding energy and reported experimental inhibitory IC_{50} values of the flavonoids set, was considered to explore their molecular inhibitory mechanism.

Results: The quality assessment methods and simultaneous docking studies on interaction of quercetin (as the most studied flavonoids) with BSA and Human serum albumin (HAS), confirm the accuracy of simulation and the second stage of docking results which were in close agreement with experimental observations, suggest that the potential residues in flavonoids binding sites (which were place neighbor of tryptophan 212 within 5Å) cannot be considered as one of glycation sites.

Conclusions: Based on the results, flavonoids don't participate in inhibitory interference mechanism, and also, the differentiation between complexes of flavonoids with BSA and HSA could destroy the speculation of using them as an exchangeable model protein in study of serum albumin and flavonoids interactions.

Keywords: Homology modeling, Molecular dynamics simulation, Correlation analyzes, Glycation sites, Flavonoids, BSA

Background

Diabetes is considered as one of the main threat to human health, according to WHO report, it is predicted that diabetes will exceed to 300 million in the years of 2025. Diabetes has a devastating effect on almost every organ in body. The hyperglycemia in diabetic conditions causes non-enzymatic glycation of proteins [1]. This reaction initiates the formation of reversible Schiff base between glucose and ε-amino group of lysine residues in proteins which by consequent intermolecular rearrangements leading to a formation of ketamine adduct. Then, the potent precursors of protein cross-linkers such as glucosone, 5-hydroxymethyl-2-furaldehyde, and 3-deoxyglucosone are formed due to the initial reaction. Next, those intermediates are oxidized, and cross linked, and fluorescent heterogeneous group of protein-bound moieties (called advanced glycated end products or AGEs) are detected in the last stage of glycation [2,3]. With body of evidence, formation and accumulation of advanced glycation products can be considered as a major factor

* Correspondence: amanlou@tums.ac.ir
[1]Department of Medicinal Chemistry, Faculty of Pharmacy and Pharmaceutical Sciences Research Center, Tehran University of Medical Sciences, Tehran, Iran
Full list of author information is available at the end of the article

in development of diabetic complication, Alzheimer's disease, and normal aging process. Therefore, the considerable efforts have been made to propose and discover inhibitors of glycation for therapeutic application in treatment of diseases that advanced glycation end product could be responsible for their pathogenesis [4].

Serum albumin is the most abundant protein in body which has a tremendous interest for binding to various natural or synthetic small-molecules such as glucose and related compounds. In diabetic condition, serum albumin undergoes glycation [5]. This character, continually expose serum albumin to altering factors which can participate in serum albumin modifications and biological compound formation that can be considered as a causative agent for some diseases [6]. Among the wide variety of interaction, the none-enzymatic interaction of serum albumin with glucose is one of the most important underlying modification factors, which are in associated with various alterations of albumin's structure and functions [7,8].

Among the glycation inhibitors' which were examined on bovine serum albumin (BSA) as a model protein, specific considerations were given to dietary natural products such as several phenolic compounds [9,10]. Researches on a limited number of flavonoids compounds indicated their ability to prevention both stage of glycation reaction [7]. In the late stage, the inhibition mechanisms of flavonoids are that, they may act as a both metal chelator and radical scavenger [11,12]. However, the inhibitory mechanism of flavonoids in the early stage completely remains unclear [7]. For some anti-glycation agent such as α-lipoate or non-steroidal anti-inflammatory drugs such as diclofenac and aspirin, hydrophobic hindrance or binding near the glycation site was considered as possible mechanism of anti-glycation activity [9,13]. Although we have no evidence that flavonoids react with the glycation site [7], in the present study, the attentions are drawn to binding behavior of flavonoids to clarifying the inhibition mechanism of them for the early stage of glycation.

Since, docking simulation results can be used to understanding the molecular interaction and analyze biological presses, rapidly and efficiently [2], in the present study, we explored the series of flavonoids' binding behavior with BSA through docking studies.

However, in the case of BSA which was considered here as a model protein (such as studies mentioned above by Morimitsu, Y., et al. and Matsuda, H., et al. [3,12]). When this study was started nobody has succeeded in obtaining crystals of intact BSA [14]. However, simultaneous with our study the importance of this protein draws the other researchers' attention to solving the tertiary structure of BSA. However, the new crystals also haven't been at high resolution (<2 Å resolution limit) [15], which can be satisfactory resolution for using in docking simulation. In this study, simulation, homology modeling was employed. While, it is generally recognized that homology modeling of proteins could be considered as accurate methods for 3D structure prediction while a model and related template sharing high sequence identity [16,17].

In present work, the model was refined with energy minimization and molecular dynamic simulation. Then, different assessment tools were adapted for checking the proper folding of constructed BSA 3D structure.

Consequently, by docking methods the validity of the model protein was examined and for getting better insight into the flavonoids' inhibitory mechanism. Firstly, the predicted binding affinity and reported IC_{50} [12] was subjected to correlation analyzes and secondly, the flavonoids binding location was studied for tracing the relation among participated amino acids in the flavonoids' binding site with ones proposed as the glycation site of BSA [18].

In addition, according to docking results, the comparison is made between obtained 3D structure of BSA and crystallographic structure of HSA for understanding their specificity in flavonoids binding location and the verification of using BSA and HSA as an exchangeable mode protein for the same case of investigation.

Methods

Amino acid sequence alignment and homology modeling of bovine serum albumin

In the first step, Amino acid sequence of BSA (UniProt ID: P02769) was retrieved from Swiss-Prot (http://www.uniprot.org/uniprot). And then, Blastp matrix blosum62 against PDB database was used to find out the best homologous structure with a known 3D structure, for applying as a template in homology modeling. Finally, among the HSA structures, the structure with a highest resolution at 1.9 Å [19] that belong to HSA (PDB ID: 1N5U) was adopted as the final target.

Sequence alignment was generated using 2d alignment function of MODELLER 9v8 program (www.salilab.org/modeller). Align 2d is based on a dynamic programming algorithm, considering the template structural information for constructing an alignment, this advantages is more significant as the similarity between the sequences decrease and the number of gaps increase [20]. After alignment, the 3D structure of fifty models were calculated completely automatically with MODELLER 9v8 [21].

Refinement of homology model by minimization and MD simulation

Molecular dynamic simulation were carried out using the parallel version of GROMACS 4.5.3 [22] In the AMBER99SB force field [23] to monitor stability and conformation of the selected model. The starting coordinates were taken from the best model that was retrieved from MODELLER and for prediction of non-standard ionization state of residues PROPKA 2.0 was applied [24]. Among the whole residues that may be adapted standard ionization state, lysine 219 was deprotonated and six histidine residues (histidine 16, histidine 37, histidine 143, histidine 239, histidine 335, and histidine 332) were completely protonated.

After assigning charge state, the protein was put into a suitable sized simulation cubic box and immersed in 41760 simple point charges (SPC) water model. Then, appropriate number of Na^+ ions were added to neutralize the charge of the system. The first energy minimization, which targeted water molecules and ions alone while configuration of protein was kept, fixed, followed by 20 ps MD simulation which again, the protein was kept fixed and the water molecules and ions were allowed to evolve. The second minimization step began with 1000 steepest descent and conjugate gradient of 9000 steps afterward. For equilibrating further the system v-rescale thermostat [25] was applied by using coupling constant (τ_t) of 0.1 ps to keep the system at the constant temperature in 100 ps at 100 K and 200 K respectively. While the pressure of the system maintained at 1 atm by using the Berendsen weak coupling algorithm [26] with coupling constant (τ_p) of 0.5 ps. For obtaining the stable system at 300 K and 1 atm, the same aforementioned parameters were determined for heating the system.

In this simulation, the non-bonded interactions were calculated by applying a 14 Å cut off and periodic boundary conditions were also applied in all directions. The Electrostatic interactions were calculated using the Particle Mesh Ewald (PME) [27]. During simulation, the frame was stored at every 1.000 ps.

Subsequently, all the analysis was performed by taking advantage of Gromacs tools and the structure which was retrieved after system stabilization was subject to evaluate the protein geometry.

Assessment of the homology model

To verify the quality of the model after molecular dynamic refinement, using different tools, which include: PRoQ, as a neural network based predictor [28], verify 3D, which analyzes the compatibility of an atomic model (3D) with its own amino acid sequence (1D) [29], PROSA program, which evaluate the energy of using a distance based pair potential [30] as well PROCHECK for checking the detailed stereochemical properties [31].

Docking analysis

Autodock 4.0 [32] was used for docking studies and for adding charges and active torsions to the ligands and assign Kollman charges to protein AutoDockTools (ADT) was employed. The rectangular lattice (100 × 100 × 100) with points separated by 0.375 Å was built by AutoGrid that was superposed on subdomin IIA of serum albumin (proposed as a primarily binding site of flavonoids) [33]. The Lamarckian genetic algorithm (LGA) was used with 100 runs for docking simulation, while an initial population size of 100, and the maximum number of 2500000 energy evaluations. All other parameters were set to default values, and the results were ranked according to Autodock scoring function and the final conformation of each structure was selected based on the highest dock score.

The chemical structures of interested flavonoids were optimized at MM+ level of molecular mechanic methods using HYPERCHEM software program (version 8.0.3 Hypercube, Inc) [34]. The geometry optimization was preceded by Polak-Ribiere algorithm to reach the 0.01 root mean square gradient. Then all these refinement structures were subject to docking simulations.

MD simulation after docking

All MD simulations were performed using the Gromacs 4.5.3 program together with the 43a2 force field [35-37] for each simulation to study the complex of BSA-quercetin, while the topology of quercetin was generated by the PRODRG 2.5 beta server [38].

Then, the protein was solvated by simple point charge water molecule in the cubic box with minimal distance of protein from its wall being 1.0 nm and the system was neutralized by adding appropriate counter ions. After performing energy minimization of the entire system, it was equilibrated under NVT ensemble for 100 ps and the periodic boundary conditions were used in tree-coordinate direction, whereas, position restrains were placed on ligand using force restraint of 1000 kcal/mol. NVT equilibration is followed by isothermal–isobaric (NPT) which was performed for 100 ps. The pressure of the system was regulated by Berendsen barostat with a relaxation time (τp) of 2.0 ps. The position restraints and simulation parameter which was applied in the NPT ensemble was the same as the ones which have been used during NPT equilibration. After convergence had been reached, the protein-ligand and water-ions groups were coupled in separate temperature baths, and v-rescale thermostat was used to keep the temperature constant at 300 k during the 2 ns simulation. Lennard-Jones interactions were calculated within a cut-off distance of 1.0 nm, and electrostatic interactions were treated with the particle mesh Ewald's method. Ultimately, from 2 ns MD simulation, the structure with low RMSD value was selected for analyzing the local conformational changes of BSA- quercetin complex.

Computational resources

The computational studies were performed on computer cluster 4 HP Prolient ML370-G5 Tower servers equipped with 2 Quad Core Intel Xeon processors E5355, 2.66 GHz and 4GB of RAM on a Linux platform.

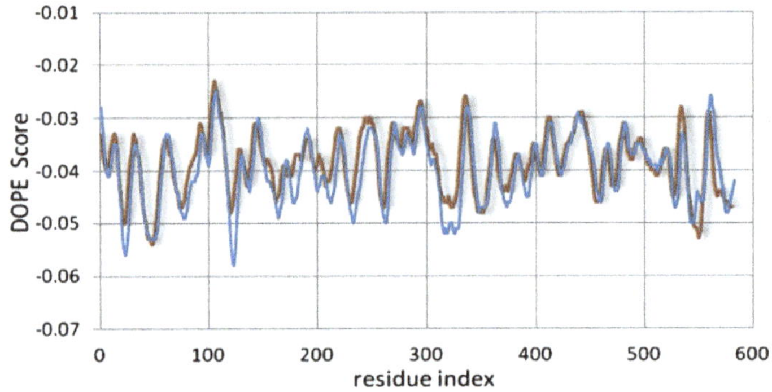

Figure 1 Analysis of DOPE score profile (obtained from Modeller). The Blue line indicates, energy profile of HSA (PDB ID: 1N5U) which used as a model and the red line indicates energy profile of target, which constructed by Modeller.

Results

Sequence alignment and modeling building

Based on the highest similarity and the lowest D-value, human serum albumin (HSA) can be considered the best homologues structure for BSA. The Sequence alignment of BSA (UniProt ID: P02769) and HSA (UniProt ID: P02768) which was generated by ClustalX program shows 76% identity between them [39]. The precursor proteins of BSA and HSA have 603 and 607 amino acid in length, respectively. Though all the crystallographic structures of HSA which were reported, only consist of 583 amino acids. This can be referred to the fact that during a secretion and maturation process of serum albumins, the 25 N-terminal amino acids were cleaved [40]. Therefore, the 25 N –terminal amino acids, which are placed out of the chain, were separated from the HSA amino acids sequence and the rest of them used as a target for homology modeling.

After alignment, the 3D structure of fifty models was calculated completely automatically with modeler 9v8. In this process, the population of the constructed model was increased for improving the DOPE energy assessment

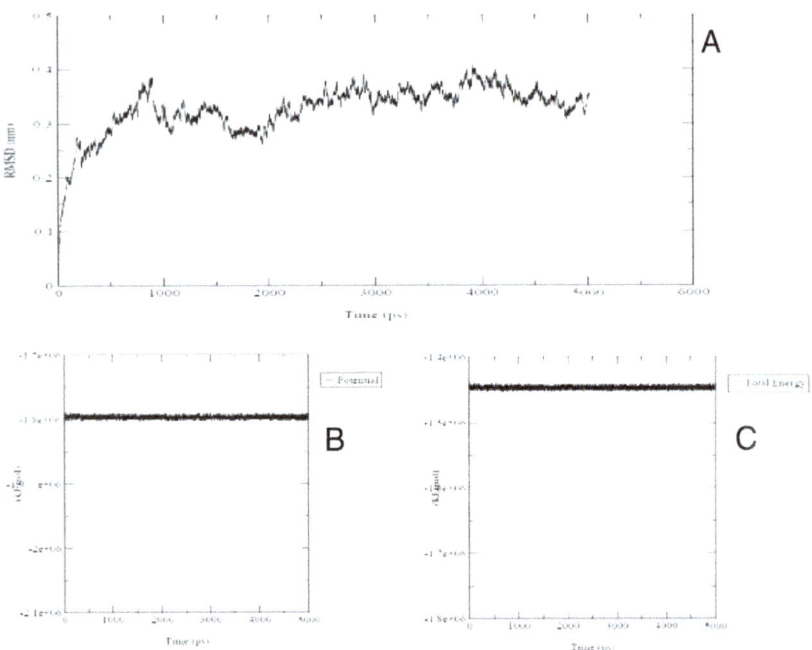

Figure 2 Analysis of a molecular dynamics simulation trajectory during 5ns generated by Gromacs. (A) The backbone root mean square deviation (RMSD) plot of the model, during 5ns simulation. **(B)** The variation of potential around constant value. **(C)** The fluctuation of total energy.

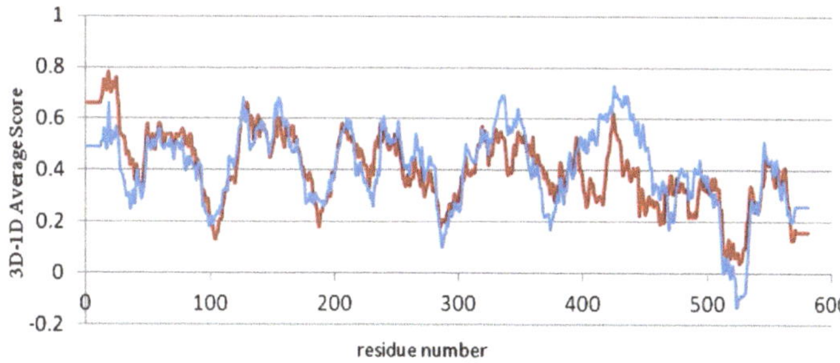

Figure 3 The Verify-3D analysis is shown for all residues. The blue line belongs to molecular structure after MD, and red one belongs to model that constructed by the Modeller. The refinement model after MD was validated by positive scores of Verify-3D.

and MODELLER objective function calculation and then the best model was selected based on the lowest DOPE score. Next, for gave an idea about the quality of input alignment the DOPE score profile (Figure 1) was calculated with "assess_dope" function of MODELLER. It can be seen in Figure 1, that in the whole range of residues, the DOPE score of both proteins converges and the results aren't showing any problematic regions.

Analysis the trajectory of the molecular dynamics simulation

During 5 ns MD simulation, the system was analyzed for its stability. The deviation plot of potential, and root mean square deviation (Figure 2) were derived from the respective trajectory by Gromacs software output. The low degree of RMSD fluctuation during last 2 ns indicates that the system tends to be converging and therefore, it is become stable. According to what illustrated in Figure 2, the total energy of the complex was observed within the range from −1.4 to −1.5 kJ/mol, which can be a reasonable value.

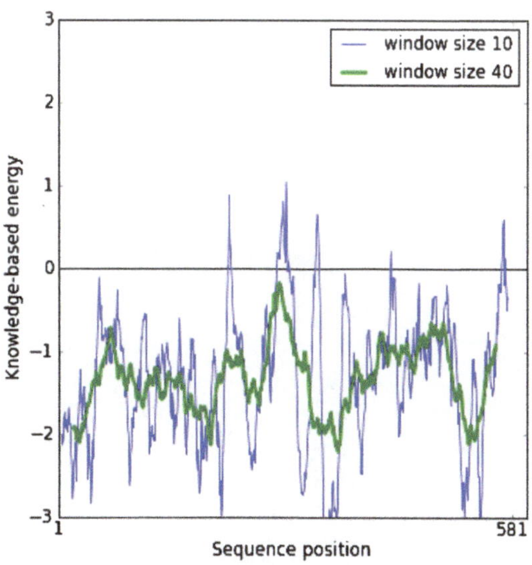

Figure 4 Energy plot from ProSA program, all residues have negative ProSA energies which confirms the reliability of the model.

Assess the validity of generated model after MD

In present work two statistical approaches such as verify3D and PROSA confirm a reliability of the constructed model.

In the first approach, the Verify 3D profile (Figure 3) represents that 3D-1D average score of the most residues in the model proteins both before and after MD, given a score over 0.2 except the ones rage 514–532. In the model protein that refined after MD, the whole residues have a positive score, whereas in the model that constructed by the modeler the amino acids in the range of 518–530 have a negative score. Therefore, based on these results, the sign of model folding improvement after molecular dynamic simulation is traceable.

The second statistical assessment method was processed with ProSA program. The Normalized Z-score calculation indicates standard deviation value is found in the range of native conformation of crystallographic structure and also according to Figure 4, ProSA score, which was calculated interaction energy per residues, has a negative score across the most of the residues' length.

After performing those earlier methodologies based on statistical approaches (Verify3D, ProSA), the PRoQ was applied to compare the validity of the model before and after MD simulation. This program is based on a neural

Table 1 Ramachandran plot statistics

% residues in most favored regions	90.8%
% residues in additional allowed regions	8.8%
% residues in generously allowed regions	0.4%
% residues in disallowed regions	0.0%
% Num. of non-glycine and non-proline residues	100.0%

Table 2 Main chain parameters plot statistics

Stereochemical parameter	No. of data pts	Parameter value	Comparison values Typical value	Comparison values Band width	No. of band widths from mean	
%-tage residues in A,B,L	535	90.8	84.9	10.0	0.6	Inside
Omega angle Std. dev.	380	7.0	6.0	3.0	0.3	Inside
Bad contacts/100 residues	0	0.0	3.3	10.0	−0.3	Inside
Zeta angle Std. dev.	565	1.3	3.1	1.6	−1.1	Better
H-bond energy Std. dev.	400	0.7	0.8	0.2	0.5	Inside
Overall G-factor	581	0.0	−0.3	0.3	1.0	Better

network that by considering the Wallner and Elofsson's study it is indeed superior to statistics-based methods [41]. In this method two quality measures are predicted, LG score and MaxSub score. Based on their range of qualities; predicted LG score and MaxSub score of the model after MD is 4.14 (which is within the range of a 'extremely good') and 0.45(which are within the range of 'good'), while values of 2.915 and 0.304 were obtained for LG score and MaxSub score, respectively in the model before MD simulation. These scores indicate the refinement of the model after MD simulation.

Ultimately, the validity of the model was evaluated by PROCHECK, and stereochemical properties of protein structure were listed in Tables 1 and 2 [31,42]. In the Figure 5, phi and psi distribution of Ramachandran plot indicate that 100% of residues were present in favored and allowed regions, which confirm that the structure is comparable with good homology model [43]. Also the main chain parameters which consist of six properties plotted are all well within the established limit of reliable structures (Table 2).

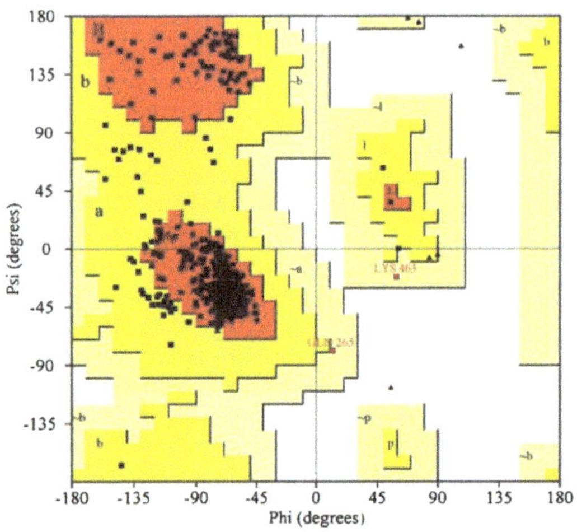

Figure 5 Ramachandran plot for 3D structural model of bovine serum albumin.

In brief, according to all applied evaluated methods, it can be concluded that obtained 3.D structural model has an acceptable geometry for further study by docking approach.

Docking studies

With the interest of comparability of docking result with experimental data (which studied the interaction among flavonoids and BSA), and also shedding the light at an ambiguous point of experimental observation in molecular level, with respect to Dufour and Dangles work [33] one stage of docking simulation was designed. Therefore, the binding interaction of quercetin (as the most studied flavonoid) and warfarin (as a site marker of subdomain IIA HSA) was subject to docking simulation.

First of all, in this process, the accuracy of applied docking protocol was examined. So, warfarin as a probe of HSA (whose high affinity binding site was known as a subdomain IIA) was docked into HSA (PDB ID: 1H9Z), which co-crystallized with it. Docking results demonstrates that the warfarin docks back into the experimental binding location which was retrieved based on the crystallographic study (Figure 6).Therefore; this protocol was confirmed and consequently, applied in docking simulation for complexes of quercetin with HSA and BSA.

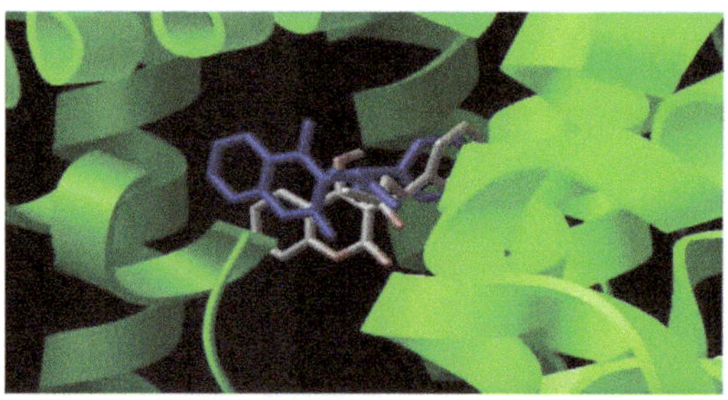

Figure 6 The docking conformation and location of warfarin on the Human serum albumin (PDB ID: 1H9Z). The conformation of warfarin after docking indicates with DG colored sketch (David Goodsell's scheme) and what was retrieved from the crystallographic study indicate as a blue sketch.

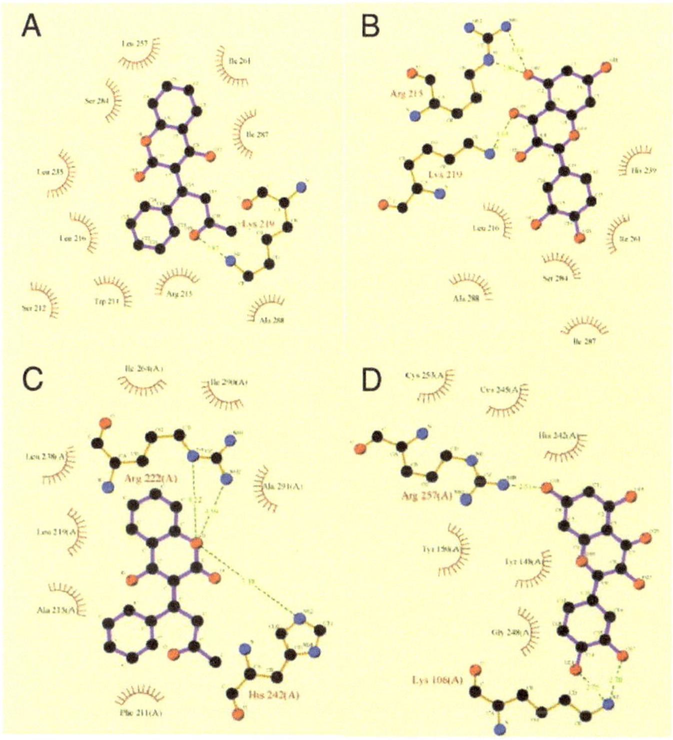

Figure 7 The structure of bovine serum albumin complexes with warfarin and quercetin (A, B), consequently (C) The structure of human serum albumin complexes with warfarin and quercetin, (D) was analyzed using the Ligplot 4.22 program. The hydrogen bonds are shown as dash lines and hydrophobic contacts are indicated with half-moon.

For analyzing the specific contact and indicating the participated amino acids in biding sites the Ligplot program was employed [44]. It is indicated in Figure 7, That in the binding site of bovine serum albumin, serine 284, isoleucine 261 and 287, alanine 288 involve in hydrophobic interaction with quercetin and warfarin, and also arginine 219 contribute in a hydrogen bond with both, this means that in the case of BSA, the warfarin and quercetin binding sites completely overlap, while these ligands are bonded in different location in HSA.

The Dufour and Dangles fluorescence spectroscopy study had shown that fluorescence of BSA-quercetin complex (protein/marker molar ratio of 1) is affected by constant concentration of warfarin (site marker of subdomain IIA),

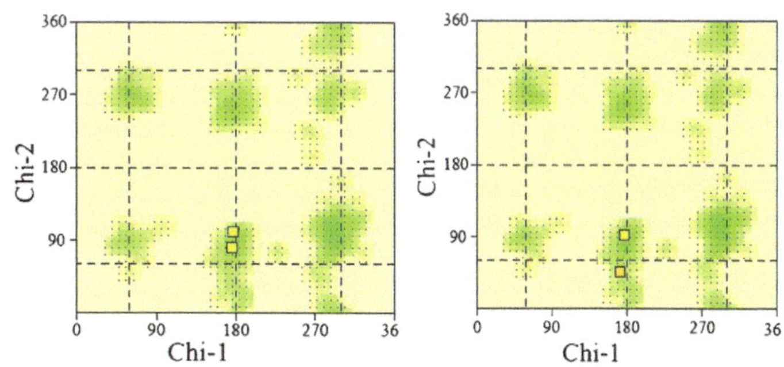

Figure 8 The χ_1/χ_2 plots are obtained from PROCHECK program. Each square represents one residue. The color coding of the squares is corresponding the range of yellow to red which is reflects the degree to which the orientation is favored; therefore, yellow indicate the residue is in a favored and red indicate the residue is an unflavored region. Two tryptophan of bovine serum albumin was indicated in both plots. The left plot indicate χ_1/χ_2 coordinate of tryptophans before MD (Left). The right plot indicates the χ_1/χ_2 coordinates of tryptophans after MD (Right). How it is shown, trp 134 remains constant while the χ_1/χ_2 coordinates of trp 212 is changed and located in unflavored region.

but fluorescence of HSA-quercetin complex is independent of warfarin presence [33].

For better understanding of the relation between experimental observations and what was retrieved from docking calculations. The more investigations were taken to visualization the effect of BSA-flavonoids interaction on local conformational changes, which leads to fluorescence quenching.

First notable issue which was considered is that the amino acids lining in the common binding site of quercetin and warfarin, are neighbors of tryptophan 212 within 5Å. This is important because the intrinsic fluorescence of BSA with excitation at 295 nm is due to the tryptophan residues (BSA has two tryptophan, tryptophan 212 and tryptophan 134) and quercetin actually promoted a strong quenching of the tryptophan emission at 340 nm

Table 3 The free energy of binding between, 12 Flavones, 12 Flavonols, 3 Flavanones, 2 Flavan-3-ols and bovine serum albumin obtained from docking study, and their AGEs inhibitions' IC_{50} (in regard to Matsuda, H., et al. [12])

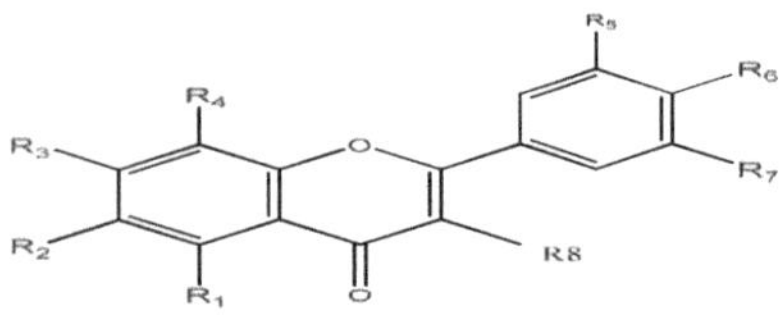

Num	Name	R^1	R^2	R^3	R^4	R^5	R^6	R^7	R^8	ΔG (Kcal/mol)	AGEs inhibition IC_{50} (% in 200 μM)
1	Flavone	H	H	H	H	H	H	H	H	−7.09	5%
2	7-Hydroxyflavone	H	H	OH	H	H	H	H	H	−6.96	27%
3	Chrysin	OH	H	OH	H	H	H	H	H	−7.56	43%
4	4,7-Dihydroxyflavone	H	H	OH	H	H	OH	H	H	−7.0	44%
5	3,4,7-Trihydroxyflavone	H	H	OH	H	OH	OH	H	H	−7.53	44%
6	Apigenin	OH	H	OH	H	H	OH	H	H	−7.52	53%
7	Luteolin	OH	H	OH	H	OH	OH	H	H	−7.53	64%
8	Diosmetin	OH	H	OH	H	OH	OCH_3	H	H	−7.05	27%
9	Pilloin	OH	H	OCH_3	H	OH	OCH_3	H	H	−7.9	29%
10	10 F	OH	H	OCH_3	H	OCH_3	OCH_3	H	H	−7.0	29%
11	Wogonin	OH	H	OH	OCH_3	H	H	H	H	−7.03	50%
12	Baicalin	OH	OH	OH	H	H	H	H	H	−7.75	79%
13	3-Hydroxyflavone	H	H	H	H	H	H	H	OH	−7.1	3%
14	Kaempferol	OH	H	OH	H	H	OH	H	OH	−7.47	46%
15	Quercetin	OH	H	OH	H	OH	OH	H	OH	−7.67	57%
16	Rhamnetin	OH	H	OCH_3	H	OH	OH	H	OH	−7.57	55%
17	Tamarixetin	OH	H	OH	H	OH	OCH_3	H	OH	−7.89	45%
18	F18	OH	H	OCH_3	H	OH	OH	H	OCH_3	−7.4	57%
19	Ombuine	OH	H	OCH_3	H	OH	OCH_3	H	OH	−7.66	27%
20	Ayanin	OH	H	OCH_3	H	OH	OCH_3	H	OCH_3	−7.66	40%
21	21 F	OH	H	OCH_3	H	OCH_3	OCH_3	H	OH	−7.69	13%
22	Myricetin	H	H	H	H	H	H	H	OH	−7.48	61%
23	Mearnsetin	H	H	H	H	H	CH3	H	OH	−7.51	10%
24	24 F	H	H	CH_3	H	H	H	H	OH	- 7.81	42%
25	Liquiritigenin	H	H	OH	H	H	OH	H	H	−7.16	40%
26	26 F	H	H	OCH_3	H	H	OH	H	H	−6.74	44%
27	Eriodictyol	OH	H	OH	H	OH	OH	H	H	−7.46	46%
28	(+)-Catechin	OH	H	OH	H	OH	OH	H	β-OH	−7.74	69%
29	(−)-Epigallocatechin	OH	H	OH	H	OH	OH	OH	α-OH	−7.06	4%

[33]. These observations lead to further study of checking the tryptophan flexibility after interaction between the quercetin and BSA complex.

So, the complex of BSA model and quercetin (best conformation after docking) was subjected to molecular dynamic simulation for 2 ns. After the stability of the system, for describing the side chain conformational changes the dihedral angles of our interested aromatic residue, χ_1 / χ_2 plot was provided by PROCHECK program [31]. The results represent the significant shuffling between side-chain conformations of tryptophan 212 before and after the refinement of BSA-quercetin complex with molecular dynamic simulation. Figure 8 indicates that the BSA residues which were involved in interaction with quercetin, pushing the tryptophan 212 side chain conformations to unflavored regions.

Discussion

In present work, based on docking calculation and molecular dynamic simulation, the detailed understanding was obtained about the interaction of quercetin (as a typical flavonoids) and BSA, which is in consistence with previous experimental data [33]. In addition, these calculations in molecular levels demonstrate its ability to providing the interpretation for experimental observation.

The first-stage docking results confirm on one hand the reliability of obtained 3D structural model, and on the other hand, by showing the significant specificity between high homologous BSA and HSA proteins, indicate the necessity of constructing BSA model's for analyzing the interaction flavonoids with it.

According to visualization of the predicted binding site of quercetin, any interventions are not observed between the quercetin binding site and reported glycation site of BSA [18]. However, for the more reliable conclusion, a number of flavonoids which introduced as an inhibitor of BSA glycation [3,12] were employed for the further docking studies.

By the speculation that the radical scavenging activity in physiological condition could inhibit oxidative fragmentation of Amadori rearrangement product and subsequently prevented the AGEs formation, the number of flavonoids was studied to find a correlation between the experimental anti glycation activity and radical scavenging activity of them [12]. In the present investigation with respect to their works, interested flavonoids was selected and by considering an interference reaction in the glycation site as the possible inhibitory mechanism [9,45,46], the theoretical binding energies of flavonoids in the complex with BSA were calculated by docking methods(calculated free energy of binding were listed in Tables 3 and 4). Then, analytical methods were performed by SPSS software (version 15). The correlation analyzes between the experimental activity (IC_{50}) and predicted binding energy reveal that there is no significant correlation between these values ($p > 0.3$).

Besides the statistical analyzes, the AutoDockTools (ADT) was used for visualization the relationship between the predicted flavonoids' binding site and the reported glycation site on BSA. Interestingly, despite the structural differentiations which exist among these flavonoids, the most likely conformation of each one of them, were placed in the same binding site (consist of lysine 219, arginine 215, isoleucine 287, and serine 284) (Figure 9) which can't be considered as any glycation sites of BSA (in respect to aforementioned Hinton and Ames study). Therefore, by considering these results, maybe it can be concluded that the hydrophobic hindrances in the glycation site can't be considered as an inhibitory mechanism for flavonoids.

Conclusion

In previous experimental studies, the high homology between BSA and HSA has invoked speculation that they have a similar structure and so share similar capability in some of their properties like ligands binding [45]. However, simulating the quercetin (as the most studied flavonoids) interactions with both BSA and HSA show significant differences between them, which confirms our speculation about the necessity of providing the affordable BSA 3D structural model for analyzing its specific

Table 4 The free energy of binding between 3 isoflavones and bovine Serum albumin obtained from docking study, and their AGEs inhibitions' IC_{50}

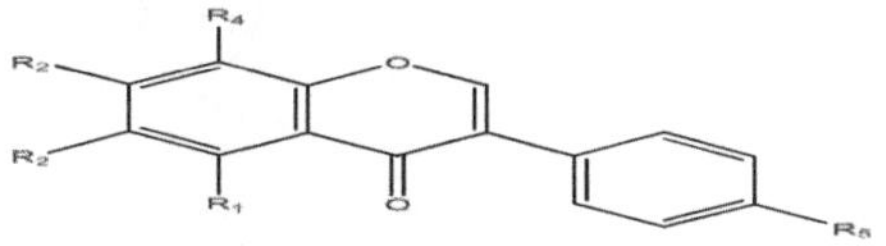

Num.	Name	R1	R2	R3	R4	R5	ΔG (Kcal/mol)	AGEs inhibition IC_{50} (% in 200 μM)
30	Daidzein	H	H	OH	H	OH	−7.05	33%
31	Genistein	OH	H	OH	H	OH	−6.44	34%
32	Biochanin A	OH	H	OH	H	OCH_3	−7.68	36%

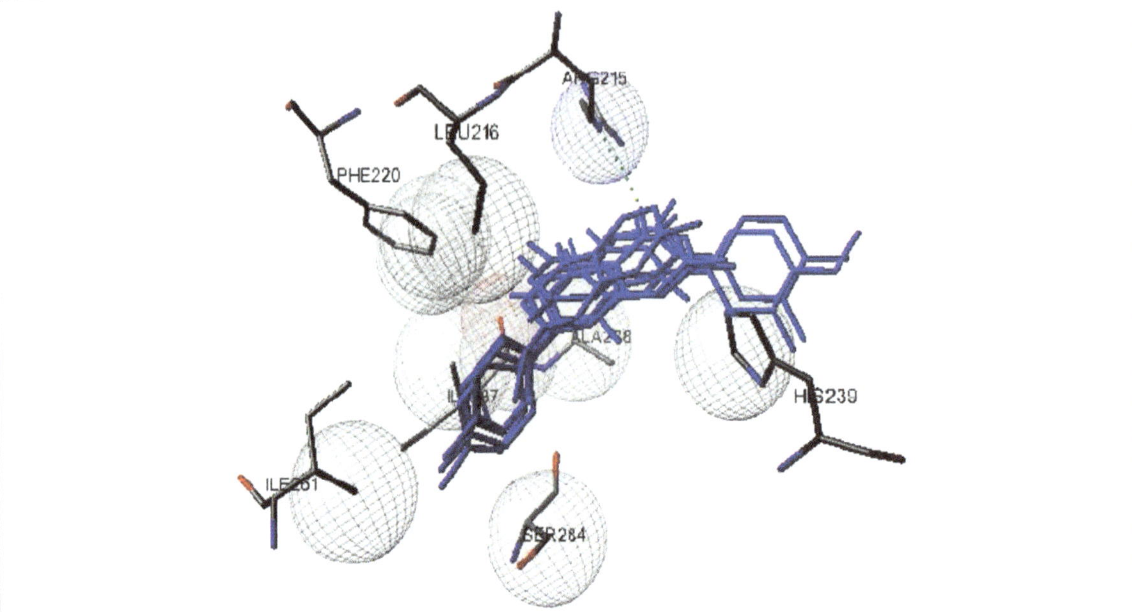

Figure 9 The superimposition of docked complex. The most likely conformation of representative flavonoids of under study groups (Flavones, flavonols, flavanones, flavan-3-ols, isoflavones), is represented in their binding site.

binding location and binding affinity for our interested ligands.

Interestingly, in the present study, the consistency between docking results and experimental data not only indicate the validity of our simulation but also become helpful in interpreting about experimental observation in molecular levels [33].

Thus different aspect of results was considered, on one hand the visualization of quercetin binding site leads to find the relationship between the binding site residues and tryptophan 212, and also by employing the MD simulation it is revealed that participated residues in flavonoids interaction site affect on tryptophan local conformational change, which at last is observed as fluorescence quenching.

On the other hand, according to our obtained results, the possibility of relation between the flavonoids binding site and glycation sites was investigated, while the correlation analyzes was adopted between binding affinity of flavonoids to BSA and IC_{50} of AGE inhibition. How was mentioned before based on the results, the flavonoids can't be considered as an intervention agent for glycation site and therefore, the possibility of this inhibitory mechanism is unacceptable in the case of flavonoids.

Ultimately, the other interesting outcome of this study is laid beneath the final examination. Coincident with our study the crystallographic structure of bovine serum albumin was determined [15]. Therefore, the comparison has been made between our calculated 3D structural models of BSA with the reported model which retrieved from crystallographic technique to get insight into their distinctive difference. These two structures were superimposed with Swiss PDB viewer software (Figure 10) [47]. And strong correlation (RMSD: 1.9) between them shades a light in the hypothesis that applied methods in this study are accurate and reliable.

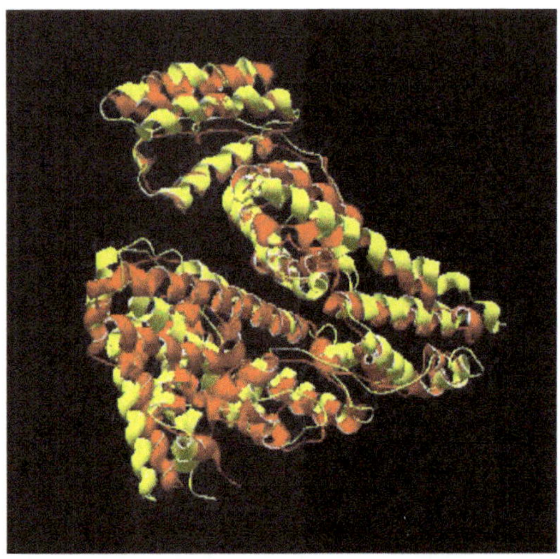

Figure 10 The superimposition between crystallographic structure of bovine serum albumin (PDB ID: 4F5S) (orange) and calculated 3D structure model (yellow), obtained with Swiss PDB viewer software.

Competing interests

The authors declare that they have no competing interests.

Authors' contributions

All authors contributed to the concept and design of study. AJ and MA performed all computational experiments and analyzed the data. MA is responsible for the study registration, financial and administrative support. AJ, MA and AAMM wrote the manuscript and all authors read and approved the final manuscript.

Acknowledgements

This work was financially supported by grants from Research Council of Tehran University of Medical Science and UNESCO Chair on Interdisciplinary Research in Diabetes, University of Tehran, Iran.

Author details

[1]Department of Medicinal Chemistry, Faculty of Pharmacy and Pharmaceutical Sciences Research Center, Tehran University of Medical Sciences, Tehran, Iran. [2]Institute of Biochemistry and Biophysics, University of Tehran, Tehran, Iran.

References

1. Nawale RB, Mourya VK, Bhise SB: **Non-enzymatic glycation of proteins: a cause for complications in diabetes.** *Indian J Biochem Biophys* 2006, **43:**337–344.
2. Iberg N, Fluckiger R: **Nonenzymatic glycosylation of albumin in vivo. identification of multiple glycosylated sites.** *J Biol Chem* 1986, **261:**13542–13545.
3. Morimitsu Y, Yoshida K, Esaki S, Hirota A: **Protein glycation inhibitors from thyme (*Thymus vulgaris*).** *Biosci Biotechnol Biochem* 1995, **59:**2018–2021.
4. Rahbar S, Figarola JL: **Novel inhibitors of advanced glycation endproducts.** *Arch Biochem Biophys* 2003, **419:**63–79.
5. Deeb O, Rosales-Hernández MC, Gómez-Castro C, Garduño-Juárez R, Correa-Basurto J: **Exploration of human serum albumin binding sites by docking and molecular dynamics flexible ligand–protein interactions.** *Biopolymers* 2010, **93:**161–170.
6. Cŕdova J, Ryan JD, Boonyaratanakornkit BB, Clark DS: **Esterase activity of bovine serum albumin up to 160°C: a new benchmark for biocatalysis.** *Enzyme Microb Techno* 2008, **42:**278–283.
7. Rondeau P, Bourdon E: **The glycation of albumin: structural and functional impacts.** *Biochimie* 2011, **93:**645–658.
8. Bousova I, Vukasovic D, Juretic D, Palicka V, Drsata J: **Enzyme activity and AGE formation in a model of AST glycoxidation by D-fructose in vitro.** *Acta Pharm* 2005, **55:**107–114.
9. Kawabata T, Packer L: **[alpha]-lipoate can protect against glycation of serum albumin, but not low-density lipoprotein.** *Biochem Biophys Res Commun* 1994, **203:**99–104.
10. Gutiérrez RMP, Diaz SL, Reyese IC, Gonzalez AMN: **Anti-glycation effect of spices and chilies uses in traditional mexican cuisine.** *J Nat Prod* 2010, **3:**95–102.
11. Bors W, Heller W, Michel C, Saran M: **Flavonoids as antioxidants: determination of radical-scavenging efficiencies.** *Methods Enzymol* 1990, **186:**343–355.
12. Matsuda H, Wang T, Managi H, Yoshikawa M: **Structural requirements of flavonoids for inhibition of protein glycation and radical scavenging activities.** *Bioorg Med Chem* 2003, **11:**5317–5323.
13. Van Boekel MA, van den Bergh PJ, Honders HJ: **Glycation of human serum albumin: inhibition by Diclofenac.** *Biochim Biophys Acta* 1992, **1120:**201–204.
14. Tai HC: *X-ray Crystallographic Studies of Bovine Serum Albumin and Helicobacter Pylori Thioredoxin-2.* Saskatoon, Canada: Thesis, University of Saskatchewan; 2004.
15. Bujacz A: **Structures of bovine, equine and leporine serum albumin.** *Acta Crystallogr Sect D Biol Crystallogr* 2012, **68:**1278–1289.
16. Ginalski K: **Comparative modeling for protein structure prediction.** *Curr Opin Struct Biol* 2006, **16:**172–177.
17. Azizian H, Bahrami H, Pasalar P, Amanlou M: **Molecular modeling of Helicobacter pylori arginase and the inhibitor coordination interactions.** *J Mol Graph Model* 2010, **28:**626–635.
18. Hinton DJS, Ames JM: **Site specificity of glycation and carboxymethylation of bovine serum albumin by fructose.** *Amino Acids* 2006, **30:**425–434.
19. Wardell M, Wang Z, Ho JX, Robert J, Ruker F, Ruble J, Carter DC: **The atomic structure of human methemalbumin at 1.9 A.** *Biochem Biophys Res Commun* 2002, **291:**813–819.
20. Sali A, Blundell TL: **Comparative protein modelling by satisfaction of spatial restraints.** *J Mol Biol* 1993, **234:**779–815.
21. Laurie AT, Jackson RM: **Q-SiteFinder: an energy-based method for the prediction of protein-ligand binding sites.** *Bioinformatics* 2005, **21:**1908–1916.
22. Hess B, Kutzner C, van der Spoel D, Lindahl E: **GROMACS 4: algorithms for highly efficient, load-balanced, and scalable molecular simulation.** *J Chem Theory Comput* 2008, **4:**435–447.
23. Hornak V, Abel R, Okur A, Strockbine B, Roitberg A, Simmerling C: **Comparison of multiple Amber force fields and development of improved protein backbone parameters.** *Proteins* 2006, **65:**712–725.
24. Bas DC, Rogers DM, Jensen JH: **Very fast prediction and rationalization of pKa values for protein–ligand complexes.** *Proteins Struct Funct Bioinf* 2008, **73:**765–783.
25. Bussi G, Donadio D, Parrinello M: **Canonical sampling through velocity rescaling.** *J Chem Phys* 2007, **126:**014101.
26. Berendsen H, Postma J, van Gunsteren W, DiNola A, Haak J: **Molecular dynamics with coupling to an external bath.** *J Chem Phys* 1984, **81:**3684–3690.
27. Essmann U, Perera L, Berkowitz ML, Darden T, Lee H, Pedersen LG: **A smooth particle mesh ewald method.** *J Chem Phys* 1995, **103:**8577–8593.
28. Wallner B, Elofsson A: **Can correct protein models be identified?** *Protein Sci* 2003, **12:**1073–1086.
29. Luthy R, Bowie JU, Eisenberg D: **Assessment of protein models with three-dimensional profiles.** *Nature* 1992, **356:**83–85.
30. Wiederstein M, Sippl MJ: **ProSA-web: interactive web service for the recognition of errors in three-dimensional structures of proteins.** *Nucleic Acids Res* 2007, **35:**W407–W410.
31. Laskowski RA, MacArthur MW, Moss DS, Thornton JM: **PROCHECK: a program to check the stereochemical quality of protein structures.** *J Appl Crystallogr* 1993, **26:**283–291.
32. Morris GM, Goodsell DS, Halliday RS, Huey R, Hart WE, Belew RK, Olson AJ: **Automated docking using a Lamarckian genetic algorithm and an empirical binding free energy function.** *J Comput Chem* 1998, **19:**1639–1662.
33. Dufour C, Dangles O: **Flavonoid-serum albumin complexation: determination of binding constants and binding sites by fluorescence spectroscopy.** *Biochim Biophys Acta* 2005, **1721:**164–173.
34. Froimowitz M: **HyperChem: a software package for computational chemistry and molecular modeling.** *Biotechniques* 1993, **14:**1010–1013.
35. Bekker H, Berendsen H, Dijkstra E, Achterop S, van Drunen R: **Gromacs method of virial calculation using a single sum.** In *Physics Computing.* 1993:257–26.
36. Lindahl E, Hess B, van der Spoel D: **GROMACS 3.0: a package for molecular simulation and trajectory analysis.** *J Mol Mod* 2001, **7:**306–317.
37. Berendsen H, van der Spoel D, van Drunen R: **GROMACS: a message-passing parallel molecular dynamics implementation.** *Comp Phys Comm* 1995, **91:**43–56.
38. Schuttelkopf AW, Van Aalten DM: **PRODRG: a tool for high-throughput crystallography of protein-ligand complexes.** *Acta Crystallogr Sect D Biol Crystallogr* 2004, **60:**1355–1363.
39. Thompson JD, Gibson TJ, Plewniak F, Jeanmougin F, Higgins DG: **The CLUSTAL_X windows interface: flexible strategies for multiple sequence alignment aided by quality analysis tools.** *Nucleic Acids Res* 1997, **25:**4876–4882.
40. Hirayama K, Akashi S, Furuya M, Fukuhara K: **Rapid confirmation and revision of the primary structure of bovine serum albumin by ESIMS and Frit-FAB LC/MS.** *Biochem Biophys Res Commun* 1990, **14:**639–646.
41. Fasnacht M, Zhu J, Honig B: **Local quality assessment in homology models using statistical potentials and support vector machines.** *Protein Sci* 2007, **16:**1557–1568.
42. Sakkiah S, Thangapandian S, John S, Lee KW: **Identification of critical chemical features for Aurora kinase-B inhibitors using Hip-Hop, virtual screening and molecular docking.** *J Mol Struct* 2011, **985:**14–26.

43. Xu Y, Colletier JP, Weik M, Jiang H, Moult J, Silman I, Sussman JL: **Flexibility of aromatic residues in the active-site gorge of acetylcholinesterase: X-ray versus molecular dynamics.** *Biophys J* 2008, **95:**2500–2511.
44. Wallace AC, Laskowski RA, Thornton JM: **L{IGPLOT}: a program to generate schematic diagrams of protein-ligand interactions.** *Protein Eng* 1995, **8:**127–134.
45. Hosseinzadeh R, Maleki R, Matin AA: **Interaction of diclofenac with bovine serum albumin investigated by diclofenac-selective electrode.** *Acta Chim Slov* 2007, **54:**126–130.
46. Hamilton JA1, Era S, Bhamidipati SP, Reed RG: **Locations of the three primary binding sites for long-chain fatty acids on bovine serum albumin.** *Proc Natl Acad Sci* 1991, **88:**2051–2054.
47. Guex N, Peitsch MC: **SWISS-MODEL and the Swiss-Pdb viewer: an environment for comparative protein modeling.** *Electrophoresis* 1997, **18:**2714–2723.

Label-free LC-MS analysis of HER2+ breast cancer cell line response to HER2 inhibitor treatment

Alessio Di Luca[1*], Michael Henry[1], Paula Meleady[1] and Robert O'Connor[1,2]

Abstract

Background: Human epidermal growth-factor receptor (HER)-2 is overexpressed in 25 % of breast-cancers and is associated with an aggressive form of the disease with significantly shortened disease free and overall survival. In recent years, the use of HER2-targeted therapies, monoclonal-antibodies and small molecule tyrosine-kinase inhibitors has significantly improved the clinical outcome for HER2-positive breast-cancer patients. However, only a fraction of HER2-amplified patients will respond to therapy and the use of these treatments is often limited by tumour drug insensitivity or resistance and drug toxicities. Currently there is no way to identify likely responders or rational combinations with the potential to improve HER2-focussed treatment outcome.

Methods: In order to further understand the molecular mechanisms of treatment-response with HER2-inhibitors, we used a highly-optimised and reproducible quantitative label-free LC-MS strategy to characterize the proteomes of HER2-overexpressing breast-cancer cell-lines (SKBR3, BT474 and HCC1954) in response to drug-treatment with HER2-inhibitors (lapatinib, neratinib or afatinib).

Results: Following 12 hours treatment with different HER2-inhibitors in the BT474 cell-line; compared to the untreated cells, 16 proteins changed significantly in abundance following lapatinib treatment (1 μM), 21 proteins changed significantly following neratinib treatment (150 nM) and 38 proteins changed significantly following afatinib treatment (150 nM). Whereas following 24 hours treatment with neratinib (200 nM) 46 proteins changed significantly in abundance in the HCC1954 cell-line and 23 proteins in the SKBR3 cell-line compared to the untreated cells. Analysing the data we found that, proteins like trifunctional-enzyme subunit-alpha, mitochondrial; heterogeneous nuclear ribonucleoprotein-R and lamina-associated polypeptide 2, isoform alpha were up-regulated whereas heat shock cognate 71 kDa protein was down-regulated in 3 or more comparisons.

Conclusion: This proteomic study highlights several proteins that are closely associated with early HER2-inhibitor response and will provide a valuable resource for further investigation of ways to improve efficacy of breast-cancer treatment.

Keywords: Afatinib, Breast cancer, HER2, Label-free LC-MS Proteomics, Lapatinib, Neratinib

Background

Breast cancer remains a leading cause of death among women in the Western World. Epidermal growth factor receptor 2 (HER2)-gene amplification or overexpression occurs in approximately 25 % of breast cancers and is associated with poor prognosis [1]. Tyrosine kinases play a critical role in the modulation of growth factor signalling and activated forms of these enzymes plays a crucial role in breast cancer pathogenesis [2]. In spite of the efforts that are underway to develop and improve HER-targeted therapies, *de novo* and acquired resistance remain major obstacles in the clinic; therefore, new drug treatments and methods of accurately predicting drug sensitivity are urgently needed [3].

Lapatinib, neratinib and afatinib are tyrosine kinase inhibitors of HER2 and EGFR (epidermal growth factor receptor) growth factor receptors which prevent the activation of the receptor tyrosine kinase, inhibiting the activation of the pathways that would promote tumour cell growth and proliferation [4]. Lapatinib is an orally active small molecule, it is a first-generation dual tyrosine

* Correspondence: alessiodiluca@gmail.com
[1]National Institute for Cellular Biotechnology, DCU, Glasnevin, Dublin 9, Dublin, Ireland
Full list of author information is available at the end of the article

kinase inhibitors that reversibly binds EGFR and HER2 [5] that has been approved in combination with capecitabine for the treatment of refractory breast cancer [6]. Although lapatinib does not cross the blood–brain barrier, it can reach therapeutic levels in brain tumours and brain metastases [7]. Neratinib and afatinib, two second-generation tyrosine kinase inhibitors that irreversibly bind to multiple HER receptors, are being investigated in clinical trials with promising results either as monotherapy or in combination [8, 9]. Both neratinib and afatinib have the ability to penetrate the blood–brain barrier and, as seen also with lapatinib, these small molecule tyrosine kinase inhibitors have minimal adverse effects on the heart [10].

Proteomics has great potentiality to guide the discovery of biomarkers with clinical utility for the diagnosis, treatment and management of breast cancer. Indeed, the identification of proteins that are differentially expressed as result of exposure to drug treatments such as lapatinib, neratinib and afatinib may provide novel drug targets for improved therapeutic action, and/or predict therapeutic outcome [11]. Mass-spectrometry based proteomics methods, such as label-free LC-MS (liquid chromatography-mass spectrometry), have become more popular for analysing quantitative changes in protein expression between samples [12, 13] though there is a lack of studies investigating the proteomic profile of lapatinib, neratinib or afatinib response in breast cancer.

To identify markers which might be useful in predicting treatment response and/or potential targets for rational additional drug treatments for increasing efficacy, a systematic approach is required. Difficulties in studying hydrophobic proteins or proteins with low or high molecular weights are common inherent proteomic challenges [14]. A method like label-free LC-MS proteomic is ideal for such analyses as it is less impacted by many of these limitations [12, 13]. In this study we have used a quantitative label-free LC-MS proteomic approach to characterize the proteomes of cell line models of HER2-inhibitor response in HER2-positive breast cancer cell lines models, SKBR3, BT474 and HCC1954, in order to further understand the molecular contributors to treatment response.

Methods

Cell culture and drug treatment

HER2-overexpressing breast cancer cell lines BT474, SKBR3 and HCC1954 were examined. The BT474 cell line was maintained in antibiotic-free Dulbeccos Modified Eagles medium (DMEM) supplemented with 10 % fetal bovine serum (PAA Labs, Austria), 2 % L-glutamine (Sigma-Aldrich, Germany) and 1 % sodium pyruvate (Sigma-Aldrich, Germany). SKBR3 and HCC1954 breast cancer cell lines were maintained in Roswell Park Memorial Institute (RPMI) 1640 medium supplemented with 10 % fetal bovine serum (PAA Labs, Austria). All cell lines were kept at 37 °C in 5 % CO2/95 % air humidified incubators. Biological replicates, for each cell line, were within 10 passages of each other. All cultures were tested routinely and were mycoplasma-free.

Drug treatments were prepared in dimethyl sulfoxide [(DMSO) Sigma-Aldrich, Germany] at a final concentration of 0.03 % (v/v) and applied as follows lapatinib 1 μM (Sequoia Sciences, Saint Louis, MO, USA), 150 nM afatinib (Sequoia Sciences, Saint Louis, MO, USA) and 150 nM or 200 nM neratinib (Sequoia Sciences, Saint Louis, MO, USA) for 12 or 24 hours of exposure. The drug treatment control consisted of the same cell line treated with the same amount of DMSO used to dilute the drug and for the same exposure time (12 or 24 hours). Three or four biological samples were prepared for each cell lines.

Protein extraction

Due to the inherent variability of protein fractionation, it was decided to analyse whole cell lysates to minimise differences between the multiple cell lines analysed. After 12 or 24 hours of drug exposure, cells were harvested for LC-MS analysis, following five washes in cold phosphate-buffered saline (PBS) by scraping into cold PBS. Approximately 3×10^6 cells were centrifuged at 200 g and the cell pellet snap frozen in liquid nitrogen.

Sample preparation for label-free LC-MS analysis

Cell pellets were lysed with lysis buffer {7 M Urea, 2 M Thiourea, 30 mM Tris, 4 % 3-[(3-cholamidopropyl)dimethylamonio]-1-propanesulfonate (CHAPS); pH 8.5} (Sigma-Aldrich, Germany) and then were cleaned up using the Ready Prep 2-D clean up kit (Bio-Rad, Hercules, CA, USA). Protein concentration was determined using the Quick Start Bradford assay (Bio-Rad, Hercules, CA, USA). Ten micrograms of protein sample were resuspended in 40 μl of 50 mM ammonium bicarbonate (Sigma-Aldrich, Germany). Reduction was performed by adding to the samples an amount of dithiothreitol (DTT) (0.5 M) (Sigma-Aldrich, Germany) to reach the concentration of 10 mM at 56 °C for 20 min, and allowed to cool to room temperature. Samples were alkylated by adding to the samples an amount of iodoacetamide (0.55 M) (Sigma-Aldrich, Germany) to reach the concentration of 55 mM and then incubated for 15 min in the dark at room temperature. Digestion with Trypsin Gold, Mass Spectrometry Grade (Promega, Madison, NJ, USA) was carried out at a ratio of 1:19 (Trypsin/Protein) at 37 °C overnight. To stop the digestion, trifluoroacetic acid (TFA) (Sigma-Aldrich, Germany) was add to the samples (0.5 % final concentration) at 37 °C for 15 min. Samples were then cleaned up using Pierce C18 Spin Columns (Thermo Fisher Scientific, USA), dried under a vacuum and stored at −20 °C. Prior to mass spectrometry analysis dried peptides were resuspended in 50 µl of 0.1 % formic acid (FA) in 2 % acetonitrile (ACN) (Sigma-Aldrich, Germany), vortexed to ensure an even suspension.

Mass spectrometry using LC-MS/MS

Nano LC-MS/MS analysis was carried out using an Ultimate 3000 nanoLC system (Dionex, USA) coupled to a hybrid linear ion trap/Orbitrap mass spectrometer (LTQ Orbitrap XL; Thermo Fisher Scientific, USA). Five µl of digest were loaded onto a C18 trap column (C18 PepMap, 300 m ID × 5 mm, 5 µm particle size, 100 Å pore size; Dionex, USA) and desalted for 10 min using a flow rate of 25 µl/min in 0.1 % TFA in 2 % ACN. The trap column was then switched online with the analytical column [PepMap C18, 75 µm ID × 500 mm, 3 µm particle and 100 Å pore size; (Dionex, USA)] and peptides were eluted with the following binary gradients of solvent A and B: 0–25 % solvent B in 240 min and 25–50 % solvent B in a further 60 min, where solvent A consisted of 2 % ACN and 0.1 % formic acid in water and solvent B consisted of 80 % ACN and 0.08 % formic acid in water. Column flow rate was set to 350 nl/min. Data were acquired in data-dependent mode and externally calibrated with Xcalibur software, version 2.0.7 (Thermo Fisher Scientific, USA). Survey MS scans were acquired in the Orbitrap in the 400–1800 m/z (mass-to-charge ratio) range with the resolution set to a value of 30000 at m/z 400. Up to three of the most intense multiply charged ions (1+, 2+ and 3+) per scan were collision-induced dissociation (CID) fragmented in the linear ion trap. A dynamic exclusion window was applied within 40 s. All tandem mass spectra were collected using a normalised collision energy of 35 %, an isolation window of 3 m/z, and one microscan.

Label-free LC-MS quantitative profiling

Label-free LC-MS analysis was carried out using Progenesis QI for proteomics software version 4.1 (NonLinear Dynamics, UK), as recommended by the manufacturer (see www.nonlinear.com for further background to alignment, normalisation, calculation of peptide abundance, etc.). As already described by Meleady et al. [15] the software processed the raw data in two steps. Firstly each sample run was subjected to alignment which involved aligning the data based on the LC retention time of each sample; this allows for any drift in retention time giving an adjusted retention time for all runs in the analysis. The sample run that yielded most features (i.e. peptide ions) was used as the reference run, to which retention time of all of the other runs were aligned and peak intensities were normalised. The Progenesis peptide quantification algorithm calculates peptide abundance as the sum of the peak areas within its isotope boundaries. Each abundance value is then transformed to a normalised abundance value by applying a global scaling factor. Protein abundance was calculated as the sum of the abundances of all peptide ions which have been identified as coming from the same protein. A number of criteria were used to filter the data before exporting the MS/MS output files to MASCOT (www.matrixscience.com) for protein identification; peptide features with ANOVA (analysis of variance) p-value ≤0.05 between experimental groups, mass peaks (features) with charge states from +1 to +3, and greater than 3 isotopes per peptide. All MS/MS spectra were exported from Progenesis software as a MASCOT generic file (mgf) and used for peptide identification with MASCOT (version 2.3) searched against the UniProtKB–SwissProt database (taxonomy, *homo sapiens*). The search parameters used were as follows: peptide mass tolerance set to 20 ppm, MS/MS mass tolerance set at 0.6 Da; up to two missed cleavages were allowed, carbamidomethylation set as a fixed modification and methionine oxidation set as a variable modification. Only peptides with ion scores of 40 and above were considered and re-imported back into Progenesis QI for proteomics software for further analysis. A number of criteria were applied to assign a protein as identified; proteins with ≥2 peptides matched, a ≥1.5 fold difference in abundance and an ANOVA between experimental groups of ≤0.05.

The biological function of the proteins identified was assigned using ontology tools in PANTHER [16].

Results

The different concentrations employed for the three different drug treatments (afatinib, neratinib or lapatinib) were chosen to reflect published clinically relevant concentrations [5, 17, 18]. As the aim of the current study was to investigate proteins that are closely associated with early treatment response and, as a short time (12 hours) exposure to drug treatments may allow identification of a proportionally small number of proteins that are associated with drugs response, another time point (24 hours) and a higher drug concentration were used to ensure that the proteins identified had a higher likelihood of a real association with drug response.

Proteomic analysis of the HER2-overexpressing breast cancer cell lines

Label-free proteomic analysis was performed in HER2-overexpressing breast cancer cell lines to reveal the proteins that were significantly different in the BT474 cell line in response to afatinib, neratinib or lapatinib treatments and also in the breast cancer cell lines SKBR3 and HCC1954 in response to neratinib treatments. Following analysis of the phenotypes using the software incorporated in Progenesis QI for proteomics, all proteins were ranked by p value derived from one-way ANOVA ($p \leq 0.05$), fold change (≥1.5) and number of peptides (≥2) matched to the protein.

38 significant ($p \leq 0.05$) proteins whose abundance changed significantly in the BT474 between afatinib-treated and control cells were identified. Of these, 16 demonstrated an increased abundance (Table 1a) and 22 a decreased abundance in the treated cells (Table 1b). Details of the significant variation between phenotypes are presented in Table 1. 21 and 16 proteins differed in abundance respectively between the BT474 cell lines neratinib or lapatinib-treated compared to untreated cells (Tables 2 and 3). In the comparison with the neratinib treated cell lines 18 proteins demonstrated an increased abundance (Table 2a) and three a decreased abundance in the treated cells (Table 2b). Of the 16 proteins identified in the comparison with the lapatinib treated cell lines 11 proteins demonstrated an increased abundance (Table 3a) and five a decreased abundance in the treated cells (Table 3b). Figure 1 show a Venn diagram highlighting the proteins that were in common between the proteins that were significantly different in the BT474 cell line in response to afatinib, neratinib or lapatinib treatments. The diagrams shows that 33, ten and eight proteins identified respectively in afatinib, neratinib or lapatinib treated cell line were unique in each comparison. Two proteins were common among all three comparisons, three and six were in common respectively between afatinib and neratinib and between neratinib and lapatinib-treated cells. There were no proteins common between afatinib and lapatinib-treated cells.

23 proteins were observed to vary significantly ($p \leq 0.05$) in abundance between the SKBR3 cell line neratinib-treated compared to untreated cells (Table 4). Out of these 23 proteins, 17 demonstrated an increased abundance (Table 4a) and six a decreased abundance in the treated cells (Table 4b).

46 proteins were observed to vary significantly ($p \leq 0.05$) in abundance between the HCC1954 cell line neratinib-treated compared to untreated cells (Table 5). Of these, 22 demonstrated an increased abundance (Table 5a) and 24 a decreased abundance in the treated cells (Table 5b).

Figure 2 show a Venn diagram highlighting the proteins that were in common between the proteins that were significantly different in the three different cell lines (BT474, HCC1954 or SKBR3) in response to neratinib treatments. The diagrams shows that 18, 42 and 18 proteins identified respectively in BT474, HCC1954 or SKBR3 treated cell line were unique in each comparison. There were no proteins in common in all three comparisons. One, three and two proteins were in common respectively between BT474 and HCC1954, between HCC1954 and SKBR3 and between BT474 and SKBR3 neratinib treated cell lines.

Following label-free proteomic analysis 194 and 228 proteins were observed to vary significantly ($p \leq 0.05$) in abundance respectively between SKBR3 and HCC1954 cell lines or between SKBR3 and HCC1954 cell lines both treated with neratinib. 123 were in common between the two comparisons. In the comparison between SKBR3 and HCC1954 cell lines 104 proteins demonstrated an increased abundance and 90 a decreased abundance in HCC1954 cell line. Of the 228 proteins identified in the comparisons between SKBR3 and HCC1954 cell lines both treated with neratinib 105 proteins demonstrated an increased abundance and 123 a decreased abundance in HCC1954 cell line treated with neratinib.

Table 6 shows a list of 17 proteins that were identified in more than one comparisons between the identified proteins with altered levels in response to afatinib, lapatinib or neratinib treatment compared to control in BT474 cell line and also in neratinib treatment compared to control in HCC1954 and SKBR3 cell lines. There were no proteins in common in all five comparisons. Trifunctional enzyme subunit alpha, mitochondrial was in common and up-regulated among four comparison whereas, heterogeneous nuclear ribonucleoprotein R and lamina-associated polypeptide 2, isoform alpha were in common and up-regulated between three comparisons. 11 proteins are in common between two comparisons, of these eight were up-regulated and three down-regulated among comparisons. Moreover, three proteins showed an irregular abundance pattern in response to different drugs treatment and/or cell line, phosphoglycerate kinase 1 was down-regulated in response to afatinib in BT474 cell line and in response to neratinib in HCC1954 cell line, but was up-regulated in response to neratinib in SKBR3 cell line. Ubiquitin-like modifier-activating enzyme 1 and heterogeneous nuclear ribonucleoprotein Q showed both an opposite abundance pattern in response to afatinib in BT474 cell line and in response to neratinib in HCC1954 cell line. Details are presented in Table 6.

Discussion

Despite the improvements in diagnosis and treatment of breast cancer, novel and more efficient tools are needed to guide diagnosis and individualise therapy to improve patient-outcomes and overall survival-rates [19]. In this study, we used label-free LC-MS proteomics to identify proteins associated with HER2-inhibitor drugs response in HER2-positive cell lines. To achieve this we characterised the proteomic response of three HER2-targeting tyrosine kinase inhibitors (lapatinib, neratinib and afatinib) in the overexpressing HER2 BT474 cell line. In addition, because of the complexity of breast cancer and to get a broader perspective in multiple breast cancer cell lines, we characterised the proteomic response to

Table 1 38 proteins identified as differentially expressed between the afatinib treated BT474 cell line and the control following label-free MS/MS analysis (Progenesis QI for proteomics)

UniProt*)	Identification	Peptides†)	Score‡)	ANOVA (*p*)	Fold change	Highest condition§)
a						
O14979;Q14103	Heterogeneous nuclear ribonucleoprotein D-like	4	216.49	0.000367	2.37	Afatinib
Q00839	Heterogeneous nuclear ribonucleoprotein U	3	151.34	0.001436	1.61	Afatinib
P31943	Heterogeneous nuclear ribonucleoprotein H	2	140.67	0.002201	1.58	Afatinib
P40939	Trifunctional enzyme subunit alpha, mitochondrial	2	190.67	0.007201	2.05	Afatinib
Q9Y2X3	Nucleolar protein 58	2	114.49	0.008894	1.86	Afatinib
Q09666	Neuroblast differentiation-associated protein AHNAK	2	90.42	0.008936	1.56	Afatinib
Q8NBS9	Thioredoxin domain-containing protein 5	2	110.22	0.013371	1.56	Afatinib
Q12906	Interleukin enhancer-binding factor 3	2	133.56	0.015709	1.62	Afatinib
P68431	Histone H3.1	2	199.81	0.019319	1.61	Afatinib
P55084	Trifunctional enzyme subunit beta, mitochondrial	1	146.98	0.023507	1.6	Afatinib
O60506	Heterogeneous nuclear ribonucleoprotein Q	1	187.85	0.024443	2.81	Afatinib
P10809	60 kDa heat shock protein, mitochondrial	2	132.64	0.026205	5.23	Afatinib
P09429	High mobility group protein B1	1	140.79	0.027432	1.58	Afatinib
P62937	Peptidyl-prolyl cis-trans isomerase A	3	193.48	0.034894	1.75	Afatinib
A6NMY6	Putative annexin A2-like protein	2	127.79	0.03901	1.69	Afatinib
O43390	Heterogeneous nuclear ribonucleoprotein R	1	217.31	0.049038	2.27	Afatinib
b						
P08133	Annexin A6	2	88.25	0.004506	1.61	Control
A6NEC2	Puromycin-sensitive aminopeptidase-like protein	2	114.96	0.004836	1.75	Control
P48735	Isocitrate dehydrogenase [NADP], mitochondrial	2	100.11	0.005263	1.65	Control
P15531	Nucleoside diphosphate kinase A	2	116.29	0.005349	2.05	Control
P12268	Inosine-5'-monophosphate dehydrogenase 2	2	123.5	0.007421	1.52	Control
P22314	Ubiquitin-like modifier-activating enzyme 1	3	162.89	0.00852	1.58	Control
P00558	Phosphoglycerate kinase 1	3	135.58	0.008782	1.62	Control
P11216	Glycogen phosphorylase, brain form	2	97.04	0.009668	1.67	Control
P61204	ADP-ribosylation factor 3	2	190.14	0.010494	1.64	Control
P50570;Q05193	Dynamin-2	2	115.29	0.011594	1.99	Control
P21796;Q9Y277	Voltage-dependent anion-selective channel protein 1	3	215.59	0.014497	1.58	Control
Q9Y5B9	FACT complex subunit SPT16	2	114.74	0.014521	2.14	Control
P07384	Calpain-1 catalytic subunit	5	261.15	0.015632	1.59	Control
P50395	Rab GDP dissociation inhibitor beta	4	193.14	0.016052	1.55	Control
O43776	Asparagine–tRNA ligase, cytoplasmic	2	84.46	0.019422	1.56	Control
Q14566	DNA replication licensing factor MCM6	3	153.97	0.022003	1.59	Control
P35579	Myosin-9	3	153.68	0.02416	1.68	Control
P49189	4-trimethylaminobutyraldehyde dehydrogenase	2	108.57	0.027635	1.56	Control
Q86VP6	Cullin-associated NEDD8-dissociated protein 1	2	100.91	0.029028	1.67	Control
P04792	Heat shock protein beta-1	3	162.14	0.032666	1.73	Control
P31948	Stress-induced-phosphoprotein 1	2	102.57	0.032815	1.84	Control
Q9NUU7	ATP-dependent RNA helicase DDX19A	2	128.15	0.042435	1.72	Control

16 proteins were up regulated in the cells treated with afatinib (Table 1a) and 22 proteins were up regulated in the untreated cells (control) (Table 1b). *) Accession number in the UniProt database; †) Peptides used for quantitation; ‡) MASCOT score. §) Indicates if the proteins were up regulated in the treated cells (afatinib) or in the not treated cells (control)

Table 2 21 proteins identified as differentially expressed between the neratinib treated BT474 cell line and the control following label-free MS/MS analysis (Progenesis QI for proteomics)

UniProt*)	Identification	Peptides†)	Score‡)	ANOVA (p)	Fold change	Highest condition§)
a						
P33121	Long-chain-fatty-acid–CoA ligase 1	2	113.74	5.94E-05	1.56	Neratinib
P40939	Trifunctional enzyme subunit alpha, mitochondrial	3	182.37	0.002972	1.51	Neratinib
P0C0S8	Histone H2A type 1	1	138.51	0.003414	3.51	Neratinib
P11021	78 kDa glucose-regulated protein	1	150.58	0.004321	2.87	Neratinib
P78527	DNA-dependent protein kinase catalytic subunit	7	374.79	0.007306	3.89	Neratinib
P0C0S5	Histone H2A.Z	1	151.7	0.007686	2.08	Neratinib
P09874	Poly [ADP-ribose] polymerase 1	5	283.35	0.008246	3.63	Neratinib
P19367	Hexokinase-1	2	130.52	0.009371	1.6	Neratinib
Q12906	Interleukin enhancer-binding factor 3	4	200.23	0.010842	1.59	Neratinib
O43390	Heterogeneous nuclear ribonucleoprotein R	2	116.88	0.011383	1.54	Neratinib
P36542	ATP synthase subunit gamma, mitochondrial	2	95.75	0.011427	1.52	Neratinib
P12956	X-ray repair cross-complementing protein 6	5	275.69	0.014417	1.94	Neratinib
P55084	Trifunctional enzyme subunit beta, mitochondrial	2	99.86	0.015542	1.52	Neratinib
Q99623	Prohibitin-2	2	121.16	0.015667	1.72	Neratinib
P42166	Lamina-associated polypeptide 2, isoform alpha	2	117	0.020737	1.65	Neratinib
P31943	Heterogeneous nuclear ribonucleoprotein H	1	135.7	0.026364	1.61	Neratinib
P80723	Brain acid soluble protein 1	2	112.84	0.029049	3.50	Neratinib
P50416	Carnitine O-palmitoyltransferase 1, liver isoform	2	135.07	0.029912	1.51	Neratinib
b						
Q16643	Drebrin	2	153.59	2.19E-05	1.62	Control
P29966	Myristoylated alanine-rich C-kinase substrate	2	142.02	0.006012	1.59	Control
O95994	Anterior gradient protein 2 homolog	2	199.76	0.011444	1.56	Control

18 proteins were up regulated in the cells treated with neretinib (Table 2a) and three proteins were up regulated in the untreated cells (control) (Table 2a). *) Accession number in the UniProt database; †) Peptides used for quantitation; ‡) MASCOT score. §) Indicates if the proteins were up regulated in the treated cells (neratinib) or in the not treated cells (control)

neratinib treatment in two other overexpressing HER2 cell lines (HCC1954 and SKBR3). The different concentrations employed for the three different drug treatments represented the typical pharmacokinetic trough concentration that has been reported from patient trials [5, 17, 18]. This approach allowed us to identify a short list of 14 proteins whose expression level alters with a similar abundance patterns between different comparisons (11 up-regulated and three down-regulated) and that appear to be strongly involved in early treatment response.

Breast cancer cell lines have been widely used to investigate different aspect of the disease, generating reproducible and quantifiable results [20], although several problems may arise when using such models. Firstly, protein expression may differ from cell line to cell line within a single organism [21]. In our study, a high number of proteins (194) were shown to change significantly in abundance between SKBR3 and HCC1954 cell lines. Secondly, no single cell line is truly representative of a primary breast cancer, however, when a panel of cell lines are used as a system they can provide powerful information [22]. This study highlighted several proteins (in the three different cell lines) that had altered abundance in response to neratinib treatment, namely, trifunctional enzyme subunit alpha, mitochondrial; lamina-associated polypeptide 2, isoform alpha; carnitine O-palmitoyltransferase 1, liver isoform and 6-phosphogluconate dehydrogenase, decarboxylating. These proteins are generally involved in the fatty acid metabolism and glycolysis and were up-regulated in response to the drug treatment. Heat shock cognate 71 kDa protein that is involved in stress response was down-regulated in response to neratinib treatment. These proteins were in common between BT474 and SKBR3, between BT474 and HCC1954 or between SKBR3 and HCC1954.

In the current study, we also investigated the protein response to lapatinib, neratinib or afatinib, emerging HER2-inhibitor in BT474 cell lines. Interestingly, trifunctional enzyme subunit alpha, mitochondrial and heterogeneous nuclear ribonucleoprotein R were altered in abundance in all treatments, whereas seven proteins were altered in abundance in two drugs treatments (afatinib and neratinib

Table 3 16 proteins identified as differentially expressed between the lapatinib treated BT474 cell line and the control following label-free MS/MS analysis (Progenesis QI for proteomics)

UniProt*)	Identification	Peptides†)	Score‡)	ANOVA (p)	Fold change	Highest condition§)
a						
P78527	DNA-dependent protein kinase catalytic subunit	2	90.99	0.001596	3.82	Lapatinib
P40939	Trifunctional enzyme subunit alpha, mitochondrial	2	120.25	0.004413	1.66	Lapatinib
O43143	Putative pre-mRNA-splicing factor ATP-dependent RNA helicase DHX15	3	173.99	0.005281	1.57	Lapatinib
P45880	Voltage-dependent anion-selective channel protein 2	2	290.14	0.006264	1.69	Lapatinib
P11021	78 kDa glucose-regulated protein	1	148.58	0.009818	1.94	Lapatinib
P09874	Poly [ADP-ribose] polymerase 1	4	236.21	0.016504	4.24	Lapatinib
P82979	SAP domain-containing ribonucleoprotein	2	150.9	0.020883	1.60	Lapatinib
P42166	Lamina-associated polypeptide 2, isoform alpha	2	127.83	0.026885	1.94	Lapatinib
P62805	Histone H4	3	301.11	0.030621	2.10	Lapatinib
Q92522	Histone H1x	2	136.5	0.037085	1.74	Lapatinib
O43390	Heterogeneous nuclear ribonucleoprotein R	2	111.08	0.048527	1.74	Lapatinib
b						
Q32MZ4	Leucine-rich repeat flightless-interacting protein 1	3	247.18	0.000444	1.62	Control
Q16643	Drebrin	2	149.36	0.001646	1.57	Control
P29966	Myristoylated alanine-rich C-kinase substrate	3	233.58	0.00855	1.64	Control
Q27J81	Inverted formin-2	2	130.65	0.0251	1.79	Control
P04155	Trefoil factor 1	2	126.83	0.026548	1.66	Control

11 proteins were up regulated in the cells treated with lapatinib (Table 3a) and five proteins were up regulated in the untreated cells (control) (Table 3a). *) Accession number in the UniProt database; †) Peptides used for quantitation; ‡) MASCOT score. §) Indicates if the proteins were up regulated in the treated cells (lapatinib) or in the not treated cells (control)

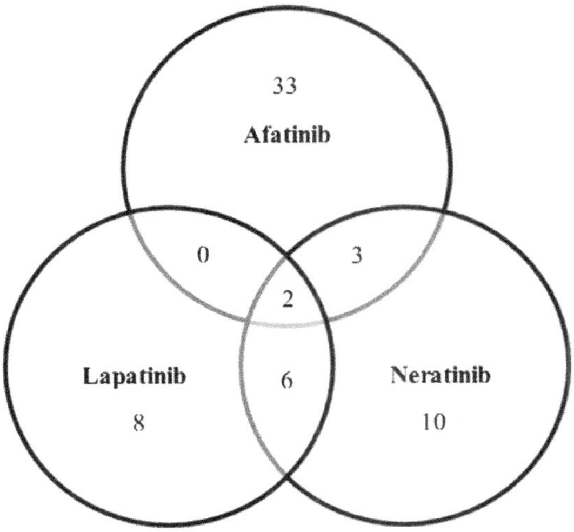

Fig. 1 Venn diagrams showing the number of identified proteins with altered levels in response to afatinib, lapatinib or neratinib treatment compared to control in BT474 cell line. The full lists of proteins and the indication if they are up or down regulate are in Tables 1, 2 and 3. Details of the proteins that were in common between different comparisons are in Table 6

or neratinib and lapatinib). All these proteins were up-regulated in response to the drugs treatment and are generally involved in the fatty acid metabolism, DNA replication and glycolysis. Drebrin and myristoylated alanine-rich C-kinase substrate were down-regulated in response to neratinib and lapatinib treatment, both proteins are involved in cell mobility.

Interestingly, within the 14 highlighted proteins a higher number (11) were up-regulated in response to drug treatments, these proteins are generally involved in the fatty acid metabolism, DNA replication and glycolysis. It is known that cancer cells are different from those of normal cells, showing an increment of aerobic glycolysis, fatty acid synthesis and glutamine metabolism that are needed for proliferation. Cancer cells reprogram their metabolism in order to satisfy their bioenergetic and biosynthetic requirements. Increased aerobic glycolysis, fatty acid synthesis and glutamine metabolism has been linked to therapeutic resistance in cancer [23]. Several studies highlighted that targeting cellular metabolism may improve the response to cancer therapeutics and the combination of chemotherapeutic drugs with cellular metabolism inhibitors may represent a promising strategy to overcome drug resistance in cancer therapy [23, 24]. In the current study, an up-regulation of these proteins was observed following drugs treatments and may be potential targets to enhances therapeutic efficacy or

Table 4 23 proteins identified as differentially expressed between the neratinib treated SKBR3 cell line and the control following label-free MS/MS analysis (Progenesis QI for proteomics)

UniProt[*)]	Identification	Peptides[†)]	Score[‡)]	ANOVA (*p*)	Fold change	Highest condition[§)]
a						
P13489	Ribonuclease inhibitor	4	310.49	0.000561	1.55	Neratinib
Q52LJ0	Protein FAM98B	2	90.26	0.000932	1.62	Neratinib
P49411	Elongation factor Tu, mitochondrial	3	201.31	0.001	1.52	Neratinib
P35232	Prohibitin	2	118.62	0.002224	1.64	Neratinib
Q8WUM4	Programmed cell death 6-interacting protein	2	105.79	0.004641	1.93	Neratinib
P00558	Phosphoglycerate kinase 1	2	201.12	0.00734	1.54	Neratinib
P27348	14-3-3 protein theta	1	151.89	0.008363	1.54	Neratinib
Q00610	Clathrin heavy chain 1	4	233.02	0.00934	1.70	Neratinib
P11177	Pyruvate dehydrogenase E1 component subunit beta, mitochondrial	2	96.98	0.010597	1.73	Neratinib
P50416	Carnitine O-palmitoyltransferase 1, liver isoform	2	126.77	0.010865	1.95	Neratinib
Q00325	Phosphate carrier protein, mitochondrial	2	106.39	0.011586	1.58	Neratinib
Q12931	Heat shock protein 75 kDa, mitochondrial	2	113.29	0.014076	1.77	Neratinib
P31040	Succinate dehydrogenase [ubiquinone] flavoprotein subunit, mitochondrial	2	100.63	0.017419	1.69	Neratinib
P40939	Trifunctional enzyme subunit alpha, mitochondrial	6	423	0.020319	1.71	Neratinib
Q13938	Calcyphosin	3	146.37	0.026178	1.98	Neratinib
P52209	6-phosphogluconate dehydrogenase, decarboxylating	3	152.09	0.035964	4.28	Neratinib
P05091	Aldehyde dehydrogenase, mitochondrial	6	351.3	0.045267	1.80	Neratinib
b						
P11142	Heat shock cognate 71 kDa protein	6	500.28	0.003207	1.59	Control
P06703	Protein S100-A6	2	114.09	0.005483	1.72	Control
P39019	40S ribosomal protein S19	4	213.75	0.005586	1.8	Control
P63220	40S ribosomal protein S21	2	166.6	0.012224	2.43	Control
Q9UNZ2	NSFL1 cofactor p47	2	135.38	0.014751	1.51	Control
P16989	DNA-binding protein A	1	136.69	0.016278	1.53	Control

17 proteins were up regulated in the cells treated with neratinib (Table 4a) and six proteins were up regulated in the untreated cells (control) (Table 4b). [*)] Accession number in the UniProt database; [†)] Peptides used for quantitation; [‡)] MASCOT score. [§)] Indicates if the proteins were up regulated in the treated cells (neratinib) or in the not treated cells (control)

combats drug resistance. The three proteins down-regulated that were identified, are involved in stress response, cell mobility and in different studies have been shown to be up-regulated in tumours of varied origins [25, 26]. In the current study, following drugs treatments a down-regulation of these proteins was observed, this could probably be due to several reasons like alterations in cell morphology, modulation of the immune response, toxicity of certain drugs [25, 26].

Few proteomics studies have been published to date characterising an extensive drugs response in breast cancer. In a previous study from our group [27], 67 proteins showed a significant change in abundance in response to lapatinib in SKBR3 cell line. Of these, inverted formin-2 was identified in our study in the BT474 cell line treated with lapatinib and was down-regulated in response to drug treatments in both studies, whereas histone H2A type 1 and histone H3.1 were respectively identified as well in the neratinib and afatinib treatment in BT474 cell line with a different abundance pattern between the two studies. Heat shock cognate 71 kDa (HSC70) protein was identified in the neratinib treatment of the SKBR3 and HCC1954 cell lines and was up-regulated in response to drug treatments in both studies.

Of the 17 proteins identified in the current study, some were generally involved in the fatty acid metabolism, of these, as previously mentioned, trifunctional enzyme subunit alpha, mitochondrial was altered in abundance in all three drugs treatments (lapatinib, neratinib or afatinib) in BT474 and in SKBR3 cell line treated with neratinib. Interestingly, the subunit beta was also identified in two comparisons. In all treatments and cell lines both subunit (alpha and beta) identified show a higher abundance in the samples with treatments compared to the control. This is to our knowledge, the first study to report differential abundance of trifunctional enzyme in relation to

Table 5 46 proteins identified as differentially expressed between the neratinib treated HCC1954 cell line and the control following label-free MS/MS analysis (Progenesis QI for proteomics)

UniProt[*)]	Identification	Peptides[†)]	Score[‡)]	ANOVA (p)	Fold change	Highest condition[§)]
a						
P23141;Q9UKY3	Liver carboxylesterase 1	5	325.17	1.42E-06	42.37	Neratinib
Q07000	HLA class I histocompatibility antigen, Cw-15 alpha chain	3	177.55	0.000129	2.38	Neratinib
P19971	Thymidine phosphorylase	2	106.97	0.000245	24.47	Neratinib
P42224	Signal transducer and activator of transcription 1-alpha/beta	2	188.79	0.000677	3.17	Neratinib
P42330	Aldo-keto reductase family 1 member C3	1	197.69	0.004702	4.75	Neratinib
P16401	Histone H1.5	2	125.54	0.005291	1.91	Neratinib
Q9P2E9	Ribosome-binding protein 1	3	160.16	0.007391	1.75	Neratinib
P42166	Lamina-associated polypeptide 2, isoform alpha	2	181.9	0.009199	1.81	Neratinib
Q04828;P51857	Aldo-keto reductase family 1 member C1	1	154	0.009747	3.28	Neratinib
P00966	Argininosuccinate synthase	2	86.9	0.010658	3.2	Neratinib
P22314	Ubiquitin-like modifier-activating enzyme 1	11	865.85	0.010735	2.32	Neratinib
O00151	PDZ and LIM domain protein 1	2	125.36	0.011806	1.89	Neratinib
Q7Z406	Myosin-14	2	115.9	0.011847	1.84	Neratinib
P52209	6-phosphogluconate dehydrogenase, decarboxylating	7	460.35	0.012246	2.06	Neratinib
P11413	Glucose-6-phosphate 1-dehydrogenase	3	219.9	0.013282	3.65	Neratinib
P21333	Filamin-A	6	427.66	0.018947	1.90	Neratinib
P30101	Protein disulfide-isomerase A3	2	103.92	0.020008	1.56	Neratinib
O43175	D-3-phosphoglycerate dehydrogenase	2	130.68	0.021376	1.56	Neratinib
Q9BRT3	Migration and invasion enhancer 1	2	101.46	0.021575	1.61	Neratinib
O75874	Isocitrate dehydrogenase [NADP] cytoplasmic	2	141.9	0.027272	1.83	Neratinib
O43707	Alpha-actinin-4	4	261.47	0.035891	1.96	Neratinib
P55327	Tumor protein D52	2	157.9	0.047466	8.1	Neratinib
b						
P40926	Malate dehydrogenase, mitochondrial	4	253.25	0.000516	1.68	Control
P11142	Heat shock cognate 71 kDa protein	4	259.61	0.000586	1.65	Control
Q5VTE0	Putative elongation factor 1-alpha-like 3	2	133.8	0.001037	1.60	Control
O60506	Heterogeneous nuclear ribonucleoprotein Q	3	190.1	0.001168	1.78	Control
P19338	Nucleolin	8	505.63	0.001194	1.7	Control
P53999	Activated RNA polymerase II transcriptional coactivator p15	2	116.09	0.001608	1.54	Control
P63244	Guanine nucleotide-binding protein subunit beta-2-like 1	6	388.91	0.001903	1.68	Control
P04083	Annexin A1	4	237.64	0.00211	1.67	Control
P04406	Glyceraldehyde-3-phosphate dehydrogenase	7	764.51	0.002767	1.75	Control
Q02790	Peptidyl-prolyl cis-trans isomerase FKBP4	4	220.23	0.003155	1.93	Control
P06748	Nucleophosmin	3	269.16	0.003382	1.78	Control
P00558	Phosphoglycerate kinase 1	5	330.19	0.004101	1.51	Control
P05120	Plasminogen activator inhibitor 2	2	125.82	0.004534	23.82	Control
P22234	Multifunctional protein ADE2	3	145.9	0.004729	1.75	Control
Q7KZF4	Staphylococcal nuclease domain-containing protein 1	2	103.98	0.005343	1.62	Control
P17301	Integrin alpha-2	2	123.5	0.006948	6.18	Control
P48643	T-complex protein 1 subunit epsilon	2	88.36	0.008121	1.67	Control
P25705	ATP synthase subunit alpha, mitochondrial	2	100.47	0.008561	1.62	Control
P16070	CD44 antigen	2	117.19	0.010439	3.57	Control

Table 5 46 proteins identified as differentially expressed between the neratinib treated HCC1954 cell line and the control following label-free MS/MS analysis (Progenesis QI for proteomics) *(Continued)*

P17987	T-complex protein 1 subunit alpha	2	113.87	0.015235	1.75	Control
P50990	T-complex protein 1 subunit theta	3	157.18	0.018346	2.22	Control
P08238	Heat shock protein HSP 90-beta	2	153.98	0.019861	3.16	Control
P48047	ATP synthase subunit O, mitochondrial	2	94.06	0.033513	2.54	Control
Q9UHD8	Septin-9	2	85.27	0.037332	1.61	Control

22 proteins were up regulated in the cells treated with neratinib (Table 5a) and 24 proteins were up regulated in the untreated cells (control) (Table 5b). [*)] Accession number in the UniProt database; [†)] Peptides used for quantitation; [‡)] MASCOT score. [§)] Indicates if the proteins were up regulated in the treated cells (neratinib) or in the not treated cells (control)

HER2-positive response breast cancer. This protein is a heterooctamer of four alpha- and four beta-subunits that catalyses three steps in the beta-oxidation spiral of long chain fatty acids. Deficiency of this proteins may cause, vomiting, lethargy, irregular heart rate or sudden, unexpected death [28, 29]. It is known that the use of HER2-targeted monoclonal antibodies like trastuzumab increase the incidence of cardiac dysfunction. A significant reduction of this problem was firstly observed with the use of HER2-targeted small-molecule inhibitors lapatinib and then further decreased incidences evident with the use of neratinib and afatinib second-generation tyrosine kinase inhibitors [30]. The higher abundance of trifunctional enzyme subunit alpha, mitochondrial observed in the current study following the use of novel HER2-targeted therapies may suggest a role for this protein as a marker for testing the toxicity of new HER2-inhibitors.

Heterogeneous nuclear ribonucleoproteins (hnRNPs) are among the most abundant proteins in the eukaryotic nucleus and comprise a family of RNA-binding proteins. These proteins are involved in various steps of messenger RNA (mRNA) biogenesis such as splicing and transport to the cytoplasm [31, 32]. Deregulation of individual hnRNPs was involved in tumour development and progression, including inhibition of apoptosis, angiogenesis and cell invasion [33]. In a study by Chen et al. [34] investigating proteins that are associated with the resistance to paclitaxel in human breast cancer cells, an overexpression of hnRNP C1/C2 was associated with drug resistance. In other studies about lung carcinogenesis a different hnRNP subtype (A2/B1) has been proposed as a marker for early detection [35, 36]. In the current study, different subtypes of this protein (D-like, U, H, Q and R) increased in abundance in one or more drugs treatments (lapatinib, neratinib or afatinib) in BT474 cell line. In particular the R subtypes was identified in all the treatments and may so be useful in predicting an early cellular response in HER2-targetting therapies.

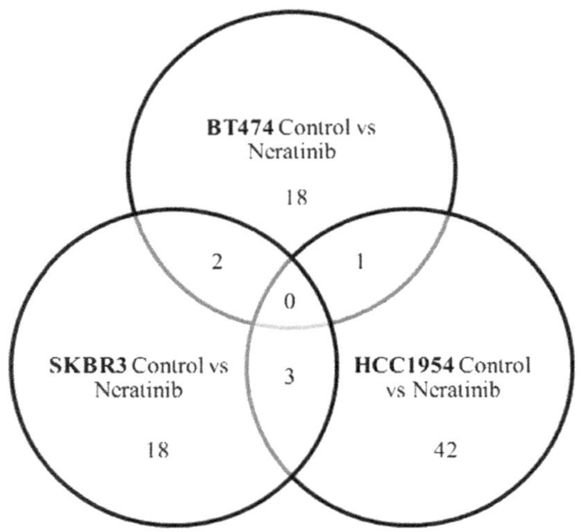

Fig. 2 Venn diagrams showing the number of identified proteins with altered levels in response to neratinib treatment compared to control in BT474, SKBR3 and HCC1954 cell lines. The full lists of proteins and the indication if they are up or down regulate are in Tables 2, 4 and 5. Details of the proteins that were in common between different comparisons are in Table 6

Lamina-associated polypeptide 2, isoform alpha (LAP2α) was up-regulated in two cell lines (BT474 and HCC1954) in response to neratinib and in response to lapatinib in BT474 cell line. LAP2α is one of six splice variants of the mammalian LAP2 gene. LAP2α is a non-membrane protein uniformly distributed throughout the nucleoplasm [37]. Several studies highlighted that this protein may be involved in cancer development or may serve as useful diagnostic and prognostic markers for some types of cancers [38–40]. However, the complex mechanisms of the involvement of this protein in the genesis of the tumour remains to be elucidated, and the contradictory reports in literature regarding its potential role in cell proliferation highlight the need for further work [38, 40]. The up-regulation observed in the current study in the treated cells may provide useful information to predict an early cellular response in HER2-targetting therapies and this information could pave the way to novel strategy to control the development of the cancer.

Proteins involved in the immune system process such as HSC70 were also identified in this study. Stress-related proteins are known as heat-shock proteins (HSP), their role is to protect, preserve or recover the proper functional conformation of proteins, they are divided into families according to their molecular weight. The 70 kDa HSP family is composed of heat inducible proteins (HSP70)

Table 6 Proteins differentially expressed that have been identified in more than one comparisons between the identified proteins with altered levels in response to afatinib, lapatinib or neratinib treatment compared to control in BT474 cell line and in neratinib treatment compared to control in HCC1954 and SKBR3 cell lines

Protein	Biological process[a)]	BT474 afatinib vs untreated	BT474 neratinib vs untreated	BT474 lapatinib vs untreated	SKBR3 neratinib vs untreated	HCC1954 neratinib vs untreated
Trifunctional enzyme subunit alpha, mitochondrial	fatty acid metabolism; carbohydrate metabolic process	↑	↑	↑	↑	-
Heterogeneous nuclear ribonucleoprotein R	DNA replication; RNA splicing; mRNA splicing; protein metabolic process	↑	↑	↑	-	-
Lamina-associated polypeptide 2, isoform alpha	immune system process; cellular defense response	-	↑	↑	-	↑
Phosphoglycerate kinase 1	Glycolysis	↓	-	-	↑	↓
Heterogeneous nuclear ribonucleoprotein H	mRNA splicing	↑	↑	-	-	-
Ubiquitin-like modifier-activating enzyme 1	coenzyme metabolic process; cellular protein modification process; proteolysis; cell communication; intracellular protein transport; nuclear transport	↓	-	-	-	↑
Interleukin enhancer-binding factor 3	apoptotic process; purine nucleobase metabolic process; protein metabolic process; cell cycle; neurological system process; response to stimulus; RNA localization	↑	↑	-	-	-
Trifunctional enzyme subunit beta, mitochondrial	protein acetylation	↑	↑	-	-	-
Heterogeneous nuclear ribonucleoprotein Q	DNA replication; RNA splicing; protein metabolic process; cell cycle	↑	-	-	-	↓
DNA-dependent protein kinase catalytic subunit	immune system process; induction of apoptosis; DNA repair; DNA recombination; protein phosphorylation; response to stress	-	↑	↑	-	-
Drebrin	cellular process; cellular component morphogenesis	-	↓	↓	-	-
Myristoylated alanine-rich C-kinase substrate	cell communication	-	↓	↓	-	-
78 kDa glucose-regulated protein	protein folding; response to stress; protein complex biogenesis	-	↑	↑	-	-
Poly [ADP-ribose] polymerase 1	DNA repair; protein ADP-ribosylation; response to stress	-	↑	↑	-	-
Carnitine O-palmitoyltransferase 1, liver isoform	cellular amino acid metabolic process; fatty acid metabolic process	-	↑	-	↑	-
Heat shock cognate 71 kDa protein	immune system process; protein folding; response to stress; protein complex biogenesis	-	-	-	↓	↓
6-phosphogluconate dehydrogenase, decarboxylating	pentose-phosphate shunt	-	-	-	↑	↑

The full lists of proteins are in Tables 1, 2, 3, 4 and 5. [a)]Biological process of the proteins obtained using PANTHER analysis [16]. Arrows indicate if the proteins were up (↑) or down (↓) regulated in the treated cells vs. control

that are expressed under cellular stress conditions, and heat shock cognate proteins (HSC70) that are constitutively expressed without any stress stimulation [41]. HSP are overexpressed in patients with malignant tumours, the expression of HSC70 has been reported on breast cancer cells and the overexpression of HSP/HSC70 in chemoresistant cancer cells highlight these proteins as possible clinical markers [25, 42, 43]. In the current study HSC70 was lower in abundance in the cell lines (SKBR3 and HCC1954) treated with neratinib compared to the control. It is known that that the inhibition of HSPs could be related to the toxicity of certain drugs [43] highlighting the chemotherapeutic implications of this protein and the potentiality as a marker to evaluate the potential importance of further treatment options. Similar data were also obtained in response to lapatinib in SKBR3 cell line in a previous study from our group [27].

Taken together, our findings highlight several proteins that are closely associated with early HER2-inhibitor response, complementary studies need to be conducted to validate the importance of our findings and this could have implication for new strategies to improve the efficacy of breast-cancer treatment.

Conclusion

In conclusion, we have identified several proteins that were differentially expressed following exposure to clinically relevant concentrations of different HER2-inhibitors drug treatments in HER2-overexpressing breast cancer cell lines, lapatinib, neratinib or afatinib in BT474 and in response to neratinib treatment in two other cell lines (HCC1954 and SKBR3). Of these, 14 proteins showed a similar abundance pattern following different drug treatments and/or in different cell lines. In particular, we have identified proteins like trifunctional enzyme subunit alpha, mitochondrial; heterogeneous nuclear ribonucleoprotein R; LAP2α and HSC70 that were altered in abundance in three or more comparisons and may be strongly involved in an early treatment response to HER2-inhibition. These may warrant further investigation for example applying siRNA knockdown protocols to reduce the protein levels in cells and to study the functional consequences of their removal, this likely could have implication for improve efficacy of HER2-inhibitor based breast-cancer treatment.

Competing interests

The authors declare that they have no competing interests.

Authors' contribution

ROC and ADL conceived and designed the study. ADL carried out laboratory work, collation of data, data analysis and wrote the manuscript. PM and MH provided expertise in proteomic analysis and helped with the bioinformatic analysis of data. ROC supervised and coordinated the study and helped writing the manuscript. All authors agreed with the last version of the manuscript.

Acknowledgement

The authors wish to thank the Science Foundation Ireland, Strategic Research Cluster award 08/SRC/B1410 for funding this work.

Author details

[1]National Institute for Cellular Biotechnology, DCU, Glasnevin, Dublin 9, Dublin, Ireland. [2]School of Nursing and Human Sciences, DCU, Glasnevin, Dublin 9, Dublin, Ireland.

References

1. Slamon DJ, Leyland-Jones B, Shak S, Fuchs H, Paton V, Bajamonde A, et al. Use of chemotherapy plus a monoclonal antibody against HER2 for metastatic breast cancer that overexpresses HER2. N Engl J Med. 2001;344(11):783–92.
2. Arora A, Scholar EM. Role of tyrosine kinase inhibitors in cancer therapy. J Pharmacol Exp Ther. 2005;315(3):971–9.
3. Nahta R, Esteva FJ. Trastuzumab: triumphs and tribulations. Oncogene. 2007;26:3637–43.
4. Rabindran SK. Antitumor activity of HER-2 inhibitors. Cancer Lett. 2005;227(1):9–23.
5. Burris HA, Hurwitz HI, Dees EC, Dowlati A, Blackwell KL, O'Neil B, et al. Phase I safety, pharmacokinetics, and clinical activity study of lapatinib (GW572016), a reversible dual inhibitor of epidermal growth factor receptor tyrosine kinases, in heavily pretreated patients with metastatic carcinomas. J Clin Oncol. 2005;23(23):5305–13.
6. Cameron D, Casey M, Oliva C, Newstat B, Imwalle B, Geyer CE. Lapatinib plus capecitabine in women with HER-2–positive advanced breast cancer: Final Survival Analysis of a Phase III Randomized Trial. The Oncologist. 2010;15(9):924–34.
7. Nancy UL. Breast cancer brain metastases: new directions in systemic therapy. Ecancermedicalscience. 2013;7:307.
8. Tsou HR, Overbeek-Klumpers E, Hallett WA, Reich MF, Floyd MB, Johnson BD, et al. Optimization of 6,7-disubstituted-4-(arylamino)quinoline-3-carbonitriles as orally active, irreversible inhibitors of human epidermal growth factor receptor-2 kinase activity. J Med Chem. 2005;48(4):1107–31.
9. Yap TA, Vidal L, Adam J, Stephens P, Spicer J, Shaw H, et al. Phase I trial of the irreversible EGFR and HER2 kinase inhibitor BIBW 2992 in patients with advanced solid tumors. J Clin Oncol. 2010;28(25):3965–72.
10. Zhang X, Munster PN. New protein kinase inhibitors in breast cancer: afatinib and neratinib. Expert Opin Pharmacother. 2014;15(9):1277–88.
11. Lau TY, O'Connor DP, Brennan DJ, Duffy MJ, Pennington SR, Gallagher WM. Breast cancer proteomics: clinical perspectives. Expert Opin Biol Ther. 2007;7(2):209–19.
12. Becker CH, Bern M. Recent developments in quantitative proteomics. Mutat Res. 2011;722(2):171–82.
13. Neilson KA, Naveid AA, Muralidharan S, Mirzaei M, Mariani M, Assadourian G, et al. Less label, more free: approaches in label-free quantitative mass spectrometry. Proteomics. 2011;11(4):535–53.
14. Panchaud A, Affolter M, Moreillon P, Kussmann M. Experimental and computational approaches to quantitative proteomics: status quo and outlook. J Proteomics. 2008;71(1):19–33.
15. Meleady P, Gallagher M, Clarke C, Henry M, Sanchez N, Barron N, et al. Impact of miR-7 over-expression on the proteome of Chinese hamster ovary cells. J Biotec. 2012;160:251–62.
16. Mi H, Muruganujan A, Thomas PD. PANTHER in 2013: modeling the evolution of gene function, and other gene attributes, in the context of phylogenetic trees. Nucleic Acids Res. 2013;41(D1):D377–86.
17. Abbas R, Hug BA, Leister C, Burns J, Sonnichsen D. Pharmacokinetics of oral neratinib during co-administration of ketoconazole in healthy subjects. Br J Clin Pharmacol. 2011;71(4):522–7.
18. Murakami H, Tamura T, Takahashi T, Nokihara H, Naito T, Nakamura Y, et al. Phase I study of continuous afatinib (BIBW 2992) in patients with advanced non-small cell lung cancer after prior chemotherapy/erlotinib/gefitinib (LUX-Lung 4). Cancer Chemother Pharmacol. 2012;69(4):891–9.
19. Metodiev M, Alldridge L. Phosphoproteomics: a possible route to novel biomarkers of breast cancer. Proteomics Clin Appl. 2008;2(2):181–94.
20. Lacroix M, Leclercq G. Relevance of breast cancer cell lines as models for breast tumours: an update. Breast Cancer Res Treat. 2004;83:249–89.

21. Geiger T, Wehner A, Schaab C, Cox J, Mann M. Comparative proteomic analysis of eleven common cell lines reveals ubiquitous but varying expression of most proteins. Mol Cell Proteomics. 2012;11:3.
22. Neve RM, Chin K, Fridlyand J, Yeh J, Baehner FL, Fevr T, et al. A collection of breast cancer cell lines for the study of functionally distinct cancer subtypes. Cancer cell. 2006;10(6):515–27.
23. Zhao Y, Butler EB, Tan M. Targeting cellular metabolism to improve cancer therapeutics. Cell Death and Disease. 2013;4, e532.
24. Vander Heiden MG, Cantley LC, Thompson CB. Understanding the Warburg effect: the metabolic requirements of cell proliferation. Science. 2009;324(5930):1029–33.
25. Torronteguy C, Frasson A, Zerwes F, Winnikov E, da Silva VD, Menoret A, et al. Inducible heat shock protein 70 expression as a potential predictive marker of metastasis in breast tumors. Cell Stress Chaperones. 2006;11(1):34–43.
26. Terakawa Y, Agnihotri S, Golbourn B, Nadi M, Sabha N, Smith CA, et al. The role of drebrin in glioma migration and invasion. Exp Cell Res. 2013;319(4):517–28.
27. O'Connell K, Li J, Engler F, Hennessy K, O'Neill F, Straubinger RM, et al. Determination of the proteomic response to lapatinib treatment using a comprehensive and reproducible ion-current-based proteomics strategy. JPGR. 2013;1(3):1–16.
28. Hum DW, Bell AW, Rozen R, MacKenzie RE. Primary structure of a human trifunctional enzyme. Isolation of a cDNA encoding methylenetetrahydrofolate dehydrogenase-methenyltetrahydrofolate cyclohydrolase-formyltetrahydrofolate synthetase. J Biol Chem. 1988;263(31):15946–50.
29. Ushikubo S, Aoyama T, Kamijo T, Wanders RJ, Rinaldo P, Vockley J, et al. Molecular characterization of mitochondrial trifunctional protein deficiency: formation of the enzyme complex is important for stabilization of both alpha- and beta-subunits. Am J Hum Genet. 1996;58(5):979–88.
30. Sendur MA, Aksoy S, Altundag K. Cardiotoxicity of novel HER2-targeted therapies. Curr Med Res Opin. 2013;29(8):1015–24.
31. Dreyfuss G, Phflipson L, Mattaj IW. Ribonucleoprotein particles in cellular processes. J Cell Biol. 1988;106(5):1419–25.
32. Chaudhury A, Chander P, Howe PH. Heterogeneous nuclear ribonucleoproteins (hnRNPs) in cellular processes: Focus on hnRNP E1's multifunctional regulatory roles. RNA. 2010;16(8):1449–62.
33. Carpenter B, MacKay C, Alnabulsi A, MacKay M, Telfer C, Melvin WT, et al. The roles of heterogeneous nuclear ribonucleoproteins in tumour development and progression. Biochim Biophys Acta. 2005;1765(2):85–100.
34. Chen S, Dong Q, Hu S, Cai J, Zhang W, Sun J, et al. Proteomic analysis of the proteins that are associated with the resistance to paclitaxel in human breast cancer cells. Mol BioSyst. 2014;10(2):294–303.
35. Montuenga LM, Zhou J, Avis I, Vos M, Martinez A, Cuttitta F, et al. Expression of heterogeneous nuclear ribonucleoprotein A2/B1 changes with critical stages of mammalian lung development. Am J Respir Cell Mol Biol. 1998;19(4):554–62.
36. Zhou J, Nong L, Wloch M, Cantor A, Mulshine JL, Tockman MS. Expression of early lung cancer detection marker: hnRNP-A2/B1 and its relation to microsatellite alteration in non-small cell lung cancer. Lung Cancer. 2001;34(3):341–50.
37. Dechat T, Gajewski A, Korbei B, Gerlich D, Daigle N, Haraguchi T, et al. LAP2alpha and BAF transiently localize to telomeres and specific regions on chromatin during nuclear assembly. J Cell Sci. 2004;117:6117–28.
38. Ward MC, van der Watt PJ, Tzoneva G, Leaner VD. Deregulated LAP2α expression in cervical cancer associates with aberrant E2F and p53 activities. IUBMB Life. 2011;63(11):1018–26.
39. de Las Heras JI, Batrakou DG, Schirmer EC. Cancer biology and the nuclear envelope: a convoluted relationship. Semin Cancer Biol. 2013;23(2):125–37.
40. Brachner A, Foisner R. Lamina-associated polypeptide (LAP)2α and other LEM proteins in cancer biology. Adv Exp Med Biol. 2014;773:143–63.
41. Dwornczak B, Mirault ME. Structure and expression of a human gene coding for a 71 kd heat shock 'cognate' protein. Nucleic Acids Res. 1987;15(13):5181–97.
42. Conroy SE, Latchman DS. Do heat shock proteins have a role in breast cancer? Br J Cancer. 1996;74(5):717–21.
43. Lazaris AC, Chatzigianni EB, Panoussopoulos D, Tzimas GN, Davaris PS, Golematis BC. Proliferating cell nuclear antigen and heat shock protein 70 immuno-localization in invasive ductal breast cancer not otherwise specified. Breast Cancer Res Treat. 1997;43(1):43–51.

Two COX-2 inhibitors induce apoptosis in human erythroleukemia K562cells by modulating NF-κB and FHC pathways

Shaghayegh Norouzi[1], Mahnaz Norouzi[1], Mohsen Amini[2], Amir Amanzadeh[3], Mohamad Nabiuni[1], Saeed Irian[1*] and Mona Salimi[4*]

Abstract

Background: Leukemia is distinguished by abnormal proliferation of leukocytes. Although there has been some progress in developing novel cancer therapies, no significant improvement was observed in the overall survival rate over the last decade. Selective cyclooxygenase-2 (COX-2) inhibitors are known to inhibit tumor growth by exerting antimetastatic and antiangiogenic effects through inhibition of COX –dependent and independent pathways. The ability of two new triaryl-oxadiazole derivatives, compounds **A** (3-(4-chlorophenyl) -5-(4-flurophenyl)-4-Phenyl-4,5-dihydro-1,2,4-oxadiazole) and **B** (3,5-bis(4-chlorophenyl)-4-Phenyl-4,5-dihydro-1,2,4-oxadiazole), to induce apoptosis in human erythroleukemia K562 cells was evaluated and the upstream mechanism was investigated.

Methods: K562 cells were treated with compounds **A** and **B** at their IC_{50} concentrations and analyzed by DAPI staining and Annexin-V-FLUOS labelling solution. Nuclear factor kappa-B (NF-κB) activation was evaluated by TransAM kit. Cyclooxygenase-2 (COX-2), Caspase-3, Bax, Bcl-2, ferritin heavy chain (FHC), extra cellular signal-regulated kinase (ERK), p-ERK and early growth response protein-1 (Egr1) levels were determined using Western blotting, while c-Myc mRNA level was investigated by RT-PCR.

Results: Changes in nuclear morphology and the increased annexin-V/PI staining revealed the apoptotic cell death in compounds **A**- and **B**-treated K562 cells. A significant reduction in NF-κB activity as well as FHC and p-ERK levels were detected in these cells. No change was observed in the levels of Bax, Bcl-2, Caspase-3, COX-2, c-Myc and Egr1, following treatment with the two compounds. Collectively, compounds **A** and **B** potentiate apoptosis as shown by DAPI staining, flowcytometry, FHC and p-ERK downregulation and NF-κB inactivation.

Conclusion: Two compounds induce apoptosis in a COX-2-independent manner which also appears to be independent from mitochondria, caspase and c-Myc/Egr1 pathways.

Keywords: Leukemia, Apoptosis, COX-2, FHC, NF-κB

Background

Leukemia, a cancer of the body's blood-forming tissues, including the bone marrow and the lymphatic system, is distinguished by abnormal proliferation of leukocytes. Based on the International Classification of Childhood Cancer, leukemia represents one of the largest diagnostic groups among individuals under 15 years of age with incidence of 34 % [1]. Although there has been some progress in developing novel cancer therapies, no significant improvement was observed in the overall survival rate over the last decade [2]. Nonsteroidal anti-inflammatory drugs (NSAIDs) with their pain relief and anti-inflammation properties have also been the focus of attention as anticancer agents [3]. The targets of traditional NSAIDs are cyclooxygenases 1 and 2 (COX-1 and COX-2), enzymes involved in the production of prostaglandins from arachidonic acid [4]. In this regard, NSAIDs are known to inhibit tumor growth by exerting antimetastatic and

* Correspondence: irian@khu.ac.ir; salimimona@pasteur.ac.ir; salimi_mona@yahoo.com
[1]Department of Cell and Molecular Biology, Faculty of Biological Sciences, Kharazmi University, P.O. Box 1481765544 Tehran, Iran
[4]Department of Physiology and Pharmacology, Pasteur Institute of Iran, P.O. Box 13164 Tehran, Iran
Full list of author information is available at the end of the article

antiangiogenic effects through inhibition of COX activity, however, a COX-independent pathway has also been suggested [3, 5].

In addition to common NSAIDs, the newly developed selective COX-2 inhibitor, celecoxib, with a better gastrointestinal risk profile, has been considered as a cost-effective alternative [6]. Celecoxib has been proven as a potent candidate for treating cancer, with several ongoing clinical trials as well as in various animal tumor models [5, 7]. Celecoxib has also been demonstrated to have inhibitory effect on the growth of K562 cells, and induce apoptosis [5, 8].

Celecoxib represents a 1, 2-di-aryl heterocyclic structure and used as an ideal lead compound for developing novel derivatives with potent apoptosis-inducing activity [9, 10]. We have recently reported that two compounds with triaryl-oxadiazole structures known as compounds **A** (3- (4-chlorophenyl) -5-(4-flurophenyl)-4-Phenyl-4,5-dihydro-1,2,4-oxadiazole) and **B** (3,5-bis(4- chlorophenyl)-4-Phenyl-4,5-dihydro-1,2,4-oxadiazole) (Fig. 1) show significant biological features such as antiproliferative activity with considerable IC_{50} values (21.66 and 22.23 μM) in human erythroleukemia (K562) cell line after a 24 h treatment [11]. In the present investigation, we examined the mechanism leading to apoptosis during treatment of K562 cell line with the two new celecoxib derivatives, compounds **A** and **B**.

Methods

Drugs and reagents

Compounds **A** and **B** were synthesized by the Department of Medicinal Chemistry, Tehran University of Medical Science (Tehran, Iran). Dulbecco's Modified Eagle's Medium (DMEM) and fetal bovine serum (FBS) were purchased from Gibco-BRL (Rockville, IN, USA). Annexin-V-FLUOS kit was prepared from Roche Applied Science (Indianapolis, USA). Polyclonal anti–caspase-3 (1:500), anti-Bcl-2 (1:500), anti-Bax (1:500), anti-COX-2 (1:1000), anti-GAPDH (1:1000) antibodies and monoclonal anti-ERK (1:1000), anti-Phospho-ERK (1:1000), anti-FHC (1:100) and anti-Egr-1 (1:200) antibodies were purchased from Abcam (Cambridge MA, USA). Anti-rabbit IgG horseradish peroxidase (HRP) antibody (1:5000) was obtained from Cell Signaling Technology (Beverly, MA, USA). All other chemicals were in high purity and prepared from Merck (Darmstadt, Germany).

Cell culture

K562 cells were obtained from the cell bank of Pasture Institute of Iran (NCBI). Cells were cultured in DMEM medium containing 10 % FBS, 100 U/mL penicillin and 100 μg/mL streptomycin. These cells were incubated at 37 °C and 5 % CO2 in a humidified atmosphere and then were treated with compounds **A** and **B** at the IC_{50} concentrations (21.66 and 22.23 μM) for 8 and 16 h.

Analysis of cell morphology by DAPI staining

The treated and untreated cells were stained by DAPI 4',6-diamido-2-phenylindole hydro chloride) (Roche Applied Science, Indianapolis, USA), and their morphology was observed under a Zeiss fluorescence microscope (Zeiss, Germany). Photomicrographs were taken with an Olympus digital camera (Tokyo, Japan).

Identification of apoptosis by Annexin-V/PI staining

Following treatment, 10^6 cells were washed in PBS and resuspended in 100 μL of annexin-V-FLUOS labeling solution containing 2 μL annexin-V-FLUOS labeling agent, 2 μL Propidium Iodide (PI) solution and 1 mL incubation buffer to achieve a concentration of 10^6 cells/mL. Following incubation at 37 °C for 15 minutes, cells were analyzed by flowcytometry. Annexin-V binds to cells expressing phosphatidyl serine on the outer layer of the cell membrane, and PI stains the cellular DNA of those with a compromised cell membrane [12]. This allows for the discrimination of live cells (unstained with either fluorochrome or PI) from apoptotic (stained with annexin-V) and necrotic cells (stained with PI).

Western blotting

K562 cells were treated with compounds **A** and **B** at their IC_{50} concentrations for 16 h. Proteins were extracted from distinctively treated cells, collected and lysed in lysis buffer (Tris 62.5 mM (pH 6.8), DTT 50 mM, SDS

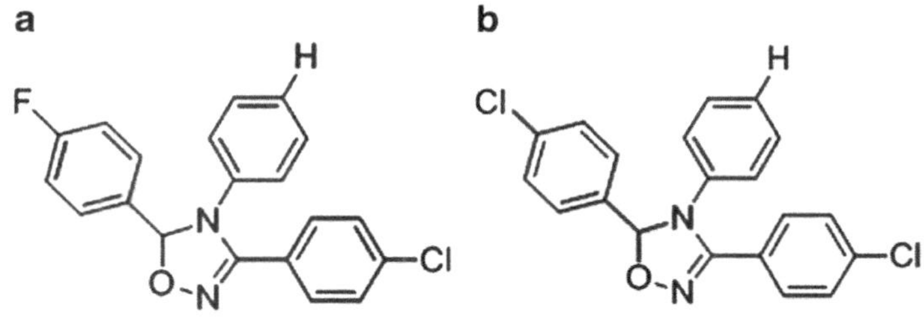

Fig. 1 Structure of the two new celecoxib derivatives

10 %, glycerol) in the presence of protease inhibitors. Then, equal amounts of protein were heated to 95 °C, separated in 12 % SDS-polyacrylamide gels and transferred to PVDF membranes. The membrane was then blocked for 2 h in TBST (50 mmol/L Tris-Cl, pH 7.6, 150 mmol/L NaCl and 0.1 % Tween 20) containing 1 % (w/v) casein, and then incubated with primary antibodies overnight, followed by incubation with HRP conjugated goat anti-rabbit IgG for 2 h. Blots were then developed using ECL advance western blotting detection kit. The signals from each protein band were normalized against the GAPDH (Glyceraldehyde Phosphate Dehydrogenase) content using the polyclonal anti-GAPDH antibody. The expression level of control was designated value "1", and thereby the expression ratios of the treatments were expressed in relation to the control.

ELISA-based TransAM assay

K562 cells were treated with compounds **A** and **B** at their IC_{50} concentrations for 16 h. Proteins of treated cells were extracted. The experiments were performed according to manufacturer's instructions for the ELISA-based TransAM p65 kit (TransAM NF-κB p65 TranscriptionFactor Assay kit). Briefly, 20 μg of protein extract per well was added to a 96-well plate coated with the immobilized oligonucleotide containing the NF-κB consensus sequence (5'-GGGACTTTCC-3') and incubated for 1 h at room temperature with mild agitation. p65 protein present in the extract will specifically bind to this sequence. Next, anti-p65 antibody (100 μL, at a 1:1000 dilution) was added to each well and incubated for 1 h, followed by the addition of 100 μL of horseradish peroxidase (HRP)-conjugated antibody (1:1000 dilution) for yet another 1 h. After adding 100 μL of the developing solution for up to 5 min, colorimetric reaction was stopped and ELISA reader was used to quantify the difference between the intensity of NF-κB p65 by reading absorbance at 450 nm with a correction wavelength of 630 nm.

Semiquantitative RT-PCR

For analysis of c-Myc mRNA expression levels, cells were treated or not treated with compounds **A** and **B** for 16 hours, and total RNA was extracted with RNX-Plus (CinnaGen, Iran) following the manufacturer's protocol. 1 μg of total RNA was used to perform reverse transcription with the RevertAid first strand cDNA synthesis Kit (Thermo, Lithuania) following the manufacturer's protocol. The resulting reverse transcription products were stored at −70 °C until use.

Reaction products were quantified by RT-PCR using a 2X TaqPreMix (Master Mix) PCR Kit (CinnaGen, Iran) according to the manufacturer's instructions. PCR of GAPDH that was chosen as an internal control was carried out in the same tubes as for the genes. The PCR primers of GAPDH and c-myc were synthesized according to the references [13, 14]. Sequences of the primers were as follows: c-myc (Forward: 5'- TGGTGCTCCATGAGGA GACA-3'; Reverse: 5'-GTGTTTCAACTGTTCTCGTC-3'), GAPDH (Forward: 5'-GAGCCCGCAGCCTCCCGCT T-3'; Reverse: 5'- CCCGCGGCCATCACGCCACAG-3').

Statistical analysis

Each experiment was performed at least three times and representative data were shown. Data in the graph are given as mean values ± standard error (SE) of the mean. Significant differences among groups were determined using a one-way ANOVA followed by the posttest tukey.

Results

Apoptosis induction in K562 cells following compounds A and B treatments

In order to examine whether compounds **A** and **B** exhibit cytotoxicity in K562 cells through apoptosis, DAPI staining analysis was undertaken in order to observe morphological changes in K562 cells following treatment with compounds **A**(21.66 μM) and **B**(22.23 μM) for 8 and 16 h (Fig. 2). Morphological evidence of apoptosis was detected as chromatin condensation and nuclear fragmentation following 8 h (Fig. 2d) and to a greater extent at 16 h (Fig. 2h) treatment with compound **B**, whereas compound **A**-treated K562 cells showed slight morphological changes at 8 h (Fig. 2c) and to a greater extent at 16 h (Fig. 2g).

Apoptosis induced by compounds **A** and **B** in K562 cells was confirmed by staining cells with Annexin-V/PI and subjecting them to flowcytometry. In the dual parameter fluorescent dot plots, the number of cells in early (annexin V+/PI−, the lower right quadrant) and late (annexin V+/PI+, the upper right quadrant) apoptosis were counted (Fig. 3). As shown in Table 1, 95.02 % of untreated cells were viable. However, treatment with compounds **A** (IC_{50}) and **B** (IC_{50}) for 16 h resulted in a reduction in the number of viable cells to 90.48 % and 85.95 %, respectively, whereas, the percentage of annexin V+/PI− cells (early apoptosis) increased significantly. These results demonstrate that compounds **A** and **B** show antitumor activities in K562 cells, mainly through the induction of apoptotic cell death.

Effect of compounds A and B on Bax, Bcl-2 and caspase-3 levels

In order to determine the possible involvement of the caspase cascade in the execution phase of apoptosis, caspase-3 level was investigated following treatment of cells with the IC_{50} concentration of compounds **A** and **B** by Western blot analysis. As shown in Fig. 4a, treatment with either compound had no effect on the cleavage of caspase-3 in K562 cell line after 8 and 16 h. In addition,

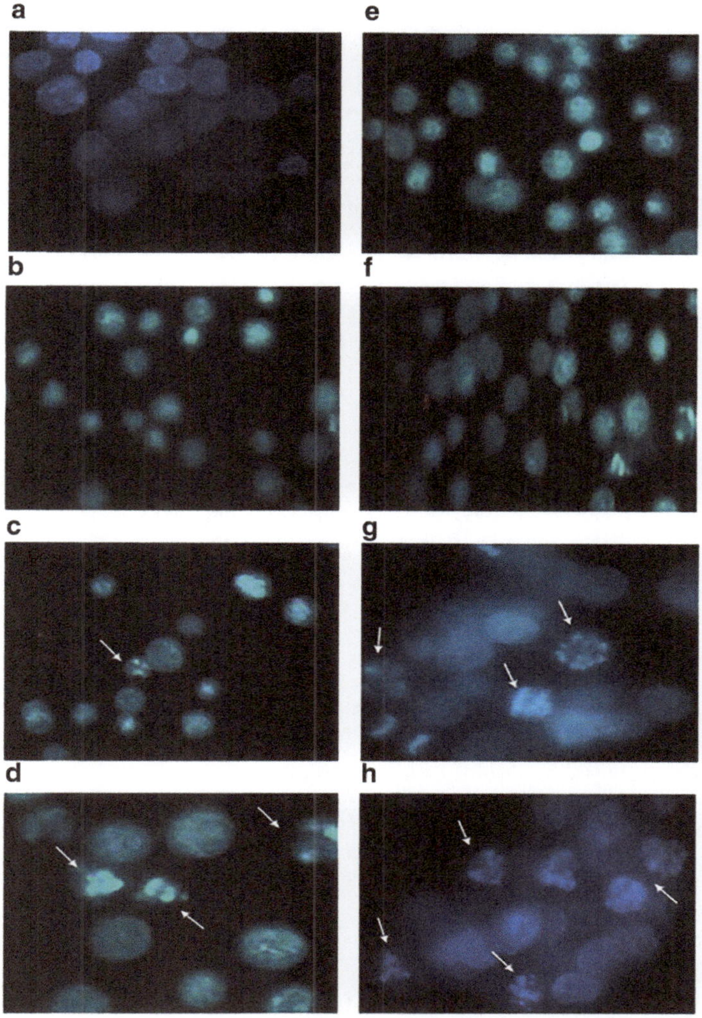

Fig. 2 Apoptotic morphological changes in K562 cells. **a** K562 control cells after 8 h. **b** K562 cells treated with DMSO for 8 h. **c** K562 cells treated with compound A at 21.66 μM for 8 h. **d** K562 cells treated with compound B at 22.23 μM for 8 h. **e** K562 control cells after 16 h. **f** K562 cells treated with DMSO for 16 h. **g** K562 cells treated with compound A at 21.66 μM for 16 h. **h** K562 cells treated with compound B at 22.23 μM for 16 h. Cells were stained with DAPI and observed by fluorescent microscopy

the expression of Bcl-2 and Bax, measured by Western blot analysis, revealed no apparent change in Bax/Bcl-2 ratio at 8 and 16 h (Fig. 4b and c).

Effect of compounds A and B on COX-2 levels

In order to determine the possible involvement of the COX-2 pathway in apoptosis induced by compounds **A** and **B**, COX-2 level was investigated following treatment of cells with the IC_{50} concentrations of the two compounds. As shown in Fig. 5a and b, neither of the compounds had any significant effect on the expression of COX-2 following a 16 h treatment of K562 cells.

Effect of compounds A and B on NF-κB activity

As NF-κB plays a critical role in the apoptosis process [15], the effects of compounds **A** and **B** on NF-κB p65 activity was assessed. As shown in Fig. 6, following a 16 h treatment of cells with compounds **A** and **B**(IC_{50}), a significant ($p < 0.05$) reduction in the concentration of nuclear p65 subunit was observed.

Effect of compounds A and B on FHC, p-ERK, c-Myc and Egr1 levels

To reveal upstream mechanism of apoptosis induction following treatment with celecoxib derivatives, levels of certain factors, located downstream of NF-κB in the

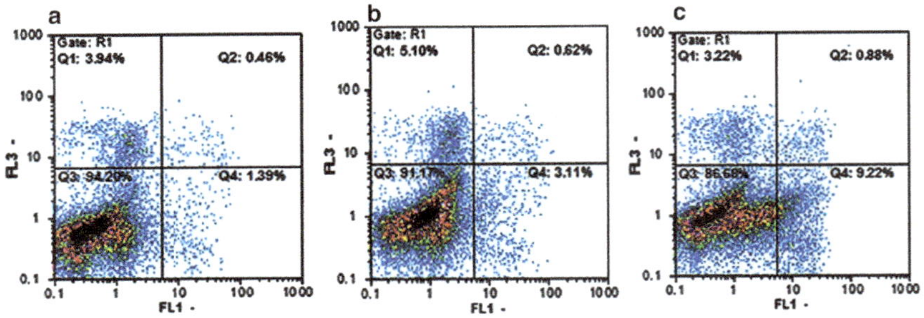

Fig. 3 Flowcytometry analysis to quantify apoptosis in K562 cells. **a** Untreated control K562 cells. **b** Cells treated with compound A (21.66 μM). **c** Cells treated with compound B (22.23 μM). Cells were stained with annexin V and propidiumiodide. The results shown are representative of three independent experiments. Quadrant 3, living cells An−/PI−; Quadrant 4, early apoptotic cells An+/PI−; Quadrant 2, late apoptotic cells An+/PI+; Quadrant 1, necrotic cells An−/PI+

apoptosis signaling pathway, including FHC, p-ERK, c-Myc and Egr1 were determined through Western and RT- PCR analysis (Fig. 5 and 7).

Administration of compounds **A** and **B** to K562 cells resulted in a reduction in FHC protein level, which was significant ($p < 0.01$) following 16 h of treatment (Fig. 5a and c). Treatment of cells with the two compounds **A** and **B** also revealed a significant ($p < 0.01$ and $p < 0.001$, respectively) reduction in the levels of p-ERK which coincided with a lack of change in those of ERK after 16 h of treatment (Fig. 5a, d and e). Collectively, these results demonstrate that treatment with compounds **A** and **B** lead to a reduction in both ERK phosphorylation and FHC levels. Finally, Semi-quantitative RT-PCR analysis revealed no change in c-Myc mRNA levels in cells treated with compounds **A** or **B** (IC_{50}) after 16 h (Fig. 7). Furthermore, consistent with the transcript levels of c-Myc, protein levels of Egr1 were not altered by compounds **A** and **B** after 16 h (Fig. 5a and f).

Discussion

To study the cytotoxicity of compounds **A** and **B**, as two new triaryl-oxadiazole derivatives which well fitted to COX-2 active site [11], their effects on the induction of "programmed cell death" in K562 cells, and the mechanisms by which these compounds induce apoptosis were investigated. K562 cells are a human cancer blood cell line derived from the chronic myeloid leukemia (CML) tumor lineage, which has been considered as a good model to study the cancer inhibitory effects of celecoxib derivatives [5, 8]. Celecoxib, as a first generation of COX-2 inhibitors, has gained a great deal of attention in cancer studies. Although, the cardiotoxic effect has been established in long period treatment of patients with celecoxib, and for this reason, its application in chemoprevention has been restrained [16]. In this regard, the two new compounds **A** and **B** show significant antiproliferative activity with considerable IC_{50} values (21.66 and 22.23 μM) in K562 cell line after a 24 h treatment [11].

The main mechanism that attributes to the observed effects of COX-2 inhibitors against different types of cancer is apoptosis [17]. Apoptosis is a kind of cell death known as "programmed cell death" that occurs in different physiological and pathological situations and marked by typical morphological and biochemical features, including cell shrinkage, nuclear DNA fragmentation and membrane blebbing [18]. Following treatment of K562 cells with compounds **A** and **B** for 16 h, the fluorescence microscopic observations demonstrated typical morphological changes indicating cell damage; however, these changes were not as much following 8 h of incubation (Fig. 2). The data obtained from annexin-V/PI analysis were in agreement with the morphological changes showing that compounds **A** and **B** induce apoptosis after 16 h (Table 1).

The two major apoptotic pathways known to operate in mammalian cells include the receptor (extrinsic) and the mitochondrial (intrinsic) pathways. Through the intrinsic pathway, members of the Bcl-2 protein family operate as regulators of survival and death during apoptosis induction [19, 20]. Although the role of

Table 1 Percentage of K562 cells in each state after treatment with compounds A (21.6 μM) and B (22.23 μM) for 16 h

Compound	Vital cells (%) An−/PI−	Early apoptosis (%) An+/PI−	Late apoptosis (%) An+/PI+	Necrosis (%) An−/PI+
A	90.48±0.38	0.427497	0.61±0.09	4.9±0.23
B	85.91±0.62	9.82±0.58	1.05±0.02	3.22±0.08
Control	95.02±1.1	1.28±0.06	0.36±0.05	3.34±0.4

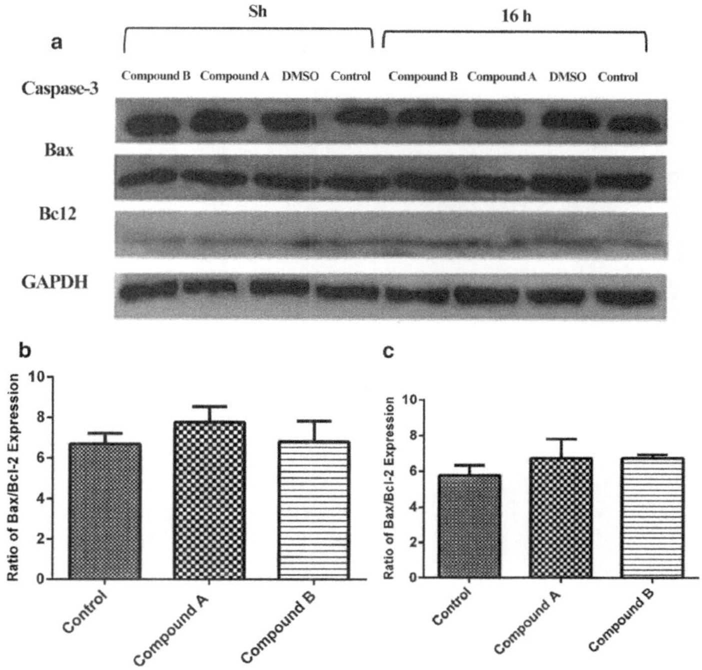

Fig. 4 Expression analysis of apoptosis associated proteins by Western blot analysis. K562 cells were treated with compounds A (21.66 μM) and B (22.23 μM). **a** Immunoblot showing the expression levels of caspase-3, Bcl-2, Bax and GADPH. **b** Ratios of Bax/Bcl-2 after 8 h. **c** Ratios of Bax/Bcl-2 after 16 h. The results of 3 independent experiments are presented as mean ± standard error

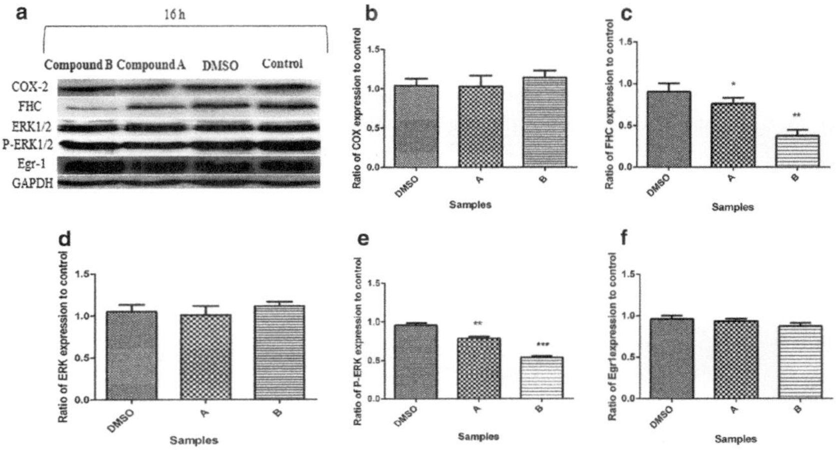

Fig. 5 Effect of compounds **A** (21.6 μM) and **B** (22.23 μM) on COX-2, FHC, ERK1/2, p-ERK1/2 and Egr1 expression in K562cells after incubation for 16 hours. **a** Immunoblot showing the expression levels of COX-2, FHC, ERK1/2, p-ERK1/2, Egr1 and GAPDH. **b** Ratios of COX-2/control. **c** Ratios of FHC/control. **d** Ratios of ERK/control. **e** Ratios of p-ERK/control. **f** Ratios of Egr1/control. The results of 3 independent experiments are presented as mean ± standard error (*$P < 0.05$, **$P < 0.01$ vs. the solvent group)

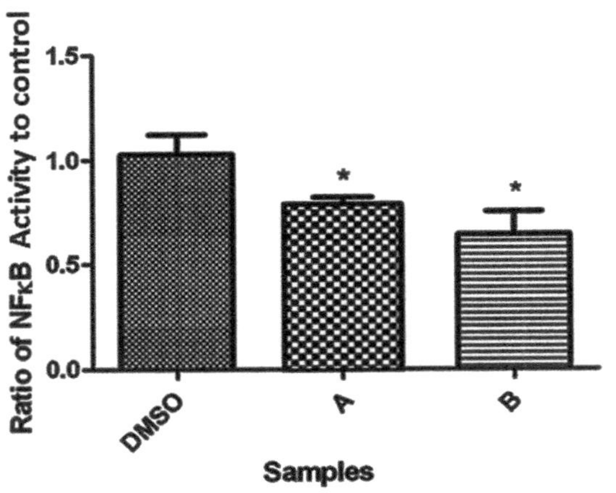

Fig. 6 Effect of compounds A (21.6 μM; IC_{50}) and B (22.23 μM; IC_{50}) on NF-κB activation in K562 cells after incubation for 16 hours. The results of 3 independent experiments are presented as mean ± standard error (*$P < 0.05$, vs. the solvent group)

mitochondria in compounds **A**- and **B**-induced apoptosis is not clear in K562 cells, several cytotoxic drugs as well as COX-2 inhibitors are known to initiate apoptosis through the mitochondrial pathway [21]. Our data clearly demonstrate that Bax and Bcl-2 do not have a critical role in the induction of apoptosis in K562 cells (Fig. 4), suggesting a mitochondria-independent apoptotic pathway induced by compounds **A** and **B**. The role of caspase-3 in the mitochondria-independent apoptotic pathway has also been well understood [22]. However, apparently compounds **A** and **B** induce apoptosis in a caspase- independent mechanism as caspase-3 levels were not altered by compounds **A** and **B** in K562 cells (Fig. 4a). Collectively these data demonstrate that compounds **A** and **B** induce apoptosis through both a mitochondria- and caspase- independent mechanism in K562 human leukemia cells. Our obtained data are in agreement with the recent report indicating the execution of apoptosis without the involvement of caspases. Indeed, apoptosis induced in these cells by compounds **A** and **B** has been shown to involve the activation of proteases other than caspases [23].

The antiproliferative and apoptotic effects of celecoxib in K562 cells are associated with COX-2 inhibition [5]. However, it is well established that tumor growth inhibition by selective COX-2 inhibitors might as well be mediated through COX-2-independent mechanisms [24]. In this study, treatment with compounds **A** and **B** were found to cause no change in COX-2 levels (Fig. 5). These findings demonstrate that the apoptotic effects of these compounds in K562 cells are mediated by a COX-2 independent pathway. Interestingly, it was recently reported that celecoxib derivatives with no COX-2 inhibitory action can be considered as anti-cancer agents without increasing the cardiovascular risk [25]. Therefore, the two compounds may have a potential in being used as chemotherapeutic agents with little or no cardiovascular side effects.

Induction of apoptosis can be triggered by a number of stimuli, activating a cell suicide program that is constitutively present in most vertebrate cells. In diverse cell types, Rel/NF-kappaB transcription factors are involved in regulation of apoptosis by either inducing or perhaps more commonly blocking it [26]. NF-κB regulates the expression of more than 400 genes involved in inflammation, cell survival, proliferation, invasion and angiogenesis. NF-κB also affects apoptosis during tumor development and progression [27], often leading to apoptosis resistance [28]. On the other hand, a reduction in NF-κB mitogenic signaling has been associated with the anticancer effects of celecoxib treatment on mouse mammary epithelial tumor cells mediated through a COX-2 independent pathway [24]. Our data also demonstrate that treatment of K562 cells with compounds **A** and **B** results in a reduction of NF-κB expression (Fig. 6) in a COX-2-independent manner.

The primary iron storage factor, FHC (Ferritin heavy chain), which mediates the antioxidant and protective activities of NF-κB, is induced downstream of NF-κB and required for TNFα-induced apoptosis [29]. Rezaie

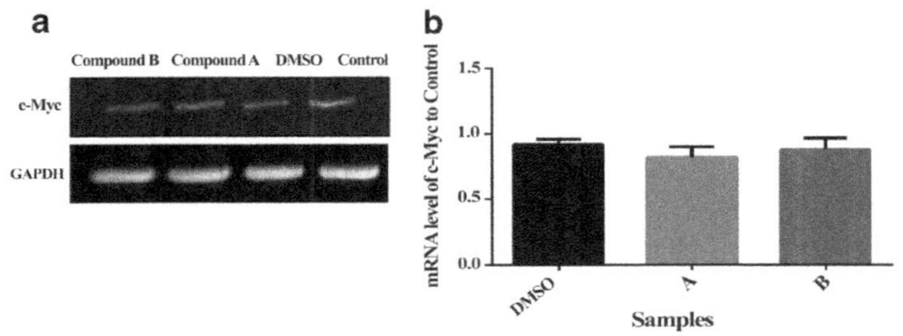

Fig. 7 Effect of compounds A (21.6 μM) and B (22.23 μM) on c-Myc mRNA levels in K562 cells after incubation for 16 hours. **a** Immunoblat showing the expression level of c-Myc. **b** Ratios of c-Myc/control. The results of 3 independent experiments are presented as mean ± standard error

et al. (2011) reported FHC down-regulation in J774.A1 macrophage-like cell lines, following celecoxib treatment [30]. Our study confirms down-regulation of FHC expression induced by compounds **A** and **B** in K562 cell line (Fig. 5). Interestingly, our data exhibit the down regulation of both NF-κB and FHC which may not be surprising as NF-κB, as a transcription factor, has been involved in the regulation of FHC expression.

Moreover, mitogen-activated protein kinase (MAPK)/ extracellular signal-regulated protein kinase (ERK) have been implied in transmitting the apoptotic signal [14]. MAPK family members are mediators of signal transduction pathways [22]. Importantly, NF-κB acts the upstream of MAPKs in the signaling of certain anticancer drugs [31]. The ERK pathway, a major player in the regulation of cell growth, survival, and differentiation, is induced in response to mitogens and growth factors [22], however, evidence for ERK pathway mediating apoptosis has also been reported [32]. According to previous studies, celecoxib has different roles in ERK1/2 activation in different cells. The present study revealed growth inhibition of K562 cells following compounds **A**- and **B**- treatment via down regulation of p-ERK1/2 (Fig. 5). These data indicate that the mechanism of antiproliferative activities of the designed compounds may be mediated through NF-κB and ERK inhibition.

Anticancer drugs induce apoptosis through different intracellular targets and cause DNA damage [21]. Another factor contributing to the regulation of apoptosis includes the early gene, c-Myc [33]. There has been conflicting reports on the regulation of c-Myc expression during NSAID-induced apoptosis. NSAID-induced apoptosis of gastric cancer cells may be mediated through the upregulation of c-Myc proto-oncogene [34], while NS-398, a COX-2 inhibitor, reduces c-Myc expression in rat colon cancer cells [35]. In the present study, RT-PCR analysis revealed no alteration in the levels of c-Myc transcript in K562 cells treated with compounds **A** or **B** compared to the control (Fig. 7b), however, compounds **A** and **B** induced apoptosis in K562 cells, suggesting the operation of a c-Myc independent apoptotic pathway. Our results are consistent with those of Ostrowski et al. (2003) who demonstrated a lack of alteration in basal and serum-stimulated c-Myc expression following treatment of rat hepatoma HTC-IR cells with aspirin or celecoxib. In addition, when treated with the selective COX-2 inhibitor, NS-398, no change was observed in c-Myc mRNA levels in rat colon mucosa as compared to untreated animals [36].

Previous studies also showed that c-Myc directly induces transcription of a noncanonical target gene, Egr1 (Early growth response-1) [37]. Egr1 can suppress the growth of a number of tumor cells, including leukemia. A diverse of anticancer agents, such as COX inhibitors, act through the modulation of Egr1 [38]. In a pancreatic cancer model, tolfenamic acid-induced Egr1 expression appears to have an essential role in the activation of apoptosis [39]. Our data revealed no change in the levels of Egr1 in K562 cell line treated with compounds **A** and **B** (Fig. 5). Therefore, the apoptosis in K562 cell line induced by compounds **A** and **B** appears to be independent from the c-myc/Egr1 pathway. These results are in line with our previous report showing an apoptosis induced by compounds **A** and **B** via a c-myc/Egr1 independent pathways in breast cancer cell line with a different mechanism [40].

Conclusion

In summary, the present study reveals that compounds **A** and **B**, as two new triaryl-oxadiazole derivatives with COX-2 inhibitory structures, induce apoptosis in K562 cells through a mitochondrial-, caspase- and COX-2-independent pathways. This COX-2-independent mechanism involves a reduction in NF-κB levels and a subsequent reduction in the downstream FHC and P-ERK1/2 signaling. Our findings also demonstrate a more pronounced apoptotic effect in response to compound **B** than compound **A** in K562 cells. Future studies need to be directed towards identifying the downstream mediators in order to reveal a more clear and detailed molecular pathway that would help in the development of compounds **A** and **B** as suitable chemotherapeutic agents against leukemia.

Competing interests

The authors declare that they have no competing interests.

Authors' contributions

SHN and MN contributed in performing laboratory experiments. MA synthesized the chemical compounds. AA contributed in cell culture techniques. SI and MN contributed in preparing manuscript and the research proposal. MS was the principle investigator who conceived the idea and helped in the preparation of the manuscript. All authors read and approved the final manuscript.

Acknowledgements

This research was financially supported by Pasteur Institute of Iran and Tehran University of Medical Sciences.

Author details

[1]Department of Cell and Molecular Biology, Faculty of Biological Sciences, Kharazmi University, P.O. Box 1481765544 Tehran, Iran. [2]Department of Medicinal Chemistry, School of Pharmacy, Tehran University of Medical Sciences, Tehran, Iran. [3]National Cell Bank of Iran, Pasteur Institute of Iran, Tehran, Iran. [4]Department of Physiology and Pharmacology, Pasteur Institute of Iran, P.O. Box 13164 Tehran, Iran.

References

1. Anjali P, Faraha S, Amit KS. Synthetic and green vegetable isothiocyanates target red blood leukemia cancers. Fitoterapia. 2012;83:255–65.
2. Shi S, Yao W, Xu J, Long J, Liu C, Yu X. Combinational therapy: New hope for pancreatic cancer. Cancer Lett. 2012;317:127–35.

3. Moon Y, Jr Bottone FG, McEntee MF, Eling TE. Suppression of tumor cell invasion by cyclooxygenase inhibitors is mediated by thrombospondin-1 via the early growth response gene Egr-1. Mol Cancer Ther. 2005;4:1551–8.
4. Hsueh CT, Chiu CF, Kelsen DP, Schwartz GK. Selective inhibition of cyclooxygenase-2 enhances mitomycin-C-induced apoptosis. Cancer Chemother Pharmacol. 2000;45:389–96.
5. Zhang GS, Liu DS, Dai CW, Li RJ. Antitumor effects of celecoxib on K562 leukemia cells are mediated by cell-cycle arrest, caspase-3 activation, and downregulation of Cox-2 expression and are synergistic with hydroxyureaor imatinib. Am J Hematol. 2006;81:242–55.
6. Wang JL, Lin KL, Chen JS, Lu YC, Jiann BP, Chang HT, et al. Effect of celecoxib on Ca2+ movement and cell proliferation in human osteoblasts. Biochem Pharmacol. 2004;67:1123–30.
7. Pyrko P, Kardosh A, Schönthal AH. Celecoxib transiently inhibits cellular protein synthesis. Biochem Pharmacol. 2008;75:395–404.
8. Subhashini J, Mahipal SV, Reddanna P. Anti proliferative and apoptotic effects of celecoxib on human chronic myeloid leukemia in vitro. Cancer Lett. 2005;224:31–43.
9. Du H, Li W, Wang Y, Chen S, Zhang Y. Celecoxib induces cell apoptosis coupled with upregulation of the expression of VEGF by a mechanism involving ER stress in human colorectal cancer cells. Oncol Rep. 2011;26:495–502.
10. Liu X, Yue P, Zhou Z, Khuri FR, Sun SY. Death receptor regulation and celecoxib-induced apoptosis in human lung cancer cells. J Natl Cancer Inst. 2004;96:1769–80.
11. Miralinaghi P, Salimi M, Amirhamzeh A, Norouzi M, MostafapourKandelousi H, Shafiee A, et al. Synthesis, molecular docking study, and anticancer activity of triaryl-1,2,4-oxadiazole. Med Chem Res. 2013;22:4253–62.
12. Van Engeland M, Nieland LJ, Ramaekers FC, Schutte B, Reutelingsperger CP. AnnexinV affinity assay: a review on an apoptosis detection system based on phosphatidylserine exposure. Cytometry. 1998;31:1–9.
13. Shi Y, Hutchinson HG, Hall DJ, Zalewski A. Downregulation of c-myc expression by antisense oligonucleotides inhibits proliferation of human smooth muscle cells. Circulation. 1993;88:1190–5.
14. Sun Y, Li Y, Luo D, Liao DJ. Pseudogenes as weaknesses of ACTB (Actb) and GAPDH (Gapdh) used as reference genes in reverse transcription and polymerase chain reactions. PLoS One. 2012;7:1–11.
15. Fan C, Yang J, Engelhardt JF. Temporal pattern of NFkappaB activation influences apoptotic cell fate in a stimuli-dependent fashion. J Cell Sci. 2002;115:4843–53.
16. Benelli R, Venè R, Minghelli S, Carlone S, Gatteschi B, Ferrari N. Celecoxib induces proliferation and Amphiregulin production in colon subepithelialmyofibroblasts, activatingerk1-2 signaling in synergy with EGRF. Cancer Lett. 2013;328:73–82.
17. Cotterchio M, Krieger N, Sloan M, Steinegart A. Non-steroidal anti-inflammatory drug use and breast cancer risk. Cancer Epidemiol Biomarkers Prev. 2001;10:1213–7.
18. Fulda S, Debatin KM. Extrinsic versus intrinsic apoptosis pathways in anticancer chemotherapy. Oncogene. 2006;25:4798–811.
19. Almeida A, Almeida J, Bolanos JP, Moncada S. Different responses of astrocytes and neurons to nitric oxide: the role of glycolytically generated ATP in astrocyte protection. Proc Natl Acad Sci U S A. 2001;98:15294–9.
20. Fujita N, Tsuruo T. Survival-signaling pathway as a promising target for cancer chemotherapy. Cancer Chemother Pharmacol. 2003;1:24–8.
21. Rudner J, Elsaesser SJ, Jendrossek V, Huber SM. Anti-apoptotic Bcl-2 fails to form efficient complexes with pro-apoptotic Bak to protect from celecoxib-induced apoptosis. Biochem Pharmacol. 2011;81:32–42.
22. Choi BK, Choi CH, Oh HL, Kim YK. Role of ERK activation in cisplatin-induced apoptosis in A172 human glioma cells. Neuro Toxicology. 2004;25:915–24.
23. Liang Y, Yan C, Schor NF. Apoptosis in the absence of caspase 3. Oncogene. 2001;20:6570–8.
24. Shirode AB, Sylvester PW. Mechanisms mediating the synergistic anticancer effects of combined γ-tocotrienol and celecoxib treatment. J Bioanal Biomed. 2011;3:1–7.
25. Dovizio M, Tacconelli S, Sostresm C, Ricciotti E, Patrignani P. Mechanistic and pharmacological issues of aspirin as an anticancer agent. Pharmaceuticals. 2012;5:1346–71.
26. Barkett M, Gilmore TD. Control of apoptosis by Rel/NF-kappaB transcription factors. Oncogene. 1999;18:6910–24.
27. Sung B, Pandey MK, Ahn KS, Yi T, Chaturvedi MM, Liu M, et al. Anacardic acid (6-nonadecyl salicylic acid), an inhibitor of histone acetyltransferase, suppresses expression of nuclear factor-kappa B regulated gene products involved in cell survival, proliferation, invasion, and inflammation through inhibition of the inhibitory subunit of nuclear factor-kappaBalph kinase, leading to potentiation of apoptosis. Blood. 2008;111:4880–91.
28. Meteoglu I, Erdogdu IH, Meydan N, Erkus M, Barutca S. NF-KAPPAb expression correlates with apoptosis and angiogenesis in clear cell renal cell carcinoma tissues. J Exp Clin Cancer Res. 2008;27:53–61.
29. Pham CG, Bubici C, Zazzeroni F, Papa S, Jones J, Alvarez K, et al. Ferritin heavy chain upregulation by NFkappa inhibits TNFalpha-induced apoptosis by suppressing reactive oxygen species. Cell. 2004;119:529–42.
30. Rezaie F, Salimi M, Ghahremani MH, Vaziri B. Potential molecular targets in chemopreventative action of celecoxib: a proteomics analysis of J774.A1 macrophage-like cell line. Mol BioSyst. 2011;7:1306–11.
31. Bava SV, Sreekanth CN, Thulasidasan AK, Anto NP, Cheriyan VT, Puliyappadamba VT, et al. Akt is upstream and MAPKs are downstream of NF-κB in paclitaxel-induced survival signaling events, which are down-regulated by curcumin contributing to their synergism. Int J Biochem Cell Biol. 2001;43:331–41.
32. Zhuang S, Schnellmann RG. A death-promoting role for extracellular signal-regulated kinase. J Pharmacol Exp Ther. 2006;319:991–7.
33. Li Q, Suen TC, Sun H, Arita A, Costa M. Nickel compounds induce apoptosis in human bronchial epithelial Beas-2B cells by activation of c-Myc through ERK pathway. Toxicol Appl Pharmacol. 2009;235:191–8.
34. Zhu GH, Wong BC, Eggo MC, Ching CK, Yuen ST, Chan EY, et al. Non-steroidal anti-inflammatory drug-induced apoptosis in gastric cancer cells is blocked by protein kinase C activation through inhibition of c-myc. Br J Cancer. 1998;79:393–400.
35. Kishimoto Y, Yashima K, Morisawa T, Shiota G, Kawasaki H, Hasegawa J. Effects of cyclooxygenase-2 inhibitor NS-398 on APC and c-myc expression in rat colon carcinogenesis induced by azoxymethane. J Gastroenterol. 2002;37:186–93.
36. Ostrowski J, Wocial T, Skurzak H, Bartnik W. Do altering in ornithine decarboxylase activity and gene expression contribute to antiproliferative properties of COX inhibitors? Br J Cancer. 2003;88:1143–51.
37. Boone DN, Ying Q, Li Z, Hann SR. Egr1 mediates p53-independent c-Myc–induced apoptosis via a noncanonical ARF-dependent transcriptional mechanism. Proc Natl Acad Sci U S A. 2011;108:632–7.
38. Liu J, Liu YG, Huang R, Yao C, Li S, Yang W, et al. Concurrent down-regulation of Egr-1 and gelsolin in the majority of human breast cancer cells. Cancer Genomics Proteomics. 2007;4:377–86.
39. Lee SH, Bahn JH, Choi CK, Whitlock NC, English AE, Safe S, et al. ESE-1/EGR-1 Pathway Plays a Role in Tolfenamic Acid-induced Apoptosis in Colorectal Cancer Cells. Mol Cancer Ther. 2008;7:3739–50.
40. Norouzi M, Norouzi SH, Amini M, Amanzadeh A, Irian S, Salimi M. Apoptotic effects of two COX-2 inhibitors on breast adenocarcinoma cells through COX-2 independent Pathway. J Cell Biochem. 2015;116:81–90.

Anti-cancer effect of *Cordyceps militaris* in human colorectal carcinoma RKO cells via cell cycle arrest and mitochondrial apoptosis

Hwan Hee Lee[1,2], Seulki Lee[1,2], Kanghyo Lee[3], Yu Su Shin[4], Hyojeung Kang[5*] and Hyosun Cho[1,2*]

Abstract

Background: *Cordyceps militaris* has been used as a traditional medicine in Asian countries for a long time. Different types of Cordyceps extract were reported to have various pharmacological activities including an anti-cancer effect. We investigated the inhibitory effect of *Cordyceps militaris* ethanol extract on a human colorectal cancer-derived cell line, RKO.

Methods: RKO cells were treated with various concentrations of nucleosides-enriched ethanol extract of *Cordyceps militaris* for 48 h and cytotoxicity was measured using a CCK-8 assay. Then, xenograft Balb/c nude mice were injected with RKO cells and subsequently orally administered with ethanol extract of *Cordyceps militaris* every day for 3 weeks to examine the inhibitory effect on tumor growth. Lastly, the effect of *Cordyceps militaris* on cell cycle as well as apoptosis was measured using flow cytometry. Also, the expression of p53, caspase 9, cleaved caspase-3, cleaved PARP, Bim, Bax, Bak, and Bad were detected using western blot assay.

Results: RKO cells were highly susceptible to the ethanol extract of *Cordyceps militaris* (CME) and the growth of RKO cells-derived tumor was significantly delayed by the treatment of *Cordyceps militaris. Cordyceps militaris* induced cell cycle arrest in G2/M phase (untreated; 20.5 %, CME 100 μg/ml; 61.67 %, CME 300 μg/ml; 66.33 %) and increased early apoptosis (untreated; 1.01 %, CME 100 μg/ml; 8.48 %, CME 300 μg/ml; 18.07 %). The expression of p53, cleaved caspase 9, cleaved caspase-3, cleaved PARP, Bim, Bak, and Bad were upregulated by the treatment of *Cordyceps militaris.*

Conclusion: Ethanol extract of *Cordyceps militaris* was highly cytotoxic to human colorectal carcinoma RKO cells and inhibited the growth of tumor in xenograft model. The anti-tumor effect of *Cordyceps militaris* was associated with an induction of cell cycle arrest and mitochondrial-mediated apoptosis.

Keywords: *Cordyceps militaris*, Human colorectal carcinoma, p53, Mitochondrial-mediated apoptosis

Background

A large number of edible mushrooms have been shown to possess various biological activities [1–5]. Edible mushrooms from Pleurotus species showed the antioxidative, antimicrobial and anrifungal properties when they were cultivated on banana agrowastes [1, 2]. Antimetastatic activity of *Hericium erinaceus* edible mushroom extracts was reported using murine colon carcinoma cells [3]. Antioxidant and cytotoxic activities of ethanolic extracts of *Phellinus Quél* were recently reported [4]. An extract of *Agaricus blazei Murill* was shown to stimulate immunocytes and regulate immune response in leukemia mice [5]. *Cordyceps* mushrooms also have received extensive attention owing to their potent pharmacological activities. *Cordyceps sinensis* and *Cordyceps militaris* are representative species for their medicinal uses in China and Korea. Both of them are fungi on the larvae of caterpillars of moths and traditional medicine involves both mushroom fruit-body and parasitized larvae. A couple of well-known active ingredients in these mushrooms include cordycepin, cordycepic acid, sterols (ergosterol), nucleosides, and polysaccharides [6, 7]. *Cordyceps militaris* is a traditional Chinese

* Correspondence: hkang72@gmail.com; hyosun1102@gmail.com
[5]College of Pharmacy, Research Institute of Pharmaceutical Sciences and Institute for Microorganisms, Kyungpook National University, Daegu 702-701, Republic of Korea
[1]College of Pharmacy, Duksung Women's University, Seoul 132-714, Republic of Korea
Full list of author information is available at the end of the article

medicine, which has been cultured successfully and has been shown to have a higher content of cordycepin and cordycepic acid than *Cordyceps sinensis* [8]. Diffferent types of extracts of *Cordyceps militaris* have been reported to exert immunomodulatory, anti-inflammatory, anti-microbial and antitumor effects although the primary pharmacological activity is a little bit different depending on the main ingredients of extract [7–10]. Recently, we found that ethanol extract of *Cordyceps militaris*, which has a couple of nucleoside analogs as the main components, had an anti-influenza effect in a DBA2 mouse model [11].

Beside the routine methods of surgery, radiotherapy and chemotherapy, traditional herb medicine is one of the major complementary and alternative medicines for treating various malignant diseases, including colorectal cancer [12–14].

Colorectal cancer is a serious health problem that has progressively increased to be one of the most common cancers in Asian countries [15]. *Cordyceps* extract has been reported to have a potent cytotoxic effect on various human cancer cells, including human lung carcinoma cells [16, 17]. However, the anti-tumor effect of *Cordyceps* extract on human colorectal cancer cells was not precisely examined *in vivo* model. Xenograft mouse model is immunocompromised animal, which could be implanted with the human tumor cells either under the skin or into any organ and does not reject the tumor. Therefore, it has been an indispensable model system for the preclinical screen and the development of novel anti-cancer agents.

p53 is known to play a critical role in the induction of cell apoptosis in response to DNA damage [18]. A typical pro-apoptotic molecule activated by p53 is Bax, a member of the Bcl-2 family [19]. The Bcl-2 family of proteins includes both pro-apoptotic members (Bak, Bax, and Bad) as well as anti-apoptotic members (Bcl-2, Bcl-xL, and Bcl-w). Mitochondria-dependent cell apoptosis is regulated mainly by the ratio of expression of Bcl-2 family proteins [20]. The activation of Bax results in the release of cytochrome c into the cytosol, which leads to the activation of caspases 9 and 3, effector caspases, in the mitochondrial pathway of cell apoptosis [21, 22].

In the present study, we investigated the cytotoxic effect of *Cordyceps militaris* ethanol extract on human colorectal carcinoma RKO cells and evaluated the anti-cancer effect of *Cordyceps militaris* in mice bearing RKO cell-derived tumors. Subsequently, the underlying mechanisms, which mediate the anti-cancer effect of *Cordyceps militaris* on human colorectal cancer, were precisely examined. We found that the anti-cancer effect of nucleosides-enriched ethanol extract of *Cordyceps militaris* was highly associated with the increased expression of p53, Bax, Bim, Bak, Bad, cleaved-caspases 9 and 3, and PARP.

Material and methods

Specimen preparation

The fungus strain *Cordyceps militaris* was from Dong-Chong-Xia-Cao Culture Collection (Mushtech, Hoengseong, Kangwondo, Reupblic of Korea). Fresh fruiting bodies or mycelia of *Cordyceps militaris* were extracted with 50 % ethanol at room temperature for 3 days. The extracts were filtered, concentrated, sterilized and dried as previously described [23]. The major compounds of extract are cordycepin, adenosine, urasil and guanosine, which structurally belong to nucleoside family (provided by Dong-a Pharm. Co., LTD, Yongin, Republic of Korea). Extracts of specimens were diluted with distilled water for RKO cell treatment as well as for oral administration in the mouse experiment.

Cell culture and treatment

Human colorectal carcinoma (RKO) cells were obtained from ATCC and cultured in Dulbecco's Modified Eagle's medium (DMEM, Gibco, USA) supplemented with 10 % heat-inactivated fetal bovine serum (FBS, Hyclone, USA), 100 U/ml penicillin and streptomycin (Gibco, USA) at 37 °C in a humidified atmosphere with 5 % CO_2.

Cell cytotoxicity

Cytotoxicity of ethanol extract of *Cordyceps militaris* on human colorectal carcinoma (RKO) cells was assessed with the Cell Counting Kit-8 (CCK-8, Dojindo, Japan) as previously described [24]. Briefly, cells were seeded in 96-well plates at a density of 3 × 103 cells/well and treated with different concentrations of ethanol extract of *Cordyceps militaris* (0, 25, 50, 100, 250, 500, and 1000 μg/ml) for 24 h or 48 h. CCK-8 solution was added to each well and incubated for another 3 h. The absorbance was measured using a microplate reader (BMG Labtech, Germany) at 450 nm.

Cell morphology

Cells were seeded at a density of 4 × 104 cells/well in 6-well plates. After incubation for 24 h, the cells were treated with different concentrations of ethanol extract of *Cordyceps militaris* (0, 100, and 300 μg/ml) and incubated for 24 h. The cells were observed by light microscopy (×200) (Nikon eclipse TS100, Japan).

Cell cycle analysis

Cells were seeded at a density of 1 × 106 cells/well in 6-well plates, and treated with different concentrations of ethanol extract of *Cordyceps militaris* (0, 100, and 300 μg/ml) for 24 h. Cells were harvested by trypsinization and fixed with 70 % ethanol at 4 °C overnight. The next day, cells were resuspended in PBS buffer containing 0.2 mg/ml RNase A (Qiagen, USA) and incubated for 1 h at 37 °C. Cells were then stained with propidium iodide for 30 min in the dark. Stained cells were analyzed using a flow cytometer (EasyCyte guava, Merck Millipore).

Annexin V-FITC and propidium iodide assay

Cell apoptosis was analyzed using the Annexin V-FITC Apoptosis Detection Kit (Roche, USA) as previously described [24]. Briefly, RKO cells were plated in 6-well plates at a density of 1 × 106 cells/well and incubated for 24 h. Cells were treated with different concentrations (0, 100, and 300 μg/ml) of ethanol extract of *Cordyceps militaris* for 24 h or 48 h and then Annexin V and PI solution were added. Cells were analyzed by flow cytometry (EasyCyte guava, Merck Millipore).

Western blot analysis

Western blot assays were performed as previously described with modification [24]. Briefly, RKO cells were treated with ethanol extract of *Cordyceps militaris* (100 and 300 μg/ml) for 48 h. Protein from cell lysates was measured using the Bradford assay, separated by electrophoresis, and transferred onto nitrocellulose membranes. Membranes were subsequently incubated with 1st and 2nd antibody, and the blots were visualized by enhanced chemiluminescent (ECL) detection solutions (GE Healthcare, USA).

Xenograft mouse model experiments

All animal experiments were conducted in accordance with recommendations in the National Research Council's Guide (IACUC, Republic of Korea) for the Care and Use of Laboratory Animals. The experimental protocol was approved by the Animal Experiments Committee of Duksung Women's University (permit number: 2014-015-007). Balb/c nude mice (female, 5 weeks old; Joong-ang Animal Experiment Company, Republic of Korea) were used as our xenograft animal model. Mice were housed individually on a 12-h day/12-h night cycle at 23 ~ 27 °C and had access to food and water. Mice were randomly divided into two groups ($n = 10$/group): (1) a drinking water group ($n = 10$): animals received oral administration of drinking water; (2) a CME group ($n = 10$): animals received oral administration of *Cordyceps militaris* ethanol extract (100 mg/kg). To produce tumors, each mouse was implanted with RKO cells (1×10^6 cells per animal), subcutaneously in the back next to the right hind leg. Next, *Cordyceps militaris* ethanol extract (100 mg/kg) or drinking water was administered orally every day for 3 weeks. Fourteen days later, the tumors were identified and then measured every 2 days with a Standard Caliper. Tumor volume was calculated as follows: tumor volume (mm^3) = [tumor length (mm) × tumor width $(mm)^2$]/2. Once tumor volume reached up to 2000 mm^3, animals were euthanized.

Statistical analysis

Data were processed using Microexcel software and were expressed as mean ± SD. Comparisons of several means were performed using one-way or two-way analysis of variance followed by the Fisher's exact test to identify significant differences between groups. P values of less than 0.05 were considered significant.

Results

Cytotoxicity of *Cordyceps* extract in RKO cells

To investigate the cytotoxic effect of ethanol extract of *Cordyceps militaris* on human colorectal carcinoma RKO cells, cells were treated with serially diluted extract of *Cordyceps militaris* (0, 25, 50, 75, 100, 250, 500, and 1000 μg/ml) for 48 h and cytotoxicity was determined by CCK-8. Figure 1a shows that ethanol extract of *Cordyceps militaris* starts to inhibit cell viability at a concentration of 75 μg/ml compared to untreated cells ($P < 0.0001$). In Fig. 1b, cell morphological changes by two different concentrations of ethanol extract of *Cordyceps militaris* (100 and 300 μg/ml) were observed. There were fewer cells in the extract-treated conditions.

In vivo evaluation of anti-cancer effect of *Cordyceps militaris* ethanol extract in a xenograft mouse model

To evaluate the anti-cancer effect of ethanol extract of *Cordyceps militaris in vivo*, mice were injected subcutaneously with human colorectal cancer RKO cells (1×10^6 cells per mouse) and then ethanol extract of *Cordyceps militaris* (100 mg/kg) or drinking water was orally administrated every day for 3 weeks. Tumor growth was detected from all 20 mice and tumor volume was measured every two days until it reached 2000 mm^3. Figure 2a displays the overall study design for animal experiment. Figure 2b shows representative photographs of xenograft mice bearing RKO cell-derived human colorectal cancer. The pictures of the extract fed and water fed groups were taken at 13 days since the tumor volume was measured. The size of tumors from the extract fed mice was smaller than that from water fed mice. In Fig. 2c, we confirmed that continuous feeding of ethanol extract of *Cordyceps militaris* (100 mg/kg) significantly inhibited the growth of RKO cell-derived tumors. We further determined whether inhibition of tumor growth directly correlates with survival rate in the xenograft animals. As expected, we observed a reduced mortality in mice administered 100 mg/kg of ethanol extract of *Cordyceps militaris* in Fig. 2d.

Evaluation of cell cycle arrest in RKO cells treated with *Cordyceps militaris* ethanol extract

To clarify the molecular mechanism of *Cordyceps militaris*, we analyzed the effect on cell cycle regulation in RKO cells using flow cytometry. Interestingly, ethanol extract of *Cordyceps militaris* (100 or 300 μg/ml) induced

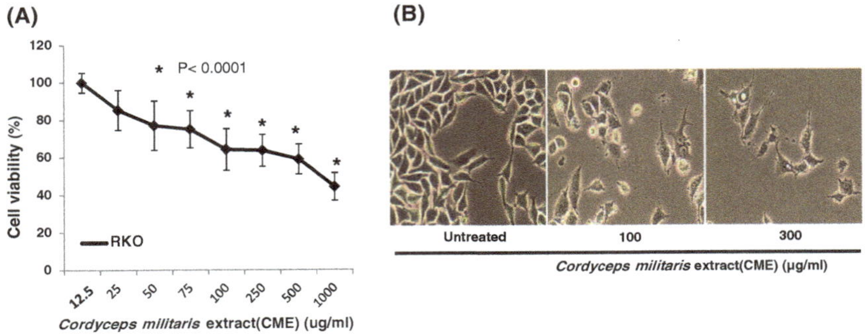

Fig. 1 Cell cytotoxicity of *Cordyceps militaris* in human colorectal carcinoma RKO cells. **a** RKO cells were treated with various concentrations (0–1000 μg/mL) of ethanol extract of *Cordyceps militaris* (CME) for 48 h, and cell viability was determined by CCK-8 assay. The results are presented as mean ± standard deviation (SD) for five independent experiments. **b** Cells were treated with or without ethanol extract of *Cordyceps militaris* (CME) for 24 h or 48 h. Cell morphology was observed by light microscopy (×200)

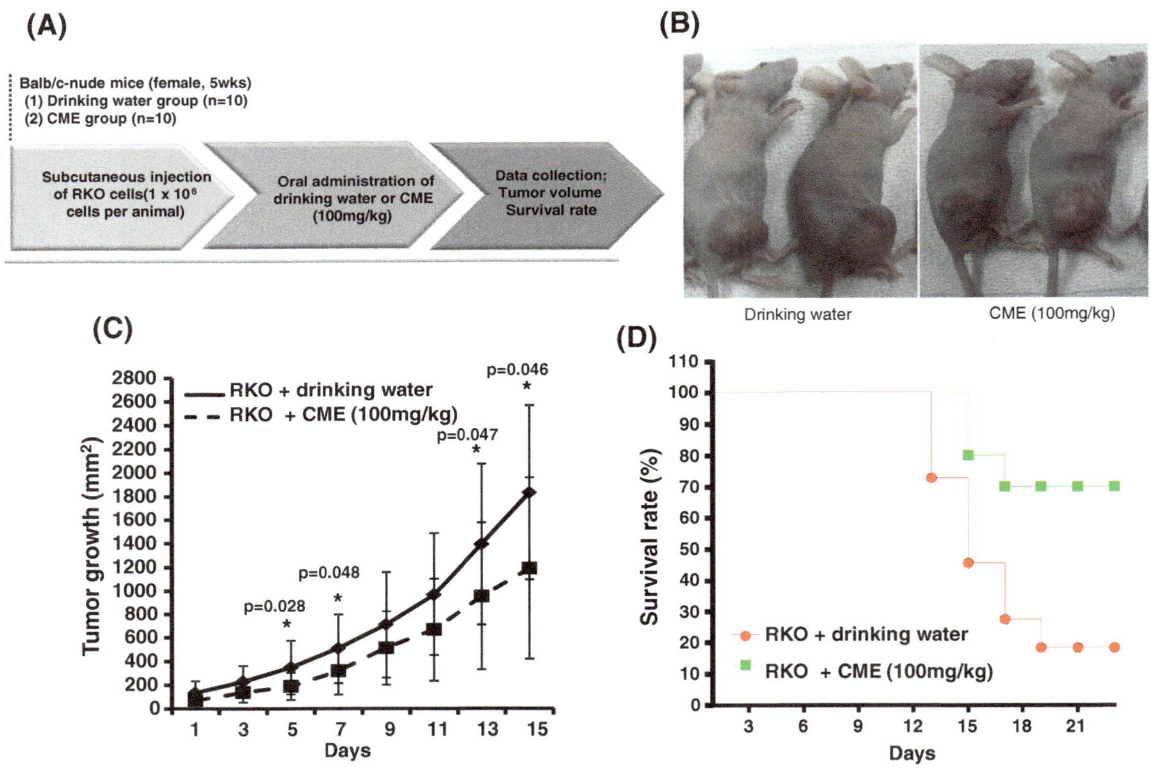

Fig. 2 Anti-cancer effect of *Cordyceps militaris* in a xenograft mouse bearing RKO cell–derived human colorectal cancer. Mice were injected with human colorectal carcinoma RKO cells (1×10^6 cells per mouse) subcutaneously into the back next to the right hind leg. Mice were sorted into 2 groups ($n = 10$/group) and orally administered ethanol extract of *Cordyceps militaris* (CME) (100 mg/kg) or drinking water. 14 days later, tumors were identified and measured every two days until the experimental endpoint. **a** Study design for animal experiment. **b** Photograph of xenograft mice bearing RKO cell-derived human colorectal cancer in right hind leg. The pictures of untreated and treated groups were taken at 13 days since the tumor volume was measured. **c** Inhibitory effect of *Cordyceps militaris* (CME) on RKO cell-derived tumor growth. Compared between drinking water group and CME group $^*P < 0.05$. **d** Correlation of survival rate of xenograft mice bearing human colorectal cancer

an increase in the G2/M phase distribution of cells (100 μg/ml; 61.67 %, 300 μg/ml; 66.33 %) as compared to untreated cells (20.5 %) (Fig. 3a). and the quantitative analysis gave a statistically significant difference (Fig. 3b).

Evaluation of cell apoptosis in RKO cells treated with *Cordyceps militaris* ethanol extract

We further examined its effect on cell apoptosis using Annexin V-FITC and propidium iodide (PI) staining. As shown in Fig. 4a, 100 or 300 μg/ml of ethanol extract of *Cordyceps militaris* induced 8.37 % or 22.5 %, respectively, early apoptosis in RKO cells. Five times of independent experiments showed that ethanol extract of *Cordyceps militaris* significantly increased early apoptosis compared to untreated cells(untreated; 1.01 %, 100 μg/ml; 8.48 %, 300 μg/ml; 18.07 %) (Fig. 4b).

Evaluation of apoptotic-related protein expression in RKO cells treated with *Cordyceps militaris* ethanol extract

To identify the responsible apoptotic-related molecules, we examined the expression of p53, Bcl-2 family proteins, caspases, and poly (ADP-ribose) polymerase (PARP) using western blot analysis. Mitochondria-mediated apoptosis involves a variety of signaling molecules including p53, caspase activators, the proapoptotic and antiapoptotic Bcl-2 family proteins [18–20]. We found increased expression of p53 and proapoptotic Bcl-2 family proteins (Bim, Bax, Bak, and Bad) in RKO cells treated with ethanol extract of *Cordyceps militaris.*

In addition, the release of cytochrome *c* is known to activate caspase-9 and caspase-3. Activation of caspase 3 triggers the cleavage of PARP (89 and 24 kDa), which functions to prevent DNA damage [25]. As shown in Fig. 5b, the extract of *Cordyceps militaris* increased the cleaved forms of caspases 9 and 3, which are final effector molecules in mitochondrial apoptosis.

Discussion

In this study, we investigated the anti-cancer effect of ethanol extract of *Cordyceps militaris* in human colorectal carcinoma RKO cells. *Cordyceps militaris* showed potent cell cytotoxicity to RKO cells (Fig. 1), which is consistent with previous studies conducted in other human cancer cell lines [26, 27]. Our *in vitro* cell cytotoxicity was correlated with inhibition of tumor growth of human colorectal cancer observed in a xenograft mouse model (Fig. 2c). A few research groups have studied the anti-cancer effect of *Cordyceps militaris* in a xenografted animal model before. Park *et al.* reported an anti-tumor effect with a water extract of *Cordyceps militaris* in lung cancer cell-derived tumors [28]. The amount of *Cordyceps militaris* extract used in that study was either 150 mg/kg or 300 mg/kg, which is slightly higher than the amount (100 mg/kg) we used in this study. Therefore, we speculate that ethanol extract of *Cordyceps militaris* is more potent than water extract [28].

We also found that the anti-cancer effect of *Cordyceps militaris* in RKO cells was directly associated with induction of cell cycle arrest and apoptosis (Figs. 3 and 4). In fact, Yang *et al.* previously reported that *Cordyceps militaris* arrested human glioblastoma cells in the G0/G1 phase of the cell cycle. Further, Mollah *et al.* reported that *Cordyceps militaris* arrested human colon cancer HT-29 cells in the G2/M phase of the cell cycle, which agrees with our results [26, 29]. Therefore, there may be a differential regulation in cell cycle progression between human glioblastoma cells and human colon-related carcinoma HT-29 or RKO cells. In terms of apoptosis, *Lee et al.* reported that cordycepin, the major ingredient of *Cordyceps militaris,* induced cell apoptosis in HT-29 cells, which is consist with our present study in RKO cells treated with ethanol extract of *Cordyceps militaris* [30]. Also, cordycepin was reported to stimulate

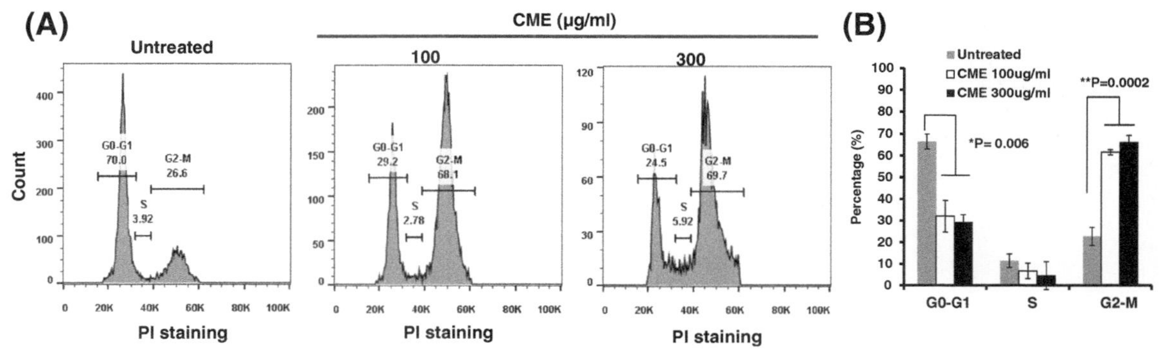

Fig. 3 Induction of cell cycle arrest by *Cordyceps militaris* in RKO cells. Cells were treated with or without ethanol extract of *Cordyceps militaris* (CME) (100 and 300 μg/ml) for 24 h. Then, cells were harvested for PI staining, which was measured by flow cytometry. **a** Representative PI staining for cell cycle progress in RKO cells. **b** The percentage of cell cycle distribution is presented as mean ± standard deviation (SD) for five independent experiments. Compared with other groups *P =0.006, **p = 0.0002

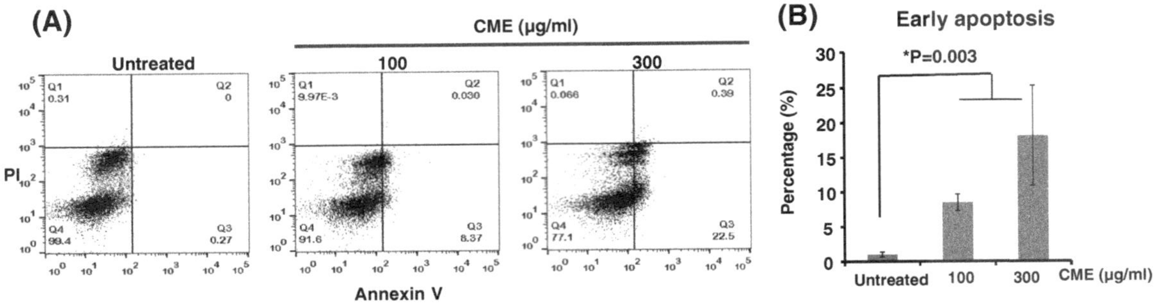

Fig. 4 Induction of cell apoptosis by *Cordyceps militaris* in RKO cells. Cells were treated with or without ethanol extract of *Cordyceps militaris* (CME) (100 and 300 μg/mL) for 48 h and then stained with Annexin V and propidium iodide (PI). Apoptosis of RKO cells was analyzed by flow cytometry. **a** Representative Annexin V and PI staining for cell apoptosis in RKO cells. **b** The percentage of early apoptosis is presented as mean ± standard deviation (SD) for five independent experiments. Compared with other groups $^{*}P = 0.003$

Hep3B human hepatocellular carcinoma cells to TRAIL-mediated apoptosis [31]. In addition, Cordycepol C, one of sesquiterpene compounds from Cordyceps extract, showed to cause poly(ADP-ribose)polymerase-1 (PARP-1) cleavage and triggered the loss of mitochondrial membrane potential ($\Delta\Psi_m$) in HepG2 cells in a time- and dose-dependent manner [32].

Finally, we identified that the responsible molecules for cell apoptosis by *Cordyceps militaris* are caspases 3 and 9, Bim, Bax, Bak, and Bad, which are critical components in the mitochondrial pathway of cell apoptosis. This result is consistent with a recent study by Zhang *et al.* [33]. Interestingly, we also found increased expression of cleaved PARP (89 kDa) in RKO cells treated with

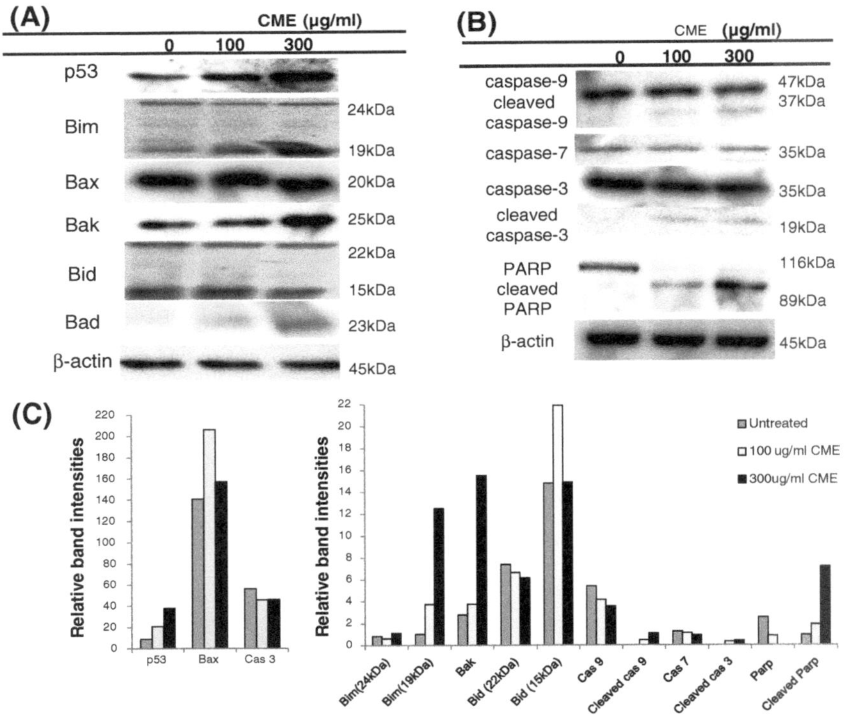

Fig. 5 Induction of mitochondrial-mediated apoptosis by *Cordyceps militaris* in a p53-dependent manner. Cells were treated with or without ethanol extract of *Cordyceps militaris* (CME) (0, 100, and 300 μg/ml) for 48 h and then western blot analysis for various apoptotic related molecules were performed. β-actin served as the loading control. **a** Expression of p53 and Bcl-2 family proteins. **b** Expression of caspases 9, 7, and 3, and PARP proteins. **c** The relative intensity of each band compared to the loading control

ethanol extract of *Cordyceps militaris* (Fig. 5b). As mentioned earlier, the activation of caspase-3 is known to trigger the cleavage of PARP, which indicates the halt of PARP function [25]. Therefore, *Cordyceps militaris* induces mitochondria-dependent apoptosis in RKO cells, which involves an increase of pro-apoptotic Bcl-2 family proteins, activation of caspases 9 and 3 and cleavage of PARP.

As mentioned early, traditional herbal medicines have become one of the most important alternative treatments for cancer therapy. These days, publics are also aware of the significance of prophylactic medications to complement or prevent various cancers. Therefore, we consider our ethanol extract of *Cordyceps militaris* could be a good nutritional supplement for cancer therapy. We will further characterize the active compounds from our extract for anti-cancer effect and investigate the responsible molecular mechanisms in detail.

Conclusions

Ethanol extract of *Cordyceps militaris* inhibited the growth of human colorectal carcinoma RKO cells as well as the *in vivo* growth of tumor in xenograft mice. The inhibitory effect on human colorectal carcinoma cells was highly connected with cell cycle arrest and p53-dependent, mitochondrial mediated apoptosis.

Abbreviations

CME: Extract of *Cordyceps militaris*; ATCC: American type culture collection; ECL: Enhanced chemiluminescene; FITC: Fluorescein isothiocyanate.

Competing interests

The authors declare that they have no competing interests.

Authors' contributions

HHL, HK and HC conceived and designed the study. HHL, SL, HK and HC carried out the study and the data analysis. HHL and HC wrote the manuscript. KL, YS, and HK revised the manuscript. All authors read and approved the final version of the manuscript.

Acknowledgements

This work was carried out with the support of "Cooperative Research Program for Agriculture Science & Technology Development (Project No. PJ0092412015)" Rural Development Administration, Republic of Korea.

Author details

[1]College of Pharmacy, Duksung Women's University, Seoul 132-714, Republic of Korea. [2]Innovative Drug Center, Duksung Women's University, Seoul 132-714, Republic of Korea. [3]Mushroom Research Division, National Institute of Horticultural and Herbal Science, Rural Development Administration, Eumseong 369-873, Republic of Korea. [4]Department of Medicinal Crop Research, National Institute of Horticultural and Herbal Science, Rural Development Administration, Eumseong 369-873, Republic of Korea. [5]College of Pharmacy, Research Institute of Pharmaceutical Sciences and Institute for Microorganisms, Kyungpook National University, Daegu 702-701, Republic of Korea.

References

1. Kunjadia PD, Nagee A, Pandya PY, Mukhopadhyaya PN, Sanghvi GV, Dave GS. Medicinal and antimicrobial role of the oyster culinary-medicinal mushroom Pleurotus ostreatus (higher Basidiomycetes) cultivated on banana agrowastes in India. Int J Med Mushrooms. 2014;16:227–38.
2. Phan CW, Lee GS, Macreadie IG, Malek SN, Pamela D. Lipid constituents of the edible mushroom, Pleurotus giganteus demonstrate anti-Candida activity. Nat Prod Commun. 2013;8:1763–5.
3. Kim SP, Nam SH, Friedman MJ. Hericium erinaceus (Lion's Mane) mushroom extracts inhibit metastasis of cancer cells to the lung in CT-26 colon cancer-tansplanted mice. Agric Food Chem. 2013;61:4898–904.
4. Yang Y, Hu J, Liu Y, Feng N, Chen H, Tang Q, et al. Antioxidant and cytotoxic activities of ethanolic extracts and isolated fractions of species of the genus Phellinus Quél. (Aphyllophoromycetideae). Int J Med Mushrooms. 2011;13:145–52.
5. Lin JG, Fan MJ, Tang NY, Yang JS, Hsia TC, Lin JJ, et al. An extract of Agaricus blazei Murill administered orally promotes immune responses in murine leukemia BALB/c mice in vivo. Integr Cancer Ther. 2012;11:29–36.
6. Tuli HS, Sharma AK, Sandhu SS, Kashyap D. Cordycepin: a bioactive metabolite with therapeutic potential. Life Sci. 2013;93:863–9.
7. Yue K, Ye M, Zhou Z, Sun W, Lin X. The genus Cordyceps: a chemical and pharmacological review. J Pharm Pharmacol. 2013;65:474–93.
8. Zhou X, Gong Z, Su Y, Lin J, Tang K. Cordyceps fungi: natural products, pharmacological functions and developmental products. J Pharm Pharmacol. 2009;61:279–91.
9. Park C, Hong SH, Lee JY. Growth inhibition of U937 leukemia cells by aqueous extract of *Cordyceps militaris* through induction of apoptosis. Oncol Rep. 2005;13:1211–6.
10. Lee H, Kim YJ, Kim HW, Lee DH, Sung MK, Park T. Induction of apoptosis by *Cordyceps militaris* through activation of caspase-3 in leukemiaHL-60 cells. Biol Pharm Bull. 2006;29:670–4.
11. Lee HH, Park H, Sung GH, Lee K, Lee T, Cho H. Anti-influenza effect of Cordyceps militaris through immunomodulation in a DBA/2 mouse model. J Microbiol. 2014;52:696–701.
12. Zhai XF, Chen ZB, Shen LF, Fan J, Zhou WP, Yang YK, et al. Traditional herbal medicine in preventing recurrence after resection of small hepatocellular carcinoma: a multicenter randomized controlled trial. J Integr Med. 2013;11:90–100.
13. Ling CQ, Yue XQ, Ling C. Three advantages of using traditional Chinese medicine to prevent and treat tumor. J Integr Med. 2014;12:331–5.
14. Li ZP, Zeng JQ, Hu AM. Clinical study on the qi and xue dual-supply therapy with chemotherapy to prevent the recurrence and metastasis from colorectal carcinoma. Shi Yong Ai Zheng Za Zhi. 2010;25:618–20.
15. John A, Kaabi SA, Dweik N, Yakoub R, Abdulla F. Emerging role for colorectal cancer screening in Asian countries. Trop Gastroenterol. 2014;35:21–4.
16. Lim HW, Kwon YM, Cho SM, Kim JH, Yoon GH. Antitumor activity of *Cordyceps militaris* on human cancer cell line. Korean J Pharmacogn. 2009;35:364–7.
17. Park SE, Yoo HS, Jin CY, Hong SH, Lee YW, Kim BM. Induction of apoptosis and inhibition of telomerase activity in human lung carcinoma cells by the water extract of *Cordyceps militaris*. Food Chem Toxicol. 2009;47:1667–75.
18. Lakin ND, Jackson SP. Regulation of p53 in response to DNA damage. Oncogene. 1999;18:7644–55.
19. Wu X, Deng Y. Bax and BH3-domain-only proteins in p53-mediated apoptosis. Front Biosci. 2002;7:151–6.
20. Murphy KM, Ranganathan V, Farnsworth M, Kavallaris LM, Lock RB. Bcl-2 inhibits Bax translocation from cytosol to mitochondria during drug-induced apoptosis of human tumor cells. Cell Death Differ. 2000;7:102–11.
21. Cain K, Brown DG, Langlais C, Cohen GM. Caspase activation involves the formation of the aposome, a large (approximately 700 kDa) caspase-activating complex. J Biol Chem. 1999;274:22686–92.
22. Adrain C, Slee EA, Harte MT, Martin SJ. Regulation of apoptotic protease activating factor-1 oligomerization and apoptosis by the WD-40 repeat region. J Biol Chem. 1999;274:20855–60.
23. Won SY, Park EH. Anti-inflammatory and related pharmacological activities of cultured mycelia and fruiting bodies of *Cordyceps militaris*. J Ethnopharmacol. 2005;96:555–61.
24. Son M, Lee M, Ryu E, Moon A, Jeong CS, Jung YW, et al. Genipin as a novel chemical activator of EBV lytic cycle. J Microbiol. 2015;53:155–65.
25. Boulares AH, Yakovlev AG, Ivanova V, Stoica BA, Wang G, Iyer S, et al. Role of poly(ADP-ribose) polymerase (PARP) cleavage in apoptosis; Caspase 3-resistant PARP mutant increases rates of apoptosis in transfected cells. J Biol Chem. 1999;274:22932–40.

26. Yang CH, Kao YH, Huang KS, Wang CY, Lin W. *Cordyceps militaris* and mycelial fermentation induced apoptosis and autophagy of human glioblastoma cells. Cell Death Dis. 2012;3, e431. doi:10.1038/cddis.
27. Park BT, Na KH, Jung EC, Par JW, Kim HH. Antifungal and anticancer activities of a protein from the mushroom cordyceps militaris. Korean J Physiol Pharmacol. 2009;1:49–54. doi:10.4196/kjpp.
28. Park SE, Kim JS, Lee YW, Yoo HS, Cho CK. Antitumor activity of water extracts from *Cordyceps Militaris* in NCI-H460 cell xenografted nude mice. J Acupunct Meridian Stud. 2009;2:294–300.
29. Mollah ML, Park DL, Park HJ. *Cordyceps militaris* grown on germinated soybean induces G2/M cell cycle arrest through down regulation of Cyclin B1 and Cdc25c in human colon cancer HT-29 Cells. Evid Based Complement Alternat Med. 2012;2012:249217.
30. Lee SY, Debnath T, Kim SK, Lim BO. Anti-cancer effect and apoptosis induction of cordycepin through DR3 pathway in the human colonic cancer cell HT-29. Food Chem Toxicol. 2013;60:439–47.
31. Lee HH, Jeong JW, Lee JH, Kim GY, Cheong J, Jeong YK, et al. Cordycepin increases sensitivity of hep3b human hepatocellular carcinoma cells to trail-mediated apoptosis by inactivating the jnk signaling pathway. Oncol Rep. 2013;30:1257–64.
32. Sun YS, Lv LX, Zhao Z, He X, You L, Liu JK, et al. Cordycepol c induces caspase-independent apoptosis in human hepatocellular carcinoma hepg2 cells. Biol Pharm Bull. 2014;37:608–17.
33. Zhang Y, Bao YL, Wu Y, Yu CL, Huang YX, Sun Y, et al. Alantolactone induces apoptosis in RKO cells through the generation of reactive oxygen species and the mitochondrial pathway. Mol Med Rep. 2013;4:967–72.

Dehydroandrographolide enhances innate immunity of intestinal tract through up-regulation the expression of hBD-2

Wen-Bi Xiong†, Zhen-Jun Shao†, Yao Xiong, Jian Chen, Yun Sun, Ling Zhu* and Li-Ming Zhou*

Abstract

Background: Dehydroandrographolide (DA) is one of major active components in the well-known oriental herbal medicine *Andrographis paniculata* (Burm.f) Nees which belongs to the Acanthaceae family. DA is used for the treatment of infections in China. However, DA has not been found to significantly inhibit bacterial and viral growth directly. The current study investigates the effect of DA on the expression of human β –defensin-2 (hBD-2) in human intestinal epithelial cells and the possible signaling pathways.

Methods: Human intestinal epithelial HCT-116 cells were incubated with 1–100 μM DA for 2–24 h. RT–PCR and Western blot were used to assess the expression of hBD-2. The specific inhibitors were used and the levels of phosphorylation of signaling molecules were detected for dissecting the signaling pathways leading to the induction of hBD-2.

Results: MTT assay showed there was no obvious cytotoxicity for HCT-116 cells by 1–100 μM DA treatment. RT-PCR and Western blot assays showed that DA (1–100 μM) could up-regulate the expression of hBD-2, and the effect lasted longer than 24 h. By using SB203580 and SB202190 (inhibitors of p38), the enhancement of hBD-2 expression were significantly attenuated. However, inhibitor of ERK and inhibitor of JNK could not block the effect of DA. Furthermore, Western blot found activation of p38 but not ERK and JNK in DA-treated HCT-116 cells.

Conclusion: The results suggested that DA enhanced innate immunity of intestinal tract by up-regulating the expression of hBD-2 through the p38 MAPK pathways.

Keywords: Innate immunity, Dehydroandrographolide, hBD-2, Antimicrobial peptide, defensin, p38 MAPK

Background

Andrographis paniculata (Burm. f) Nees, which belongs to the Acanthaceae family, is an oriental herbal medicine that has been widely used in China, India, and other Southeastern Asian countries for hundreds of years due to its significant antipyretic and anti-inflammatory effect. In China, *A. paniculata* is often used for treatment of chronic or repeated onset infection and inflammation, especially for the upper respiratory tract infection and gut diarrhea [1–3]. Both andrographolide (Androg) and dehydroandrographolide (DA) are main active components in *A. paniculata*, which have been demonstrated to contribute anti-infectious property of the *A. paniculata*. Contemporary laboratory tests have exhibited their anti-inflammatory, antipyretic, antimicrobial, antiviral and immunostimulant capability [4–6]. In China, Androg and DA are called "Natural Antibiotics" [7]. However, the mechanism has not been fully clarified and Androg and DA have not been found to significantly inhibit bacterium and virus growth directly [8]. Our recent work demonstrated that DA could enhance innate immune function by up-regulating the expression of human β –defensin (hBD-1) of human lung epithelial cells [9].

Innate immunity plays a very important role for mucous membranes in defense against invading pathogenic microbes. The human gut harbors trillions of microbes which are essential for mediating physiology, metabolism and host immune responses. In normal condition, the microbes could coexist peacefully with the body owing to the innate immunity despite the intestinal mucosal

* Correspondence: zhuling529@163.com; zhou108@163.com
†Equal contributors
Department of Pharmacology, West China Medical Center, Preclinical and Forensic Medical College, Sichuan University, Chengdu 610041, P.R. China

surface acting as a primary barrier [10]. Hence, it is a good choice to enhance intestinal innate immune function for treatment of intestinal infection rather than using antibiotic for less antibiotic resistance and dysbacteriosis, and it is an alternative strategy to look for active ingredients to enhance the body's innate immunity from natural products such as ellagic acid [11], paeoniflorin [12], avocado sugar [13] etc.

Defensins, one of the 3 major antimicrobial peptides (AMPs) families, are important moleculars in innate immune system. Defensins are small (Mr 2 000 ~ 6 000 Da), cationic peptides containing disulfide bonds, so can interact with the membrane of invading microbes and active against many Gram-negative and Gram-positive bacteria, fungi, and enveloped viruses [14]. According to the position of their disulfide bonds human defensins are further classified as α- and β-defensins. Human β-Defensin (hBD) has six members which are expressed by many types of epithelial cells, including enterocytes. hBD-1, firstly discovered in 1995, is an important antimicrobial peptide against infection in human prostate, kidney and urogenital tract luminal epithelium [15]. hBD-2, discovered in 1997 [16], is the first discovered inducible human antimicrobial protein. Moreover, it was shown that hBD-2 had a broad spectrum of antimicrobial activity *in vitro* [17]. Therefore, in this study, we investigated the role of DA in hBD-2 expression in HCT-116 intestinal epithelial cells and the possible mechanism.

Materials and methods

Specific reagents

DA (Fig. 1) was obtained from the Sichuan Academy of Chinese Medical Sciences. The purity was 99.97 % as determined by high-performance liquid chromatography. DA was dissolved in dimethylsulphoxide (DMSO) at a concentration of 200 mmol/L. The final concentration of DMSO in the medium was not more than 0.1 % (v/v). The inhibitors PD98059 (an inhibitor of ERK), SB203580 and SB202190 (two different inhibitors of p38), SP600125 (an inhibitor of JNK) were purchased from Beyotime (Jiangsu, China). SB203580 is a pyridinyl imidazole derivative that specifically suppresses phosphorylation of p38. SB202190 is a highly potent and cell-permeable inhibitor of p38 that selectively inhibits the p38 a and b isoforms. Each inhibitor was reconstituted in DMSO and added to the culture medium so that the final concentration of DMSO was less than 0.1 % of the total volume.

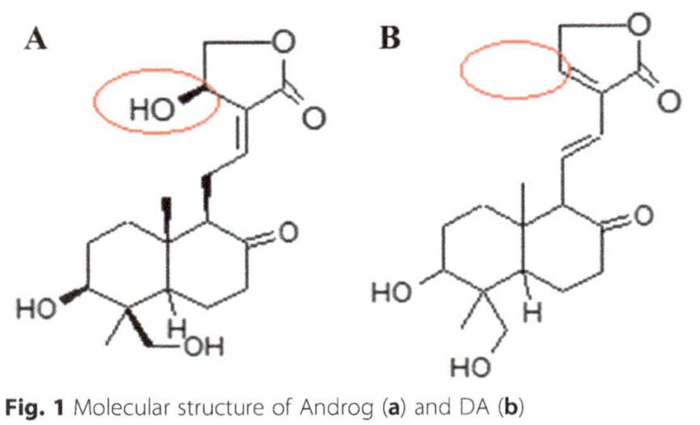

Fig. 1 Molecular structure of Androg (**a**) and DA (**b**)

Cell line and culture

HCT-116 intestinal cells, a human cell line derived from the colonic epithelial cell line, were maintained at 37 °C in a humidified atmosphere of 95 % air and 5 % CO_2 in RPMI 1640 medium (Gibco-BRL, Grand Island, NY). The medium mixture contains 10 % fetal bovine serum, 100 U/ml penicillin G and 100 μg/ml streptomycin. After reaching confluence, cells were seeded onto six well plates and incubated with DA. For all experiments, DA were added to cells on ice and incubated for 10 min, allowing DA to settle onto the cells, and then incubated at 37 °C in 5 % CO_2 for the specified intervals. Cells treated with lipopolysaccharide (LPS, Sigma-Aldrich, St. Louis, Mo., USA) were employed as positive control. Vehicle control with equal concentration of DMSO was always included. HCT-116 intestinal cells were exposed to the specified concentrations of each inhibitor for 30 min prior to stimulation with DA.

MTT assay

3-(4,5-Dimethylthiazol-zyl)-2,5-diphenyltetrazolium bromide (MTT) assay was used to evaluate the effect of DA on cell viability and to determine the non-cytotoxic concentrations. Briefly, HCT-116 cells (10^5) were seeded on 96 well plates and incubated with DA at various concentrations (0, 1, 20, 40, 80 and 100 μM) for 48 h. Thereafter, the medium was changed and MTT (1 mg/ml) was added to each well and incubated in the CO_2 incubator for 4 h. The viable cell number was directly proportional to the production of formazan crystals which, following adding isopropanol 100 μl to dissolve and the absorbance of each well was obtained using a Bio-Rad Microplate reader at wavelength of 490 nm.

Semi-quantitative RT-PCR

Semi-quantitative RT-PCR was performed as described previously [15]. Total RNA was isolated from cells using Trizol (BBI, Kitchener, Ont., Canada), and samples of total RNA were quantified by reading optical density at 260 nm. mRNA was reverse transcribed using a first strand cDNA synthesis kit (Fermentas, Glenn Burnie, Md., USA) according to the manufacturer's instructions. One microgram of cDNA was amplified in the standard reaction mixture using 2× PCR MasterMix (TIANGEN, China) and the forward and reverse primers for hBD-2 and β-actin, an internal standard. The forward and reverse primers and product sizes were as follows: hBD-2 (255 bp) forward: 5′-CCAGCCATCAGCCATGAGG GT- 3′; reverse: 5′-GGAGCCCTTTCTGAATCCGC A- 3′. For β-actin (300 bp), forward: 5′-TCACCCAC ACTGTGCCCATCTACGA- 3′; reverse: 5′-CAGCGG AACCGCTCATTGCCAATGG- 3′. Amplification proceeded in a PCR Thermal Cycler (Takara PCR Thermal Cycler MP; Takara Bio, Otsu-shi, Japan) using 32 cycles consisting of 94 °C for 60 s, 62 °C for 30 s, and 72 °C for 120 s. The PCR products were verified by electrophoresis in a 1.2 % agarose gel and detected by ethidium bromide staining. Detectable fluorescent bands were visualized with an ultraviolet transill. The values of densitometry of the mRNA bands were acquired using ImageJ software (National Institutes of Health, USA) and then normalized with β-actin.

Western blot analysis

After cells were treated with DA or inhibitors, total cell extracts were prepared in ice-cold lysis buffer (150 mmol/L NaCl, 1 mmol/L phenylmethylsulfonyl fluoride, 1 mg/mL aprotinin, 1 mg/mL pepstatin, 1 mmol/L pervanadate,1 mmol/L EDTA, 1 % igepal, 0.25 % deoxycholic acid,1 mmol/L NaF, and 50 mmol/L Tris–HCl (pH 7.4)). The lysates were centrifuged at 12 000 r/min for 10 min, and the resulting supernatants were assessed with a Bio-Rad assay kit using bovine serum albumin as the standard. Equal amounts of protein (40 μg/lane) were separated by SDS PAGE and blotted onto 0.22 μm polyvinylidene difluoride membranes (Bio-Rad Laboratories, Hercules, Calif., USA). The membranes were blocked in TBST (Tris-buffered solution, pH 7.6, 0.05 % Tween 20) containing 5 % nonfat dried milk. Membranes were probed overnight at 4 °C with specific primary antibodies including anti-hBD-2, anti-p-p38 (Thr180/182), p38 and anti-β-actin (Santa Cruz, Calif., USA); anti-ERK1/2, anti-p-ERK1/2, anti-JNK, anti-p-JNK (Cell Signaling Technology Inc, USA) . After 3 washes, the blots were subsequently incubated with appropriate secondary antibodies with horseradish peroxidase (HRP, ZSGB-BIO) at room temperature for 1 h and developed in the ECL Western blot detection reagents (Beyotime, Jiangsu, China). The values of densitometry of the protein bands were acquired using ImageJ software (National Institutes of Health, USA) and then normalized with β-actin.

Statistics

Results were presented as mean ± SD. Data were statistically evaluated using one-way analysis of variance (ANOVA) followed by Dunnett's test by SPSS 13.0 software (SPSS, Chicago, USA). A P value < 0.05 was considered as statistically significant.

Results

Cytotoxicity of DA on HCT-116 intestinal epithelial cells

First, we determined the cytotoxicity of DA by treating HCT-116 intestinal epithelial cells (10^5 cells) with DA at various concentrations (0–100 μM) for 48 h followed by MTT assay. In comparison with that of vehicle control (DMSO), the viability of HCT-116 cells was a little decreased with increased DA. The viability of 100 μM group was only 14 % less than control group, and the difference between DA treatment groups and control group had no statistical significance (Fig. 2). Therefore 0–100 μM was applied in all subsequent experiments.

Expression of hBD-2 mRNA

In this study, we used different concentrations of DA (0, 1, 25, 50 and 100 μM) to stimulate the HCT-116 intestinal epithelial cells for 16 h and 100 μM DA for different time intervals (0, 2, 8, 16 and 24 h), the results revealed that the DA can up-regulate the expression of the hBD-2 mRNA. The optimal concentration 100 μM, the maximal expression of hBD-2 mRNA occurred after 24 h (Fig. 3). There was a dose-dependent and time-dependent enhancement expression of hBD-2 mRNA upon treatment with DA. It was important to note that expression of the housekeeping gene β -actin was not affected by DA.

Expression of hBD-2 protein

As revealed in Fig. 4, hBD-2 protein expression was detected by Western blot correlated with the hBD-2 mRNA expression. The expression of hBD-2 protein was

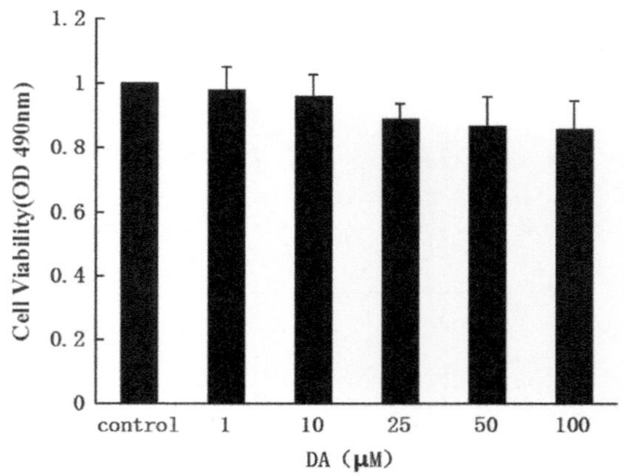

Fig. 2 Effects of DA on HCT-116 intestinal epithelial cell viability. HCT-116 intestinal epithelial cells were treated with various concentrations (1, 10, 25, 50, 100 μM) of DA for 48 h. Cell viability was analyzed by MTT assay. DMSO served as the vehicle control. Data were shown as mean ± SD by six parallel experiments. Statistical analysis was performed with one-way ANOVA and Dunnett's test

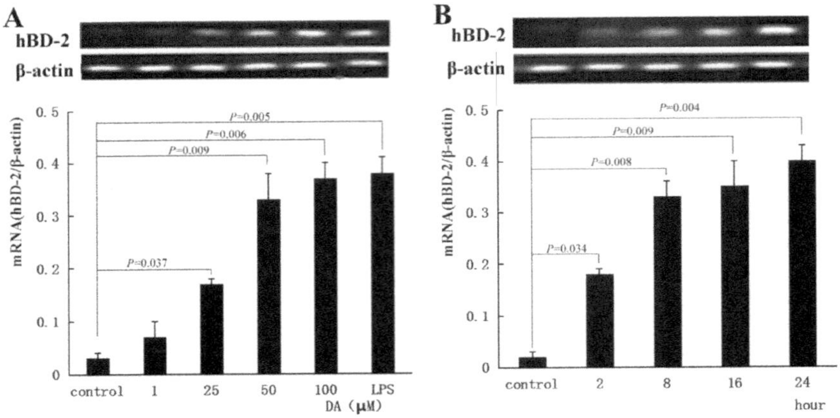

Fig. 3 Effects of DA on HCT-116 intestinal epithelial cells hBD-2 mRNA expression. Intestinal epithelial HCT-116 cells were treated with or without different concentrations of DA (1, 25, 50, 100 μM) for 16 h (**a**), or DA 100 μM for different time (**b**). DMSO was used as the vehicle control. LPS (5 μg/ml) was used as the positive control. The total RNA was extracted from cells and analyzed for *hBD-2* or *β-actin*, an internal control by RT-PCR. The results of the RT-PCR were depicted as mean ± SD of three independent experiments. Statistical analysis was performed with one-way ANOVA and Dunnett's test

significantly enhanced by DA, the optimal concentration was 100 μM and the maximal expression of hBD-2 protein occurred after 24 h.

Mechanism of hBD-2 expression induced by DA

The previous results showed DA could induce the expression of hBD-2 mRNA and protein in a dose- and time-dependent manner. So we further investigate the possible mechanism of hBD-2 up-regulating in HCT-116 intestinal epithelial cells. Both mRNA and protein expression in responsive to DA was attenuated by pretreatment with two p38 inhibitors (SB203580 and SB202190) respectively, but not by ERK inhibitor PD98059, or JNK inhibitor SP600125. Moreover, we found the phospho-p38 but not phospho-ERK and phospho-JNK was increased in DA treated HCT-116 intestinal epithelial than control (Fig. 5).

Discussion

Both DA and Androg are main active components in *A. paniculata* which are popular used for all kinds of infection and inflammation in Asia. They have the similar structure and both are labdane diterpenoids. The only difference is the dehydroxylation in C-14 for DA comparing

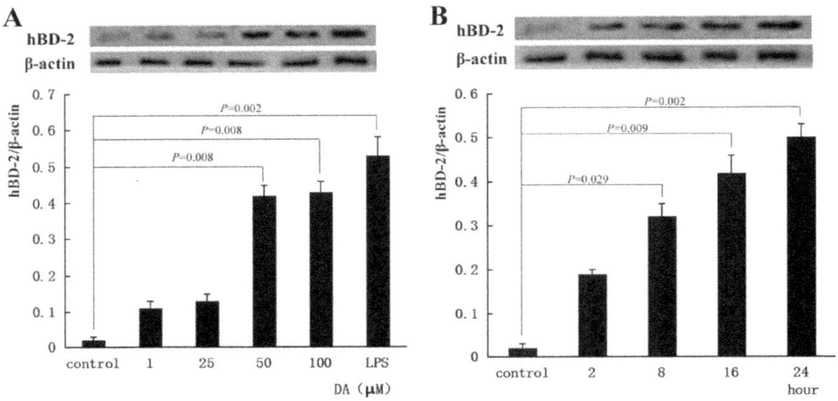

Fig. 4 Effects of DA on HCT-116 intestinal epithelial cells hBD-2 protein expression. HCT-116 intestinal epithelial cells were treated with or without different concentration of DA (1, 25, 50, 100 μM) for 16 h (**a**), or DA 100 μM for different time (**b**). DMSO was used as the vehicle control. LPS (5 μg/ml) was used as the positive control. Whole cell lysates were prepared and used for western blot with anti-hBD-2 antibody. β-actin served as an internal control. The values of densitometry of the protein bands were acquired using ImageJ software (National Institutes of Health) and then normalized with β-actin and expressed as relative signal intensity. All values were expressed as mean ± SD of three independent experiments. Statistical analysis was performed with one-way ANOVA and Dunnett's test

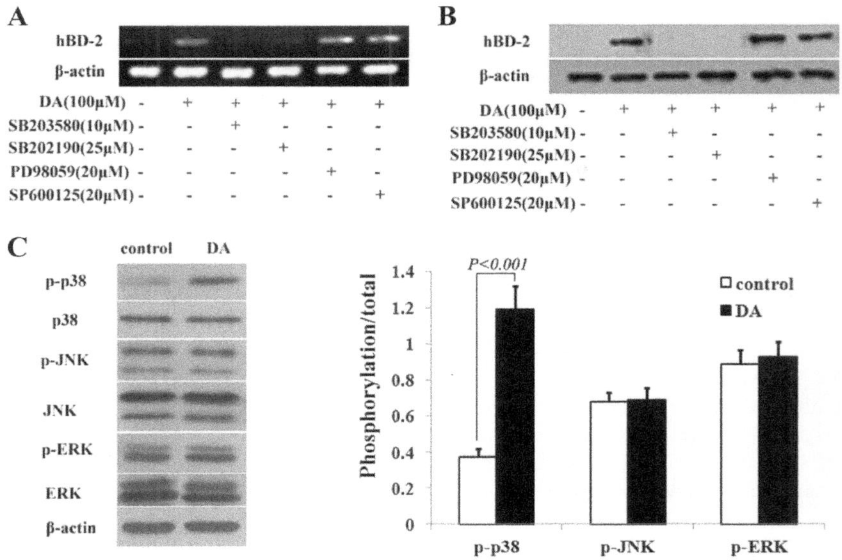

Fig. 5 Role of MAPK signaling pathway in DA-induced hBD-2 expression. HCT-116 intestinal epithelial cells were pretreated with indicated concentrations of chemical inhibitors for 30 min, and then treated with 100 μM DA for 16 h, *β-actin* served as an internal control. Total RNA was extracted from cells and analyzed for *hBD-2* by RT-PCR (**a**). In addition, whole cell lysates were prepared and used for western blot with antibodies *hBD-2* (**b**). HCT-116 intestinal epithelial cells were treated with 100 μM DA for 30 min, cell lysates were harvested for the detection of phospho-p38 MARP, ERK, and JNK by western blot, *β-actin* served as an internal control. 'p' indicates the phosphorylated form of the protein. The values were expressed as mean ± SD of three independent experiments (**c**)

to Androg (Fig. 1). Consequently, they have the similar actions in many conditions [18, 19]. We have found that both Androg and DA could enhance innate immunity by stimulate hBD-1 and hBD-2 expression in respiratory tract epithelial cells [20]. However, it has remained unclear whether they have the same effect in intestinal epithelial cells. Therefore, we first added different concentrations of Androg and DA into culture HCT-116 cells, found DA had less cytotoxic effect for HCT-116 cells than Androg (IC_{50} DA >200 μM vs IC_{50} Androg 10.67 μM for HCT-116 cells 48 h). As the lower toxicity of DA, DA succinate (trade name: Yan-Hu-Ning Injection)) is more popular used for injection in clinical for the treatment of viral pneumonia and upper respiratory tract infections in China [21, 22]. Therefore we focused on observing the effect of DA on hBD-2 expression in HCT-116 cells in this study. We found the level of mRNA and protein of hBD-2 increased 11 and 20 times comparing with control respectively in DA treatment group at non-toxic concentration 100 μM. The effect of DA induction hBD-2 expression was maintained for 24 h, which longer than human lung epithelial cells expression hBD-1.

hBD-2 plays important roles in innate defence system at gastrointestinal (GI) tract mucosal surfaces. Unlike hBD-1 constitutively expression within GI tract and mostly remain stable during inflammation and infection, hBD-2 is induced upon pathogen [23–25]. hBD-2 is seldom expressed in normal colon but its expression is significantly increased in inflamed colonic epithelium [26]. It has been shown that certain probiotic strains can induce the secretion of antimicrobial peptides (such as hBD-2) by intestinal cells and probiotics have already been used as "ecological treatments" in gastrointestinal infections such as diarrhoea, dysentery [27]. At the same time, scientists pay attention to looking for defensins inducer from Chinese herbal medicines such as *Astragalus membranaceus (Fisch.) Bunge., Coptis chinensis Franch, Houttuynia cordata Thunb., Isatis tinctoria* and Lentinan, which will also appear as attractive strategies for these diseases. From our results, DA was proved to be a defensins inducer and would be beneficial for the rehabilitation of intestinal infection.

For the promoter region of the hBD-2 gene contains binding sites for AP-1, and AP-1 is a transcription factor that can be activated by different MAPK pathways, including the p38, ERK and JNK pathway [28], we investigated whether MAPK signalling pathways were involved in DA induced hBD-2 expression in human intestinal epithelial cells. The results showed that it was the specific inhibitors of p38 MAPK but not the inhibitors of ERK and JNK significantly attenuated DA-induced hBD-2 gene expression. When measured the p-p38 (p38 active form) we found the p-p38 increased in DA treated HCT-116 cells, however the p-ERK (ERK active form) and p-JNK (JNK active form) had no significant change. Our findings on the signal passway of DA induced hBD-2 expression in human intestinal epithelial cells are partial consistent with that of a previous study by Gan et al. [12], which reported that paeoniflorin, a substance came from herbal plant peony upregulates β-defensin-2 expression in human bronchial epithelial cell through the p38 MAPK, ERK, and NF-κB signaling pathways. Several studies revealed different inducer may induce hBD-2 expression through different signalling pathways in different cells. *Bacteroides fragilis* enterotoxin induces hBD-2 expression in intestinal epithelial cells via p38/NF-κB-dependent pathway [29]. *Escherichia coli* Nissle 1917 induces hBD-2 expression in intestinal epithelial cells via NF-κB and AP-1 signalling pathways [30]. Avocado sugar modulates the hBD-2 expression through toll-like receptor-2 and ERK/MAPK activation in human keratinocytes [13]. As DA is a potential NF-κB inhibitor [31, 32], whether NF-κB is involved in hBD-2 expression in intestinal epithelial cells need to further confirm. It is still a question whether DA will lead to more serious inflammatory for upregulation hBD-2. Especially for those associated with a high level of hBD-2 gut inflammation such as Crohn's disease [33, 34]. Immune mediators often have dual-direction regulation like the water extract of *Houttuynia cordata* Thunb [35] and paeoniflorin,which could upregulate β-defensin-2 expression in human bronchial epithelial cell at the same time downregulated β-defensin-2 expression in mice colonic mucosa with oxazolone-induced colitis [36]. The existing evidences have described DA is a immune mediator. DA could significantly reduce the level of IL-1β, IL-6 and TNF-α in the bronchoalveolar lavage fluid of the LPS-induced acute lung injury mouse [37]. DA could dose-dependently inhibited ovalbumin-induced increases in total and eosinophil counts, IL-4, IL-5, and IL-13 levels in lavage fluid in a mouse asthma model [31]. Therefore, DA may not enhance inflammatory at the same time of hBD-2 inducing in GI tract.

Conclusions

In summary, we have demonstrated that exposure of intestinal epithelial cells to DA caused the activation of a signaling cascade involving p38 MAPK up-regulation expression of hBD-2 in intestinal epithelial cells. This is one main reason why DA could be used for intestinal infection.

Abbreviations

DA: Dehydroandrographolide; hBD-2: human β –defensin-2; RT-PCR: Reverse transcription polymerase chain reaction; MAPK: Mitogen-activated protein kinase; ERK: Extracellular regulated protein kinases; JNK: c-Jun N-terminal k inase; DMSO: Dimethylsulphoxide; NF-κB: Nuclear factor kappa-light-chain-enhancer of activated B cells.

Competing interests

This research was sponsored by the Chinese National Natural Science Foundation (grant No. 30672650). The authors declare that they have no conflict of interest.

Authors' contributions

LZ and LMZ conceived and designed the study. WBX, ZJS, YX, JC and YS performed the experiments. WBX performed the statistical analysis and wrote the manuscript. All authors read and approved the final manuscript.

References

1. Parichatikanond W, Suthisisang C, Dhepakson P, Herunsalee A. Study of anti-inflammatory activities of the pure compounds from *Andrographis paniculata* (burm.f.) Nees and their effects on gene expression. Int Immunopharmacol. 2010;10(11):1361–73.
2. Chandrasekaran CV, Murali B, Deepak M, Agarwal A. In vitro comparative evaluation of non-leaves and leaves extracts of *Andrographis paniculata* on modulation of inflammatory mediators. Antiinflamm Antiallergy Agents Med Chem. 2012;11(2):191–7.
3. Jayakumar T, Hsieh CY, Lee JJ, Sheu JR. Experimental and clinical pharmacology of andrographis paniculata and its major bioactive phytoconstituent andrographolide. Evid Based Complement Alternat Med. 2013;2013:846740.
4. Lim JC, Chan TK, Ng DS, Sagineedu SR, Stanslas J, Wong WS. Andrographolide and its analogues: Versatile bioactive molecules for combating inflammation and cancer. Clin Exp Pharmacol Physiol. 2012;39(3):300–10.
5. Wen L, Xia N, Chen X, Li Y, Hong Y, Liu Y, et al. Activity of antibacterial, antiviral, anti-inflammatory in compounds andrographolide salt. Eur J Pharmacol. 2014;740:421–7.
6. Yan YY, Shi GX, Shao J, Wang TM, Wang CZ. Advance in studies on anti-infection of andrographolide and its derivatives in past 10 years. Zhongguo Zhong Yao Za Zhi. 2013;38(22):3819–24.
7. Chen Q, Liu Y, Liu YM, Liu GY, Zhang MQ, Jia JY, et al. Pharmacokinetics and tolerance of dehydroandrographolide succinate injection after intravenous administration in healthy Chinese volunteers. Acta Pharmacol Sin. 2012;33(10):1332–6.
8. Wang Z, Yu P, Zhang G, Xu L, Wang D, Wang L, et al. Design, synthesis and antibacterial activity of novel andrographolide derivatives. Bioorg Med Chem. 2010;18(12):4269–74.
9. Shao ZJ, Li XP, Wu YY, Zheng XW, Huang J, Deng WL, et al. Expression of the human β-defensin-1 induced by dehydroandrographolide in human pulmonary gland epithelial cells. Food and Agricultural Immunology. 2010;21(4):361–7.
10. Pott J, Hornef M. Innate immune signalling at the intestinal epithelium in homeostasis and disease. EMBO Rep. 2012;13(8):684–98.
11. Promsong A, Chung WO, Satthakarn S, Nittayananta W. Ellagic acid modulates the expression of oral innate immune mediators: potential role in mucosal protection. J Oral Pathol Med. 2015;44(3):214–21.
12. Gan Y, Cui X, Ma T, Liu Y, Li A, Huang M. Paeoniflorin upregulates β-defensin-2 expression in human bronchial epithelial cell through the p38 MAPK, ERK, and NF-κB signaling pathways. Inflammation. 2014;37(5):1468–75.
13. Paoletti I, Buommino E, Fusco A, Baudouin C, Msika P, Tufano MA, et al. Patented natural avocado sugar modulates the HBD-2 and HBD-3 expression in human keratinocytes through toll-like receptor-2 and ERK/MAPK activation. Arch Dermatol Res. 2012;304(8):619–25.
14. De Smet K, Contreras R. Human antimicrobial peptides: Defensins, cathelicidins and histatins. Biotechnol Lett. 2005;27(18):1337–47.
15. Menendez A, Brett FB. Defensins in the immunology of bacterial infections. Curr Opin Immunol. 2007;19(4):385–91.
16. Harder J, Bartels J, Christophers E, Schröder JM. A peptide antibiotic from human skin. Nature. 1997;387(6636):861.
17. Scharf S, Hippenstiel S, Flieger A, Suttorp N, N"Guessan PD. Induction of human β-defensin-2 in pulmonary gland epithelial cells by *Legionella pneumophlia*: Involvement of TLR2 and TLR5, p38 MAPK, JNK, NF-κB and AP-1. Am J Physiol Lung Cell Mol Physiol. 2010;298(5):687–95.

18. Shao ZJ, Zheng XW, Feng T, Huang J, Chen J, Wu YY, et al. Andrographolide exerted its antimicrobial effects by upregulation of human β-defensin-2 induced through p38 MAPK and NF-κB pathway in human lung epithelial cells. Can J Physiol Pharmacol. 2012;90(5):647–53.
19. Suebsasana S, Pongnaratorn P, Sattayasai J, Arkaravichien T, Tiamkao S, Aromdee C. Analgesic, antipyretic, antiinflammatory and toxic effects of andrographolide derivatives in experimental animals. Arch Pharm Res. 2009;32(9):1191–200.
20. Tzeng YM, Lee YC, Cheng WT, Shih HN, Wang HC, Rao YK, et al. Effects of andrographolide and 14-deoxy-11,12-didehydroandrographolide on cultured primary astrocytes and PC12 cells. Life Sci. 2012;90(7–8):257–66.
21. Coon JT, Ernst E. Andrographis paniculata in the treatment of upper respiratory tract infections: a systematic review of safety and efficacy. Planta Med. 2004;70(4):293–8.
22. Zhu T, Guan X, Zhang W, Wang D. Dehydroandrographolide succinate inhibits oxidative stress in mice with lipopolysaccharide-induced acute lung injury by inactivating iNOS. Nan Fang Yi Ke Da Xue Xue Bao. 2012;32(9):1238–41.
23. Klotman ME, Chang TL. Defensins in innate antiviral immunity. Nat Rev Immunol. 2006;6:447–56.
24. Ng TB, Cheung RC, Wong JH, Ye XJ. Antimicrobial activity of defensins and defensin-like peptides with special emphasis on those from fungi and invertebrate animals. Curr Protein Pept Sci. 2013;14(6):515–31.
25. Jarczak J, Kościuczuk EM, Lisowski P, Strzałkowska N, Jóźwik A, Horbańczuk J, et al. Defensins: Natural component of human innate immunity. Hum Immunol. 2013;74(9):1069–79.
26. Ayala-Sumuano JT, Téllez-López VM, Domínguez-Robles Mdel C, Shibayama-Salas M, Meza I. (). Toll-like receptor signaling activation by Entamoeba histolytica induces beta defensin 2 in human colonic epithelial cells: Its possible role as an element of the innate immune response. PLoS Negl Trop Dis. 2013;7(2), e2083.
27. Hamanaka Y, Nakashima M, Wada A, Ito M, Kurazono H, Hojo H, et al. Expression of human beta-defensin 2 (hBD-2) in Helicobacter pylori induced gastritis: antibacterial effect of hBD-2 against Helicobacter pylori. Gut. 2001;49:481–7.
28. Liu L, Wang L, Jia HP, Zhao C, Heng HH, Schutte BC, et al. Structure and mapping of the human β-defensin HBD-2 gene and its expression at sites of inflammation. Gene. 1998;222(2):237–44.
29. Yoon YM, Lee JY, Yoo D, Sim YS, Kim YJ, Oh YK, et al. Bacteroides fragilis enterotoxin induces human β-defensin-2 expression in intestinal epithelial cells via a mitogen-activated protein kinase/IκB kinase/NF-κB-dependent pathway. Infect Immun. 2010;78(5):2024–33.
30. Wehkamp J, Harder J, Wehkamp K, Wehkamp-von Meissner B, Schlee M, Enders C, et al. NF-kappaB- and AP-1-mediated induction of human beta defensin-2 in intestinal epithelial cells by Escherichia coli Nissle 1917: a novel effect of a probiotic bacterium. Infect Immun. 2004;72(10):5750–8.
31. Guan SP, Kong LR, Cheng C, Lim JC, Wong WS. Protective role of 14-deoxy-11,12-didehydroandrographolide, a noncytotoxic analogue of andrographolide, in allergic airway inflammation. J Nat Prod. 2011;74(6):1484–90.
32. Wang W, Wang J, Dong SF, Liu CH, Italiani P, Sun SH, et al. Immunomodulatory activity of andrographolide on macrophage activation and specific antibody response. Acta Pharmacol Sin. 2010;31(2):191–201.
33. Salzman NH, Underwood MA, Bevins CL. Paneth cells, defensins, and the commensal microbiota: a hypothesis on intimate interplay at the intestinal mucosa. Semin Immunol. 2007;19(2):70–83.
34. Ho S, Pothoulakis C, Koon HW. Antimicrobial peptides and colitis. Curr Pharm Des. 2013;19(1):40–7.
35. Satthakarn S, Hladik F, Promsong A, Nittayananta W. Vaginal innate immune mediators are modulated by a water extract of Houttuynia cordata Thunb. BMC Complement Altern Med. 2015;15(1):183–90.
36. Zhou Y, Wang H, Li YS, Tao YW, Zhang JY, Zhang ZQ. Paeoniflorin increases beta-defensin expression and attenuates lesion in the colonic mucosa from mice with oxazolone-induced colitis. Yao Xue Xue Bao. 2010;45(1):37–42.
37. Salim E, Kumolosasi E, Jantan I. Inhibitory effect of selected medicinal plants on the release of pro-inflammatory cytokines in lipopolysaccharide-stimulated human peripheral blood mononuclear cells. J Nat Med. 2014;68(3):647–53.

The emergence of plasmid mediated quinolone resistance *qnrA*2 in extended spectrum β-lactamase producing *Klebsiella pneumoniae* in the Middle East

Leila Vali*, Ali A. Dashti, Mehrez M. Jadaon and Sherief El-Shazly

Abstract

Background: *Klebsiella pneumoniae* is one of the most important opportunistic pathogens causing serious complications in patients in hospitals and community. The clinical significance of *K. pneumoniae* is mainly due to its ability to acquire multiple antibiotic resistance genes. In this study we report the findings of a survey of plasmid mediated quinolone resistance in Extended-Spectrum β-lactamase (ESBL)-producing *K. pneumoniae* in Kuwait.

Methods: Clinical samples were collected from the microbiology laboratories of three major hospitals. Isolates were confirmed as ESBL-producers by disc diffusion method and PCR for the presence of *bla* genes. Antimicrobial susceptibility testing and genetic analysis were performed to detect the presence of a number of genes conferring resistance to β-lactam and fluoroquinolone antimicrobial agents including bla_{SHV}, bla_{TEM}, *aac* (6')-*Ib-cr*, *qnrA*, *qnrB* and *qnrS*. Pulsed-field gel electrophoresis (PFGE) was used for typing the isolates.

Results: In total 173 ESBL-producing *K. pneumoniae* were detected. *qnr* genes were identified in 27 (15.6 %) isolates and *aac(6')-Ib Ib-cr* gene in 26 (96 %). One (3.7 %) contained *qnrA*2, 21 harbored *qnrB*1 (78 %) and 5 (18.5 %) contained *qnrS*. Twenty one (78 %) isolates contained all three *bla* genes. PFGE showed diverse profiles.

Conclusion: We identified for the first time the emergence of the mobile fluoroquinolone resistance *qnrA*2 in a clinical isolate in the middle east and also showed the dissemination of *aac* (6')-*Ib-cr*, *qnr*B, and *qnr*S genes among ESBL-producing *K. pneumoniae* in Kuwait. The abundance of plasmid mediated resistance to fluoroquinolones among ESBL-producing *K. pneumoniae* is alarming as it facilitates therapy failure. Preventing the spread of these isolates is crucial if we are to sustain the effectiveness of the limited choices we have left in antimicrobial therapy.

Keywords: *Klebsiella pneumoniae*, Fluoroquinolones, *qnr*, Pulsed-field gel electrophoresis, Extended spectrum β-lactamase

Background

Members of the *Enterobacteriaceae* family in particular the multi-drug resistant *Klebsiella pneumoniae* are amongst the opportunistic pathogens. *K. pneumoniae* causes a wide range of infections from urinary and respiratory tract infections to bacteraemia, particularly in elderly or debilitated patients. Antibiotic resistance is an important factor that hinders therapy and delays improvement in patients' health. In *K. pneumoniae* resistance to antimicrobial agents is caused by different mechanisms however the production of extended spectrum β-lactamases (ESBLs) such as CTX-M and other enzymes including TEM-1, TEM-24, SHV-12 and the plasmid-mediated AmpC (CMY-2) are considered highly important [1–3]. CTX-M-15 producing strains can often contain variants of an aminoglycoside-modifying enzyme expressed by *aac(6')-Ib-cr* genes. Aminoglycoside-modifying enzymes cause reduced susceptibility to aminoglycosides and to some fluoroquinolones [4]. Fluoroquinolone resistance in *K. pneumoniae* can arise by mutations in the chromosomal type II topoisomerases and changes in the expression of efflux pumps and porins. Furthermore fluoroquinolone resistance can also be

* Correspondence: leila@hsc.edu.kw
Department of Medical Laboratory Sciences, Faculty of Allied Health, Sciences, Kuwait University, P.O. Box 31470-Sulaibekhat, 90805 Sulaibekhat, Kuwait

facilitated by plasmid-mediated resistance determinants *qnr* that express the pentapeptide repeat proteins. These proteins protect the quinolone targets (DNA gyrase or topoisomaerase IV enzymes) from the inhibitory activity of fluoroquinolone antibiotics [5, 6]. In view of the genetic heterogeneity variants of *qnrA*, *B* and *S*-like genes share 94 % to 99 %, 85 % to 99 % and 90 % nucleotide identity respectively [7].

In addition *K. pneumoniae* has been reported to produce clinically important carbapenemases; such as Ambler class B metallo-β-lactamases (NDM), the class A enzymes (KPC) and the class D oxacillinase enzymes (OXA-48) [8, 9].

Following the rise in the use of cephalosporins in hospitals; the incidence of infections caused by ESBL-producing *K. pneumoniae* has soared [2, 10]. Resistance to 3rd generation cephalosporins is predominantly associated with the presence of bla_{CTX-M} genes located on plasmids [11]. Therefore plasmid mediated resistance to fluoroquinolones among ESBL producing *K. pneumoniae* is alarming as it facilitates therapy failure. Moreover; the exchange of the genetic information among bacterial species threatens the efficacy of fluoroquinolones and increases the dependency on carbapenem antibiotics for treatment. The purpose of the present study was to determine the prevalence of plasmid-mediated fluoroquinolone resistance in ESBL-producing *K. pneumoniae* in hospitalized patients in Kuwait.

Material and methods

Bacterial isolates

In-patient clinical samples were collected from the microbiology laboratories of three major governmental hospitals that serve the six governorates of Kuwait, namely Al-Ahmadi hospital, Al-Amiri hospital and Adan hospital. All three hospitals are tertiary health care providers with bed capacities of 300, 500 and 600, respectively. The average number of specimens processed every day in each hospital varies from 500 to 700 which includes samples from out-patient and in-patient specialists units. A table was created based on the patients' records containing information such as age, gender, hospital, and type of specimen. Specimens were processed by clinical staff members of the diagnostic microbiology laboratories using standard protocols. The species identification was carried out by the API (bioMérieux, Marcy l'Etoile, France) and the VITEK 2 systems (Vitek AMS; bioMérieux Vitek Systems Inc., Hazelwood, MO, USA). The results were analyzed according to the Clinical and Laboratory Standards Institute (CLSI) (2012) guidelines [12]. The isolates were stored in 10 % skim milk at −70 °C.

Susceptibility testing

Antibiotic susceptibility tests were performed by the Kirby-Bauer method disc diffusion test following the CLSI (2012) criteria and recommendations [12]. The antibiotics tested were ampicillin, ampicillin/sulbactam, amoxicillin, amoxicillin/clavulanic acid, piperacillin/tazobactam, ceftazidime, cefepime, ceftriaxone, cefazolin and cefuroxime. The Minimum Inhibitory Concentration (MIC) was determined by agar dilution method and E-test when available for the following antibiotics: trimethoprim gentamicin, cefotaxime, imipenem, meropenem, ciprofloxacin, levofloxacin and tetracycline. Isolates that showed resistance to at least three classes of antibiotics were considered as MDR. Isolates that were detected as resistant to cefoxitin were further investigated for the presence of an *amp*C β-lactamase by using multiplex PCR [13, 14].

Double-disc synergy method

ESBLs were detected as previously described using the disc approximation and double-disc synergy methods and confirmed with cefotaxime and ceftazidime E-test ESBL strips (AB Biodisk, Biomerieux-diagnostics, Durham, NC, USA) [2]. For the disc approximation test, clavulanate diffusion from an amoxicillin–clavulanate (AMC30) disc was used to test for synergy with cefotaxime, ceftazidime, cefuroxime, cefepime and cefixime (Oxoid) as described previously [15]. For the double-disc synergy test, a ceftazidime disc (30 μg) was placed 30 mm away from a disc containing amoxicillin–clavulanate (60/10 μg). ESBL production was considered positive when an enhanced zone of inhibition was visible between the β-lactam and β-lactamase inhibitor-containing discs. For the E-test, ESBL strips containing ceftazidime and ceftazidime–clavulanate and strips containing cefotaxime and cefotaxime–clavulanate were used to determine the MIC ratio according to the manufacturer's instructions (AB Biodisk, Biomerieux-diagnostics, Durham, NC, USA). Cultures were incubated aerobically at 37 °C for 18–24 h. CTX-M-15 β-lactamase enzyme displays a catalytic activity toward ceftazidime.

Detection of *bla* genes and other resistance determinants

The presence of resistant genes (listed below) were investigated by PCR assays as previously reported [16]. PCR was conducted in a GeneAmp 9700 (Perkin-Elmer, Illinois, USA) system using the conditions specified for each primer; corresponding to the source references. The resistant genes investigated were bla_{TEM-1}, bla_{SHV}, $bla_{CTX-M-like}$, bla_{NDM}, bla_{OXA-1}, *qnr*A, *qnr*B, *qnr*S, *aac(6')-Ib Ib-cr*, *gyr*A, *par*C, *gyr*B, *par*E, *intI*1, *intI*2, bla_{KPC}, bla_{VIM}, bla_{IMP}, bla_{OXA-48}, and *amp*C. The detection of bla_{PER}, bla_{GES} and bla_{VEB} was performed by PCR according to Opazo *et al.* [17].

Isolates resistant to ciprofloxacin and for which the ceftaxidime or cefotaxime MICs were >8 mg/L were screened for ESBLs and *qnr* genes. Double disc and combination disc tests were used for ESBLs confirmation.

Amplified PCR products were purified with Qiagen purification kit (Qiagen, Limburg Netherlands) according to the

Table 1 The total number of ESBL producing *Enterobacteriaceae* isolates containing *qnr* genes during this study

Hospital	Enterobacteriaceae (ESBL producers)	*Escherichia coli*	*Enterobacter cloacae*	*Proteus mirabilis*	*Klebseilla oxytoca*	*Klebsiella pneumoniae*	*qnr* positive *K. pneumoniae*
Amiri	480	383 (80 %)	1 (0.2 %)	18 (3.8 %)	6 (1 %)	72 (15 %)	5 (6.9 %)
KOC	137	83 (61 %)	6 (4 %)	7 (5 %)	4 (3 %)	37 (27 %)	10 (2.7 %)
Adan	215	140 (65 %)	4 (1.8 %)	3 (1.4 %)	4 (1.8 %)	64 (30 %)	12 (18.8 %)
Total	832	606 (73 %)	11 (1.3 %)	28 (3 %)	14 (1.7 %)	173 (21 %)	27 (15.6 %)

manufacturer's instructions and both strands were sequenced by automated ABI3100 DNA sequencer (Applied Biosystems, Foster City, CA, USA). The BLAST program of the National Centre for Biotechnology Information (http://www.ncbi.nlm.nih.gov) was used to search and compare databases for similar nucleotide sequences.

Pulsed-Field Gel Electrophoresis (PFGE)

PFGE was performed by using the restriction enzyme *Xba*I [18], with a run time of 20 h and switch times of 5 to 50 and 5 to 35 s at 14 °C and 6 V/cm (CHEF-DR II System; Bio-Rad, Hercules, CA, USA). The PFGE profiles were analyzed by using BioNumerics software version 7.1 (Applied Maths, Sint-Martens-Latem, Belgium). Statistics was added at the end of the methods section.

Statistical analysis

Out of the total number of isolates included hereby, the percentage of the different ESBL-producing bacteria were calculated in each of the three hospitals participating in the study.

Table 2 The list of *K. pneumoniae* isolates

Hospital	Isolate number	Specimen	Gender	Age	Species
Adan	ADA-17	Urine	M	NA	K. pneumoniae
	ADA-28	Urine	M	NA	K. pneumoniae
	ADA-30	Urine	M	NA	K. pneumoniae
	ADA-39	Bile	F	33	K. pneumoniae
	ADA-45	Urine	M	76	K. pneumoniae
	ADA-49	Bile	F	33	K. pneumoniae
	ADA-69	Urine	F	78	K. pneumoniae
	ADA-89	Urine	M	84	K. pneumoniae
	ADA-111	Urine	M	77	K. pneumoniae
	ADA-140	Urine	F	77	K. pneumoniae
	ADA-214	Urine	M	79	K. pneumoniae
	ADA-215	Urine	F	8	K. pneumoniae
Ahmadi	KOC-2	Urine	M	82	K. pneumoniae
	KOC-7	Urine	F	47	K. pneumoniae
	KOC-12	Catheter Tip	F	14	K. pneumoniae
	KOC-32	Urine	F	36	K. pneumoniae
	KOC-37	Urine	F	36	K. pneumoniae
	KOC-63	Urine	F	90	K. pneumoniae
	KOC-64	Urine	F	58	K. pneumoniae
	KOC-66	Catheter Tip	F	72	K. pneumoniae
	KOC-74	Urine	F	60	K. pneumoniae
	KOC-105	Diabetic Foot	M	59	K. pneumoniae
Al-Amiri	Y-2	Diabetic Foot	M	52	K. pneumoniae
	Y-4	Urine	M	78	K. pneumoniae
	Y-12	Bedsore Swab	F	65	K. pneumoniae
	Y-15	Penile Swab	M	81	K. pneumoniae

NA Not available

Table 3 The profiles of *qnr* positive *K. pneumoniae* isolates and other resistance genes studied

Profiles of the antibiotic resistance genes	No. of isolates
*qnr*B1, *bla* $_{CTX-M-15}$	2
*qnr*B1, *bla* $_{CTX-M-2}$, *bla* $_{SHV}$, *aac(6')-Ib-cr*	1
*qnr*B1, *bla* $_{CTX-M-15}$, *bla* $_{SHV}$, *aac(6')-Ib-cr*	3
*qnr*S, *bla* $_{CTX-M-2}$, *bla* $_{TEM-1}$, *bla* $_{SHV}$, *aac(6')-Ib-cr*	1
*qnr*S, *bla* $_{CTX-M-15}$, *bla* $_{TEM-1}$, *bla* $_{SHV}$, *aac(6')-Ib-cr*	4
*qnr*A2, *bla* $_{CTX-M-15}$, *bla* $_{TEM-1}$, *bla* $_{SHV}$, *aac(6')-Ib-cr*	1
*qnr*B1, *bla* $_{CTX-M-15}$, *bla* $_{TEM-1}$, *bla* $_{SHV}$, *aac(6')-Ib-cr*	15
Total	27

DNA profiles were analysed by the unweighted pair method with arithmetic average (UPGMA) using BioNumerics v.7.1. The development of the algorithms necessary for the comparison of fingerprinting profiles of isolates was based on the Dice correlation coefficient. The hierarchic Cluster analysis and phylogenetic trees were subsequently analysed with an optimization of 1.0 % and a tolerance of 1 %. Isolates were considered to belong to the same PFGE clone if their Dice similarity index was ≥85 %.

Results

Bacterial isolates

All three governmental hospitals participated during our study period from 2010 to 2012; however there were inconsistencies in the level of strain contribution from each hospital. Therefore under-representation of ESBL-mediated *K. pneumoniae* might exist. A total of 832 ESBL-producing *Enterobacteriaceae* isolates were obtained Table 1. They comprised of 606 *Escherichia coli* (73 %), 11 *Enterobacter cloacae* (1.3 %), 28 *Proteus mirabilis* (3 %), 14 *Klebsiella oxytoca* (1.7 %) *and* 173 *Klebsiella pneumoniae* (21 %).

The antibiotic sensitivity testing for *K. pneumoniae* isolates was performed followed by double-disc synergy tests. The results were confirmed with PCR and sequencing the product.

From the total of 173 (21 %) ESBL-producing *K. pneumoniae qnr* genes were identified in 27 (15.6 %) isolates. The distribution of the isolates is presented in Table 2.

Sensitivity to antimicrobial agents

All the 27 *qnr* positive isolates were resistant to ampicillin (MIC > 16), ciproflaxoacin (MIC > 4), cefotaxime (MIC > 4), ceftazidime (MIC > 4), ceftriaxone (MIC > 4), and gentamicin (MIC > 16); but sensitive to imipenem (MIC > 1) and meropenem (MIC > 1).

Sequencing the PCR products showed the distribution of the resistance determinants (Table 3). *bla*$_{CTX-M-15}$ was detected in 25 (93 %), *bla*$_{CTXM-2}$ in 2 (7 %), *bla*$_{TEM}$ in 21 (78 %), *bla*$_{SHV}$ and *aac(6')-Ib Ib-cr* gene was found in 26 (96 %) isolates. Twenty one (78 %) isolates contained all three *bla* genes. From the 27 *K. pneumonia* isolates only 1 (3.7 %) contained *qnrA2*, 21 harbored *qnrB*1 (78 %) and 5 (18.5 %) contained *qnrS*. Class I integrons (*intI*1) was detected in 25 (93 %) isolates but class II integrons (*intI*2) was not found in any of the isolates tested. *bla*$_{KPC}$, *bla*$_{VIM}$, *bla*$_{PER}$, *bla*$_{GES}$, *bla*$_{VEB}$, *bla*$_{IMP}$, *bla*$_{OXA1}$, *bla*$_{OXA48}$ and *amp*C were not detected in this study. No mutations were found in *gyr*A and *par*C.

PFGE

PFGE showed diverse profiles among the isolates tested (Fig. 1). Only two isolates (KOC 7 and KOC 64) from urinary tract infection had identical PFGE patterns. The majority of isolates with similar *qnr* genes; displayed similar antimicrobial resistance phenotypes but their PFGE profiles were not identical. In total three isolates (ADA-45, ADA-49 and KOC-37) were not typable by PFGE.

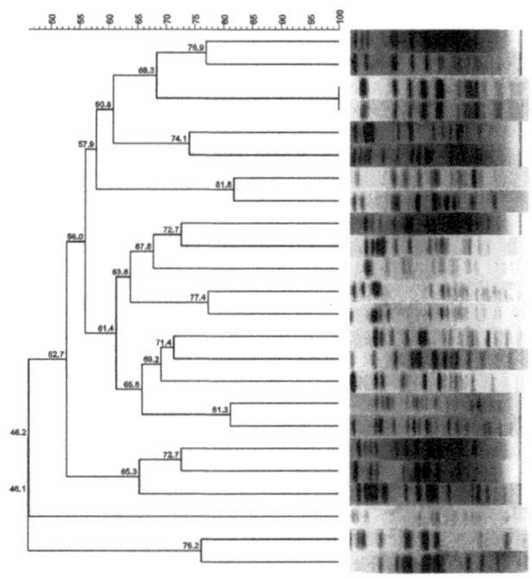

Key	Qnr	CTX-M	SHV	TEM-1	aac	INTG-1	SOURCE
ADA-17	B1	15	+	+	+	+	Urine
Y-12	B1	15	-	-	+	-	Bedsore Swab
KOC-7	B1	15	+	-	+	+	Urine
KOC-64	B1	15	+	-	+	+	Urine
Y-15	B1	15	+	+	+	+	Penile Swab
Y-31	B1	15	+	+	+	+	Wound Swab (Diabetic Foot)
KOC-32	B1	15	+	+	+	+	Urine
KOC-66	B1	15	+	+	+	+	Catheter Tip
ADA-30	S	15	+	+	+	+	Urine
ADA-140	S	15	+	+	+	+	Urine
ADA-214	B1	15	+	+	+	+	Urine
ADA-69	B1	15	+	+	+	+	Urine
ADA-215	B1	15	+	+	+	+	Urine
ADA-111	S	15	+	+	+	+	Urine
KOC-63	B1	15	+	+	+	+	Urine
ADA-89	B1	15	+	+	+	+	Urine
KOC-105	B1	15	-	-	+	+	Wound Swab (Diabetic Foot)
Y-2	S	15	+	+	+	+	Wound Swab (Diabetic Foot)
ADA-28	B1	15	+	-	-	-	Urine
ADA-39	B1	15	+	+	+	+	Bile Swab
Y-4	B1	15	+	+	+	+	Urine
KOC-2	B1	15	+	+	+	+	Urine
KOC-12	A2	15	+	+	+	+	Catheter Tip
KOC-74	S	2	+	+	+	+	Urine

Fig. 1 PFGE showing the relationship between DNA banding patterns

Discussion

In the present study we detected a similar rate of ESBL-producing *K. pneumoniae* (21 %) as previously reported (28 %) [19]. However, we found 15.6 % (27/173) of ESBL-producing *K. pneumoniae* contained a plasmid mediated *qnr* gene. Previous research undertaken in Kuwait in 2007 did not identify either *qnr*A or *qnr*S in ESBL-producing Enterobacteriaceae and reported a low prevalence of 4.7 % (3 out of 64 isolates) of *qnrB* in *E. coli* [7]. Here we identified *qnr A*, *B* and *S* in ESBL-producing *K. pneumonia.* The incidence rate of 15.6 % *qnr* in Kuwait compared to other countries in Asia such as Iran (30.4 %) [20]. Thailand (34.6 %) [21], Malaysia (37 %) [22], India (67 %) [23] and Saudi Arabia (44 %) [24] is considerably lower.

The key findings in our study are the emergence of *qnrA*2 in the Middle East for the first time and also the spread of *qnrS* among the clinical ESBL-producing *K. pneumonia* isolates in Kuwait. *qnrA* is the first plasmid-mediated quinolone resistance identified however, in *K. pneumoniae* it is not as widespread as *qnrB* [25]. *qnrA* confers resistance to quinolones such as nalidixic acid and increases minimum inhibitory concentration (MIC) values of fluoroquinolone up to 20-folds [26]. It has also been shown that when both *qnrA* and *aac- (6`)-Ib-cr* are present in the same cell, the level of ciprofloxacin resistance is increased fourfold more than that conferred by *qnrA* alone [5]. Therefore the detection of *qnrA*2 gene in an ESBL producing *K. pneumoniae* from the catheter tip of a 14 year old female patient was alarming and a challenge for empirical antibiotic therapy such as fluoroquinolones in clinical settings. The rise of plasmid-mediated fluoroquinolone resistance is concerning for antimicrobial treatment of *K. pneumoniae* whereby the only option left will be carbapenems.

In this study $bla_{CTX\text{-}M\text{-}15}$ was the predominant β-lactamase and in 93 % of the cases (25 out of 27 isolates) it was associated with the presence of *aac(6)-1b-cr*. We also identified *qnr*B1 and *qnr*S in isolates harbouring *aac(6`)-Ib Ib-cr* and $bla_{CTX\text{-}M}$. These isolates were resistant to penicillins, most cephalosproins, β-lactamase inhibitors as well as fluoroquinolones posing a risk to combination β-lactam/β-lactamase inhibitor therapy. The correlation between ESBL and ciprofloxacin resistance is an indication of the important contribution of the plasmid-mediated resistance to fluoroquinolone resistance in this region.

Urine samples comprised 67 % (18/27) of the specimens followed by wound swabs 15 % (4/27). We did not find any correlation between antimicrobial resistance characteristics or specimen type and PFGE profiles. In fact overall the PFGE profiles of the tested isolates were diverse implying that the spread of *qnr* genes is not concentrated to only a specific clonal lineage. A detailed longitudinal study is required to identify the clonal identity of ESBL-producing *qnr*-positive *K. pneumonia* isolates.

Conclusion

This manuscript reports the genotypic variation among strains of *qnr* positive K. pneumonieae in hospitalized patients in Kuwait. The presence of *qnr* and *aac-(6`)-Ib-cr* genes especially when they co-exist in ESBL-producing isolates contribute to the increase in fluoroquinolone resistance.

In conclusion the clinical importance of our findings is that the circulating MDR plasmids that contain *qnr, aac-(6`)-Ib-cr* and *bla* genes are concerning in hospitals as they increase the chances of *K. pneumoniae* adaptability to environmental pressures such as antibiotics. If guidelines are not in place regarding the strict use of antibiotics we will face antimicrobial therapy failure in hospitalized patients. Continuous monitoring of plasmid mediated fluoroquinolone ESBL-producing *Enterobactericeae* in clinical settings is crucial.

Abbreviations

ESBL: Extended-Spectrum β-lactamase; *K. pneumoniae*: *Klebsiella pneumoniae*; *qnr*: Plasmid-mediated quinolone resistance gene; *bla*: β-lactamase gene; PFGE: Pulsed-field gel electrophoresis; MIC: Minimum Inhibitory Concentration; MDR: Multi-drug Resistant; PCR: Polymerase Chain Reaction; AMC: Amoxicillin/Clavulanic acid.

Competing interests

The authors declare that they have no competing interests.

Authors' contributions

LV, AAD, MMJ and SE all participated equally in the design of the study, processing the samples, laboratory experiments and analysing the data. LV drafted the manuscript. All authors read and approved the final manuscript.

Acknowledgement

The authors would like to thank Miss Shorooq Barrak Al-Inizi for her technical support. The authors would also like to acknowledge the Research Unit for Genomics, Proteomics and Cellomics Studies (OMICS) of the Health Sciences Centre, Kuwait University (Project No. SRUL02/13) for assisting in DNA sequencing.

Funding

This work was supported by Kuwait University Research Administration Grant number NM02/10 and the Kuwait Foundation for Advancement of Science (KFAS), Grant no. 2011130204.

References

1. Karisik E, Ellington MJ, Pike R, Warren RE, Livermore DM, Woodford N. Molecular characterization of plasmids encoding CTX-M-15 β-lactamases from *Escherichia coli* strains in the United States. J Antimicrob Chemother. 2006;58:665–8.
2. Dashti AA, Jadaon MM, Gomaa HH, Noronha B, Udo EE. Transmission of a Klebsiella pneumoniae clone harbouring genes for CTX-M-15-like and SHV-112 enzymes in a neonatal intensive care unit of a Kuwaiti hospital. J Med Microbiol. 2010;59:687–92.
3. Munier GK, Johnson CL, Snyder JW, Moland ES, Hanson ND, Thomson KS. Positive extended-spectrum-beta-lactamase (ESBL) screening results may be due to AmpC beta-lactamases more often than to ESBLs. J Clin Microbiol. 2010;48:673–4. http://www.ncbi.nlm.nih.gov/pubmed/19955269.
4. Park CH, Rovicsek A, Jacoby GA, Sahm D, Hooper DC. Prevalence in the United States of aac(6')-Ib-cr encoding a ciprofloxacin-modifying enzyme. Antimicrob Agent Chermother. 2006;50:3953–5.

5. Mammeri H, Van De Loo M, Poirel L, Martinez-Martinez L, Nordmann P. Emergence of plasmid-mediated quinolone resistance in *Escherichia coli* in Europe. Antimicrobio Agents Chemother. 2005;49:71–6.
6. Vetting MW, Hegde SS, Fajardo JE, Fiser A, Roderick SL, Takiff HE, et al. Pentapeptide repeat proteins. Biogeosciences. 2006;45:1–10.
7. Cattoir V, Poirel L, Rotimi V, Soussy CJ, Nordmann P. Multiplex PCR for detection of plasmid-mediated quinolone resistance *qnr* genes in ESBL-producing enterobacterial isolates. J Antimicrob Chemother. 2007;60:394–7.
8. Poirel L, Hombrouck-Alet C, Freneaux C, Bernabeu S, Nordmann P. Global spread of New Delhi metallo-β-lactamase 1. Lancet Infect Dis. 2010;10:832.
9. Poirel L, Carbonnelle E, Bernabeu S, Gutmann L, Rotimi V, Nordmann P. Importation of OXA-48-producing Klebsiella pneumoniae from Kuwait. J Antimicrob Chemother. 2012;67:2051–2.
10. Jacoby TS, Kuchenbecker RS, Dos Santos RP, Magedanz L, Guzatto P, Moreira LB. Impact of hospital-wide infection rate, invasive procedures use and antimicrobial consumption on bacterial resistance inside an intensive care unit. J Hosp Infect. 2010;75:23–7.
11. Peirano G, Pitout JDD. Molecular epidemiology of *Escherichia coli* producing CTX-M beta-lactamases: the worldwide emergence of clone ST131 O25:H4. Int J Antimicrob Agents. 2010;35:316–21.
12. Clinical and Laboratory Standards Institute. Performance standards for antimicrobial susceptibility testing; twenty-first informational supplement. Document M100-S21. Wayne, PA: CLSI; 2012.
13. Pérez-Pérez FJ, Hanson ND. Detection of plasmid-mediated AmpC β-lactamase genes in clinical isolates by using multiplex PCR. J Clin Microbiol. 2002;40:2153–62.
14. Pitout JD, Gregson DB, Church DL, Laupland KB. Population-based laboratory surveillance for AmpC beta-lactamase-producing *Escherichia coli*, Calgary. Emerg Infect Dis. 2007;13:443–8.
15. Sonnevend A, Al Dhaheri K, Mag T, Herpay M, Kolodziejek J, Nowotny N, et al. CTX-M-15-producing multidrug-resistant enteroaggregative *Escherichia coli* in the United Arab Emirates. Clin Microbiol Infect. 2006;12:582–5.
16. Dashti AA, Vali L, El-Shazly S, Jadaon MM. The characterization and antibiotic resistance profiles of clinical Escherichia coli O25b-B2-ST131 isolates in Kuwait. BMC Microbiol. 2014;14:214.
17. Opazo A, Vali L, Al Obaid K, Dashti AA, Amyes SG. Novel genetic structure harbouring bla_{PER-1} in ceftazidime-resistant *Acinetobacter baumannii* isolated from Kuwait. Int J Antimicrob Agents. 2014;43:383–4.
18. Ribot FM, Fair NA, Gautom R, Carmeron DN, Hunter SB, Swaminathan B, et al. Standardization of pulsed-field gel electrophoresis protocols for the subtyping of *Escherichia coli* O157, Salmonella and Shigella for pulsenet. Foodborne Path Dis. 2006;3:59–67.
19. Al Benwan K, Al Sweih N, Rotimi VO. Etiology and antibiotic susceptibility patterns of community- and hospital-acquired urinary tract infections in a general hospital in Kuwait. Med Princ Pract. 2010;19:440–6.
20. Seyedpour SM, Eftekhar F. Quinolone susceptibility and detection of *qnr* and *aac(6')-Ib-cr* genes in community isolates of *Klebsiella pneumoniae*. Jundishapur J Microbiol. 2014. doi:10.5812/jjm.11136.
21. Pasom W, Chanawong A, Lulitanond A, Wilailuckana C, Kenprom S, Puang-Ngern P. Plasmid-mediated quinolone resistance genes, *aac(6')-Ib-cr*, *qnrS*, *qnrB*, and *qnrA*, in urinary isolates of *Escherichia coli* and *Klebsiella pneumoniae* at a teaching hospital, Thailand. Jpn J Infect Dis. 2013;66:428–32.
22. Al-Marzooq F, Mohd Yusof MY, Tay ST. Molecular analysis of ciprofloxacin resistance mechanisms in Malaysian ESBL-producing *Klebsiella pneumoniae* isolates and development of mismatch amplification mutation assays (MAMA) for rapid detection of *gyrA* and *parC* mutations. Biomed Res Int. 2014. doi:10.1155/2014/601630.
23. Tripathi A, Dutta SK, Majumdar M, Dhara L, Banerjee D, Roy K. High prevalence and significant association of ESBL and QNR genes in pathogenic *Klebsiella pneumoniae* isolates of patients from Kolkata, India. Indian J Microbiol. 2012;52:557–64.
24. Shibl AM, Al-Agamy MH, Khubnani H, Senok AC, Tawfik AF, Livermore DM. High prevalence of acquired quinolone-resistance genes among Enterobacteriaceae from Saudi Arabia with CTX-M-15 β-lactamase. Diagn Microbiol Infect Dis. 2012;73:350–3.
25. Martı´nez-Martı´nez L, Pascual A, Jacoby GA. Quinolone resistance from a transferable plasmid. Lancet. 1998;351:797–9.
26. Robicsek A, Jacoby GA, Hooper DC. The worldwide emergence of plasmid-mediated quinolone resistance. Lancet Infect Dis. 2006;6:629–40.

Thallium exists in opioid poisoned patients

Amir Ghaderi[1], Naser Vahdati-Mashhadian[2], Zohreh Oghabian[3], Valiallah Moradi[2], Reza Afshari[4,5*] and Omid Mehrpour[6]

Abstract

Background: Thallium (Tl) is a toxic heavy metal that exists in nature. Tl poisoning (thallotoxicosis) may occur in opioid addicts. This study was designed to evaluate the frequency and level of urinary Tl in opioid abusers. In addition, clinical findings were evaluated.

Methods: A total of 150 subjects were examined. Cases with a history of at least 3 years of abuse were admitted in the Imam Reza Hospital as the case group; 50 non-opioid abusers from the target population were included as the control group. Twenty-four hour urinary qualitative and quantitative Tl analyses were performed on both groups.

Results: Out of the 150 subjects, 128 (85 %) were negative for qualitative urinary Tl, followed by 5 % (trace), 7 % (1+), 2 % (2+), and 1 % (3+). Mean (standard error (SE), Min–Max) quantitative urinary Tl level was 14 μg/L (3.5 μg/L, 0–346 μg/L). Mean urinary Tl level in the case group was 21 μg/L (5 μg/L, 0–346 μg/L) and that in the controls was 1 μg/L (0.14 μg/L, 0–26 μg/L), which were significantly different ($P = 0.001$). The most frequent clinical findings were ataxia (86 %), sweating (81 %), and constipation (54 %). In all cases ($n = 150$), the mean (SE) value for cases with positive qualitative urinary Tl was 26.8 μg/L (0.9 μg/L) and that in the negative cases was 2.3 μg/L (0.2 μg/L), which were significantly different ($P = 0.002$).

Conclusions: This study showed that long-term opioid abuse may lead to Tl exposure. In opioid abusers with the clinical manifestation of thallotoxicosis, urinary Tl should be determined.

Keywords: Thallium, Opioid, Poisoning

Background

Thallium (Tl) is a highly toxic heavy metal with atomic number 81 and a molecular weight of 204.37 discovered by Sir William Crookes in 1861 [1]. It is a soft, bluish-white or gray water-insoluble metal but the salt forms are colorless, tasteless, and odorless. Tl is readily absorbed via ingestion, inhalation, and dermal contact [1–3]. Tl does not have any biological function in the body and the fatal dose is more than 10–15 mg/kg of body weight [4]. In the past, Tl was used as a hair remover and rodenticide because of its toxicity, but presently Tl administration is restricted to industrial usage such as optic lenses, and the radioisotope forms are used for medical purposes such as diagnosis of malignancies (such as melanoma) and tissue scintigraphy (such as cardiac scanning) [5]. Any amount of Tl in the body is abnormal [1]. In humans, Tl toxicity may occur occupationally (industrial exposure), accidentally (contact with Tl-containing material), or in cases of homicide; oral ingestion is the main route of Tl entrance in the body [1]. The clinical manifestation of thallotoxicosis has a wide spectrum but painful ascending peripheral neuropathy (both motor and sensory), gastrointestinal, and dermatologic manifestations (particularly alopecia) are major characteristics in Tl toxicity [5]. The exact mechanism of toxicity is still unclear, but because Tl ions are similar to potassium (K) ions, Tl may alter the number of K-dependent systems and enzymes in the body such as sulfhydryl groups, essential enzymes in the Krebs cycle, succinate dehydrogenase, and interactions with sodium-potassium ATPase and riboflavin [3, 6, 7]. Treatment includes early gastrointestinal decontamination, Prussian blue therapy (potassium ferric hexacyanoferrate), activated charcoal, laxatives, and enhanced elimination via forced diuresis and hemodialysis [3, 6, 8]. In Tl poisoning, early diagnosis and treatment is necessary for complete recovery; any

* Correspondence: AfshariR@mums.ac.ir
[4]Addiction Research Centre, Mashhad University of Medical Sciences, Imam Reza Hospital, Ibn-e-Sina Street, Mashhad 91735-348, Iran
[5]British Columbia Center for Disease Control, Vancouver, Canada
Full list of author information is available at the end of the article

delay may lead to permanent neurological disorders [6, 9]. Illicit opium may be adulterated with various substances such as sugars, quinine, caffeine, lactose, strychnine, paracetamol, and heavy metals such as lead [10, 11]. In fact, salesmen and smugglers may add any kind of heavy metals to opium to increase its weight for more profit. Recently, there have been reports of Tl toxicity in illicit opium users [12, 13]. We decided to evaluate Tl as an adulterant in opioid-like compounds from opium users, for the early diagnosis and treatment of thallotoxicosis.

Methods

Study design

This is a case–control study. One-hundred opioid-like abusers, raw opium, opium residue, crystal heroin, or mixed abusers for more than 3 years, aged 18–65 years, were recruited following admission to Imam Reza Hospital because of poisoning or rehabilitation as the case group. Controls were 50 non-abuser subjects with no history of drug use in the previous year. Urinary morphine tests using immunoassay tests were used to determine positive cases. Controls were verified to be opioid naïve via verbal conversation. All ethical approvals were considered and the aim of the study was explained to all subjects in both groups. Twenty-four hour urinary samples were taken on admission for qualitative and quantitative Tl analyses, and other data including demographic, neurological, dermal, and gastrointestinal clinical findings were entered into a predesigned checklist. Diphenoxylate, acetaminophen codeine, and tramadol users were excluded from the study.

Laboratory assessment

In acute poisoning, high concentrations of Tl appear in the kidney; thus, urine is the fluid of choice for Tl detection [14]. The normal concentration is <5 μg/L (<24.5 nmol/L) in a 24-h urine sample. The urine samples were placed in 100 mL urine collection containers (polyethylene) and stored at −20 °C until analysis [15]. The first 24-h urinary samples in the two groups were examined for Tl using a qualitative (semi-quantitative) survey. Reagents included: 1) cyanide reagent: 1.6 g of sodium hydroxide, 1.2 g of sodium-potassium tartrate, and 1.36 g of potassium cyanide dissolved in 10 mL of water. 2) Dithizone solution (250 mg/L) in chloroform prepared fresh: 12 mL urine sample and 1 mL cyanide reagent to dithizone solution (dithizone + chloroform) were combined, shaken for 2 min, and left for 3–5 min. Two-phase formation occurred, consisting of an upper urine phase and a lower chloroform phase. A pink-red color in the lower chloroform phase indicates the presence of Tl and indicates a positive result. According to semi-quantitative Tl-screening tests, <50 μg/L is considered negative, trace (50–100 μg/L), 1+ (100–200 μg/L), 2+ (200–300 μg/L), 3+ (300–400 μg/L), and 4+ (>400 μg/L) [16]. In the second step, quantitative analysis via graphite furnace atomic absorption spectrometry (Perkin Elmer, Model 3030 with HGA 400 Programmer), which is a highly sensitive spectroscopic technique that provides excellent detection limits for measuring concentrations of Tl in urine, was performed on all samples [17]. In this test, we applied a Tl standard solution, traceable to standard reference materials from National Institute of Standards and Technology thallium(I) nitrate in nitric acid 0.5 mol/L (1000 mg/L) TlCertipur®, provided from Merck. To measure TL in urine, after extraction with nitric acid, sulfuric acid, and Triton X- 100, the liquid phases were separated from the sediment. Next, 2 % ammonium monovanadate in 1 % sodium hydroxide was then added to neutralize acidity to prevent graphite tube damage. The solution was centrifuged at high speed for 5 min, and 25 μL from the upper layer was injected into the graphite. A thermal program was selected for drying; 130 °C, 300 °C for organic solvents, and 800 °C for inorganic solvents and ash removal, and 1700 °C for atomization. Absorbance was measured at 276.8 nm [18, 19]. Detection limits were 0.2 μg/L, precision 3.65 %, and accuracy 97.4 % of analyses were determined by repeated analyses of biological reference material (SERONORM urine trace element level 2, lot 1011645) [20]. We evaluated both qualitative and quantitative urinary Tl because they complement each other.

Statistical analysis

Data were analyzed with SPSS software (version 16). Student's t test and Spearman's coefficient test were used to analyze the data. P value was considered to be less than 0.05 throughout the study.

Results

Demographic findings

In total, 150 subjects, including 100 cases and 50 controls, were recruited. Among them, 134 (89 %) were male. Mean (standard error (SE), Min–Max) age was 41 (1.2, 19–85) years. Mean (SE) age in cases was 41 years (1.6) and in controls was 41 years (0.3), which were similar. Among cases, raw opium or opium residues were used by 66 % cases, followed by mixed (28 %), and crystal heroin (6 %). Cases only smoking were 49 %, those smoking and ingesting were 45 %, those only injecting were 3 %, and those using a mixture of methods were 3 %.

Clinical findings

Neurological

Frequency of ataxia in cases (n = 100) was 86 %, followed by tremor (85 %), insomnia (83 %), depression (82 %), blurred vision (79 %), memory deficits (78 %), weakness (77 %), fatigue (77 %), aggressiveness (77 %), jerking movements (76 %), vertigo (73 %), emotional liability

Table 1 Qualitative urinary thallium results ($n = 150$)

Qualitative Urinary Thallium Results	Cases n (%)	Controls n (%)	Total n (%)
Negative	80 (80)	48 (96)	128 (85)
Trace	6 (6)	1 (2)	7 (5)
1+	10 (10)	1 (2)	11 (7)
2+	3 (3)	0 (0)	3 (2)
3+	1 (1)	0 (0)	1 (1)
Total	100 (100)	50 (100)	150 (100)

(65 %), headache (59 %), paresthesia (40 %), tinnitus (38 %), seizure (36 %), delirium-psychosis-coma (30 %), and choreoathetosis (0 %).

Dermal: Frequency of sweating in cases ($n = 100$) was 81 %, followed by scalp hair loss (45 %), dry skin (36 %), acne (8 %), rashes (6 %), body hair loss (5 %), Mees' lines (0 %), and palmar erythema (0 %).

Gastrointestinal: Frequency of constipation in cases ($n = 100$) was 54 %, followed by nausea (20 %), vomiting (20 %), abdominal pain (16 %), and diarrhea (14 %).

Qualitative urinary Tl results

For all subjects, 128 (85 %) were negative for qualitative urinary Tl, followed by 5 % (trace), 7 % (1+), 2 % (2+), and 1 % (3+). The distribution of qualitative results is shown in Table 1. The two groups were significantly different ($P = 0.01$).

Quantitative urinary Tl level

The mean (SE, Min–Max) quantitative urinary Tl level was 14 μg/L (3.5 μg/L, 0–346 μg/L). Mean urinary Tl levels in the case group were 21 μg/L (5 μg/L, 0–346 μg/L) and in controls were 1 μg/L (0.14 μg/L, 0–26 μg/L), which were significantly different ($P = 0.001$).

Comparison of qualitative and quantitative results

In all cases ($n = 150$), the mean (SE) value for cases with positive qualitative urinary Tl levels was 26.8 μg/L (1 μg/L) and in negative cases was 2.3 μg/L (0.4 μg/L), which were significantly different ($P = 0.002$).

Duration of abuse was not associated with Tl levels ($r = 0.329$, $P = 0.099$). Positive Tl results were significantly higher for raw opium abusers in comparison with heroin abusers ($P < 0.001$). Table 2 summarizes these differences. Positive Tl results were significantly higher for smoke and ingestion compared with ingestion alone ($P = 0.001$). Table 2 summarizes these differences.

Discussion

Our results indicate that contaminated opiates could be a source of Tl poisoning. Substance abuse is one of the most preventable health hazards worldwide. Iran appears to have both traditional and modern drug use and abuse problems, and it appears to play an important transit role in the transfer of opium and other drugs from Afghanistan to western countries [21, 22]. Adding heavy metals such as lead adulterant to the drugs is already described [23, 24]. Opium is still a most frequently abused drug. Informal, and often illegal, laboratories refine opium into a sticky, brown paste, which is pressed into bricks and sun dried. This material can then be ingested or smoked. This process results in introduction of impurities such as lead into the product [25]. Salesmen and smugglers may add any number of heavy metals to opium to increase the weight for more profit. Although the amount of Tl in opium is usually small, when taken in large amounts, opium adulterated with Tl can produce clinical toxicity. However, very few reports describe unusual and exotic causes of chronic Tl poisoning as an adulterant to illicit drugs [12–14]. Afshari *et al.* reported three cases of suspected Tl poisoning after heroin abuse. Urine qualitative tests resulted in a range from negative to 4+ Tl, and three months after substitution of heroin, signs and symptoms of thallotoxicos returned; they concluded that contaminated heroin was responsible [13]. Questel *et al.* also reported two cases of Tl poisoning in heroin users [12].

In our study, the most frequent symptoms were ataxia, tremor, insomnia, neuropathy (both sensory and motor), sweating, scalp hair loss, dry skin, constipation, nausea, and vomiting, which were slightly different from previous studies that emphasized on polyneuropathy, paresis, abdominal pain, and alopecia [4, 6, 9, 21]. This dissimilarity may be because of the amount of Tl used or less severity of toxicity. There were significant differences in urinary Tl tests between case and control groups in addition to clinical findings. Surprisingly, nearly one-third of our patients had a history of seizure, possibly

Table 2 Comparison of qualitative urinary thallium results in different type of abused drugs ($n = 100$)

type of abused drugs	Qualitative test						Total
	Negative	Trace	1+	2+	3+	Positive	
(Crystal) Heroin	5(83 %)	0(0 %)	1(16 %)	0(0 %)	0(0 %)	1(16 %)	6(100 %)
Opium	51(77 %)	5(7 %)	7(10 %)	2(3 %)	1(1 %)	15(21 %)	66(100 %)
Mixed user	24(85 %)	1(3 %)	2(7 %)	1(3 %)	0(0 %)	4(13 %)	28(100 %)
Total	80(80 %)	6(6 %)	10(10 %)	3(3 %)	1(1 %)	20(20 %)	100(100 %)

because of abuse of tramadol or other unknown abuse of illicit drugs. In Iran, opium addicts have a great affinity for tramadol because of the euphoria experience or because of replacement of opiates [26–27]. Our study showed the most frequent illicit substance was raw opium and opium residue (66 %), and positive Tl results were significantly higher in this group in comparison with other abusers. In addition, ingestion and smoking was the most frequent route of consumption in the positive Tl group. Comparison between qualitative and quantitative results indicated that for exact diagnosis, it is better to incorporate both qualitative and quantitative analyses. Tl poisoning has a wide spectrum of clinical manifestation and any amount of Tl in the human body is abnormal. Moreover, it acts as a silent disease and diagnosis is sometimes difficult without suspicion. Our study showed that opium is a source of Tl in Iran and maybe in other parts of the world, so physicians should be aware of Tl exposure in opioid abusers, and they should be notified of its clinical symptoms. Although our findings suggested chronic Tl poisoning as an adulterant to illicit drugs, it should be noted that the findings may also result from cultivating opium poppies in Tl-contaminated soils or water.

Conclusion

As Tl is an accumulative poison [9], any illicit abuser subject with neuropathy, gastrointestinal complaints, and alopecia should be suspected of thallotoxicosis, and both urinary qualitative and quantitative Tl analyses would be helpful for exact diagnosis.

Limitations

This study is subjected to certain limitations because of the incontinency of opioid concentration and dose in the street drug abusers.

Competing interests

The authors declare that they have no competing interests.

Authors' contributions

AG clinical work and data collection. ZO drafting the manuscript NV and VM: Data collection RA: Research design, data interpretation, revising the manuscript. OM darafting the manuscript and revising the manuscript. All authors read and approved the final manuscript.

Acknowledgement

This research was supported by Addiction Research Center, Mashhad University of Medical Science (MUMS/2013–920441).

Author details

[1]Department of Addiction studies, School of Medical Kashan University of Medical Sciences, Kashan, Iran. [2]Departments of Pharmacodynamics and Toxicology, School of Pharmacy, Mashhad University of Medical Sciences, Mashhad, Iran. [3]Department of Clinical Toxicology, Kerman University of Medical Sciences, Kerman, Iran. [4]Addiction Research Centre, Mashhad University of Medical Sciences, Imam Reza Hospital, Ibn-e-Sina Street, Mashhad 91735-348, Iran. [5]British Columbia Center for Disease Control, Vancouver, Canada. [6]Atherosclerosis and Coronary Artery Research Center, Birjand University of Medical Science, Birjand, Iran.

References

1. Galván-Arzate S, Santamaría A. Thallium toxicity. Toxicol Lett. 1998;99(1):1–13.
2. Cvjetko P, Cvjetko I, Pavlica M. Thallium toxicity in humans. Arh Hig Rada Toksikol. 2010;61(1):111–9.
3. Mulkey JP, Oehme FW. A review of thallium toxicity. Vet Hum Toxicol. 1993;35(5):445–53.
4. Lech T, Sadlik JK. Thallium intoxication in humans. Toxicol Lett. 2007;172:S85.
5. Ibrahim D, Froberg B, Wolf A, Rusyniak DE. Heavy metal poisoning: clinical presentations and pathophysiology. Clin Lab Med. 2006;26(1):67–97. viii.
6. Misra UK, Kalita J, Yadav RK, Ranjan P. Thallium poisoning: emphasis on early diagnosis and response to haemodialysis. Postgrad Med J. 2003;79(928):103–5.
7. Hasan M, Chandra SV, Dua PR, Raghubir R, Ali SF. Biochemical and electrophysiologic effects of thallium poisoning on the rat corpus striatum. Toxicol Appl Pharmacol. 1977;41(2):353–9.
8. Ghannoum M, Nolin TD, Goldfarb DS, Roberts DM, Mactier R, Mowry JB, et al. Extracorporeal treatment for thallium poisoning: recommendations from the EXTRIP Workgroup. Clin J Am Soc Nephrol. 2012;7(10):1682–90.
9. Jha S, Kumar R, Kumar R. Thallium poisoning presenting as paresthesias, paresis, psychosis and pain in abdomen. J Assoc Physicians India. 2006;54:53–5.
10. Afshari R, Emadzadeh A. Short communication: case report on adulterated opium-induced severe lead toxicity. Drug Chem Toxicol. 2010;33(1):48–9.
11. Aghaee-Afshar M, Khazaeli P, Behnam B, Rezazadehkermani M, Ashraf-Ganjooei N. Presence of lead in opium. Arch Iran Med. 2008;11(5):553–4.
12. Questel F, Dugarin J, Dally S. Thallium-contaminated heroin. Ann Intern Med. 1996;124(6):616.
13. Afshari R, Mégarbane B, Zavar A. Thallium poisoning: one additional and unexpected risk of heroin abuse. Clin Toxicol. 2012;50(8):791–2.
14. Thallium health monitoring guidelines,PN10474 Version 2. Last updated June 2012.accessed 2014 April www.deir.qld.gov.au/workplace/…/ddp-thalliumguide.pdf.
15. Ćurković M, Sipos L, Puntarić D, Dodig-Ćurković K, Pivac N, Kralik K. Detection of thallium and uranium in well water and biological specimens of an eastern Croatian population. Arch Ind Hyg Toxicol. 2013;64(3):385–94.
16. Flanagan RJ, Braithwaite RA, Brown SS, Widdop B, Wolff FA. Basic Analytical Toxicology. 1st ed. Geneva: World Health Organization; 1995.
17. Ediger R. Atomic absorption analysis with the graphite furnace using matrix modification. Atomic Absorption Newsletter. 1975;14(5):127–30.
18. Christian G, Purdy W. Coulometric determination of thallium in blood and urine. Am J Clin Pathol. 1966;46(2):185.
19. Savory J, Roszel N, Mushak P, Sunderman F. Measurements of thallium in biologic materials by atomic absorption spectrometry. Am J Clin Pathol. 1968;50(4):505.
20. Fuller C. The effect of acids on the determination of thallium by atomic absorption spectrometry with a graphite furnace. Anal Chim Acta. 1976;81(1):199–202.
21. Karrari P, Mehrpour O, Afshari R, Keyler D. Pattern of illicit drug use in patients referredto addiction treatment centres in Birjand, Eastern Iran. J Pak Med Assoc. 2013;63(6):711–6.
22. Mehrpour O, Karrari P, Sheikhazadi A. Survey of factors related to criminal behavior in a sample of Iranian substance abusers. J Forensic Leg Med. 2013;20(8):1078–81.
23. Mehrpour O, Karrari P, Abdollahi M. Chronic lead poisoning in Iran; a silent disease. Daru. 2012;20(1):8.
24. Karrari P, Mehrpour O, Abdollahi M. A systematic review on status of lead pollution and toxicity in Iran: Guidance for preventive measures. Daru. 2012;20(1):2.
25. Jalili M, Azizkhani R. Lead toxicity resulting from chronic ingestion of opium. West J Emerg Med. 2009;10(4):244–146.
26. Mehrpour O. Addiction and seizure ability oftramadol in high-risk patients. Indian J Anaesth. 2013;57(1):86–7.
27. Taghaddosinejad F, Mehrpour O, Afshari R, Seghatoleslami A, Abdollahi M, Dart RC. Factors related to seizure in tramadol poisoning and its blood concentration. J Med Toxicol. 2011;7(3):183–8.

Phthalimide analogs as probable 15-lipoxygenase-1 inhibitors: synthesis, biological evaluation and docking studies

Alireza Aliabadi[1,2*], Ahmad Mohammadi-Farani[1,3], Zeinab Hosseinzadeh[2,4], Hamid Nadri[5], Alireza Moradi[5] and Farahnaz Ahmadi[1,3]

Abstract

Background: Recent studies have been explained the role of lipoxygenases (LOX) in the origin of cancer. Among the lipoxygenases, the 5-LOX, 12-LOX and 15-LOX are more important in the cause of neoplastic disorders. In the present investigation, a new series of anticancer agents with 1,3,4-thiadiazole and phthalimide substructures were synthesized and their *in vitro* cytotoxicity was evaluated by MTT assay. Moreover, enzyme inhibitory potency was also assessed by enzymatic protocol towards 15-LOX-1. Molecular docking was performed to explore *in silico* binding mode of the target compounds.

Results: Tested compounds showed a better cytotoxic activity against HT29 cell line (colorectal cancer) in comparison with other cell lines (PC3: prostate carcinoma; SKNMC: neuroblastoma). Unfortunately, all of the tested derivatives rendered lower inhibitory potency than quercetin towards 15-LOX-1. Four hydrogen bonds were detected in docking studies for compound **4d** as the most potent derivative in enzymatic assay.

Conclusions: The biological results of reported compounds in this research were not so satisfactory. But, further structural modifications are necessary to improve the bioactivity of these derivatives.

Keywords: Synthesis, Phthalimide, 1,3,4-Thiadiazole, Lipoxygenase, Anticancer

Background

Arachidonic acid is a fatty acid released from membrane phospholipids during cell stimulation. Arachidonic acid is metabolized mainly by two groups of enzymes consist of lipoxygenases (LOX, which includes 5-LOX, 12-LOX, and 15-LOX) and cyclooxygenase (COX). Inhibition of cyclooxygenases delays tumorigenesis in animals and humans [1, 2]. Various epidemiological and animal studies have confirmed that there is a close relationship between high fat consumption with an increased incidence and growth of tumors at several specific organ sites like breast. More recent studies also presented that patients with consumption of diets with a high proportion of polyunsaturated ω-6 fatty acid (n-6 PUFA), such as arachidonic acid and linoleic acid are associated with a more advanced disease stage at the time of diagnosis of breast cancer [2]. The LOXs convert polyunsaturated fatty acids like arachidonic and linoleic acids into biologically active metabolites that affects various cellular events such as signaling, structure and metabolism. According to the later tumorigenesis studies, it is likely that polyunsaturated fatty acids may enhance tumorigenesis via oxidative metabolism. Eicosanoids derived from the arachidonic acid cascade have been implicated in the pathogenesis of a variety of human diseases, including cancer, and are now believed to play important roles in tumor promotion, progression, and metastatic disease [3–5]. Vigorous expression of the enzymes (LOXs & COXs) that synthesize bioactive lipid metabolites from unsaturated fatty acids (arachidonic acid and linoleic acid) appears to be related to the development of prostate carcinoma remarkably. Other research have also reported that 15-LO-2 is expressed in normal prostate tissue, but poorly expressed in prostate tumors. Thus, 15-LO-1 is highly expressed in prostate tumors while 15-LO-2 is highly expressed in normal tissue. 15-LO-1 in prostate cancer tumors

* Correspondence: aliabadi.alireza@gmail.com
[1]Pharmaceutical Sciences Research Center, School of Pharmacy, Kermanshah University of Medical Sciences, Kermanshah, Iran
[2]Department of Medicinal Chemistry, Faculty of Pharmacy, Kermanshah University of Medical Sciences, Kermanshah, Iran
Full list of author information is available at the end of the article

converts linoleic acid, its preferred substrate to 13-*S*-hydroxy-octadecadienoic acid (13-(*S*)-HODE) and other metabolites. These metabolites appear to alter cellular signaling pathways, and thus the inappropriate expression might alter biological events and contribute to tumor development [6–8]. On the basis of this information, the drugs with capability of interaction with pathways related to the production of lipoxygenases metabolites or signaling functions of lipoxygenases products may be effective pharmaceutical agents in prevention or treatment of cancer.

Literature reviews declare that 1,3,4-thiadiazole ring as 5-membered heterocycle have diverse biological effects such as anti-inflammatory, anticonvulsant, antibacterial, antileshmanial, antioxidant and anticancer [9–20]. On the other hands, phthalimide moiety is another heterocyclic residue derived from the isoindole ring. This moiety has also exhibited several pharmacological activities like anticonvulsant, antitubercular, anti-inflammatory, anti-acetylcholinesterase as well as anticancer effects [21–31]. In the current investigation, we encouraged to synthesize a new series of chemical entities bearing 1,3,4-thiadiazole and phthalimide (isoindoline-1,3-dione) residues as potential anticancer agents.

Methods

Chemistry

The corresponding chemical reagents and starting materials were purchased from the commercial companies such as Merck and Sigma-Aldrich. The purification of the prepared compounds was carried out by column chromatography using ethyl acetate/petroleum ether. Spectroscopic methods were applied for characterization of the synthesized compounds. ^{1}H NMR spectra were acquired by Bruker 250 MHz in deutrated chloroform ($CDCl_3$) and the obtained data were expressed as δ (ppm) compared to tetramethylsilane (TMS) as internal standard. Infrared (IR) spectra of the prepared compounds were obtained by Shimadzu 470 with preparing potassium bromide (KBr) disk. The mass spectra were run on a Finigan TSQ-70 spectrometer (Finigan, USA) at 70 eV. Melting points were determined using electrothermal 9001 melting point analyzer apparatus and are uncorrected.

Synthesis of 2-(1,3-Dioxoisoindolin-2-yl)acetic acid (2)

5 g (33.8 mmol) of phthalic anhydride, 2.53 g (33.8 mmol) glycine and 4.67 ml (33.8 mmol) triethylamine (Et_3N) were mixed in toluene (100 ml) and the reaction mixture was refluxed overnight (Scheme 1). The reaction was monitored by thin layer chromatography (TLC). Toluene was evaporated by rotary evaporator apparatus under reduced pressure. The obtained residue was washed by diethyl ether (Et_2O) and *n*-hexane. The obtained white powder was used for the next step without any extra purification [32].

^{1}HNMR ($CDCl_3$, 250 MHz) δ (ppm): 4.3 (s, 2H, $-CH_2-$), 7.70 (dd, 2H, $J = 8.4$ Hz, $J = 2.4$ Hz, $H_{5,6}$-Phthalimide), 7.85

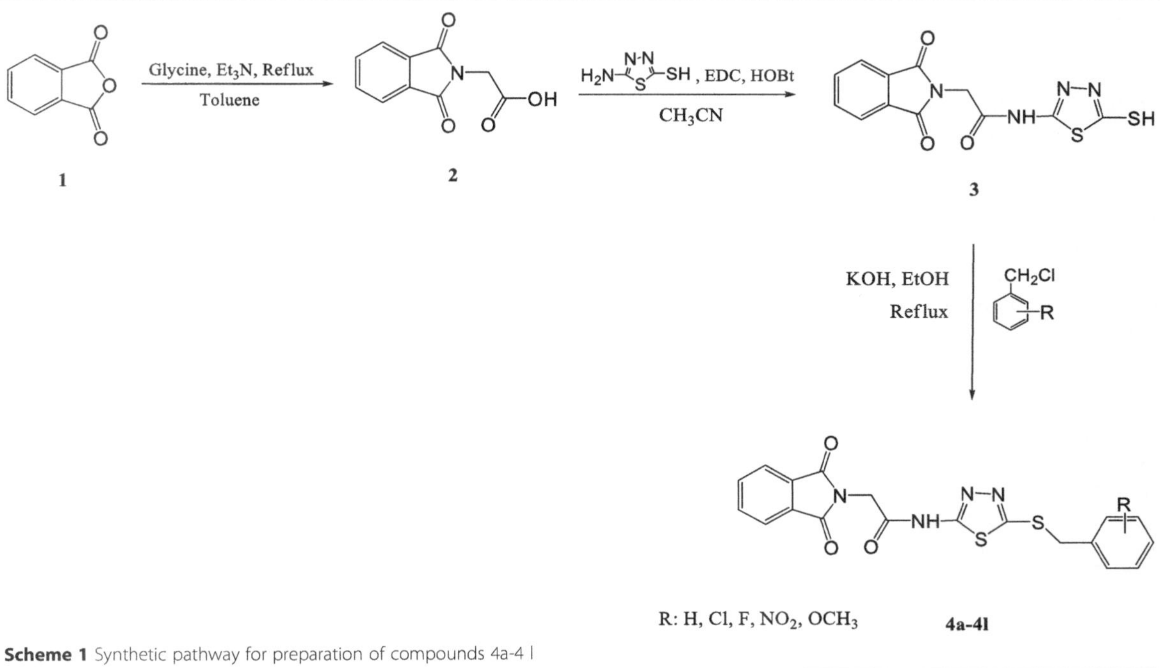

Scheme 1 Synthetic pathway for preparation of compounds 4a-4 l

(dd, 2H, $J = 8.4$ Hz, $J = 2.4$ Hz, $H_{4,7}$-Phthalimide), 11.97 (brs, –COOH). IR (KBr, cm^{-1}) ῡ: 3468 (OH, acid), 3155, 2989, 2939, 1705 (C=O, acid). MS (*m/z*, %): 205 (M^+, weak), 160 (100), 133 (20), 104 (40), 76 (35), 50 (20).

***Synthesis of 2-(1,3-Dioxoisoindolin-2-yl)-N-(5-mercapto-1,3,4-thiadiazol-2-yl)acetamide* (3)**

3 g (14.63 mmol) of 2-(1,3-dioxoisoindolin-2-yl)acetic acid (compound **2**), 2.80 g (14.63 mmol) *N*-ethyl-*N*-dimethylaminopropyl carbodiimide (EDC) and 1.98 g (14.63 mmol) hydroxybenzotriazole (HOBt) were mixed in 70 ml acetonitrile (CH_3CN) and the obtained mixture was stirred for 30 min. Then, 1.95 g (14.63 mmol) of 5-amino-1,3,4-thiadiazole-2-thiol was added to the reaction mixture and the stirring was continued for 24 h. The reaction end was proved by thin layer chromatography (TLC). Then, acetonitrile was evaporated using rotary evaporator and the residue was washed by diethyl ether and *n*-hexane. More purification was done by column chromatogaraphy (petroleum ether/ethyl acetate 70/30) to afford a yellowish powder [33–35].

^{1}HNMR ($CDCl_3$, 250 MHz) δ (ppm): 4.81 (s, 2H, $-CH_2$-CO-), 3.82 (s, 1H, SH), 7.89 (dd, 2H, $J = 8.4$ Hz, $J = 2.4$ Hz, $H_{5,6}$-Phthalimide), 7.94 (dd, 2H, $J = 8.4$ Hz, $J = 2.4$ Hz, $H_{5,6}$-Phthalimide), 13.81 (brs, NH). IR (KBr, cm^{-1}) ῡ: 3201, 3070, 2924, 1739, 1608, 1554, 1465, 1377, 1307, 1053, 717. MS (*m/z*, %): 320 (10), 287 (80), 263 (60), 231 (100), 160 (80), 159 (60), 121 (40), 104 (40), 76 (45).

***General procedure for synthesis of compounds* 4a-4 l**

In a flat bottom flask, 0.2 g (0.625 mmol) of 2-(1,3-dioxoisoindolin-2-yl)-*N*-(5-mercapto-1,3,4-thiadiazol-2-yl)acetamide (compound **3**) was treated with 0.035 g (0.625 mmol) potassium hydroxide in absolute ethanol and heated for 5 min, then equimolar (0.625 mmol) quantity of appropriate benzyl chloride derivative was added to the reaction medium and reflux condition was performed for 24 h. Thin layer chromatography (TLC) was carried out to determine the reaction end. Then, crushed ice was added to the reaction flask and the formed precipitate was filtered and collected. Crystallization was performed using ethanol [35].

***2-(1,3-Dioxoisoindolin-2-yl)-N-(5-(2-nitrobenzylthio)-1,3,4-thiadiazol-2-yl)acetamide* (4a)**

^{1}HNMR ($CDCl_3$, 250 MHz) δ (ppm): 4.79 (s, 2H, –S-CH_2-), 4.89 (s, 2H, $-CH_2$-CO-), 7.45 (t, 1H, H_4-2-Nitrophenyl), 7.57 (m, 2H, $H_{5,6}$-2-Nitrophenyl), 7.81 (dd, 2H, $J = 8.4$ Hz, $J = 2.4$ Hz, $H_{5,6}$-Phthalimide), 7.95 (dd, 2H, $J = 8.4$ Hz, $J = 2.4$ Hz, $H_{5,6}$-Phthalimide), 8.06 (d, 1H, $J = 10$ Hz, H_3-2-Nitrophenyl). IR (KBr, cm^{-1}) ῡ: 3414, 3325, 3170, 3035, 2927, 2854, 2742, 1774, 1720, 1573, 1523, 1415, 1346, 1303, 1195, 952, 713.

***2-(1,3-Dioxoisoindolin-2-yl)-N-(5-(3-nitrobenzylthio)-1,3,4-thiadiazol-2-yl)acetamide* (4b)**

^{1}HNMR ($CDCl_3$, 250 MHz) δ (ppm): 4.45 (s, 2H, –S-CH_2-), 4.77 (s, 2H, $-CH_2$-CO-), 7.48-7.59 (m, 2H, 3-Nitrophenyl), 7.73 (dd, 2H, $J = 8.4$ Hz, $J = 2.4$ Hz, $H_{5,6}$-Phthalimide), 7.92 (d, 1H, $J = 7.5$ Hz, H_4-3-Nitrophenyl), 8.24 (dd, 2H, $J = 8.4$ Hz, $J = 2.4$ Hz, $H_{4,7}$-Phthalimide), 8.36 (s, 1H, H_2-3-Nitrophenyl). IR (KBr, cm^{-1}) ῡ: 3429, 3209, 3066, 2924, 2854, 1774, 1708, 1527, 1411, 1350, 1296, 1195, 1053, 952, 717. MS (*m/z*, %): 455 (M^+, Weak), 398 (15), 268 (100), 235 (35), 193 (45), 136 (55), 109 (15), 89 (30), 60 (35).

***2-(1,3-Dioxoisoindolin-2-yl)-N-(5-(4-nitrobenzylthio)-1,3,4-thiadiazol-2-yl)acetamide* (4c)**

^{1}HNMR ($CDCl_3$, 250 MHz) δ (ppm): 4.42 (s, 2H, –S-CH_2-), 4.79 (s, 2H, $-CH_2$-CO-), 7.52 (d, 2H, $J = 10$ Hz, $H_{2,6}$-4-Nitrophenyl), 7.79 (dd, 2H, $J = 8.4$ Hz, $J = 2.4$ Hz, $H_{5,6}$-Phthalimide), 7.91 (dd, 2H, $J = 8.4$ Hz, $J = 2.4$ Hz, $H_{4,7}$-Phthalimide), 8.2 (d, 2H, $J = 10$ Hz, $H_{2,6}$-4-Nitrophenyl). IR (KBr, cm^{-1}) ῡ: 3421, 3352, 3113, 2927, 2850, 1774, 1720, 1519, 1415, 1346, 1303, 1107, 952, 713. MS (*m/z*, %): 455 (M^+, Weak), 398 (12), 268 (100), 235 (20), 193 (90), 136 (30), 109 (25), 89 (60), 60 (40).

***2-(1,3-Dioxoisoindolin-2-yl)-N-(5-(3-methoxybenzylthio)-1,3,4-thiadiazol-2-yl)acetamide* (4d)**

^{1}HNMR ($CDCl_3$, 250 MHz) δ (ppm): 3.74 (s, 3H, $-OCH_3$), 4.38 (s, 2H, –S-CH_2-), 4.86 (s, 2H, $-CH_2$-CO-), 6.77 (d, 1H, $J = 10$ Hz, H_4-3-Methoxyphenyl), 6.92 (m, 2H, H_2, H_6 -3-Methoxyphenyl), 7.20 (t, 1H, $J = 7.5$ Hz, H_5-3-Methoxyphenyl), 7.77 (dd, 2H, $J = 8.4$ Hz, $J = 2.4$ Hz, $H_{5,6}$-Phthalimide), 7.92 (dd, 2H, $J = 8.4$ Hz, $J = 2.4$ Hz, $H_{4,7}$-Phthalimide). IR (KBr, cm^{-1}) ῡ: 3425, 3329, 3170, 3035, 2927, 2850, 1720, 1624, 1577, 1415, 1303, 1269, 1159, 1049, 952, 713. MS (*m/z*, %): 440 (M^+, 10), 160 (40), 121 (100), 104 (45), 92 (20), 76 (35), 65 (60), 52 (55).

***2-(1,3-Dioxoisoindolin-2-yl)-N-(5-(4-methoxybenzylthio)-1,3,4-thiadiazol-2-yl)acetamide* (4e)**

^{1}HNMR ($CDCl_3$, 250 MHz) δ (ppm): 3.76 (s, 3H, $-OCH_3$), 4.35 (s, 2H, –S-CH_2-), 4.85 (s, 2H, $-CH_2$-CO-), 6.82 (d, 2H, $J = 7.5$ Hz, $H_{3,5}$-4-Mehoxyphenyl), 7.28 (d, 2H, $J = 7.5$ Hz, $H_{2,6}$-4-Mehoxyphenyl), 7.77 (dd, $J = 8.4$ Hz, $J = 2.4$ Hz, 2H, $H_{5,6}$-Phthalimide), 7.92 (dd, 2H, $J = 8.4$ Hz, $J = 2.4$ Hz, $H_{5,6}$-Phthalimide). IR (KBr, cm^{-1}) ῡ: 3325, 3248, 3132, 3035, 2927, 2850, 1774, 1705, 1627, 1577, 1419, 1307, 1246, 1195, 1180, 1064, 952. MS (*m/z*, %): 440 (M^+, Weak), 249 (10), 193 (10), 160 (60), 121 (100), 104 (30), 92 (40), 76 (75), 65 (70), 52 (45).

2-(1,3-Dioxoisoindolin-2-yl)-N-(5-(2-fluorobenzylthio)-1,3,4-thiadiazol-2-yl)acetamide **(4f)**

^{1}HNMR ($CDCl_3$, 250 MHz) δ (ppm): 4.47 (s, 2H, S-CH_2-), 4.83 (s, –CH_2-CO-), 7.04-7.09 (m, 4H, 2-Fluorophenyl), 7.79 (dd, 2H, J = 8.4 Hz, J = 2.4 Hz, $H_{5,6}$-Phthalimide), 7.91 (dd, 2H, J = 8.4 Hz, J = 2.4 Hz, $H_{4,7}$-Phthalimide). IR (KBr, cm^{-1}) ῡ: 3429, 3329, 3170, 2924, 2854, 2738, 1774, 1720, 1624, 1573, 1492, 1415, 1303, 1195, 952, 759. MS (*m/z*, %): 428 (M^+, 12), 371 (25), 241 (20), 166 (30), 109 (100), 83 (10).

2-(1,3-Dioxoisoindolin-2-yl)-N-(5-(3-fluorobenzylthio)-1,3,4-thiadiazol-2-yl)acetamide **(4 g)**

^{1}HNMR ($CDCl_3$, 250 MHz) δ (ppm): 4.39 (s, 2H, –S-CH_2-), 4.85 (s, 2H, –CH_2-CO-), 6.92 (t, 1H, J = 7.5 Hz, H_5-3-Fluorophenyl), 7.11 (m, 2H, H_4, H_6 -3-Fluorophenyl), 7.24 (m, 1H, H_2-3-Fluorophenyl), 7.77 (dd, 2H, J = 8.4 Hz, J = 2.4 Hz, $H_{5,6}$-Phthalimide), 7.92 (dd, 2H, J = 8.4 Hz, J = 2.4 Hz, $H_{5,6}$-Phthalimide), 13.70 (brs, NH). IR (KBr, cm^{-1}) ῡ: 3444, 3170, 3035, 2924, 2854, 1774, 1720, 1566, 1415, 1300, 952, 713. MS (*m/z*, %): 428 (M^+, 15), 371 (30), 241 (40), 166 (25), 109 (100), 83 (10).

2-(1,3-Dioxoisoindolin-2-yl)-N-(5-(4-fluorobenzylthio)-1,3,4-thiadiazol-2-yl)acetamide **(4 h)**

^{1}HNMR ($CDCl_3$, 250 MHz) δ (ppm): 4.36 (s, 2H, –S-CH_2-), 4.86 (s, 2H, –CH_2-CO-), 6.99 (t, 2H, $H_{2,6}$-4-Fluorophenyl), 7.32 (t, 2H, $H_{3,5}$-4-Fluorophenyl), 7.77 (dd, 2H, J = 8.4 Hz, J = 2.4 Hz, $H_{5,6}$-Phthalimide), 7.92 (dd, 2H, J = 8.4 Hz, J = 2.4 Hz, $H_{4,7}$-Phthalimide). IR (KBr, cm^{-1}) ῡ: 3433, 3329, 3159, 3039, 2927, 2850, 1774, 1720, 1624, 1573, 1508, 1415, 1303, 1226, 1087, 952, 831, 713. MS (*m/z*, %): 428 (10), 371 (20), 241 (10), 166 (40), 109 (100), 83 (12).

N-(5-(2-Chlorobenzylthio)-1,3,4-thiadiazol-2-yl)-2-(1,3-dioxoisoindolin-2-yl)acetamide **(4i)**

^{1}HNMR ($CDCl_3$, 250 MHz) δ (ppm): 4.54 (s, 2H, –S-CH_2-), 4.87 (s, 2H, –CH_2-CO-), 7.20 (m, 2H, $H_{3,6}$-2-Chlorophenyl), 7.35 (t, 1H, H_4-2-Chlorophenyl), 7.43 (t, 1H, H_5-2-Chlorophenyl), 7.77 (dd, 2H, J = 8.4 Hz, J = 2.4 Hz, $H_{5,6}$-Phthalimide), 7.92 (dd, 2H, J = 8.4 Hz, J = 2.4 Hz, $H_{4,7}$-Phthalimide). IR (KBr, cm^{-1}) ῡ: 3475, 3429, 3170, 3051, 2927, 2858, 2738, 1774, 1720, 1566, 1469, 1415, 1300, 1195, 952, 713. MS (*m/z*, %): 446 (M^++2, 4), 444 (M^+, 10), 284 (12), 162 (10), 160 (85), 125 (100), 104 (10), 76 (15).

N-(5-(3-Chlorobenzylthio)-1,3,4-thiadiazol-2-yl)-2-(1,3-dioxoisoindolin-2-yl)acetamide **(4j)**

^{1}HNMR ($CDCl_3$, 250 MHz) δ (ppm): 4.37 (s, 2H, –S-CH_2-), 4.85 (s, 2H, –CH_2-CO-), 7.24 (m, 3H, 3-Chlorophenyl), 7.41 (s, 1H, H_2-3-Chlorophenyl), 7.77 (dd, 2H, J = 8.4 Hz, J = 2.4 Hz, $H_{5,6}$-Phthalimide), 7.92 (dd, 2H, J = 8.4 Hz, J = 2.4 Hz, $H_{4,7}$-Phthalimide). IR (KBr, cm^{-1}) ῡ: 3325, 3170, 3055, 2927, 2850, 1720, 1627, 1573, 1400, 1300, 1203, 1111, 1083, 1049, 956, 713, 648. MS (*m/z*, %): 446 (M^++2, 5), 444 (M^+, 15), 162 (25), 160 (50), 125 (100), 104 (30), 76 (35).

N-(5-(4-Chlorobenzylthio)-1,3,4-thiadiazol-2-yl)-2-(1,3-dioxoisoindolin-2-yl)acetamide **(4 k)**

^{1}HNMR ($CDCl_3$, 250 MHz) δ (ppm): 4.35 (s, 2H, –S-CH_2-), 4.85 (s, 2H, –CH_2-CO-), 7.28 (dd, 4H, 4-Chlorophenyl), 7.77 (dd, 2H, J = 8.4 Hz, J = 2.4 Hz, $H_{5,6}$-Phthalimide), 7.91 (dd, 2H, J = 8.4 Hz, J = 2.4 Hz, $H_{5,6}$-Phthalimide). IR (KBr, cm^{-1}) ῡ: 3325, 3155, 3059, 3035, 2927, 2850, 1774, 1720, 1627, 1573, 1492, 1303, 1091. MS (*m/z*, %): 446 (M^++2, 5), 444 (M^+, 12), 284 (5), 162 (15), 160 (90), 125 (100), 104 (20), 76 (25).

N-(5-(Benzylthio)-1,3,4-thiadiazol-2-yl)-2-(1,3-dioxoisoindolin-2-yl)acetamide **(4 l)**

^{1}HNMR ($CDCl_3$, 250 MHz) δ (ppm): 4.39 (s, 2H, –S-CH_2-), 4.86 (s, 2H, –CH_2-CO-), 7.23-7.37 (m, 5H, Phenyl), 7.77 (dd, 2H, J = 8.4 Hz, J = 2.4 Hz, $H_{5,6}$-Phthalimide), 7.92 (dd, 2H, J = 8.4 Hz, J = 2.4 Hz, $H_{4,7}$-Phthalimde). IR (KBr, cm^{-1}) ῡ: 3425, 3329, 3170, 3032, 2927, 2850, 1720, 1627, 1573, 1546, 1415, 1396, 1303, 1195, 1111, 952, 709. MS (410, M^+), 160 (75), 91 (100), 77 (10).

MTT assay

Synthesized derivatives (compounds **4a-4 l**) were tested for cytotoxic activity at 0.1-100 μM concentration in three human cancer cell lines of PC3 (Prostate carcinoma), HT29 (Colorectal cancer) and SKNMC (Neuroblastoma). Cells were purchased from the Pasteur Institute of Iran. Cells from different cell lines were seeded in 96-well plates at the density of 8000–10,000 viable cells per well and incubated for 24 h to allow cell attachment. The cells were then incubated for another 24 h with various concentrations of compounds **4a-4 l**. Cells were then washed in PBS, and 20 μL of MTT (3–(4,5-dimethylthiazol-2-yl)-2,5-diphenyl tetrazolium bromide solution (5 mg/mL) were added to each well. An additional 4 h of incubation at 37 °C were done, and then the medium was discarded. Dimethyl sulfoxide (60 μL) was added to each well, and the solution was vigorously mixed to dissolve the purple tetrazolium crystals. The absorbance of each well was measured by plate reader (Anthous 2020; Austria) at a test wavelength of 550 nm against a standard reference solution at 690 nm. The amount of produced purple formazan is proportional to the percentage of cell viability [33–35].

15-Lipoxygenase-1 assay

The basis of this method is oxidative coupling of 3-methyl-2-benzothiazolinone hydrazone (MBTH) with 3 (dimethylamino) benzoic acid (DMAB) in a hemoglobin catalyzed reaction. This reaction is initiated in the presence of lipoxygenase reaction product, linoleic acid hydroperoxide and results in a blue color formation which has a peak absorbtion at 590 nm [36]. Quercetin was used as the reference compound. Linoleic acid and two stock solutions (A and B) were prepared first. Solution A contained 50 mM DMAB and 100 mM phosphate buffer (pH = 7.0). Solution B was prepared by mixing 10 mM MBTH (3 mL) and hemoglobin (5 mg/mL, 3 mL) in 50 mM phosphate buffer at pH 5.0 (25 mL). A linoleic acid solution (1 mg/ml) was prepared by diluting 5 mg linoleic acid (solubilised in 0.5 ml ethanol) with KOH 100 mM.

For each compound the samples were solved in ethanol (25 μl) and mixed in a test tube with SLO (4000 units/mL, prepared in 50 mM phosphate buffer pH = 7.0, 25 μL) and phosphate buffer (50 mM, pH = 7, 900 μL). After a 5 min delay at room temperature, 50 μL linoleic acid was added to the mixture to start the hydroperoxidation reaction. After 8 min, solution A (270 μL) and solution B (130 μL) were added to the above mixture. 5 min later, 200 μL of SDS solution (2 %) was added to stop the reaction. The absorbance at 590 nm was compared with control (ethanol without sample).

Docking

The related protein structure was downloaded from brookhaven protein data bank (http://RCSB.org). Namely, 15-Lipoxygenase-1 in complex with dihydroxybenzoic acid (pdb code: 1N8Q) was utilized. ArgusLab software 4.0 was used for drawing the chemical structures and then energy minimization was carried out using AM1 as semiemperical method [37]. The related ligand groups as well as binding site groups were defined. The binding location of dihydroxybenzoic aicd was defined as binding site for searching the best pose and conformation for all ligands. The geometry optimization of the protein structure was done by universal force field (UFF) as molecular mechanic method. Binding mode and related interactions of ligands with lipoxygense enzyme were explored in ArgusLab software.

Results and discussion

Chemistry

According to the Table 1 all intermediate and final compounds were prepared with an average yield. Compound **4a** with *ortho* nitro moiety obtained with a low yield (39 %) and compound **4c** with *para* nitro moiety prepared with an acceptable yield (74 %). For affording compound **2**, phthalic anhydride was reacted with glycine in the presence of triethylamine in toluene under reflux conditions to perform a Gabriel reaction. The white powder of compound **2** was treated with *N*-ethyl-*N*-dimethylaminopropyl carbodiimide (EDC) and hydroxybenzotriazole (HOBt) in acetonitrile and after 30 min, 5-amino-1,3,4-thiadiazole-2-thiol was added to form an amidic bond. The obtained thiol derivative was used for synthesis of the final products **4a–4 l** in alkaline medium that generated by potassium hydroxide in refluxing ethanol.

Synthesized compounds were characterized by spectroscopic methods such as ^1H NMR, IR and MS and corresponding melting points were also measured. Compound **4a** with *ortho* nitro moiety rendered the lowest melting point (179 °C) among the final products and compounds **4e** with *para* methoxy group demonstrated the highest melting point (259 °C) in these series. ^1H NMR spectra were acquired in deutrated chloroform ($CDCl_3$). In the most cases the acidic property of the proton of the amidic bond (NH group) was caused to not be appeared in the NMR spectra. Phthalimide group as well as 1,3,4-thiadiazole ring function as electron withdrawing groups and these have an important role in

Table 1 Properties of synthesized compounds

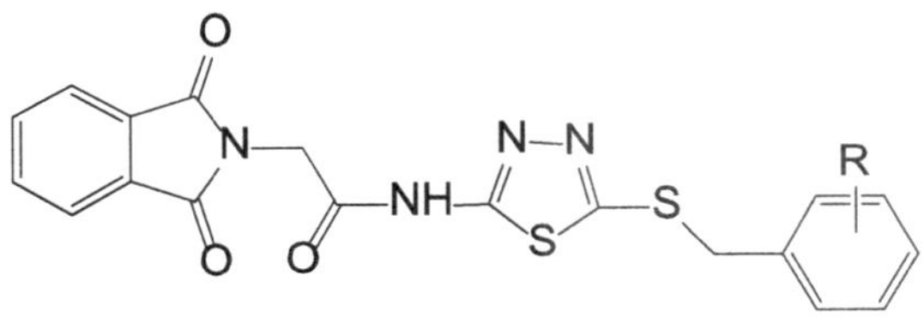

Compound	(R)	Closed formula	MW (g/mol)	m.p (°C)	Yield (%)
2	-	$C_{10}H_7NO_4$	205.4	115	70
3	-	$C_{12}H_8N_4O_3S_2$	320.3	220	48
4a	*o*-NO_2	$C_{19}H_{13}N_5O_5S_2$	455.4	179	39
4b	*m*-NO_2	$C_{19}H_{13}N_5O_5S_2$	455.4	243	46
4c	*p*-NO_2	$C_{19}H_{13}N_5O_5S_2$	455.4	204	74
4d	*m*-OCH_3	$C_{20}H_{16}N_4O_4S_2$	440.5	186	43
4e	*p*-OCH_3	$C_{20}H_{16}N_4O_4S_2$	440.5	259	41
4f	*o*-F	$C_{19}H_{13}FN_4O_3S_2$	428.4	190	48
4 g	*m*-F	$C_{19}H_{13}FN_4O_3S_2$	428.4	173	40
4 h	*p*-F	$C_{19}H_{13}FN_4O_3S_2$	428.4	154	57
4i	*o*-Cl	$C_{19}H_{13}ClN_4O_3S_2$	444.9	205	47
4j	*m*-Cl	$C_{19}H_{13}ClN_4O_3S_2$	444.9	188	57
4 k	*p*-Cl	$C_{19}H_{13}ClN_4O_3S_2$	444.9	155	45
4 l	H	$C_{19}H_{14}N_4O_3S_2$	410.4	187	53

enhancing the acidic property of the hydrogen of NH group.

Cytotoxicity evaluation

Three cancerous cell lines were used to test the anticancer activity of the final compounds **4a-4 l**. PC3 (Prostate carcinoma), HT29 (colorectal cancer) and SKNMC (neuroblastoma) was cultured and intended derivatives were assessed at concentration 0.1-100 μM and the obtained results were compared to doxorubicin as reference drug. None of the tested compounds showed superior cytotoxic effect than doxorubicin at tested concentrations towards the utilized cell lines. Generally tested derivatives exerted a better cytotoxic activity against HT29 cell line compared to other cell lines. PC3 and SKNMC cell lines were the most resistant cell lines to the tested compounds. None of the introduced moieties containing electron withdrawing groups and electron donating groups on the phenyl residue were efficacious to produce a remarkable anticancer activity.

Enzymatic assay

An enzyme inhibitory assay was performed towards 15-lipoxygenase-1 and obtained results were presented as percent of inhibition and provided in Table 2. Unfortunately, none of the tested derivatives demonstrated superior inhibitory effect than quercetin as reference compound and natural product inhibitor of the enzyme. Compound **4d** with *meta* positioning of the methoxy moiety was the most potent inhibitor in this series (38 % inhibition). Moving the position of the methoxy to the *para* decreased the inhibitory effect of the compound significantly as observed in compound **4e**. Nitro containing derivatives (**4a, 4b, 4c**) and compound **4 k** with *para* positioning of the chlorine substituent did not show any inhibitory activity against 15-lipoxygenase-1.

Molecular modeling

All prepared derivatives were docked by ArgusLab software into the active site of 15-lipoxygenase-1. Compound **4d** (m-OCH_3) as representative of synthesized compounds in this series that showed a superior enzyme inhibitory activity in enzymatic assay has been shown in Fig. 1. Four hydrogen bonds were detected with Ser 582, Ser 586 and Ala 587. One of the nitrogen atom of the 1,3,4-thiadiazole ring has participated in hydrogen bonding interaction with Ser 582. Amino acid Ser 586 has also formed two hydrogen bonding interactions with oxygen of the methoxy group. The first one is with oxygen atom of the hydroxyl group in the side chain of this amino acid and the second one is with related NH_2 group of the Ser 586. Finally, Ala 587 is responsible for the fourth hydrogen bond interaction. The NH of the amidic bond between Ala 587 and Ser 586 has the role of hydrogen bond donor to the oxygen of the methoxy group. This potential and probable hydrogen bonds maybe a logical reason for higher enzyme inhibitory potency of compound **4d** compared to others.

Structure activity relationship

Enzyme inhibitory effect of the final prepared compounds was investigated towards 15-lipoxygense-1 and obtained results were listed in Table 2. None of the tested derivatives exerted favorable inhibitory potency towards 15-LOX-1 at 200 μM concentration compared to quercetin as reference compound. Quercetin as

Table 2 Biological data of synthesized compounds. Results of the cytotoxicity assay were reported as $IC_{50} \pm SD$ (μM)

Compound	R	15-Lipoxygenase-1 (% of inhibition)[a]	PC3	HT29	SKNMC
4a	o-NO_2	NA[b]	100<	100<	100<
4b	m-NO_2	NA	>100	100<	100<
4c	p-NO_2	NA	100<	100<	100<
4d	m-OCH_3	38	100<	100<	100<
4e	p-OCH_3	11	100<	100<	100<
4f	*o*-F	31	100<	10.91 ± 4.1	100<
4 g	*m*-F	26	100<	100<	50.2 ± 5.4
4 h	*p*-F	35	88.83 ± 4.3	100<	100<
4i	*o*-Cl	17	81.92 ± 4.7	100<	100<
4j	*m*-Cl	18.5	89.21 ± 5.7	100<	100<
4 k	*p*-Cl	NA[a]	>100	24.06 ± 3.1	69.7 ± 3.6
4 l	H	19	>100	100<	100<
Doxorubicin	-	-	3.8 ± 0.75	2.1 ± 0.26	1.3 ± 0.4
Quercetin	-	100	-	-	-

a:The percent of inhibition was determined at 200 μM concentration
b:No activity

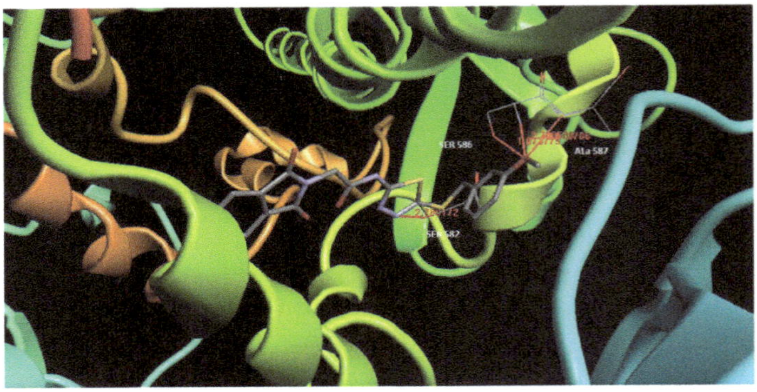

Fig. 1 Structure of docked compound 4d (m-OCH_3) into the active site of 15-lipoxygenase. Four hydrogen bonds were detected with Ser 582 (one), Ser 586 (two) and Ala 587 (one)

naturally occurring compound showed 100 % inhibition at 200 μM concentration. Among the tested derivatives, compound **4d** with *meta* positioning of the methoxy group afforded the highest inhibitory effect (38 %). Movement of the methoxy to the *para* position caused a detrimental effect and decreased the inhibitory activity. Nitro containing compounds (**4a, 4b, 4c**) as well as *para* chlorine containing compound (**4 k**) did not demonstrated any inhibitory activity at tested concentration. Fluorine containing derivatives also exhibited a high inhibitory activity compared to others. This inhibitory activity was more observable while the fluorine substituted at position *ortho* and *para*. It is probable that electron withdrawing effect of this moiety is a critical factor to increase the enzyme inhibitory effect. Replacement of the fluorine substituent with chlorine caused a decrease in activity. Chlorine atom has a greater size and lipophilicity than fluorine and it is likely that these parameters induce a negative effect on interaction of the ligands to the corresponding receptor.

Three cancerous cell lines were used to evaluate the *in vitro* cytotoxicity potency of synthesized derivatives. Unfortunately, tested compounds did not display a remarkable activity against utilized cell lines (Table 2). Only compounds **4f** (*ortho* fluorine) and **4 k** (*para* chlorine) rendered an acceptable cytotoxic potency against HT29 cell line. None of the nitro and methoxy substituted derivatives exerted an inhibitory potency (IC_{50}) up to 100 μM concentration. Substitution of the fluorine at *meta* position of the phenyl residue caused an enhancement in cytotoxic activity towards SKNMC cell line. *Para* positioning of the fluorine was also caused a brief increase in anticancer activity in PC3 cell line. A descending trend in IC_{50} was seen from compound **4i** (*o*-Cl) to **4 k** (*p*-Cl) against PC3 cell line. But, a reverse trend was demonstrated for chlorinated derivatives against HT29 and SKNMC cell lines. Steric factor and lipophilicity effects produced by chlorine atom maybe a probable reason for this observation.

Based on the above mentioned information, there is not any direct correlation between the cytotoxic activity and inhibition of lipoxygenase. According to the previously reported literature [34, 35], it could be hypothesized that inhibition of tyrosine kinases is the probable of cytotoxicity of these compounds.

Conclusions

A new series of compounds with combination of 1,3,4-thiadiazole and phthalimide substructures were synthesized and their cytotoxicity was evaluated *in vitro* using MTT protocol. Furthermore, synthesized derivatives were tested in an enzymatic assay for exploration of the inhibitory activity towards 15-lipoxygenase-1. According to the obtained results in MTT assay as well as enzymatic experiment, the investigated compounds did not show a favorable anticancer activity. Amongst them, only compounds **4f** (*ortho* fluorine) and **4 k** (*para* chlorine) exhibited an acceptable cytotoxic potency towards HT29 cell line. Hence, further structural modifications are needed to achieve derivatives with superior activity.

Competing interests

The authors declared that they have no competing interest.

Authors' contributions

AA: Synthesis Molecular Modelling. AM-F: Cytotoxicity assay. ZH: Contributor in all parts. HN: Enzymatic assay. AM: Enzymatic assay. FA: Cytotoxicity assay.

Acknowledgements

The authors are acknowledged from the research council of Kermanshah University of Medical Sciences due to financial support of the current research. This work was performed in partial fulfillment of the requirement for PharmD of Mrs Zeinab Hossseinzadeh.

Author details
[1]Pharmaceutical Sciences Research Center, School of Pharmacy, Kermanshah University of Medical Sciences, Kermanshah, Iran. [2]Department of Medicinal Chemistry, Faculty of Pharmacy, Kermanshah University of Medical Sciences, Kermanshah, Iran. [3]Department of Pharmacology, Toxicology and Medical Services, Faculty of Pharmacy, Kermanshah University of Medical Sciences, Kermanshah, Iran. [4]Students Research Committee, Kermanshah University of Medical Sciences, Kermanshah, Iran. [5]Neurobiomedical Research Center, Yazd Shahid Sadoughi University of Medical Sciences, Yazd, Iran.

References

1. Rioux N, Castonguay A. Inhibitors of lipoxygenase: a new class of cancer chemopreventive agents. Carcinogenesis. 1998;8:1393–400.
2. Tong WG, Ding XZ, Adrian TE. The mechanisms of lipoxygenase inhibitor-induced apoptosis in human breast cancer cells. Biochem Biophys Res Commun. 2002;296:942–8.
3. Steele VE, Holmes CV, Hawk ET, Kopelovich L, Lubet RA, Crowell JA. Lipoxygenase inhibitors as potential cancer chemopreventives. Cancer Epidemiol Biomarkers Prev. 1999;8:467–83.
4. Shureiqi I, Chen D, Jack Lee J, Yang P, Newman RA, Brenner DE, et al. 15-LOX-1: a novel molecular target of nonsteroidal anti-inflammatory drug-Induced apoptosis in colorectal cancer cells. J Natl Cancer Inst. 2000;14:1136–42.
5. Shureiqi I, Lippman SM. Lipoxygenase modulation to reverse carcinogenesis. Cancer Res. 2001;61:6307–12.
6. Kelavkar UP, Nixon JB, Cohen C, Dillehay D, Eling TE, Badr KF. Overexpression of 15-lipoxygenase-1 in PC-3 human prostate cancer cells increases tumorigenesis. Carcinogenesis. 2001;11:1765–73.
7. Shureiqi I, Xu X, Chen D, Lotan R, Morris JS, Fischer SM. Nonsteroidal anti-Inflammatory drugs induce apoptosis in esophageal cancer cells by restoring 15-Lipoxygenase-1 expression. Cancer Res. 2001;61:4879–84.
8. Mahdavi M, Shirazi MS, Taherkhani R, Saeedi M, Alipour E, Moghadam FH, et al. Synthesis, biological evaluation and docking study of 3-aroyl-1-(4-sulfamoylphenyl)thiourea derivatives as 15-lipoxygenase inhibitors. Eur J Med Chem. 2014;82:308–13.
9. Asadipour A, Edraki N, Nakhjiri M, Yahya-Meymandi A, Alipour E, Saniee P, et al. Anti-Helicobacter pylori activity and structure-activity relationship study of 2-Alkylthio-5-(nitroaryl)-1,3,4-thiadiazole derivatives. Iran J Pharm Res. 2013;3:281–7.
10. Mohammadhosseini N, Saniee P, Ghamaripour A, Aryapour H, Afshar F, Edraki N, et al. Synthesis and biological evaluation of novel benzyl piperazine derivatives of 5-(5-nitroaryl)-1,3,4-thiadiazoles as Anti-Helicobacter pylori agents. Daru: J Pharm Sci. 2013;1:66.
11. Moshafi MH, Sorkhi M, Emami S, Nakhjiri M, Yahya-Meymandi A, Negahbani AS, et al. 5-Nitroimidazole-based 1,3,4-thiadiazoles: heterocyclic analogs of metronidazole as anti-Helicobacter pylori agents. Arch Pharm Chem Life Sci. 2011;344(3):178–83.
12. Rajak H, Deshmukh R, Aggarwal N, Kashaw S, Kharya MD, Mishra P. Synthesis of novel 2,5-disubstituted 1,3,4-thiadiazoles for their potential anticonvulsant activity: pharmacophoric model studies. Arch Pharm Chem Life Sci. 2009;342:453–61.
13. Abdel-Aziz M, Aly OM, Khan SS, Mukherjee K, Bane S. Synthesis, Cytotoxic properties and tubulin polymerization inhibitory activity of novel 2-pyrazoline derivatives. Arch Pharm Chem Life Sci. 2012;345:535–48.
14. Mishra G, Singh AK, Jyoti K. Review article on 1,3,4-Thiadiazole derivatives and its pharmacological activities. Int J Chem Tech Res. 2011;3:1380–93.
15. Singh AK, Mishra G, Jyoti K. Review on Biological Activities of 1,3,4-Thiadiazole derivatives. J App Pharm Sci. 2011;5:44–9.
16. Kalidhar U, Kaur A. 1,3,4-Thiadiazole derivatives and their biological activities: A Review. Res J Pharm Biol Chem. 2011;4:1091–106.
17. Siddiqui N, Ahuja P, Ahsan W, Pandeya SN, Alam MS. Thiadiazoles: progress report on biological activities. J Chem Pharm Res. 2009;1:19–30.
18. Behrouzi-Fardmoghadam M, Poorrajab F, Kaboudanian Ardestani S, Emami S, Shafiee A, Foroumadi A. Synthesis and in vitro anti-leishmanial activity of 1-[5-(5-nitrofuran-2-yl)-1,3,4-thiadiazol-2-yl]- and 1-[5-(5-nitrothiophen-2-yl)-1,3,4-thiadiazol-2-yl]-4-aroylpiperazines. Bioorg Med Chem. 2008;16:4509–15.
19. Poorrajab F, Kaboudanian Ardestani S, Emami S, Behrouzi-Fardmoghadam M, Shafiee A, Foroumadi A. Nitroimidazolyl-1,3,4-thiadiazole-based anti-leishmanial agents: Synthesis and in vitro biological evaluation. Eur J Med Chem. 2009;4:1758–62.
20. Mirzaei J, Siavoshi F, Emami S, Safari F, Khoshayand MR, Shafiee A, et al. Synthesis and in vitro anti-Helicobacter pylori activity of *N*-[5-(5-nitro-2-heteroaryl)-1,3,4-thiadiazol-2-yl]thiomorpholines and related compounds. Eur J Med Chem. 2008;8:1575–80.
21. Kok SHL, Gambari R, Chui CH, Yuen MCW, Lin E, Wong RSM, et al. Synthesis and anti-cancer activity of benzothiazole containing phthalimide on human carcinoma cell lines. Bioorg Med Chem. 2008;16:3626–31.
22. Yang YJ, Yang YN, Jiang JS, Feng ZM, Liu HY, Pan XD, et al. Synthesis and cytotoxic activity of heterocycle-substituted phthalimide derivatives. Chin Chem Lett. 2010;21:902–4.
23. Machado AL, Lima LM, Araújo-Jr JX, Fraga CAM, Koatzc VLG, Barreiroa EJ. Design, synthesis and antiinflammatory activity of novel phthalimide derivatives, structurally related to thalidomide. Bioorg Med Chem Lett. 2005;15:1169–72.
24. Malgorzata W, Katarzyna K. Synthesis and anticonvulsant evaluation of some *N*-substituted phthalimides. Acta Pol Pharm. 2009;3:249–57.
25. Lee N-J, Jeong I-C, Cho M-Y, Jeon C-W, Yun B-C, Kim Y-O, et al. Synthesis and *in vitro* antitumor activity of phthalimide polymers containing podophyllotoxin. Eur Polym J. 2006;42:3352–9.
26. Lima LM, Brito FCF, Souza SD, Miranda ALP, Rodrigues CR, Fragaa CAM, et al. Novel phthalimide derivatives, designed as leukotriene D_4 receptor antagonists. Bioorg Med Chem Lett. 2002;12:1533–5.
27. Santos JL, Yamasaki PR, Chin CM, Takashi CH, Pavan FR, Leite CQF. Synthesis and in vitro anti mycobacterium tuberculosis activity of a series of phthalimide derivatives. Bioorg Med Chem. 2009;17:3795–9.
28. Mohammadi-Farani A, Ahmadi A, Nadri H, Aliabadi A. Synthesis, docking and acetylcholinesterase inhibitory assessment of 2-(2-(4-Benzylpiperazin-1-yl)ethyl)isoindoline-1,3-dione with potential anti-alzheimer effects. Daru J Pharm Sci. 2013;21:47–55.
29. Foroumadi A, Mohammadi-Farani A, Garmsiri Mahvar M, Aliabadi A. Synthesis and evaluation of anti-acetylcholinesterase activity of 2-(2-(4-(2-Oxo-2-phenylethyl)piperazin-1-yl)ethyl)isoindoline-1,3-dione derivatives with potential anti-Alzheimer effects. Iran J Basic Med Sci. 2013;10(16):1049–54.
30. Aliabadi A, Gholamine B, Karimi T. Synthesis and antiseizure evaluation of isoindoline-1,3-dione derivatives in mice. Med Chem Res. 2014;23:2736–43.
31. Aliabadi A, Foroumadi A, Safavi M, Kaboudian Ardestani S. Synthesis, molecular docking and cytotoxicity evaluation of 2-(4-substituted-benzyl)isoindoline-1,3-dione derivatives as anticancer agents. J Rep Pharm Sci. 2012;1:19–22.
32. Ragavendran JV, Sriram D, Patel SK, Reddy IV, Bharathwajan N, Stables J. Design and synthesis of anticonvulsants from a combined phthalimide-GABA-anilide and hydrazone pharmacophore. Eur J Med Chem. 2007;42:146–51.
33. Mohammadi-Farani A, Foroumadi A, Rezvani Kashani M, Aliabadi A. *N*-Phenyl-2-*p*-tolylthiazole-4-carboxamide derivatives: Synthesis and cytotoxicity evaluation as anticancer agents. Iran J Basic Med Sci. 2014;17:502–8.
34. Aliabadi A, Eghbalian E, Kiani A. Synthesis and cytotoxicity evaluation of a series of 1,3,4-thiadiazole based compounds as anticancer agents. Iran J Basic Med Sci. 2013;11:1133–8.
35. Aliabadi A, Hasanvand Z, Kiani A, Mirabdali SS. Synthesis and *in vitro* cytotoxicity assessment of *N*-(5-(Benzylthio)-1,3,4-thiadiazol-2-yl)-2-(4-(trifluoromethyl)phenyl)acetamide with potential anticancer activity. Iran J Pharm Res. 2013;4:687–93.
36. Anthon GE, Barrett DM. Colorimetric method for the determination of lipoxygenase activity. J Agric Food Chem. 2001;49:32–7.
37. ArgusLab 4.0 Mark A. Thompson Planaria Software LLC, Seattle, WA http://www.arguslab.com.

Repaglinide-loaded solid lipid nanoparticles: effect of using different surfactants/stabilizers on physicochemical properties of nanoparticles

Hossein Ali Ebrahimi[1,2,3], Yousef Javadzadeh[1,2], Mehrdad Hamidi[3,4*] and Mohammad Barzegar Jalali[2]

Abstract

Background: Repaglinide is an efficient anti-diabetic drug which is prescribed widely as multi-dosage oral daily regimens. Due to the low compliance inherent to each multi-dosage regimen, development of prolonged-release formulations could enhance the overall drug efficacy in patient populations.

Methods: Repaglinide-loaded solid lipid nanoparticles (SLNs) were developed and characterized in vitro. Various surfactants were used in this study during the nanocarrier preparation procedure and their corresponding effects on some physicochemical properties of SLNs such as size, zeta potential; drug loading parameters and drug release profiles was investigated. Stearic acid and glyceryl mono stearate (GMS) were used as lipid phase and phosphatidylcholin, Tween80, Pluronic F127, poly vinyl alcohol (PVA) and polyvinyl pyrrolidone (PVP) were used as surfactant/stabilizer.

Results: The results showed some variations between formulations; where the Tween80-based SLNs showed smallest size, the phosphatidylcholin-based SLNs indicated most prolonged drug release time and the highest loading capacity. SEM images of these formulations showed morphological variations and also confirmed the nanoscale size of these particles. The FTIR and DSC results demonstrated no interaction between drug and excipients. The *invitro* release profiles of different formulations were studied and observed slow release of drug from all formulations. However significant differences were found among them in terms of their initial burst release as well as the whole drug release profile. From fitting these data to various statistical models, the Peppas model was proposed as the best model to describe the statistical indices and, therefore, mechanism of drug release.

Conclusion: The results of this study confirmed the effect of surfactant type on SLNs physicochemical properties such as morphological features, loading parameters, particle sizes and drug release kinetic. With respect to the outcome data, the mixture of phosphatidylcholin/Pluronic F127 was selected as the best surfactant/stabilizer to coat the lipid core comprising stearic acid and GMS.

Introduction

Diabetes mellitus is a wide spread chronic disease with serious life-threatening effects on different parts/functions throughout the body. The majority of diabetic patients are found to be type II diabetes mellitus, i.e., (non-insulin-dependent). To manage this type of diabetes, different classes of oral anti-diabetic drugs are used routinely in the market [1]. Repaglinide, a drug in the class of meglitinides, is a new anti-diabetic agent which approved by FDA as an oral hypoglycemic drug in 1998. It reduces the fasting glucose concentration by stimulating the release of insulin from pancreatic beta cells. Repaglinide differs from other anti-diabetic drugs in its structure, binding profile, duration of action and mode of excretion. It is practically insoluble in water, while capable of being rapidly absorbed from GI tract after oral administration: a typical behavior in class II Biopharmaceutical Classification System (BCS II) drugs. Repaglinide undergoes extensive first pass metabolism in liver which, collectively, results in poor oral bioavailability of the drug

* Correspondence: hamidim@zums.ac.ir
[3]Zanjan Pharmaceutical Nanotechnology Research Center (ZPNRC), Zanjan University of Medical Sciences, Zanjan, Iran
[4]Department of Pharmaceutics, School of Pharmacy, Zanjan University of Medical Sciences, Zanjan, Iran
Full list of author information is available at the end of the article

(56 %). It has a high plasma protein binding (more than 98 %) and its half-life in systemic blood circulation is about 1 h. Repaglinide causes hypoglycemia following oral administration, although the extent of this feature is less than the sulphonylureas [2]. These properties have proposed the drug as a good candidate for sustain oral delivery formulations. In this way, many attempts have been made as application of different carriers such as liquisolid compacts [3], gastroretentive floating delivery system [4] and different polymeric nanoparticles [5, 6].

In the recent decades, solid lipid nanoparticles (SLNs) have attracted many attentions as nanotechnology-based drug delivery systems. Their potential advantages such as the possibility of controlled drug release and targeting, feasible incorporation of lipophilic as well as hydrophilic drugs, remarkable biocompatibility and low biotoxicity, capability of avoiding organic solvents in production cycle and ease of scale up, have provoked many research projects exploiting the possible use of these nanostructures in drug delivery. Oral administration of SLNs can potentially increase the lymphatic transport of drugs, thereby causing decreased first pass hepatic metabolism and increased oral bioavailability of the drug [7].

The two main ingredients of SLN-based formulations are lipid and surfactant/stabilizer. Surfactants reduce the interfacial tension between the hydrophobic surface of lipid core and the aqueous environment and, therefore, stabilize the SLNs structure. The effect of surfactant on the properties of SLNs has been investigated and described in several studies. Drug-independent properties of SLNs such as particle size, stability and zeta potential were studied by majority of these researches [8–20] and, to the best of our knowledge, drug-dependent properties such as drug incorporation and drug release have not yet been evaluated as a function of surfactant/stabilizer composition [12, 18]. Such study will potentially help to develop efficient carriers to deliver drug by SLNs. In addition it may shed a light on the mechanism(s) by which the physicochemical features of a drug may interact with the stabilizer in formation of a drug-loaded SLN. So in this study it was tried to investigate the effects of different surfactants on some important attributes of a typical BCS II drug like repaglinide to be formulated as a SLN-loaded nanopharmaceutical.

Materials and methods

Materials

Repaglinide was a gift from Alborz Darou Pharmaceuticals, (Qazvin, Iran); pluronic F127 was purchased from Sigma, USA. Stearic acid (Art No. 8.00673.1000, Merck, Germany), glyceryl mono stearate (GMS, MYVEROL™, KERRY, Denmark), phosphatidylcholin (Art No. E80-103, Lipoid, USA), tween80 (Art No. 601809, Titrachem, Iran), poly vinyl pyrrolidone (PVP; 30 KDa, Rahavard Tamin, Iran) and poly vinyl alcohol (PVA; 145 KDa, Art No. 1.41353.1000, Merck, Germany) were purchased and applied. Other ingredients and solvents were from HPLC or chemical laboratory purity grades, as needed, and were purchased locally.

Preparation of SLNs

SLNs were prepared by a modified solvent diffusion method, where ethanolic phase containing 150 mg stearic acid, 50 mg GMS and 50 mg repaglinide was diffused in aqueous phase under magnetic stirring condition (1000 g) at 50 °C with an addition rate of 1 ml/min and, then, the resulting dispersion was allowed cooling until the room temperature. Surfactants were added to alcoholic or aqueous phases according to their solubility. After formation, SLNs were centrifuged at 50,000 g and lyophilized. Phosphatidylcholin (100 mg), poly vinyl pyrrolidone (PVP) (1 %), Tween 80 (1 %), pluronicF127 (100 mg), poly vinyl alcohol (PVA) and a mixture of phosphatidylcholin/Tween80 (100 mg/ 1 %) and phosphatidylcholin/pluronicF127 (100 mg/100 mg) were used as stabilizer during the preparation procedure.

Particle size and zeta potential analysis

Particle size and zeta potential distribution of the prepared SLNs population were determined based on dynamic light scattering (DLS) technique using a laser scattering particle size/zeta analyzer (Malvern, model Nano ZS, UK). For particle size analysis, SLNs were diluted in water until their refractive index (RI) became to 1.4.

Repaglinide assay

High performance liquid chromatography (HPLC) analysis was applied for determination of repaglinide concentrations in samples from drug loading or in vitro drug release studies. A HPLC system (Waters, model 1515, USA) was equipped with a UV C_{18} reverse phased column (MZ analytical, 250*4.6 mm, Mainz, Germany) and the mobile phase consisted of acetonitrile: phosphate buffer, 10 mM (pH = 2.5) at a ratio of 4:1. Chromatography was performed at flow rate of 1 ml/min at room temperature and the samples absorbance was determined at 245 nm by diode array detector (Waters, dual absorbances, model 2487, USA).

Determination of drug loading and entrapment efficiency

For this purpose, an accurately weighed amount of freeze dried of repaglinide-loaded SLNs was dissolved in ethanol and the quantity of the drug was determined spectrophotometrically at wavelength of 245 nm. The drug loading efficiency (DLE) was computed as below:

$$Drug\ loading\ Efficiency = \frac{amount\ of\ drug * 100}{total\ weight\ of\ SLN}$$

To calculate the entrapment efficiency (EE), the SLNs dispersion were centrifuged at 50,000 g for 45 min and, then, the supernatant phase was decanted and the amount of drug in this phase was determined by ultraviolet spectroscopy at 245 nm. The entrapment efficiency was computed by the equation:

$$Entrapment\ efficiency = \frac{amount\ of\ drug * 100}{amount\ of\ drug\ used\ in\ formulation}$$

Morphology studies by scanning electron microscopy

The size, shape and morphological properties of the prepared nanocarriers were studied by scanning electron microscopy (SEM). Lyophilized nanoparticles were coated by gold and at acceleration voltage of 7 kV were observed by SEM (MIRA TESCAN, Czech Republic).

Fourier transform infrared (FTIR) spectroscopy

The freeze dried samples were homogenously mixed with potassium bromide and the mixture was then compressed into discs by a hydraulic compressor through applying pressure of about 10 tones in 2 min. The discs were placed in infrared light pass and the infrared spectrum was recorded in region of 400–4000 cm^{-1} using a FTIR spectroscope (Bruker, Tensor 27, Germany).

Differential scanning calorimetry

Differential scanning calorimetry (DSC) was carried out on the lyophilized samples of the nanocarriers using a differential scanning calorimeter (Mettler-Toledo Inc., STARe system, US). 2 mg of accurately weighed lyophilized samples were placed on the aluminum pan and sealed. An empty aluminum pan was used as standard. Both pans were heated from 25 °C to 300 °C at a scanning rate of 10 °C per minute under nitrogen flow. The quantity of heat flow was determined as a function of samples temperature and it was used to study the thermal behaviors of nanoparticles.

In vitro drug release profile study

The in vitro drug release test was carried out thrice using dialysis bag diffusion technique. Dialysis bags (cut-off = 12 KDa) were immersed in distilled water for 24 h before use. 3 ml of SLNs dispersion equivalent to 2 mg repaglinide was placed into the dialysis bag, sealed by double-folding on both sides, and immersed in 100 ml of phosphate buffered saline (PBS) at 37 ° C. The system was placed on continuous magnetic stirring at 50 rpm. At predetermined time intervals, 1 ml sample was taken from receiver phase and the amount of repaglinide was analyzed by HPLC method as described above. The volume of release media was kept constant by addition of rectified volumes of PBS after each sampling stage. The sink conditions were preserved at whole time of the test in such a way that the repaglinide concentration in receiver phase remained less than 15 % of its saturation concentration in the same medium. Concentration of samples was determined by HPLC method as mentioned above and the release profile of each formulation was plotted graphically as percent drug released against the time in a bi-numerical mode.

Drug release kinetic estimation

In order to determine the best model to describe the kinetic parameters of the drug release profiles, the experimental release data were fitted to multiple statistical models. The corresponding equations of each model were given in Table 1. The linear form of each equation ($y = at + b$) was fitted to the pure or transformed data (according to each equation) and the squared correlation coefficient (r^2) between time and y parameter (related to release data based on each equation) was determined in each case. The r^2 was used as a critical parameter to evaluate strength of correlation in models and also to compare each model with others. In addition, the mean relative error (MRE) was used as another critical parameter in order to overcome possible biases of r^2 [21]. MRE was calculated as follows:

$$MRE = (M-C) * 100/C$$

Where C is the experimental data and M is the calculated release data from the applied model.

Statistical analysis

All experiments and measurements were replicated thrice. The mean diameter and standard deviations were calculated by Microsoft Excel 2007. The effect of

Table 1 Applied statistical models to release data of repaglinide

Function	Equation
Zero order	$M_0 - M = kt$
First order	$lnM_0 - lnM = kt$
Higuchi	$M_0 - M = kt^{0.5}$
Peppas	$M_0 - M = kt^n$
Hixon-crowell	$M_0^{1/3} - M^{1/3} = kt$
Square root	$M_0^{1/2} - M^{1/2} = kt$
weibull	$M_0 - M = 1 - e^{-\left(\frac{t}{T_d}\right)^{\beta}}$
Linear wagner	$Z_0 - Z = kt$
Log wagner	$Z_0 - Z = klnt$

M_0 and M are the remained amounts of the drug in carrier in the time zero and t respectively. Z is the probit of surface of nanoparticles along time. K is the equation constant and β is a shape factor of the equation figure different surfactants on the release profiles properties and kinetics were compared using a one-way analysis of variance using SPSS 16. In this analysis, statistical difference was significant when $p < 0.05$.

Results and discussions

Preparation of solid lipid nanoparticles

The solvent diffusion method was applied in the current study to prepare SLNs. This method is based on the rapid diffusion of an organic miscible solvent such as ethanol or acetone in aqueous solution, which, in turn causes a remarkable change in the dielectric constant and solubility parameter of the resulting hydro-organic solvent that eventually leads to the precipitation of the lipid in the new system. This lipid particulate which constitutes the core body of the SLNs becomes limited to the nano-sized via using high shear mixing as well as the presence of stabilizers in the preparation medium [22]. The simplicity and possibility of avoidance of toxic solvents in the SLNs preparation process described earlier are the main advantages of this method. Ethanol is highly soluble in water with minimal interfacial tension, so it diffuses very quickly in aqueous phase thereby resulting in the precipitating of lipids which in the presence of a stabilizer leads to the formation of nanoparticles. In this study some modifications were applied on the characteristics of standard solvent diffusion method, where addition of ethanolic solution to the aqueous phase was performed at about 50 °C. In fact it was seen that if the temperature was upper than the melting point of the lipids, the smaller and more stable particles were produced. It may be due to more rapid evaporation of organic phase (ethanol) which causes lower tendency of lipid phase to aqueous phase. This property possibly forms smaller particles. In addition high temperatures yield more time for surfactants to adsorb on lipid particles and stabilize them.[8] In preliminary tests through using experimental design approach, it was determined that surfactant concentrations affect the production of SLNs, with their particle size being considered as the response. Other conditions such as stirring rate (in a domain of 500–2000 g), rate of ethanolic phase addition to aqueous phase and etc., have no considerable effect on the particle size as response. Hence these conditions were kept constant. Such approach for comparison of different surfactants effect has been observed in several studies [8, 10, 15, 17]. This approach will help to evaluate the effect of surfactant only and without any other interactions. The lipids, repaglinide and surfactants (except PVA which dissolves in water phase) were completely soluble in ethanol. Among the different surfactants used, the phosphatidylcholin-based SLNs showed most opalescence characteristics and the tween 80-based formulations showed least one. The PVP-based SLNs showed lowest yield of nanoparticle production, which can be attributed to its low emulsifying capability.

Effect on the particle size and zeta potential of SLNs

The particle size and zeta potential of different formulations are shown in Table 2. It has been showed that particles with submicron sizes, specially smaller than 400 nm, could improve bioavailability of drugs [23, 24] and in our study, as indicated, all the SLNs samples showed submicron sizes in a desirable range (83–326 nm). So these nanoparticles are favorable in oral drug delivery systems. However the extent of bioavailability may be dependent to nanoparticles size and usually it is increased by decreasing the size [23, 25]. Hence bioavailability measurement is useful to get a more complete perception of results of this study and it should be investigated later. It had been observed that low molecular surfactants form smaller particles [16]. The reason is their ability to cover interfacial surfaces more quickly than high molecular surfactants [10]. The results of this study agreed those observations, where tween 80, pluronic and lecithin based SLNs formed smaller particle sizes than PVA and PVP based SLNs. Schubert et al. reported that at least 10 % lecithin is necessary to form nanoparticles [18]. However in this study SLNs formed using lower percents of lecithin. The presence of a non-ionic hydrophilic surfactant like tween 80 seems to lead to smaller particles while the phospholipid and co-polymer-based stabilizers made intermediate

Table 2 The particle size, zeta potential and loading parameters of different SLNs

Stabilizer(s) used	Size (nm)	Zeta Potential (mV)	Entrapment Efficiency (percent)	Loading Efficiency (percent)
Phosphatidylcholin	203 ± 7	(−)54 ± 8	85 ± 4	7.1 ± 2
Phosphatidylcholin + tween80	91 ± 4	(−)29 ± 4	35 ± 2	4.7 ± 2
Phosphatidylcholin + Pluronic	169 ± 11	(−)46 ± 9	83 ± 4	5.4 ± 1
Pluronic	210 ± 15	(−)43 ± 8	78 ± 5	6 ± 3
PVP	326 ± 24	(−)27 ± 5	28 ± 2	2.8 ± 1
PVA	265 ± 14	(−)26 ± 7	57 ± 3	4.5 ± 2
Tween 80	83 ± 3	(−)22 ± 3	27 ± 3	3.1 ± 1

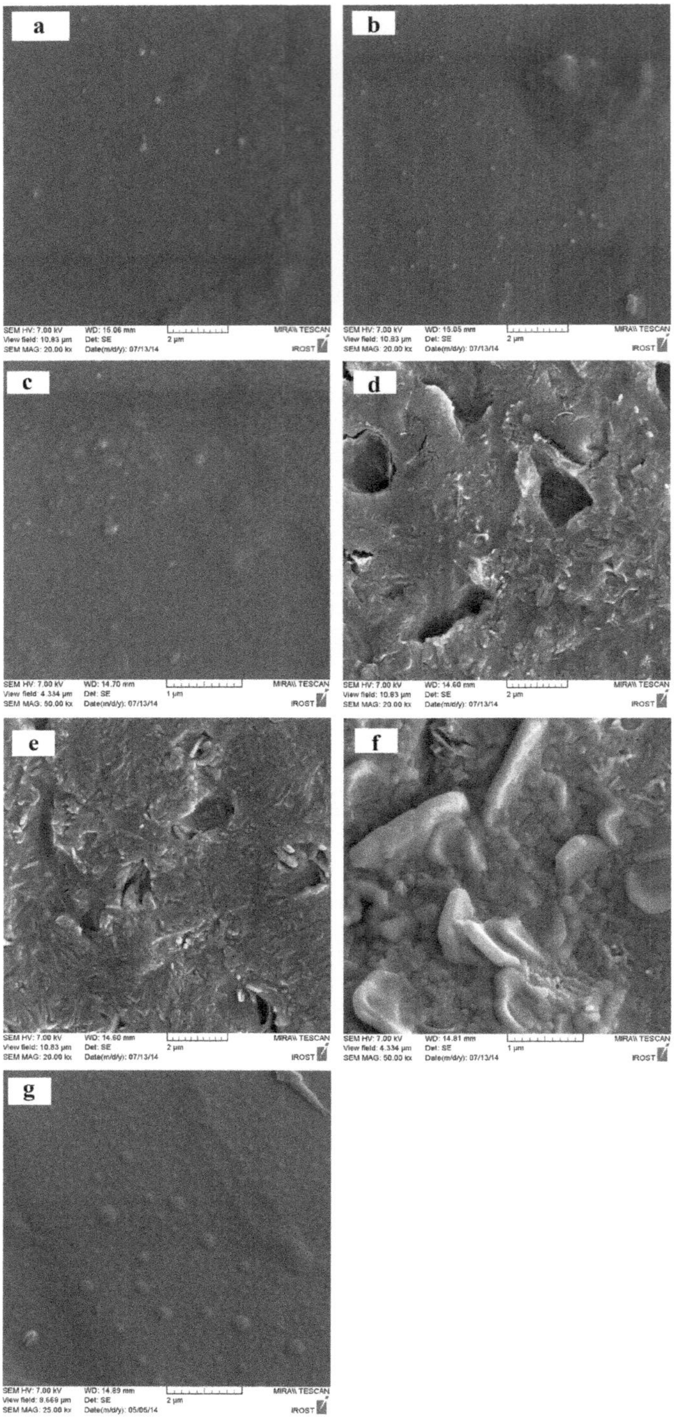

Fig. 1 SEM images of different formulations: **a**: tween 80, **b**: tween 80 + phosphatidylcholin, **c**: phosphatidylcholin, **d**: PVA, **e**: PVP, **f**: pluronic F127, **g**: phosphatidylcholin + pluronic F127

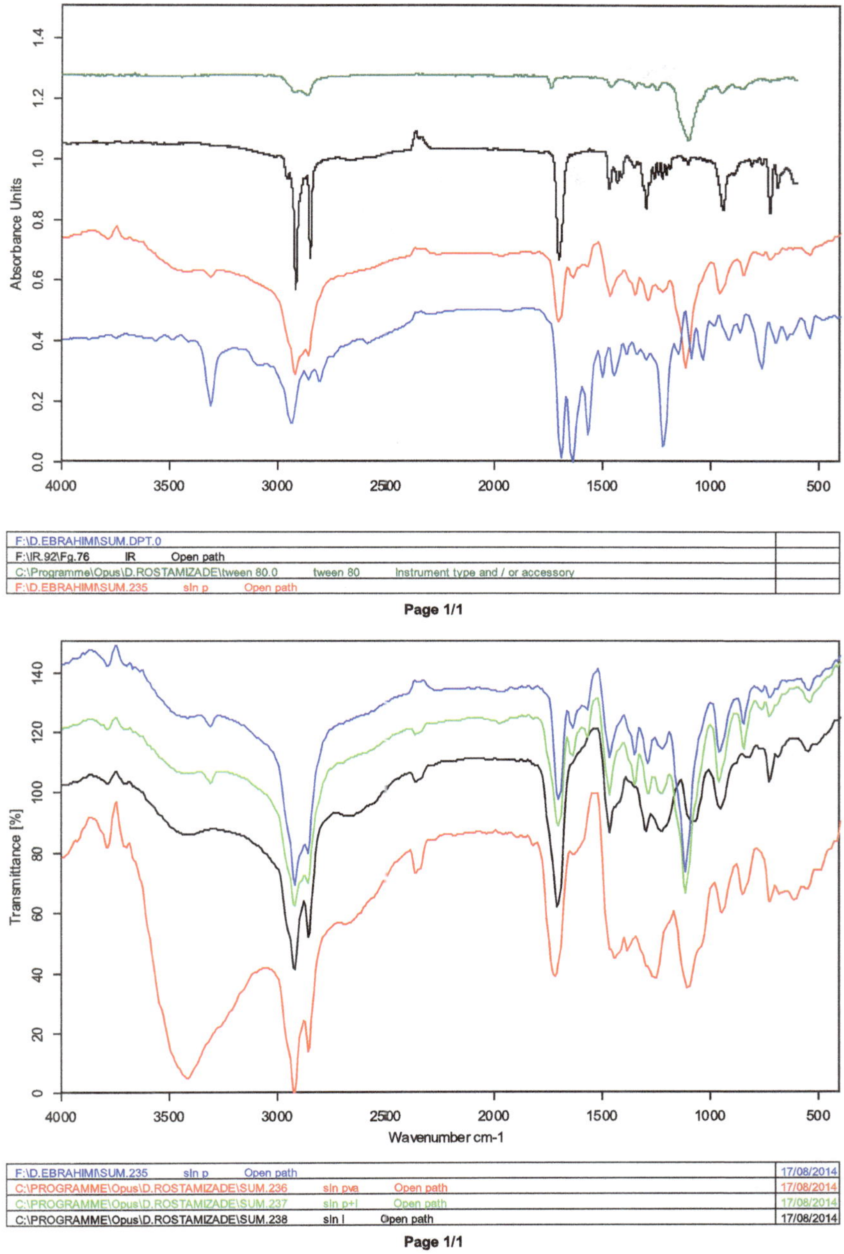

Fig. 2 FTIR spectrums of **a**: SLNs-tween80, **b**: stearic acid, **c**: SLNs-PVP, **d**: repaglinide, **e**: SLNs-pluronic, **f**: SLNs-PVA, **g**: SLNs-pluronic/phosphatidylcholin, **h**: SLNs-phosphatidylcholin

sizes and the poly-vinyl-based stabilizers led to largest particles among others. The lowest size was observed when a mixture of tween 80 and phosphatidylcholin was used. Blending of surfactants can decrease the particle size and this property was observed in several investigations [12, 16, 18–20, 26, 27]. The results of our study confirm that theory, while addition of tween 80 to phosphatidylcholin and pluronic f127 decreases the particle sizes. The zeta potentials of all formulations were in the negative region, which related to the negative charge of lipids, however, the absolute value of this parameter was dependent to the applied surfactant. This feature of SLNs has been

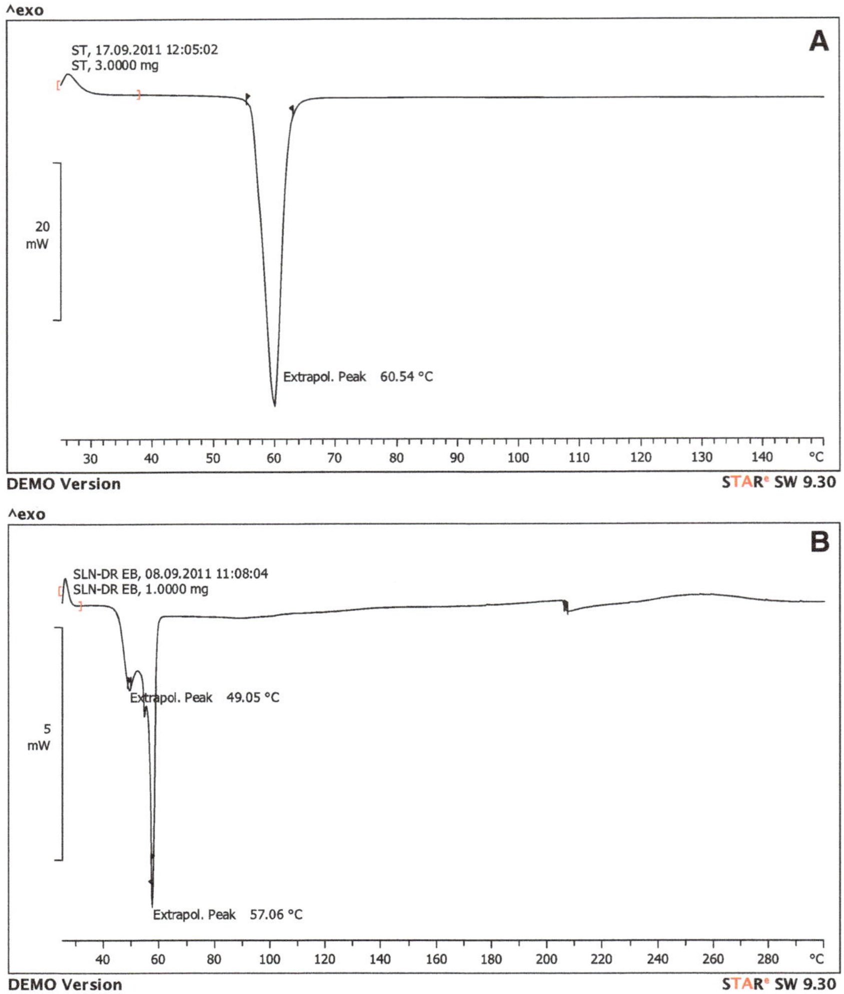

Fig. 3 DSC thermograms of **a** = stearic acid, **b** = SLNs

confirmed by various studies [19, 20, 26]. Phosphatidylcholin and mixtures containing it, due to its ionic characteristic, showed the highest surface potential. In fact phosphatidylcholin due to its ionic structure forms an electric double layer on the surface of nanoparticles and this layer increases the zeta potential [10]. Nonionic surfactants stabilize SLNs through their steric properties [19]. The mixture of ionic surfactant like phosphatidylcholin and a nonionic surfactant like pluronic f127 forms more stabilized SLNs [12, 18, 19]. It seems that the molecular weight, structure and conformation play an important role on the quantity of zeta potential of SLNs. Presence of relatively high zeta potential value led to more stable nanoparticles and overcomes the tendency of aggregation due to wander walls attraction forces [10].

Drug loading parameters

The drug loading efficiency and entrapment efficiency of different formulations have been shown in Table 2. The majority of the formulations, as shown, had remarkable drug entrapment efficiency as well as drug loading. The drug solubility in matrix solvent, miscibility in lipid phase and the lipid phase polymorphic state have shown to affect the loading quantity [4, 6, 28, 29]. Repaglinide is poorly soluble in water [30], so it causes low tendency to escape from lipid carrier and thus as indicated, generally it shows high entrapment efficiency. Stearic acid forms lipid structures with high crystalinity [31]. This polymorphic state repels the drug from SLN core to its surface and to the matrix of mixture [28]. GMS was added to lipid phase to decrease the degree of lipid phase crystalinity and to

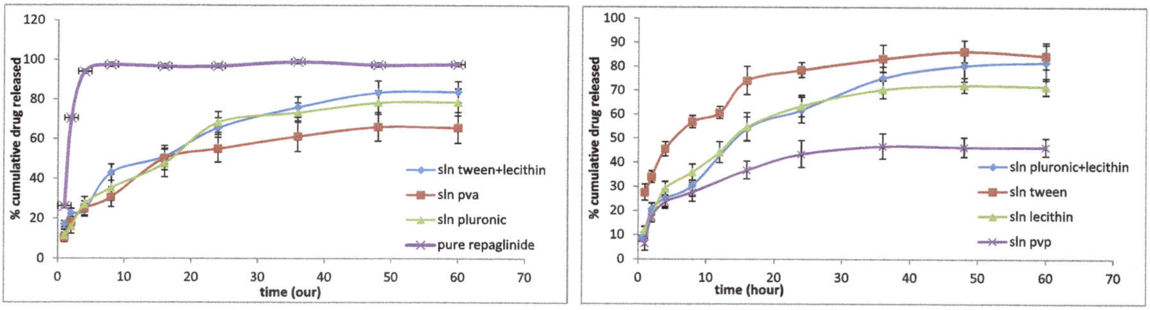

Fig. 4 Release data of different SLNs formulations

increase loading capacity. As indicated, the loading parameters show an increase by ascending the particle size from the smallest sizes (83 nm, 27 %) until medium sizes (203 nm, 85 %). More increase in the size of particles showed a decrease in loading parameters. In some previous studies, the reverse relation between particle size and loading parameters has been showed [18]. Lowering the particle size increases the specific surface area and thus increase drug loading. The latter part of our finding can be explained by this theory. However since limited number of surfactants were used by Schubert et al., extension of this theory in all conditions such as lower particle sizes in our study, is not possible. Mehnert et al., mentioned mobility of drug after incorporation in SLN through particle surfaces [16]. It is obvious that the bigger surface leads to a higher mobility and tendency of drug to escape from the carrier. So it may be concluded that in smaller particles like tween 80-based SLNs, the whole particle surface is larger and drug repulsion is higher. Therefore loading parameters in these smaller particles are lower relatively. After evaluation of the size and drug loading parameters, the phosphatidylcholin/pluronic-based SLNs which showed maximum loading efficiency (85 %) with eligible particle size (203 nm) was selected for further evaluation.

Morphological characterization of SLNs

SEM images of the nanoparticles prepared using different stabilizers are shown in Fig. 1. The nanoscale sizes of particles in all formulations are evident, though the shapes and assemblies are different among the nanoformulations. The shapes of all nanoparticles except PVP and PVA-based SLNs were spherical and in these two cases, the particles were in rod forms. The surface of phosphatidylcholin and phosphatidylcholin/pluronic-based NPs are smooth but for others are irregular.

FTIR spectroscopy analysis

FTIR spectra of repaglinide, stearic acid and solid lipid nanoparticles are shown in Fig. 2.

FTIR of pure repaglinide showed peaks at 3306 cm − 1 (NH stretching), 2938 cm − 1 (CH stretching), and 1684 cm − 1 (C = O stretching). The bands at 1040 cm − 1 and 1209 cm − 1 are related to C–O stretching in phenylalkylether structure. The bands at 1566 cm − 1 and 1638 cm − 1 are due to aromatic C = C and N–H bending respectively.

The FTIR spectrum of stearic acid showed a strong peak at 1702 cm − 1 (C = O stretching), 2918 cm − 1 (OH stretching) and 2849 cm − 1 (CH stretching). The long-chain bond is seen in 720 cm − 1 and the CH_2 and CH_3 bands are seen in around 1550 cm − 1 and 1300 cm − 1 respectively.

The FTIR spectrum of SLNs shows approximately all absorbances of stearic acid with some minor displacements for 2918 cm − 1 (OH stretching) and 2849 cm − 1 (CH stretching) which is related to inter-molecular forces and re-arrangement of molecules in SLNs structure. Additional peaks in SLNs spectrum are probably related to the applied surfactants. Therefore, these data indicate

Table 3 Particle size and release profile parameters of different surfactant formulations

Surfactant/stabilizer	Tween 80	Tween 80+ phosphatidylcholin	Pluronic F127+ phosphatidylcholin	Phosphatidylcholin	Pluronic F127	PVA	PVP
Particle size (nm)	83	91	169	203	210	265	306
Burst release (%)	27.5	17.13	8.4	11.8	11.6	10.5	6.4
Release rate (%/h)	1.49	1.55	1.49	1.63	1.4	1.16	1.12
Max. drug depletion (%)	86.42	84.14	81.68	72.21	78.44	66.14	46.8

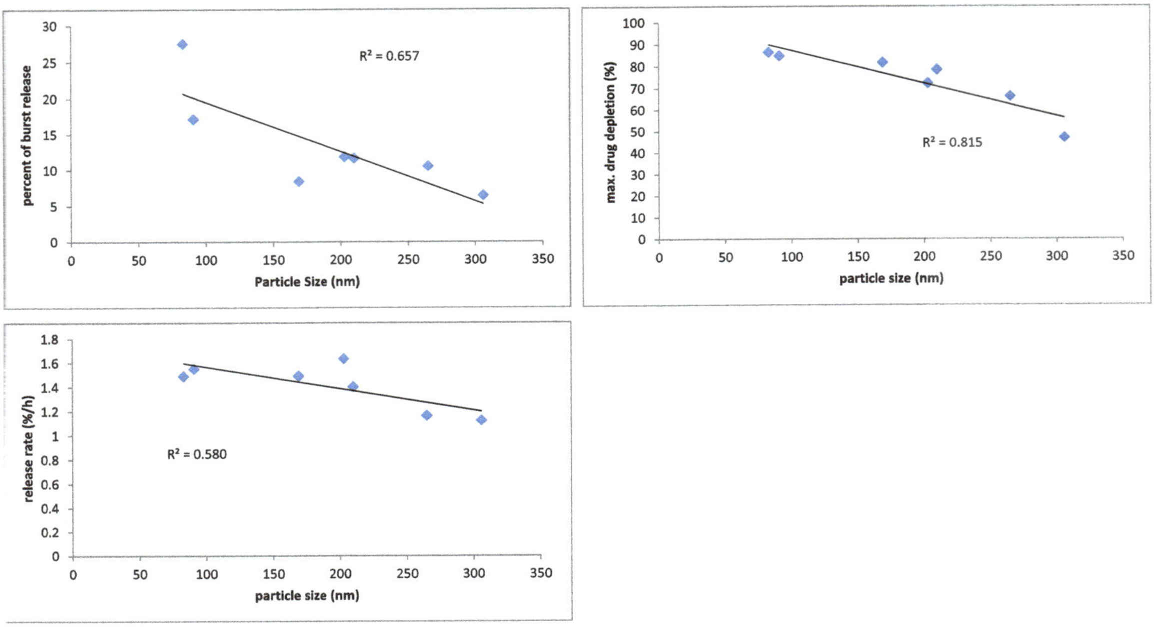

Fig. 5 Correlation between particle size and release parameters; burst release, maximum drug depletion and release rate

no formation of chemical bonds between the nanocarrier and the drug which, in turn, ensures the stability of the drug main structure during the preparation process.

Differential scanning calorimetry (DSC) analysis

DSC thermograms of stearic acid and SLNs have been shown in Fig. 3. As shown, the peak related to stearic acid melting displaced slightly from 60 °C to 57 °C. The GMS melting point is similar to stearic acid and thus maybe shows interaction with it in this area. The peak related to pluronic F127 is seen lower than 50 °C. All these findings indicate minor displacements of the ingredient peaks which imply new molecular arrangements rather than the formation new chemical bonds between ingredients, a finding supported by the FTIR data.

In vitro drug release

The dialysis bag method was used to determine the release profile of the drug from SLNs. This is an efficient method to study the drug release from nanocarriers [32]. The release profiles of the drug from seven different SLNs have been shown in Fig. 4. There are clear differences among profiles which have been described by evaluating key factors of the profiles. These key factors are: i) the burst release, ii) the release rate and iii) the maximum drug depletion quantity (MDDQ) (Table 3). The amount of burst release of the drug (total cumulative of drug released in first one hour) from different formulations was significantly different and accordingly, the formulations can be classified into three groups of: low burst release

Table 4 R-squared from fitting release data of different formulations on various models

	Phosphatidylcholin	Phosphatidylcholin/pluronic	Pluronic	PVA	PVP	Tween	Tween/phosphatidylcholin
Zero	0.78	0.88	0.85	0.82	0.72	0.73	0.89
First	0.86	0.96	0.92	0.89	0.77	0.85	0.97
Higuchi	0.93	0.98	0.96	0.94	0.88	0.89	0.97
Peppas	0.99	0.97	0.98	0.98	0.98	0.996	0.98
Hixon-crowell	0.84	0.94	0.9	0.87	0.75	0.81	0.95
Square root	0.83	0.93	0.89	0.86	0.75	0.79	0.94
weibull	0.98	0.99	0.99	0.98	0.9	0.98	0.98
Linear Wagner	0.76	0.86	0.84	0.78	0.63	0.77	0.9
Log Wagner	0.98	0.97	0.98	0.99	0.94	0.98	0.96

Table 5 The mean relative error (MRE) from empirical data to calculated data from models

	Phosphatidylcholin	Phosphatidylcholin/pluronic	Pluronic	PVA	PVP	Tween	Tween/phosphatidylchTolin
Zero	21.11	22.61	27.14	26.36	37.06	13.24	20.75
First	25.97	21.93	20.31	24.31	35.88	15.14	11.9
Higuchi	14.8	11.28	10.64	12.44	23.75	10.72	7.62
Peppas	4.49	8.49	5.03	7.63	5.03	1.53	7.8
Hixon-crowell	26.83	25.88	22.91	24.78	36.24	16.19	15.44
Square root	27.5	27.4	24.03	24.99	36.44	16.69	16.92
Weibull	4.09	5.12	5.55	6.4	16.74	2.13	7.33
Linear Wagner	42.85	41.13	25.52	25.5	36.89	36.96	18.05
Log Wagner	3.9	8.6	8.16	4.62	13.44	3.29	11.81

(PVP = 6.4 %, pluronic F127 = 11.6 %, PVA = 10.5 %, phosphatidylcholin/pluronic F127 = 8.4 %, phosphatidylcholin = 11.8 %), medium burst release (phosphatidylcholin/tween 80 = 17.13 %) and high burst release (tween 80 = 27.54 %) (Table 3). The quantity of burst release has direct relation with the amount of drug existed on the surface of nanoparticles [16, 28]. So it can be concluded that the greater the burst release, greater the drug on the particles surfaces. To explain these differences in multiple SLNs, it seems they related to variations in particle sizes since in constant mass of nanoparticles, the smaller ones contain greater particle surfaces and in our study the smaller SLNs showed greater burst release.

The second specification of release profiles is the rate of release. For this purpose, the rate of drug release from the starting point of the ascending part of the profile to reach the plateau was calculated. As it was shown in Table 3, there is no meaningful difference between these formulations in terms of the release rate.

The third factor was the maximum drug depletion quantity (MDDQ). The SLNs due to their condensed and highly ordered molecular conformation, usually retain a part of the loaded drug inside themselves [28]. As it is shown in Table 3, the amount of drug retained in SLNs differs in various formulations significantly.

In order to explore these differences, a correlation analysis was performed between these parameters and their corresponding particle sizes. As indicated in Fig. 5, there is a significant reverse correlation between particle size and the reverse amount of maximum drug depletion quantity ($r^2 = 0.815$). This quantity parameter equals to 0.657 and 0.580 for the values of burst release and release rate, respectively.

In explanation of these correlations, it seems that the higher particle sizes of PVP-based SLNs make a bigger total internal lipophilic space for the highly lipophilic drug to be accommodated which becomes smaller and smaller with decreasing particle sizes for other formulations. The higher the ratio of the internal spaces-to-interfaces, the higher the total drug retention in particles would occur. So the lipid core could detain more drugs and thus the MDDQ becomes greater. The other two parameters (burst release and release rate) showed no significant correlation with particle size, as indicated.

Drug release kinetic study

The results from substitution of the empirical data on different statistical models are shown in Tables 4 and 5. As indicated, the r^2 and MRE values of the weibull and logarithmic Wagner models showed most fitness with experimental data in most formulations. It means that there are surface and size variations in particles along release process [33, 34].

In addition the Peppas model showed high fitness with these data which indicates that the diffusion, erosion or relaxation processes probably contribute in release process [35, 36].

To determine the share of each parameter, the release exponent, n, in Peppas equation was calculated and due to its number in different formulations (Table 6), it can be argued that in tween-based and tween/phosphatidylcholin-based SLNs which $n < 0.43$, the mechanism of drug release is fickian diffusion, but in other formulations where $0.51 < n < 0.54$, the mechanism of release is a combination of fickian diffusion and non-fickian release mechanisms such as erosion and relaxation [35, 36].

Table 6 The "n" parameter from peppas equation in different formulations

	Phosphatidylcholin	Phosphatidylcholin/pluronic	Pluronic	PVA	PVP	Tween	Tween/phosphatidylcholin
n	0.54	0.52	0.52	0.51	0.52	0.36	0.41

Conclusion

The results of this study confirmed the effect of surfactant type on SLNs physicochemical properties such as morphological features, loading parameters, particle sizes and drug release kinetic. These variations due to surfactant effect have been noted in previous studies. In addition, an appropriate mixture of surfactants such as phosphatidylcholin/pluronic can modify the properties of repaglinide loaded SLNs so that convert it as a suitable candidate for delivery of repaglinide for specific purposes, e.g., improvement of the drug bioavailability.

Competing interests

This work has been supported financially by the Biotechnology Research Center, Tabriz University of Medical Sciences, Tabriz, Iran under a Ph.D. thesis proposal. The authors are also most grateful for the continuing financial support of this study by the Pharmaceutical Nanotechnology Research Center, Zanjan University of Medical Sciences, Zanjan, Iran.

Author details

[1]Biotechnology Research Center, Tabriz University of Medical Sciences, Tabriz, Iran. [2]Department of Pharmaceutics, Faculty of Pharmacy, Tabriz University of Medical Sciences, Tabriz, Iran. [3]Zanjan Pharmaceutical Nanotechnology Research Center (ZPNRC), Zanjan University of Medical Sciences, Zanjan, Iran. [4]Department of Pharmaceutics, School of Pharmacy, Zanjan University of Medical Sciences, Zanjan, Iran.

References

1. Yao J, Shi YQ, Li ZR, Jin SH. Development of a RP-HPLC method for screening potentially counterfeit anti-diabetic drugs. J Chromatogr B. 2007;853:254–9.
2. Culy JR, Jarvis B. Repaglinide: a review of its therapeutic use in type 2 diabetes mellitus. Drugs. 2001;61:1625–60.
3. El-Houssieny BM, Wahman L, Arafa NM. Bioavailability and biological activity of liquisolid compact formula of repaglinide and its effect on glucose tolerance in rabbits. BioScience Trends. 2010;4(1):17–24.
4. Jain SK, Awasthi AM, Jain NK, Agrawal GP. Calcium silicate based microspheres of repaglinide for gastroretentive floating drug delivery: Preparation and in vitro characterization. J Control Release. 2005;107:300–9.
5. Lokhande AB, Mishra S, Kulkarni RD, Naik JB. Preparation and characterization of repaglinide loaded ethylcellulose nanoparticles by solvent diffusion technique using high pressure homogenizer. J Pharm Res. 2013;7:421–6.
6. UM D I, Poovi G, Neelakanta Reddy P. In vitro characterization and in vivo toxicity studyofrepaglinideloadedpoly (methyl methacrylate)nanoparticles. Int J Pharm. 2010;396:194–203.
7. Demirel M, Yazan Y, Müller RH, Kiliç F, Bozan B. Formulation and in vitro-in vivo evaluation of piribidil solid lipid micro and nanoparticles. J Microencapsul. 2001;18(3):359–71.
8. Helgason T, Awad TS, Kristbergsson K, McClements DJ, Weiss J. Effect of surfactant surface coverage on formation of solid lipid nanoparticles (SLN). J Colloid Interface Sci. 2009;334:75–81.
9. Radomska-Soukharev A. Stability of lipid excipients in solid lipid nanoparticles. Adv Drug Deliv Rev. 2007;59:411–8.
10. Kovacevic A, Savic S, Vuleta G, Müller RH, Keck CM. Polyhydroxy surfactants for the formulation of lipid nanoparticles (SLN and NLC): Effects on size, physical stability and particle matrix structure. Int J Pharm. 2011;406:163–72.
11. Xie S, Wang S, Zhu L, Wang F, Zhou W. The effect of glycolic acid monomer ratio on the emulsifying activity of PLGA in preparation of protein-loaded SLN. Colloids and Surfaces B. Biointerfaces. 2009;74:358–61.
12. Tan SW, Billa N, Roberts CR, Burley JC. Surfactant effects on the physical characteristics of Amphotericin B-containing nanostructured lipid carriers. Colloids and Surfaces A: Physicochem. Eng Aspects. 2010;372:73–9.
13. Salminen H, Aulbach S, Leuenberger BH, Tedeschi C. Influence of surfactant composition on physical and oxidative stability of Quillaja saponin-stabilized lipid particles with encapsulated omega-3 fish oil. Colloids and Surfaces B. Biointerfaces. 2014;122:46–55.
14. Keck CM, Kovačević A, Müller RH, Savić S, Vuleta G, Milić J. Formulation of solid lipid nanoparticles (SLN): The value of different alkyl polyglucoside surfactants. Int J Pharm. 2014;474:33–41.
15. Olbrich C, Müller RH. Enzymatic degradation of SLN—effect of surfactant and surfactant mixtures. Int J Pharm. 1999;180:31–9.
16. Wolfgang Mehnert KM. Solid lipid nanoparticles production, characterization and applications. Adv Drug Deliv Rev. 2001;47:165–96.
17. Schöler N, Olbrich C, Tabatt K, Müller RH, Hahn H, Liesenfeld O. Surfactant, but not the size of solid lipid nanoparticles (SLN) influences viability and cytokine production of macrophages. Int J Pharm. 2001;221:57–67.
18. Schubert MA, Müller-Goymann CC. Characterisation of surface-modified solid lipid nanoparticles (SLN): Influence of lecithin and nonionic emulsifier. Eur J Pharm Biopharm. 2005;61:77–86.
19. Fei H, Sanming L, Ran Y, Hongzhuo L, Lu X. Effect of surfactants on the formation and characterization of a new type of colloidal drug delivery system: nanostructured lipid carriers. Colloids and surfaces a. A Physicochem Eng Asp. 2008;315:210–6.
20. Trotta M, Debernardi F, Caputo O. Preparation of solid lipid nanoparticles by a solvent emulsification-diffusion technique. Int J Pharm. 2003;257:153–60.
21. Paulo Costa JMSL. Modeling and comparison of dissolution profiles. Eur J Pharm Sci. 2001;13:123–33.
22. Niwa T, Takeuchi H, Hino T, Kunou N, Kawashima Y. Preparations of biodegradable nanospheres of water-soluble and insoluble drugs with D,L-lactide/glycolide copolymer by a novel spontaneous emulsification solvent diffusion method, and the drug release behavior. J Control Release. 1993;25(1–2):89–98.
23. Hu L, Tang X, Cui F. Solid lipid nanoparticles (SLNs) to improve oral bioavailability of poorly soluble drugs. J Pharm Pharmacol. 2004;56:1527–35.
24. Melike Üner GY. Importance of solid lipid nanoparticles (SLN) in various administration routes and future perspectives. Int J Nanomedicine. 2007;2(3):289–300.
25. Luo F, Chen DW, Ren LX, Zhao XL, Qin J. Solid lipid nanoparticles for enhancing vinpocetine's oral bioavailability. J Control Release. 2006;114:53–9.
26. Rawat MK, Jain A, Mishra A, Muthu MS, Singh S. Development of repaglinide loaded solid lipid nanocarrier: selection of fabrication method. Curr Drug Deliv. 2010;7:44–50.
27. Mulla JAS, Hiremath SP, Sharma NK. Repaglinide loaded solid lipid nanoparticles: design and characterization. RGUHS J Pharm Sci. 2012;2(4):41–9.
28. Muller RH, Mader K, Gohla S. Solid lipid nanoparticles (SLN) for controlled drug delivery - a review of the state of the art. Eur J Pharm Biopharm. 2000;50.
29. Gardouh AR, Gad S, Ghonaim HM, Ghorab MM. Design and characterization of glyceryl monostearate solid lipid nanoparticles prepared by high shear homogenization. British J Pharmaceutical Res. 2013;3(3):326–46.
30. Kavitha R, Sathali AA. Enhancement of solubility of repaglinide by solid dispersion technique. Int J Chem Sci. 2012;10(1):377–90.
31. Almeida EDP, Costa AA, Serafini MR, Rossetti FC, Marchetti JM, Sarmento VHV, et al. Preparation and characterization of chloroaluminum phthalocyanine-loaded solid lipid nanoparticles by thermal analysis and powder X-ray diffraction techniques. J Therm Anal Calorim. 2011;108:191–6.
32. Pelczarska A, Delie F, Domańska U, Carrupt PA, Martel S. New high throughput screening method for drug release measurements. Eur J Pharm Biopharm. 2013;85:151–7.
33. Barzegar-Jalali M, Adibkia K, Valizadeh H, Siahi Shadabad MR, Nokhodchi A, Omidi Y, et al. Kinetic analysis of drug release from nanoparticles. J Pharm Pharm Sci. 2008;11(1):167–77.
34. Wagner JG. Interpretation of percent dissolved-time plots derived from in vitro testing of conventional tablets and capsules. J Pharm Sci. 1969;58(10):1253–7.
35. Siepmann J, Siepmann F. Mathematical modeling of drug delivery. Int J Pharm. 2008;364:328–43.
36. Siepmanna J, Peppas NA. Modeling of drug release from delivery systems based on hydroxypropyl methylcellulose (HPMC). Adv Drug Deliv Rev. 2001;48:139–57.

26

A model for priority setting of health technology assessment: the experience of AHP-TOPSIS combination approach

Mohammadreza Mobinizadeh[1], Pouran Raeissi[2], Amir Ashkan Nasiripour[1*], Alireza Olyaeemanesh[3] and Seyed Jamaleddin Tabibi[1]

Abstract

Background: In recent times, the use of health technologies in the diagnosis and treatment of diseases experienced considerable and accelerated growth. The goal of the present study was to describe the designated pilot MCDM (Multiple Criteria Decision Making) model for priority setting of health technology assessment in Iran.

Methods: Relevant articles were sought and retrieved from the most appropriate medical databases, including the Cochrane Library, PubMed and Scopus via three separate search strategies, using MESH and free text until March, 2015. Retrieved criteria were questioned from health technology assessment experts in two rounds and the relative weight for valid criteria was finally obtained from paired wise comparison method. After extraction of relative weights based on the aforementioned procedure, TOPSIS (The Technique for Order of Preference by Similarity to Ideal Solution) priority setting model was designed. The stated model was applied for assessing three technologies (adenosine, tissue plasminogen activator and mechanical thrombectomy) which were available for projects call of Iranian health technology assessment department in order to determine applicability of the model for practical purpose.

Results: Nine criteria, including efficiency/effectiveness, safety, population size, vulnerable population size, availability of alternative technologies, cost effectiveness in other countries, budget impact, financial protection, quality of evidence, were extracted by the Iranian health technology assessment experts. The relative weights of these criteria were as follows 0.12, 0.2, 0.06, 0.08, 0.08, 0.13, 0.08, 0.09, and 0.15, respectively. Finally TOPSIS pilot model was designed by three health technologies and nine criteria relative weights. Results showed that, the applicability of the stated model was suitable and as the pilot testing, tissue plasminogen activator was the first priority, adenosine was second and mechanical thrombectomy was third for performing health technology assessment by the Iranian ministry of health and medical education.

Conclusion: According to the results of this study, this model with nine effective criteria and their relative weights and in combination with TOPSIS approach could be used with suitable applicability by health technology assessment department in deputy of curative affairs and food and drug organization for determination of research priorities in health technology assessment.

Keywords: Priority setting, Health Technology Assessment, Iran

Background

Acceptance of health technologies in health systems within the last decades has experienced some intensive changes. The belief in abiding with the acceptance of health technologies within 1960s and 1970s gradually was replaced by an increasing suspicion of society towards the credibility of advanced health technologies. Nowadays, politicians and the public have an ambiguous opinion about the use of a new health technology [1].

Within recent years, the use of health technologies for diagnosis and treatment of diseases experienced considerable and accelerated growth. The proper use of these technologies may considerably help in the diagnosis and treatment of diseases. On the other hand, unlimited and unrestricted entry of these technologies may result in induced demand by service providers [2].

Given, the number of health technologies which required assessment was more than available resources;

* Correspondence: nasiripour@srbiau.ac.ir
[1]Department of Health Services Management, Science and Research Branch, Islamic Azad University, Tehran, Iran
Full list of author information is available at the end of the article

so all health technology assessment organizations must prioritize their research projects [3]. Various studies have been applied for this purpose worldwide until now, such as Canadian Drug and Health Technologies Organization (CADTH) which utilized the analytical hierarchy process (AHP) for priority setting of health technologies [4]. Another existing model in relation to priority and selection of health technologies was EVIDEM (Evidence and Value: Impact on Decision Making) model in Canada [5]. Nonetheless, there is no consensus on appropriate priority setting between health technology assessment organizations [3]. The main goal of the present study was to describe the designated pilot MCDM model for priority setting of health technology assessment in Iran.

Methods

In order to achieve the aforementioned goal, relevant articles until March, 2015, based on three separate strategies using MESH and free text were sought for using the Cochrane Library, Pub Med and Scopus. The criteria and sub criteria (in pre assessment and assessment phase, at this stage, the criteria of assessment phase were also included, on the assumption that there may be some of these criteria which can be used in pre assessment phase in Iranian health system context) obtained from systematic review were questioned by experts of health technology assessment context via questionnaire (these expert were selected from official committee of HTA in Iranian ministry of health and medical education and during of this research just 11 ones of them were available for inclusion). At first, to determine the content validity as pilot, experts of health technology assessment were provided with questionnaire in three forms, including (a.) determination of face validity for each item (as two-options: it is clear and demonstrative or it is not clear and demonstrative), (b.) determination of content validity rate (CVR) for each item (as three-options: it is necessary, useful but not necessary or not necessary) and (c.) determination of content validity index (CVI) for each item (as five-options: completely irrelevant, irrelevant, relatively irrelevant, relevant or completely relevant). Sub criteria from which the minimum content validity was obtained was also included in the final questionnaire phase. In this questionnaire, the importance of each of these sub criteria was questioned by experts in these five options context (very slightly important, slightly important, moderately important, important, and very important). For this purpose, a 75 % cut point was used. This implied that for each one of these sub criteria, 75 % of experts who voted important or very important in the process of health technology assessment priority setting were included in the analytic hierarchy process (AHP) phase for extraction of their relative weight through paired wise comparisons. In the analytical hierarchy process, relative weight was obtained by paired comparison matrix. For a consistent paired comparison matrix, weight was calculated through normalization of elements of each column. However, if the matrix was inconsistent, to obtain the weight, four major methods were introduced, including 1 - least squares, 2 - least logarithm squares, 3 - Eigen vector, 4 - approximate methods [6]. The first three methods involve tedious calculations, thus some approximate methods have been proposed which are of lower accuracy (that is acceptable) and involve less and simpler calculations. In this study, geometric mean method was used. The geometric mean of elements of each row was calculated; later, the obtained vector was normalized to obtain the weight vector. Inconsistency rate of each matrix A was calculated based on the following steps:

1. Formation of the paired comparison matrix A;
2. Specification of the weight vector (W);
3. Is the maximum Eigen value of matrix A (λ_{max}) specified? If yes, go to forth step, otherwise (according to following steps) estimate its value.
   3-1: Obtaining a well-suited estimation of $\lambda_{max}W$ by multiplying vector W by matrix A ($AW = \lambda_{max}W$);
   3-2: Upon dividing the obtained values for $\lambda_{max}W$ by relative W, estimation of of λ_{max} is calculated;
   3-3: The obtained mean λ_{max} is calculated;
4. Calculation of inconsistency index (I.I) based on following equation:
   Formula (1)

$$I.I = \frac{\lambda_{max} - n}{n-1}$$

5. Calculation of inconsistency ratio (I.R.) based on following formula:
   Formula (2)

$$I.R = \frac{I.I}{I.I.R.}$$

In this formula I.I.R. denotes the random matrix inconsistency index. This matrix was calculated for matrices whose numbers were completely randomly selected. In each matrix, the product of dividing the inconsistency index by random matrix inconsistency matrix with the same dimension will be a suitable criterion for judgment about matrix inconsistency which is called inconsistency ratio. If this number is smaller or equal to 0.1, system consistency is acceptable; otherwise the judgments must be revised [6].

After extraction of relative weights based on the above procedure, TOPSIS priority setting model was designed. Essential principles of this method are as follows:

a. Appropriateness of each index must be uniform in ascending (descending) order (whatever r_{ij} is higher, appropriateness also higher or vice versa) so that the best existing value of an index denotes its ideal and the worst existing value thereof shows negative ideal for it.

b. The interval of an option from ideal (or negative ideal) may be calculated as Euclidean distance (from second exponent) or as the sum total of absolute value of linear distances (known as block gaps) that is dependent on the exchange and replacement rate among indices.

First step: this involves the conversion of existing decision making matrix to a matrix descaled using following formula:

Formula (3):

$$n_{ij} = \frac{r_{ij}}{\sqrt{\sum_{i=1}^{m} r_{ij}^2}}$$

Second step: this involves creating weighted descaled matrix by assumption of vector W as input to the algorithm.

Formula (4):

$$W = \{w_1, w_2, \ldots w_n\} \approx (\text{supposed of } DM)$$

$$V = N_D . W_{n \times n} = \begin{matrix} V_{11\ldots} & V_{1j\ldots} & V_{1n\ldots} \\ \vdots & \vdots & \vdots \\ V_{m1\cdots} & V_{mj\cdots} & V_{mn\cdots} \end{matrix}$$

Where N_D is a matrix having the score of indices therein descaled and comparable and $W_{n \times n}$ is a diametrical matrix having only its main elements as nonzero.

Third step: This involves determination of ideal solution and negative ideal solution

For ideal option A^+ and negative ideal A^-, the following definition is provided:

Formula (5):

$$A^+ = \left\{ (\overset{max}{i} V_{ij} | j \in J), (\overset{min}{i} V_{ij} | j \in J) | i = 1, 2, \ldots m \right\}$$

$$= \left\{ V_1^+, V_2^+, \ldots, V_j^+, \ldots, V_n^+ \right\}$$

$$A^- = \left\{ (\overset{min}{i} V_{ij} | j \in J), (\overset{max}{i} V_{ij} | j \in J) | i = 1, 2, \ldots m \right\}$$

$$= \left\{ V_1^-, V_2^-, \ldots, V_j^-, \ldots, V_n^- \right\}$$

$$J = \{j = 1, 2, \ldots, n | \text{js}) \text{ referred to the profit}\}$$

$$J = \{j = 1, 2, \ldots, n | \text{js referred to the cost}\}$$

Forth step: This involves calculation of separation size (distance).

The distance between option i and ideals based on Euclidean method is as follows:

Formula (6)

$$d_{i+} = \left\{ \sum_{j=1}^{n} \left(V_{ij} - V_j^+ \right)^2 \right\}^{0.5}, i = 1, 2, \ldots, m$$

$$d_{i-} = \left\{ \sum_{j=1}^{n} \left(V_{ij} - V_j^- \right)^2 \right\}^{0.5}, i = 1, 2, \ldots, m$$

Fifth step: This involves calculation of relative closeness of A_i to the ideal solution. This relative closeness is defined as follows:

Formula (7):

$$cl_{i+} = \frac{d_{i-}}{(d_{i+} + d_{i-})}; 0 \le cl_{i+} \le 1; i = 1, 2, \ldots, m$$

As observed, if

$$A_i = A^{\mp}$$

Then:

$$d_{i+} = 0$$

And will have:

$$cl_{i+} = 1$$

And in case:

$$A_i = A^-$$

Then:

$$d_{i-} = 0$$

And

$$cl_{i+} = 0$$

Therefore, whatever A_i is closer to the ideal solution A^+, value of cl_i will be closer to the unit.

Sixth step: This involves ranking of the options. The existing options of supposed problem can be ranked based on the descending order cl_{i+} [7, 8].

Ultimately, the first designed model was examined by pilot test using the last health technology assessment projects call of The Iranian Department of Health Technology Assessment, including 3 technologies (Adenosine, Tissue Plasminogen Activator (tPA), Mechanical Thrombectomy) and the results were provided to the experts for judgment.

Results

Systematic review

After screening of retrieved papers via PRISMA framework, from 7012 papers, 40 were left included in the final phase. Criteria for selection of health technologies (in pre-assessment and also in assessment phase) were categorized into the six main themes such as 1 - health outcomes, 2 - disease and target population, 3 - technology alternatives, 4 -economic aspects, 5 - evidence and 6 - other

Table 1 Classification of main criteria and sub criteria based on frequency in reviewed Studies (in pre-Assessment and also in Assessment phase)

Main Criteria	Health Outcomes		Disease and Target Population		Alternatives		Economic Aspects		Evidence		Other Factors	
	Sub criteria	Frequency	Sub criteria	Frequency	Sub criteria	Frequency	Sub criteria	Frequency	Sub criteria	Frequency	Sub criteria	Frequency
1	Health effects/benefits	8	Disease severity	12	Number of alternatives	2	Cost-effectiveness	15	Quality of evidence	4	Issues related to health system	11
2	Clinical effects/benefits	7	Disease burden	8	Availability of alternative	1	Costs	11	Number of evidence	3	Sporadic sub criteria	11
3	Efficacy/effectiveness	4	Target population age	7	Limitations of comparative interventions	1	Budget impact	10	Evidence relevance and validity	1	Political, social and moral issues	10
4	Individual health benefits	3	Population size	3	Lack of alternatives	1	Economic impact	6	Power of evidence	1	Benefits of beneficiaries	6
5	Safety	3	Number of potential beneficiaries	3	-	-	Poverty Reduction	4	Completeness and consistency of reporting evidence	1	Issues related to patients	5
6	Quality of life	1	Characteristics of target social groups for intervention	2	-	-	Value for money	2	Adherence to requirements of decision making body	1	Issues related to decision-making conditions	5
7	Potential changes in health consequences	1	Number of patients	2	-	-	Financial opportunity/ consequences	2	-	-	Fairness and equity	4
8	The effect of assessment on reduction of uncertainty	1	Effect of technology on reduction of disease prevalence and incidence	1	-	-	Economic productivity	2	-	-	-	-
9	Marginal benefits	1	Disease impacts	1	-	-	Financial protection	1	-	-	-	-
10	Ability to reduce own health risk	1	Effect on targeted groups	1	-	-	Subsidized Payment	1	-	-		
11	Potential to extend life	1	Size of vulnerable population	1	-	-	Society interest and demand	1	-	-	-	-
12	Potential to detect a condition which, if treated early, averts costs in the future	1	-	-	-	-	Technology price and sale volume	1	-	-	-	-

factors. Maximum frequency in health outcomes related to health effects/benefits (8 studies), maximum frequency in disease and target population was related to disease severity (12 studies), maximum frequency in alternatives was related to number of alternatives (2 studies), maximum frequency in economic aspects was related to cost-effectiveness (15 studies), maximum frequency in evidence was related to quality of evidence (4 studies) and in other factors, max frequency was related to issues concerning the health system (11 studies) (Table 1).

Phase 1: Content validity verification

Sub criteria obtained from the systematic review phase that were classified into six dimensions were designed as three questionnaires, including 54 sub criteria and one question for extraction of extra criteria. To determine the content validity of 11 health experts, technology assessment were questioned in three ways: (a.) determination of face validity for each item (as two-option: it is clear and demonstrative or it is not clear and demonstrative), (b.) determination of content validity ratio (CVR) for each item (as three-option: it is necessary, useful but not necessary or not necessary) and (c.) determination of content validity index (CVI) for each item (as five-option: completely irrelevant, irrelevant, relatively irrelevant, relevant or completely relevant). Firstly, content validity index (CVI) was calculated for each item such that out of 55 items, 21 items were obtained following a minimum of 0.79 which included health benefits, clinical impacts, efficacy/effectiveness, potential to increase the life, safety, population size, the number of potential beneficiaries, the impact on target groups, the size of vulnerable populations, the availability of alternative technologies, cost-effectiveness, costs, budget impact, financial protection, the quality of evidence, number of evidence, the issues related to the health system, the issues related to the availability of expertise, equity in better access to health care and the question of additional criteria. Shortly following this, content validity ratio was calculated for each item such that, out of 54 sub criteria, all questioned experts had consensus on the necessity of only 9 sub criteria (health benefits, clinical benefits, efficacy/effectiveness, safety, cost-effectiveness, costs, technology price, quality of the evidence and issues related to rate availability of expertise) in this framework and obtained a score higher than score of Lawshe table for 11 experts. Whereas, Lawshe clarified that each item with more than half the total population of people had consensus on its necessity, and had a level of content validity (to the same rate of people that voted to its necessity) [9]. Thus, in addition to 9 sub criteria that had obtained the required score of CVR, a sub criteria greater than 50 % of people (including 50 % itself and higher) voted to its necessity and a CVI greater than 0.79 was obtained, kept and included into the final questionnaire (for assessment of their importance). These sub criteria were as follows: clinical impacts, efficiency/effectiveness, individual health benefits, safety, population size, number of potential beneficiaries, effect on targeted group, vulnerable population size, availability of alternative technologies, quality of evidence, number of evidence, budget impact, cost effectiveness, financial protection, issues related to health system and availability rate of experience and specialty and additional question for other criteria. Based on face validity, according to the opinion of experts, 4 sub criteria including individual health benefits, clinical impacts, efficiency/effectiveness, and effect on targeted group due to their overlap were all combined in the efficiency/effectiveness sub criteria. In addition, in the same manner, sub criteria of number of potential beneficiaries was combined with the population size, costs combined with cost effectiveness while number of evidence was renamed as the adequacy of the evidence. Thus, in the final questionnaire, 13 sub criteria were included based on 6 dimensions of conceptual model of study (Table 2).

Table 2 Sub criteria obtained after first phase of question from experts

No.	Criteria	Sub criteria
Dimension 1	Health Outcomes	Efficiency/Effectiveness, Safety
Dimension 2	Disease and target population	Population Size, Vulnerable Population Size
Dimension 3	Alternatives	Availability of Alternative Technologies
Dimension 4	Economic Aspects	Budget Impact, Cost Effectiveness of Technology in Other Countries, Financial Protection
Dimension 5	Evidence	Quality of Evidence, Adequacy Number of Evidence
Dimension 6	Other criteria	Issues Related to Health System, Issues Related to Availability of Experience and Specialty about Technology and Issue Related to the Equity

Table 3 Final sub criteria obtained after two phases questioning from experts

No.	Criteria	Sub criteria
Dimension 1	Health Outcomes	Efficiency/Effectiveness, Safety
Dimension 2	Disease and target population	Population Size, Vulnerable Population Size
Dimension 3	Alternatives	Availability of Alternative Technologies
Dimension 4	Economic Aspects	Budget Impact, Cost Effectiveness of Technology in Other Countries, Financial Protection
Dimension 5	Evidence	Quality of evidence
Dimension 6	Other criteria	-

Table 4 Relative weight obtained from normalization of geometric mean of each row of final matrix

	Efficiency/ effectiveness	Safety	Population size	Vulnerable population	Availability rate of alternative technologies	Cost effectiveness in other countries	Budget impact	Financial protection	Quality of evidence
Relative Weight	0.12	0.20	0.06	0.08	0.08	0.13	0.08	0.09	0.15

Phase 2: Determining importance of each sub criteria

Thirteen obtained sub criteria in previous phase were included into the final questionnaire phase based on the same process, 9 sub criteria, including Efficiency/effectiveness, safety, Population size, vulnerable population size, availability of alternative technologies, budget Impact, cost effectiveness of technology in other countries, financial protection, quality of evidence that obtained a greater than 75 % importance as viewpoint of questioned experts, were included in the paired wise comparisons questionnaire as the final 9 effective criteria in the priority setting of health technology assessment and this finalized the extraction of relative weight (Table 3). To assess the reliability of the final questionnaire, data obtained from each sub criterion were entered into SPSS software as Likert spectrum and the Cronbach's alpha was calculated with its value at 0.697. This demonstrated an acceptable reliability of the final questionnaire. Moreover, no consensus was made between questioned experts in relation to the additional criteria individually mentioned by the experts. These criteria include Ethical issues, burden of disease, information value, the elasticity of demand for technology, procedures and methods of diagnosis and treatment, the external dependence of the use of technology, the development and application of technology in the world and the indication of technology.

Phase 3: Identification of relative weights of final criteria

Nine final effective criteria selected based on the opinion of experts were designed during the first and second phases as paired comparisons questionnaire and in another case they were presented to nine questioned experts in the first and second phases (at this phase, two experts of the previous phases were not available) in order to extract the relative weight of each one of the 9

Table 5 Coding of efficiency/effectiveness criteria [10]

Quantitative code	Status	For Technologies Related to Treatment and Rehabilitation: Clinical Benefit and Improvement of Quality of Life
5	Perfect treatment	
4	Lifetime increasing and major improvement of quality of life	
3	Lifetime increasing and low improvement of quality of life	
2	Major improvement of quality of life	
1	Low improvement of quality of life	
Quantitative code	Status	For Technologies Related to Screening and Diagnosis: Accuracy of Technology and Treatment Status of Disease under Screening and Diagnosis
5	Technology accuracy was more than 80 % and disease under screening and diagnosis may be treated.	
4	Technology accuracy was within 60–80 % and disease under screening and diagnosis may be treated.	
3	Technology accuracy was over 80 % but the disease under screening and diagnosis may not be treated.	
2	Technology accuracy was within 60–80 % and disease under screening and diagnosis may not be treated or accuracy was 60 % and disease under screening and diagnosis may be treated.	
1	Technology accuracy was less than 60 % and disease under screening and diagnosis may be treated.	
Quantitative code	Status	For Technologies Related to Prevention: Effectiveness of Technology for Prevention of Disease
5	Over 90 %	
4	81–90 %	
3	71–80 %	
2	61–70 %	
1	Less or equal to 60 %	

final criteria. After filling the 9 questionnaires aforementioned, the information of these questionnaires was entered into an excel sheet as 9 matrixes (9*9) and to extract the final weight and equalizing the data of these 9 matrixes, a final matrix was formed such that in each one of its entries was included the geometric mean of its corresponding entries in 9 matrixes (9*9). The relative weigh of each criterion was extracted from the final formed matrix through normalization of geometric mean of each line thereof. Later, the obtained inconsistency ratio for the system was calculated, which was less than the range of 0.1 (IR = 0.03) and demonstrated consistency between extracted weights (Table 4).

Phase 4: Piloting the priority setting model

According to the inquiry from health technology assessment department of ministry of health, and medical education, 3 health technologies that were requested for health technology assessment, were selected and TOPSIS priority setting pilot model was implemented on them. These technologies included the following:

a. Adenosine
b. Tissue Plasminogen Activator (tPA)
c. Mechanical Thrombectomy

Furthermore, to fill the decision matrix for execution of model pilot, values 1 to 5 were designed for each one of 9 final criteria, and data related thereto were extracted from available evidence for the three pilot technologies: (Tables 5, 6, 7, 8, 9, 10, 11, 12 and 13).

The data obtained from evidence about three abovementioned technologies

Adenosine for the treatment of supraventricular tachycardia [11] Status of efficiency/effectiveness criteria: This medication with a dose of 12 mg quickly and effectively terminated proximal episodes of the supraventricular tachycardia (relative code = 5) [12]. Status of safety criteria: The use of this medication resulted in a slightly bad side effect such as confusion, nausea, redness of face etc. (relative code = 4) [13]. Status of population size criteria: Supraventricular tachycardia prevalence was 2.25 cases in a general 1000-persons population. Therefore, the size of target population of this medication in Iran, considering its 80 million population was about 180 thousand peoples (relative code = 4) [11]. Status of vulnerable population size criteria: The probability of supraventriclar tachycardia in women was 2 times more than men, and majorly in pregnancy and fertility ages (within 15–30 years) (relative code = 4) [11]. Status of alternative technologies availability criteria: Verapamile is the alternative medication that has equal efficiency and relatively equal safety and mostly available in the health centers (relative code = 2) [11, 13]. Status of quality of evidence criteria: Concerning this medication, there is a systematic review study of randomized controlled studies of meta-analysis type with a high quality (relative code = 5) [13]. Status of cost effectiveness criteria: The data about this criterion was unspecified (relative code = 1). Status of budget impact criterion: The data about this criterion was unspecified (relative code = 1). Status of financial protection criterion: The data about this criterion was unspecified (relative code = 1).

Table 6 Coding of Safety Criteria (as qualitative estimation or using quantitative indicators available in the safety context): Improvement rate in reduction of risk or incidence of side effects arising out of utilization of technology in the target population

Quantitative code	Status
5	Completely safe (lack of side effects) (Incidence of side effects less than 1 %)
4	Relatively safe (mild and slight side effects) (Incidence of side effects between 1 to 9.9 %)
3	Proper safety (averagely side effects) (Incidence of side effects between 10 to 39 %)
2	Poor safety (much side effects) (Incidence of side effects 40 to 50 %)
1	Unsafe (major side effects) (Incidence of side effects more than 50 %)

Tissue plasminogen activator (tPA) for the treatment of stroke [14] Status of efficiency/effectiveness criteria: The use of this medication resulted in a 0.07 increase of lifetime together with 0.24 increase of QALY (relative code = 3) [15]. Status of safety status: In comparison to placebo, the use of this technology had higher risk of intracranial hemorrhage (relative code = 3) [16]. Status of population size criteria: prevalence of stroke in west countries was about 12000 per million peoples [17]. The prevalence and incidence of stroke in Iran was significantly higher than western countries [18]. Thus, in Iranian population, assuming 80 million people, the population size under impact of this disease will be higher than one million people (relative code = 5). Status

Table 7 Coding of population size criteria: number of people under effect of disease or health problem that will be treated or prevented by technology [10]

Quantitative code	Status
5	More than 500000
4	100001 to 500000
3	50001 to 100000
2	10001 to 50000
1	Less or equal to 10000

Table 8 Coding of vulnerable population criteria: share of children below 5 years old or women in fertility ages or elders over 65 years old or patients suffering from special diseases (including MS, dialysis, hemophilia and thalassemia) or patients suffering from neuropsychological diseases in the target population

Quantitative code	Status
5	More than 50 %
4	26–50 %
3	11–25 %
2	Less or equal to 10 %
1	Unspecified vulnerable population size

of vulnerable population size criteria: The incident of stroke was mostly prevalent among Iranian women (within 51–53 %) and majorly occurred within seventh decade of life (relative code = 4) [19]. Status of alternative technologies availability criteria: This technology was the first and the only effective therapeutic method for patients with stroke 3 times after its first occurrence (relative code = 5) [16]. Status of quality of evidence criteria: In relation to this technology, there was a high quality randomized multicenter controlled trial (elative code = 3) [16]. Status of cost effectiveness criteria: The incremental cost effectiveness ratio for all patients consuming this medication was about 6255 Dollars per QALY. This value was obtained for USA. Considering her per capital GDP in 2014 as equal to 53000$. This value is rather highly cost effective (relative code = 5) [15]. Status of budget impact criteria: The data in relation to this criterion was unspecified (relative code = 1). Status of financial protection criteria: The data in relation to this criterion was unspecified (relative code = 1).

Table 9 Coding of Availability rate of Alternative technologies (qualitative estimation): Availability of other alternative methods for technology in target population

Quantitative code	Status
5	Partial availability of alternative technologies with the same safety and effectiveness for target population
4	Relatively appropriate availability of alternative technologies with the same safety and effectiveness for target population
3	Appropriate availability of alternative technologies with the same safety and effectiveness for target population
2	High availability of alternative technologies with the same safety and effectiveness for target population
1	Very high availability of alternative technologies with the same safety and effectiveness for target population

Table 10 Coding of quality of evidence: quality of evidences of health technology assessment, systematic review and clinical trials on technology

Quantitative code	Status
5	Systematic reviews with high quality of randomized controlled trials or heath technology assessment with high quality therein systematic review has been performed (based on checklist of CASP and INAHTA)
4	Systematic reviews with medium or low quality of randomized controlled trials or heath technology assessment with medium or low quality therein systematic review has been performed (based on checklist of CASP and INAHTA)
3	Randomized controlled trials or clinical controlled trials with high quality or systematic review with high quality of other studies (based on CASP checklist)
2	Randomized controlled trials or clinical controlled trials with medium or low quality or systematic review with medium or low quality of other studies or cohort studies with any kind of quality (based on CASP checklist)
1	Other studies (cohort, case series and quasi-random studies etc.) with any quality

Mechanical thrombectomy for the treatment of stroke [20] Status of efficiency/effectiveness criteria: This technology resulted in a 0.68 increase of QALY (relative code = 1) [21]. Status of safety criteria: This technology was safe which could demonstrate higher rate of symptomatic bleeding than medicinal methods (relative code = 3) [20]. Status of population size criteria: Prevalence of stroke in west countries was about 12000 per million peoples [17]. The Prevalence and incidence of stroke in Iran was significantly higher than western countries [18]. Thus, in Iranian population, assuming 80 million people, the population size under impact of this disease will be higher than one million people (relative code = 5). Status of vulnerable population size criteria: The incident of stroke was mostly prevalent among Iranian women (within 51–53 %) and majorly occurred within seventh decade of life (relative code = 4) [19]. Status of alternative technologies availability criteria: This method was the only

Table 11 Coding of cost effectiveness: status of cost effectiveness of technology in other countries

Quantitative code	Status
5	very cost effective (cost per QALY lower than 1 time more than per capital GDP)
4	Reasonable cost effective (cost for QALY within 1–2 times more than per capital GDP)
3	Slightly cost effective (cost for QALY within 2–3 times more than per capital GDP)
2	Not-cost effective (cost for QALY more than 3 times more than per capital GDP)
1	Unspecified cost effectiveness status

Table 12 Coding of budget impact (as qualitative estimation): net impact of covering the technology on the budget of health system

Quantitative code	Status
5	Significant savings
4	Moderate savings
3	Very slight change in the amount of savings
2	No significant changes in the costs or additional charges
1	Unspecified budget impact status

therapeutic method for patients with incident of stroke who were not treated by clot solving medications, since the use of this method resulted in failure with respect to them (during first 3–4 h after this occurrence) (relative code = 5) [20]. Status of quality of evidence criteria: In relation to this technology, there was health technology report from randomized r controlled trial with high quality (elative code = 5) [20]. Status of cost effectiveness criteria: The incremental cost effectiveness ratio for all patients taking this medication was about 16000 Dollars per QALY. This value was obtained for USA and considering per capital GDP of this country in 2014, which equaled 53000$, this value is rather highly cost effective (relative code = 5) [21]. Status of budget impact criteria: The data in relation to this criteria was unspecified (relative code = 1). Status of financial protection criterion: The data in relation to this criterion was unspecified (relative code = 1).

Final TOPSIS pilot model

Finally TOPSIS pilot model was designed by 3 health technologies and relative weights. The results showed that tissue plasminogen activator treatment was the first priority, adenosine was second and mechanical thrombectomy was third in performing health technology assessment by Iranian ministry of health and medical education (Table 14). Finally, the pilot model was presented to an internal panel which was made up of 6 experts of health technology assessment and was approved.

Table 13 Coding of financial protection: the probability that the technology covered by the basic health insurance package and thus prevent the occurrence of catastrophic health expenditures

Quantitative code	Status
5	100 %
4	76 to 99 %
3	50 to 75 %
2	Less than 50 %
1	Unspecified financial protection status

Discussion

Generally, this study which was applied based on the combined model of analytic hierarchy process and TOPSIS, was presented for the first time in the world, in the health technology assessment priority setting context. The differences and similarities between this model and main model of Canadian Agency for Drugs and Technologies in Health are explained in terms of finalized criteria in this model. The criteria used in this model which extracted using a systematic review which included a number of alternatives and access such as, budget impact, clinical impact, controversial nature of technology, disease burden, economic impact, moral and legal issues, quality and level of evidences, expected level of interests, time period of assessment and its effect on health and clinical medicine policies, variety in direction for use and application of technology. The criteria used in the model of this study included efficiency/effectiveness, safety, population size, vulnerable population size, availability of alternative technologies, cost effectiveness in other countries, budget impact, financial protection, and quality of evidences. Efficiency/effectiveness, availability of alternative technologies, quality of evidences and budget impact as common items and controversial nature of technology, disease burden, economic impact, moral and legal issues, expected level of interests, time period of assessment and its effect on health and clinical medicine policies, variety in direction for use and application of technology in Canadian model and safety, population size, vulnerable population size, cost effectiveness in other countries and financial protection in the model of this study were assumed as differences. In relation to multi criteria decision making model used in this study, it is noteworthy that in Canadian model, overall relative weight extraction, as well as, final priority setting were performed based on analytic hierarchy process, whilst in the model of this study, only relative weight was extracted for determination of exact weight using final purpose which implied that, health technology assessment priority setting in Iran, through paired comparisons and no judgment of experts, were applied on the final model. This subject was designed in order to adhere to evidence based medicine (EBM) and its evidence pyramid using TOPSIS model and ascertain the use of codes extracted from evidence related to the technology, which can prevent the fully and unlimited interventions of medical beneficiary groups for selection of health technologies that are assumed as the stewardship scope. In fact, out of 11 criteria acquired from systematic review phase of Canadian model and mentioned earlier, 6 criteria including disease burden, clinical impact, alternative technologies, budget impact, economic impact and available evidence were selected as the main criteria by health technology assessment experts of that country.

Table 14 Final TOPSIS pilot model

Decision Matrix									
Criteria Technology	Efficiency/ effectiveness	Safety	Population size	Vulnerable population	Availability rate of alternative technologies	Cost effectiveness in other countries	Budget impact	Financial protection	Quality of evidence
Adenosine	5	4	4	4	2	1	1	1	5
Tissue Plasminogen Activator	3	3	5	4	5	5	1	1	3
Mechanical Thrombectomy	1	3	5	4	5	5	1	1	5
Weight Matrix									
	Efficiency/ effectiveness	Safety	Population size	Vulnerable population	Availability rate of alternative technologies	Cost effectiveness in other countries	Budget impact	Financial protection	Quality of evidence
RelativeWeight	0.12	0.20	0.06	0.08	0.08	0.13	0.08	0.09	0.15
Norm Matrix									
Criteria Technology	Efficiency/ effectiveness	Safety	Population size	Vulnerable population	Availability rate of alternative technologies	Cost effectiveness in other countries	Budget impact	Financial protection	Quality of evidence
Adenosine	0.85	0.69	0.49	0.58	0.27	0.14	0.58	0.58	0.65
Tissue Plasminogen Activator	0.51	0.51	0.62	0.58	0.68	0.70	0.58	0.58	0.39
Mechanical Thrombectomy	0.17	0.51	0.62	0.58	0.68	0.70	0.58	0.58	0.65
V Matrix									
	Efficiency/ effectiveness	Safety	Population size	Vulnerable population	Availability rate of alternative technologies	Cost effectiveness in other countries	Budget impact	Financial protection	Quality of evidence
Adenosine	0.11	0.14	0.03	0.05	0.02	0.02	0.05	0.05	0.10
Tissue Plasminogen Activator	0.06	0.10	0.04	0.05	0.05	0.09	0.05	0.05	0.06
Mechanical Thrombectomy	0.02	0.10	0.04	0.05	0.05	0.09	0.05	0.05	0.10
Positive Ideal									
	Efficiency/ effectiveness	Safety	Population size	Vulnerable population	Availability rate of alternative technologies	Cost effectiveness in other countries	Budget impact	Financial protection	Quality of evidence
A–	0.11	0.14	0.04	0.05	0.05	0.09	0.05	0.05	0.10
Negative Ideal									
	Efficiency/ effectiveness	Safety	Population size	Vulnerable population	Availability rate of alternative technologies	Cost effectiveness in other countries	Budget impact	Financial protection	Quality of evidence
A-	0.02	0.10	0.03	0.05	0.02	0.02	0.05	0.05	0.06
Final Priority Setting									
d1+	0.08	d1-	0.10	closeness1	0.56	2			
d2+	0.07	d2-	0.09	closeness2	0.57	1			
d3+	0.09	d3-	0.09	closeness3	0.49	3			

In relation to weight extraction phase, the following values were obtained: disease burden (0.216), clinical impact (0.258), alternative technologies (0.081), budget impact (0.143), economic impact (0.167), and available evidence (0.135) [4]. Furthermore, these values were comparable with the values obtained from the present, study including efficiency/effectiveness (0.12), safety (0.2), population size (0.06), vulnerable population size (0.08), availability of alternative technologies (0.08), cost effectiveness in other countries (0.13), budget impact (0.08), financial protection (0.09), and quality of evidence (0.15). The model designed in this study may also be compared to the health technology assessment priority setting model in Latvia. In this model, research of literature review as well as qualitative study was used in the model design, followed by a test for health technology assessment priority setting. To test the model and method, 3 round Delphi model was implemented using electronic questionnaire. Accordingly, Delphi technique was invented as a method for making consensus in the health technology assessment priority setting for Latvia. Criteria affecting this model included health benefit, evidence, assessment scheduling, expected level of policy makers' benefits, social, legal and moral concepts [22]. Two criteria of health benefit and evidence were common criteria in the model designed in the present study. The designed model of this study may be compared to the health technology assessment priority setting model in Netherlands. In this model, various methods were used for classification, scoring and weighting the policy making criteria, including actual disease burden, potential health benefit, number of patients, direct intervention costs for each patient, financial consequences of intervention implementation over time and its impact on the health system policies [23]. Three criteria, including health benefit, number of patients and financial consequences were assumed as the three common criteria in the model designed for this study. Overall, the model designed in the present study in comparison to previous models in this context had innovation in the light of effective criteria because of its additional safety, vulnerable population size, cost effectiveness of technology in other countries and financial protection to the previous models. In addition, as mentioned before, technically this is the first time that a combined model of analytic hierarchy process and TOPSIS has been used in this relation.

Conclusion

According to the results of this study, this model with nine effective criteria and their relative weights and in combination with TOPSIS approach could be used with suitable applicability by health technology assessment department in deputy of curative affairs and food and drug organization for determination of research priorities in health technology assessment. Considering the increasing growth of health technologies, ministry of health and medical education, using this model, can allocate its research budgets to health technologies assessment which are of priority and importance to the health system and society. It may promote the final impact of health technology assessment reports on the macro health policies and optimize the allocation of financial resources of health sector.

Limitations

This model is not applicable for prioritization of orphan drugs.

Competing interest

The authors declare that they have no competing interests

Authors' contribution

MRM contributed to design, data analysis and drafting. PR and AAN contributed to design, data collection, drafting and supervision. AO contributed to design and drafting. SJT contributed to design and data collection. All authors read and approved the final manuscript.

Acknowledgement

This study was part of a Ph.D. dissertation which was supported by Science and Research branch of Islamic Azad University, Tehran, Iran and Iranian Ministry of Health and Medical Education.

Author details

[1]Department of Health Services Management, Science and Research Branch, Islamic Azad University, Tehran, Iran. [2]Department of Health Services Management, School of Management and Medical Information Science, Iran University of Medical Sciences, Tehran, Iran. [3]National Institute for Health Research, Tehran University of Medical Sciences, Tehran, Iran.

References

1. Carlsson P. Health technology assessment and priority setting for health policy in Sweden. Int J Technol Assess Health Care. 2004;20(01):44–54.
2. Bridges JF, Jones C. Patient-based health technology assessment: a vision of the future. Int J Technol Assess Health Care. 2007;23(1):30–5.
3. Noorani HZ, Husereau DR, Boudreau R, Skidmore B. Priority setting for health technology assessments: a systematic review of current practical approaches. Int J Technol Assess Health Care. 2007;23(03):310–5.
4. Husereau D, Boucher M, Noorani H. Priority setting for health technology assessment at CADTH. Int J Technol Assess Health Care. 2010;26(3):341–7.
5. Goetghebeur MM, Wagner M, Khoury H, Rindress D, Grégoire JP, Deal C. Combining multicriteria decision analysis, ethics and health technology assessment: applying the EVIDEM decision making framework to growth hormone for Turner syndrome patients. Cost Eff Resour Alloc. 2010;8(1):4.
6. Ghodsi Pour. Analitical Hierarchy Process (AHP). Tehran, Iran: Amirkabir Press; 2003
7. Shirouyehzad H, Tavakoli MM. "Multi Attribute Decision Making". Tehran, Iran: Barin Press; 2014.
8. Asgharpour M. "Multi Attribute Decision Making". Tehran, Iran: TEHRAN university publication; 2004.
9. Lawshe CH. A quantitative approach to content validity. Pers Psychol. 1975;28:563–75.
10. Youngkong S, Baltussen R, Tantivess S, Mohara A, Teerawattananon Y. Multicriteria decision analysis for including health interventions in the universal health coverage benefit package in Thailand. Value Health. 2012;15(6):961–70.
11. Medi C, Kalman JM, Freedman SB. Supraventricular tachycardia. Med J Aust. 2009;190(5):255–60.
12. DiMarco JP, Miles W, Akhtar M, Milstein S, Sharma AD, Platia E, Govier WC. Adenosine for paroxysmal supraventricular tachycardia: dose ranging and comparison with verapamil: assessment in placebo-controlled, multicenter trials. Ann Intern Med. 1990;113(2):104–10.
13. Delaney B, Loy J, Kelly AM. The relative efficacy of adenosine versus verapamil for the treatment of stable paroxysmal supraventricular tachycardia in adults: a meta-analysis. Eur J Emerg Med. 2011;18(3):148–52.
14. Health Quality Ontario. Effect of a 60-minute door-to-needle tissue plasminogen activator on stroke disability: a rapid review. Toronto: Health Quality Ontario (HQO). Rapid Review. 2015. http://www.crd.york.ac.uk/crdweb/ShowRecord.asp?ID=32015000499.
15. Boudreau DM, Guzauskas G, Villa KF, Fagan SC, Veenstra DL. A model of cost-effectiveness of tissue plasminogen activator in patient subgroups 3 to 4.5 hours after onset of acute ischemic stroke. Ann Emerg Med. 2013;61(1):46–55.
16. Bluhmki E, Chamorro Á, Dávalos A, Machnig T, Sauce C, Wahlgren N, et al. Stroke treatment with alteplase given 3·0–4·5 h after onset of acute ischaemic stroke (ECASS III): additional outcomes and subgroup analysis of a randomised controlled trial. Lancet Neurol. 2009;8(12):1095–102.

17. Tubaro M, Vranckx P, Price S, Vrints C. The ESC Textbook of Intensive and Acute Cardiovascular Care. Tehran, Iran: Oxford University Press. 2014.
18. Safari R, Borhanihaghighi A, Heydari ST, Safari A, Cruz-Flores S. Stroke subtypes in southern Iran. Galen Med J. 2015;4(1):47–9.
19. Hosseini AA, Sobhani-Rad D, Ghandehari K, Benamer HT. Frequency and clinical patterns of stroke in Iran-Systematic and critical review. BMC Neurol. 2010;10(1):72.
20. Puñal-Riobóo J, Atienza G, Blanco M. Safety and efficacy of mechanical thrombectomy using stent retrievers in the endovascular treatment of acute ischaemic stroke: a systematic review. Interv Neurol. 2014;3(3-4):149–64.
21. Kim AS, Nguyen-Huynh M, Johnston SC. A cost–utility analysis of mechanical thrombectomy as an adjunct to intravenous tissue-type plasminogen activator for acute large-vessel ischemic stroke. Stroke. 2011;42(7):2013–8.
22. Jankauskiene D, Petronyte G. A model for HTA priority setting: experience in Lithuania. Int J Technol Assess Health Care. 2013;29(4):450.
23. Oortwijn WJ, Vondeling H, van Barneveld T, van Vugt C, Bouter LM. Priority setting for health technology assessment in The Netherlands: principles and practice. Health Policy. 2002;62(3):227–42.

27

A study on quantitative structure–activity relationship and molecular docking of metalloproteinase inhibitors based on L-tyrosine scaffold

Maryam Abbasi[1,2], Fatemeh Ramezani[1], Maryam Elyasi[3], Hojjat Sadeghi-Aliabadi[2] and Massoud Amanlou[1*]

Abstract

Background: MMP-2 enzyme is a kind of matrix metalloproteinases that digests the denatured collagens and gelatins. It is highly involved in the process of tumor invasion and has been considered as a promising target for cancer therapy. The structural requirements of an MMP-2 inhibitor are: (1) a functional group that binds the zinc ion, and (2) a functional group which interacts with the enzyme backbone and the side chains which undergo effective interactions with the enzyme subsites.

Methods: In the present study, a QSAR model was generated to screen new inhibitors of MMP-2 based on L–hydroxy tyrosine scaffold. Descriptors generation were done by Hyperchem 8, DRAGON and Gaussian98W programs. SPSS and MATLAB programs have been used for multiple linear regression (MLR) and genetic algorithm partial least squares (GA-PLS) analyses and for theoretical validation. Applicability domain of the model was performed to screen new compounds. The binding site potential of all inhibitors was verified by structure-based docking according to their binding energy and then the best inhibitors were selected.

Results: The best QSAR models in MLR and GA-PLS were reported, with the square correlation coefficient for leave-one-out cross-validation (Q^2_{LOO}) larger than 0.921 and 0.900 respectively. The created MLR and GA-PLS models indicated the importance of molecular size, degree of branching, flexibility, shape, three-dimensional coordination of different atoms in a molecule in inhibitory activities against MMP-2.
The docking study indicated that lipophilic and hydrogen bonding interactions among the inhibitors and the receptor are involved in a ligand-receptor interaction. The oxygen of carbonyl and sulfonyl groups is important for hydrogen bonds of ligand with Leu82 and Ala83. R_2 and R_3 substituents play a main role in hydrogen bonding interactions. R_1 is sited in the hydrophobic pocket. Methylene group can help a ligand to be fitted in the lipophilic pocket, so two methylene groups are better than one. The Phenyl group can create a π-π interaction with Phe86.

Conclusions: The QSAR and docking analyses demonstrated to be helpful tools in the prediction of anti-cancer activities and a guide to the synthesis of new metalloproteinase inhibitors based on L-tyrosine scaffold.

Keywords: GA-PLS, Metalloproteinase inhibitors, MLR, Molecular docking, QSAR

* Correspondence: amanlou@tums.ac.ir
[1]Department of Medicinal Chemistry, Faculty of Pharmacy, Pharmaceutica Science Research Center, Tehran University of Medical Science, Tehran, Iran
Full list of author information is available at the end of the article

Introduction

The matrix metalloproteinases (MMPs) function predominantly as enzymes that degrade structural components of the extracellular matrix (ECM) [1-4]. MMPs play a substantial role in tumor progression and invasion of inflammatory cells. Among MMPs, MMP-2 easily digests the denatured collagens and gelatins [5,6]. It is highly involved in the process of tumor invasion and has been considered as a promising target for cancer therapy [3,7,8]. MMP-2 has a catalytic center) zinc (II) ion (and two hydrophobic domains (S1′ pocket and S1 pocket). S1′ pocket, the key domain of MMP-2, is deeper and narrower than other MMP subtypes and S1 pocket is a solvent exposure domain [3,9,10].

The structural requirements of an MMP-2 inhibitor are: (1) a functional group that binds the zinc ion (zinc-binding group; ZBG), capable of chelating the active site zinc ion; (2) a functional group which interacts with the backbone of enzyme; (3) side chains that undergo effective interactions with the enzyme subsites, such as S1′ pocket and S1 pocket [3,11,12].

Cheng et al. studied the L–hydroxy proline scaffold-based MMP-2 inhibitors in 2008 [13], and, in order to identify more potent MMP-2 inhibitors, replaced L-hydroxy proline with the L-tyrosine scaffold to form a new integrated structural pattern. They reported that the alteration in substitution pattern at R_1, R_2 and R_3 positions alter MMP-2 inhibitory activity [1].

In 2012, 30 L–hydroxy tyrosine scaffold-based MMP-2 inhibitors were identified. It seems that finding a relationship between the structure of these compounds and their inhibitory activities in order to design structures with better activities and to predict their activity would be essential.

Quantitative structure activity relationships (QSARs), one of the most extensively used methods in chemometrics, and molecular docking are two of the helpful methods for drug design and prediction of drug activity [14-16]. QSAR models are mathematical equations which generate a communication between chemical structures and their biological activities, while molecular docking is done to specify the structural features that are important for interaction with a receptor.

In this report, we have performed a QSAR study and a molecular docking examination on 30 compounds of L-tyrosine derivatives which had been synthesized and evaluated as metalloproteinase (MMP-2) inhibitors [1].

Materials and methods

QSAR

All calculations were implemented using an Intel Core i5 2.4 GHz processor, with the windows 7 operating system. Geometry optimization was done by Hyperchem 8.0 software. Descriptor generation was performed by Hyperchem 8.0, DRAGON package and Gaussian 98 W programs. SPSS software (version 11.5) and MATLAB software (version 7.12.0) were used for model creation and validation methods.

Activity data and descriptors generation

In this study, the biological data employed is MMP-2 inhibitory activity of 30 compounds. The synthesis and determination of biological activity of these inhibitors have been reported by Cheng et al. [1]. The structure of these compounds and their biological activity are shown in Table 1. The two-dimensional structures of molecules were drawn using Hyperchem 8.0 software. At the beginning, pre-optimization was conducted using the MM + molecular mechanic force field and then a more accurate optimization was performed with the semi-empirical PM3 method. The optimization was performed using the Polak–Ribiere algorithm until the root mean square gradient reached 0.01 kcal/ (Å mol). Hyperchem 8.0 program was also used to calculate chemical descriptors including: surface area, molecular volume, hydration energy, octanol/water partition coefficient (logP), molar refractivity, molar polarisability and molar mass.

The output files of Hyperchem 8.0 software (.hin files) were transferred to DRAGON package to calculate four classes of descriptors (0D, 1D, 2D and 3D) including 28 constitutional descriptors, 10 functional groups, 18 atom-centered fragments, 216 topological descriptors, 15 molecular walk counts, 64 BCUT descriptors, 24 Galvestopol.charge indices, 96 2D autocorrelations, 14 charge descriptors, 41 Randic molecular profiles, 27 geometrical descriptors, 150 radial distribution function descriptors (RDF), 160 3D-MoRSE descriptors, 99 WHIM descriptors and 196 GETAWAY descriptors.

The z-matrix files of compounds were also provided by Hyperchem 8.0 program (.zmt files) and then were transferred as input files to the Gaussian98W program [17]. Semi-empirical molecular orbital calculation by PM3 method was performed using Gaussian98W program. Different quantum chemical descriptors were obtained by this method including highest occupied molecular orbital energy (E_{HOMO}), lowest unoccupied molecular orbital energy (E_{LUMO}), and molecular dipole moment. Local charge was obtained by PM3 method in Gaussian98W. Hardness ($\eta = 0.5$ $(E_{HOMO} + E_{LUMO})$), softness ($S = 1/\eta$), electronegativity ($\chi = 0.5$ $(E_{HOMO} - E_{LUMO})$) and electrophilicity ($\omega = \chi^2/2\eta$) were calculated according to the method proposed by Thanikaivelan et al. [18].

Data processing and models building

All calculated descriptors were collected in a data matrix, D, the number on rows was representative of molecule numbers and the numbers on columns accounted for

Table 1 Chemical structures of L-tyrosine derivatives and their experimental and predicted activity by MLR and GA-PLS models

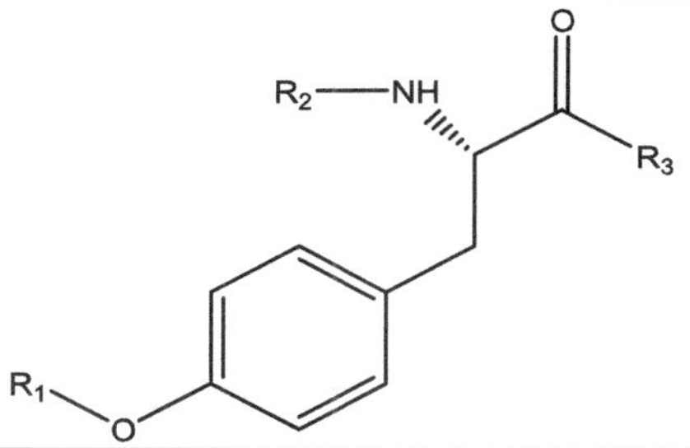

Comp.	R_1	R_2	R_3	Experimental pIC_{50}	Predicted pIC_{50}	
					MLR	GA-PLS
4a	$C_6H_5CH_2$	C_6H_5CO	OCH_3	4.17	4.01	3.90
4b	$C_6H_5CH_2$	p-$CH_3C_6H_4CO$	OCH_3	4.08	3.82	3.92
4c	$C_6H_5CH_2$	CH_3CO	OCH_3	4.56	4.42	4.61
4d	$C_6H_5CH_2$	CH_3SO_2	OCH_3	4.75	4.74	4.74
4e	$C_6H_5CH_2$	p-$CH_3C_6H_4SO_2$	OCH_3	4.97	4.75	4.86
4f	$C_6H_5CH_2CH_2$	C_6H_5CO	OCH_3	4.13	4.16	3.79
4 g	$C_6H_5CH_2CH_2$	p-$CH_3C_6H_4CO$	OCH_3	4.07	3.94	4.42
4 h	$C_6H_5CH_2CH_2$	CH_3CO	OCH_3	4.90	4.98	4.97
4i	$C_6H_5CH_2CH_2$	CH_3SO_2	OCH_3	5.62	5.82	5.98
4j	$C_6H_5CH_2CH_2$	p-$CH_3C_6H_4SO_2$	OCH_3	5.20	5.24	5.44
5a	$C_6H_5CH_2$	C_6H_5CO	OH	5.01	4.39	4.78
5b	$C_6H_5CH_2$	p-$CH_3C_6H_4CO$	OH	5.09	4.77	4.3
5c	$C_6H_5CH_2$	CH_3CO	OH	5.52	5.68	5.66
5d	$C_6H_5CH_2$	CH_3SO_2	OH	5.85	6.03	6.06
5e	$C_6H_5CH_2$	p-$CH_3C_6H_4SO_2$	OH	5.60	5.99	5.91
5f	$C_6H_5CH_2CH_2$	C_6H_5CO	OH	5.12	5.57	5.33
5 g	$C_6H_5CH_2CH_2$	p-$CH_3C_6H_4CO$	OH	5.35	5.90	5.82
5 h	$C_6H_5CH_2CH_2$	CH_3CO	OH	6.12	6.67	6.08
5i	$C_6H_5CH_2CH_2$	CH_3SO_2	OH	6.92	6.69	6.48
5j	$C_6H_5CH_2CH_2$	p-$CH_3C_6H_4SO_2$	OH	6.57	6.49	6.52
6a	$C_6H_5CH_2$	C_6H_5CO	NHOH	5.77	6.04	5.84
6b	$C_6H_5CH_2$	p-$CH_3C_6H_4CO$	NHOH	6.34	6.42	6.82
6c	$C_6H_5CH_2$	CH_3CO	NHOH	7.43	7.32	6.84
6d	$C_6H_5CH_2$	CH_3SO_2	NHOH	7.17	7.44	7.39
6e	$C_6H_5CH_2$	p-$CH_3C_6H_4SO_2$	NHOH	7.60	7.19	7.14
6f	$C_6H_5CH_2CH_2$	C_6H_5CO	NHOH	6.05	6.05	6.86
6 g	$C_6H_5CH_2CH_2$	p-$CH_3C_6H_4CO$	NHOH	5.41	5.57	5.95
6 h	$C_6H_5CH_2CH_2$	CH_3CO	NHOH	7.89	7.55	7.53
6i	$C_6H_5CH_2CH_2$	CH_3SO_2	NHOH	7.54	7.91	7.94
6j	$C_6H_5CH_2CH_2$	p-$CH_3C_6H_4SO_2$	NHOH	7.77	7.49	7.73

descriptors (30 × 1168). At the beginning, the columns which had constant and near constant values were removed from the original data matrix. Since collinear variables disrupt the models in MLR analysis, collinear descriptors needed to be detected and removed. The correlation of descriptors with one another and with activity data was then investigated. In the pairs with collinearity higher than 0.9, one which had the highest correlation versus the activity was retained and the rest were omitted. The number of total descriptors for each molecule reached 291.

The data set (30 compounds) was split into a calibration set and validation set. Validation subset was made of 20% of the total data (here, 6 biological activity data). An MLR analysis was performed by the stepwise regression SPSS (version 12.0) software and the model was built.

Since the data splitting has a considerable influence on the final selected model, a combined data splitting-feature selection (CDFS) strategy was employed [19]. In the CDFS methodology, several subdivisions of calibration and validation set were made (10 times). In each case, the best model was chosen with a correlation coefficient higher than 0.95. The created models were validated by leave-one out (LOO) cross-validation method and Y-randomization test to investigate their predictability.

Molecular docking

Molecular docking has become an increasingly main tool for drug discovery. Docking is a method which predicts the preferred orientation of one ligand when bound in an active site to form a stable complex. In this study, molecular docking of L-tyrosine derivatives with MMP-2 was studied by AutoDock 4.2 program [20] to find their binding site and the best direction based on the binding energy. Pdb file of MMP-2 was obtained from www.pdb.org (PDB: 3AYU) [21]. All water molecules were deleted, polar hydrogens were added and the Kollman charge [22] was computed. A 120 x 120 x 120 Å size was chosen for the grid box, which covers the whole protein. In all of the ligands, the same as protein, polar hydrogens were added and the Gasteiger charge was computed [23]. After preparation of ligand and protein files, the map files were created. Docking process with 50 runs and maximum number of evaluations 2500000 were performed. The final .dlg files were analyzed and the interaction between ligands and the active site of protein were studied. The ligand-protein interactions were analyzed and visualized by Discovery studio Ver. 3.

Result and discussion

Multiple linear regression analysis (MLR)

This study made use of an MLR analysis, as a simple regression method. The stepwise regression (using SPSS software) was also utilized to choose the most relevant set of descriptors for each type of the split data. The model coefficients were calculated using calibration data and then were used to predict the biological activity of validation samples. Several models were constructed by running a typical stepwise regression which is ranked based on calibration correlation coefficient (R^2c). A model with calibration correlation coefficient higher than 0.9 was selected. The created model needed to be validated. The theoretical validation is generally classified into two groups: internal and external validation. Two of the internal validation methods include Leave-one out cross validation (LOO) and Y-randomization [24]. The offered model was evaluated for both over-fitting and avoidance of chance correlations by the leave-one-out cross-validation (LOO) method and Y-randomization test respectively.

MLR method was repeated several times by different splitting data. In each case, one model was proposed. Leave-one-out cross-validation was performed and lastly, the best ten models were obtained with R^2 and Q^2_{LOO} higher than 0.9 in as reported in Table 2. The statistical qualities of models were acceptable and all of them had Q^2_{LOO} larger than 0.92; hence, the predicted models can make over 92% of variances in the inhibitory activity. In addition, results were acceptable in the prediction sets. The values of prediction correlation coefficient (R^2_p) are listed in Table 2 for the ten final models. All of the

Table 2 The best ten models were selected for future analysis in MLR

NO.	Descriptor used	R^2_c [a]	S.E [b]	R^2_p [c]	Q^2_{LOO} [d]	RMS_{CV} [e]
1	IC1, RDF135e, Mor24m, RDF035u, E3u, RDF120m, Mor15e	0.985	0.177	0.988	0.956	0.250
2	IC1, Mor24m, Mor15e, R7e0, G3p	0.989	0.154	0.90	0.967	0.218
3	IC1, Mor24m, Mor15e, dipx, GATS8p, RDF065m	0.986	0.170	0.952	0.962	0.230
4	IC1, SP20, RDF115m, RDF115e, Mor28e	0.988	0.148	0.972	0.972	0.199
5	IC1, Mor24m, Mor15e, Mor09e, G2u, Mor27u	0.976	0.228	0.951	0.940	0.300
6	IC1, Mor24m, Mor15e, Mor09e, G2u, Mor27u	0.969	0.243	0.962	0.932	0.309
7	IC1, Mor28e, HATS3p, RDF120m, RDF115m	0.987	0.152	0.974	0.969	0.203
8	IC1, Mor28e, HATS3p, RDF115m, RDF120m, G3m	0.978	0.194	0.972	0.952	0.245
9	IC1, Mor24m, RDF135e, RDF035v, RDF135m, Mor26m	0.977	0.223	0.979	0.918	0.354
10	IC1, Mor26m, G3p, GATS8p, HATS7e	0.976	0.214	0.953	0.942	0.284

[a]R^2_c = Correlation Coefficient of calibration set.
[b]S E = Standard error of regression.
[c]R^2_p = Correlation Coefficient of prediction set.
[d]Q^2_{LOO} = Leave-one-out cross-validation correlation coefficient.
[e]$RMSE_{CV}$ = Root mean square error of cross validation.

squared correlation coefficients were higher than 0.90, so the resultant linear models can predict 90% of variances in the inhibitory activity in the ten prediction sets.

The total number of descriptors, which existed in all the ten models, was 22. These descriptors are briefly described in Table 3. Among these, 3 descriptors were common. Some of the descriptors such as E3u, HATS7e, RDF065m, SP20, RDF115e, G3m and dipx were observed only in one model. The repeated descriptors were IC1, Mor24m and Mor15e. IC1 descriptor existed in all the ten models. IC1 is topological descriptor and Mor24m and Mor15e are 3D-MoRSE ones.

The repetition of IC1 in all the ten models indicated that this descriptor has a main effect on L-tyrosine scaffold-based MMP-2 inhibitors. 3D-MoRSE descriptors also have significant effects. The quantum descriptors such as (dipx) that were seen only in one model have lower effects on MMP-2 inhibitors. The observation of the models, as listed in Table 2, revealed that there is a high degree of resemblance between the subset of descriptors (without considering the difference between the chosen descriptors in different models).

To create a general model, all of the 22 descriptors were used and an MLR analysis was applied with the stepwise variable selections. Finally, one model with balance between the highest R^2, Q^2_{LOO} and the lowest number of descriptors was opted for further analysis, as reported in MLR Equation 1:

$$pIC_{50} = -13.428\ (\pm 1.720) + 5.965\ (\pm 0.488)\ IC1 + 1.464\ (\pm 0.618)\ Mor24m - 0.187\ (\pm 0.044)\ RDF115m + 0.307\ (\pm 0.067)\ SP20 + 1.284\ (\pm 0.514)\ Mor15e \quad (1)$$

$$N = 24,\ R^2_c = 0.958,\ S.E = 0.285,\ Q^2_{LOO} = 0.921,\ RMS_{CV} = 0.346$$

In this equation, N represents the number of molecules in the calibration set. R^2_c and Q^2_{LOO} are respectively the squared correlation coefficients for calibration and cross-validation. In addition, S.E is the standard error of calibration and RMS_{CV} is the root mean square error of cross-validation. This equation has three common descriptors (IC1, Mor24m and Mor15e), with high calibration statistics and prediction ability.

Topological descriptors, such as IC1, explain the size, degree of branching, flexibility and overall shape. 3D-MoRSE descriptors explain three-dimensional coordination of the different atoms in a molecule. IC1, Mor24m and Mor15e have positive signs which indicate that pIC_{50} is directly related to these descriptors. The radial distribution function (RDF) descriptors are based on the distance distribution in the molecule. RDF115m has a negative sign which indicates that pIC_{50} is inversely related to this descriptor.

For the MMP-2 inhibition activity, a higher value of molecular size, degree of branching, flexibility, shape, three-dimensional coordination of the different atoms in a molecule (IC1) and a lower value of radial distribution function, RDF115m, are beneficial to the activity.

The general model has a Q^2_{LOO} equal to 0.921; hence, the predicted model can make over 92% of variances in the inhibitory activity. The predicted values of pIC_{50} were obtained for all the molecules by MLR equation which was listed in Table 1 and were plotted against the experimental values (Figure 1A).

Table 3 Brief description of the descriptors in ten models

NO.	Name	Description
1	IC1	Information content index (neighborhood symmetry of 1-order)
2	RDF135e	Radial Distribution Function −3.5/ weighted by atomic Sanderson electronegativities
3	Mor24m	3D-MoRSE – signal 24/ weighted by atomic masses
4	RDF035u	Radial Distribution Function −3.5/ unweighted
5	E3u	3rd component accessibility directional WHIM index/ unweighted
6	RDF120m	Radial Distribution Function −12.0/ weighted by atomic masses
7	Mor15e	3D-MoRSE – signal 15/ weighted by atomic Sanderson electronegativities
8	G3p	3st component symmetry directional WHIM index/weighted by atomic polarizabilities
9	R7e0	R maximal autocorrelation of lag 7/weighted by atomic Sanderson electronegativities
10	dipx	Molecular dipole moment at X-direction
11	GATS8p	Geary autocorrelation -lag 8/ weighted by atomic polarizabilities
12	RDF065m	Radial Distribution Function −6.5/ weighted by atomic masses
13	SP20	Shape profile no. 20
14	Mor28e	3D-MoRSE – signal 28/ weighted by atomic Sanderson electronegativities
15	Mor09e	3D-MoRSE – signal 09/ weighted by atomic Sanderson electronegativities
16	G2u	2st component symmetry directional WHIM index/ unweighted
17	Mor27u	3D-MoRSE – signal 27/unweighted
18	RDF115m	Radial Distribution Function −11.5/ weighted by atomic masses
19	RDF115e	Radial Distribution Function −11.5 / weighted by atomic Sanderson electronegativities
20	HATS3p	Leverage- weighted autocorrelation of lag 3/ weighted by atomic polarizabilities
21	G3m	3st component symmetry directional WHIM index/ weighted by atomic masses
22	Mor26m	3D-MoRSE – signal 26/ weighted by atomic masses

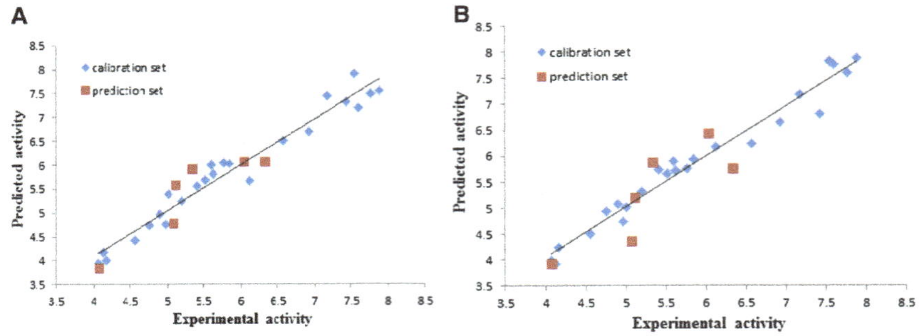

Figure 1 Plot of predicted pIC_{50} versus the experimental values for MLR model **(A)**, and GA-PLS model **(B)**.

The Y-randomization test was performed to evaluate the robustness of the general model. In the Y-randomization test, the activity data were randomly permuted in the original model and 10 models were generated. All of the models were expected to have lower R^2 and Q^2_{LOO} values than the original MLR model. If the reverse occurs, a suitable MLR model cannot be generated. The lower R^2 and Q^2_{LOO} values are shown in Table 4.

Genetic algorithm partial least squares (GA-PLS)

Since the variable selection method, that is the stepwise regression, may not be a suitable selection, variable selection methods such as the genetic algorithm, which demonstrate much better outcomes in comparison with the stepwise regression, are more favorable [25,26].

In genetic algorithm, if its corresponding descriptor is contained, a gene receives a value of 1 in the subset; otherwise, it takes a value of zero. The number of genes at each chromosome is equivalent to the number of descriptors. The population size varied between 80 and 125 for different GA runs. The number of genes with the values of 1 was relatively lower than the number of genes with the values of 0. The genes with the values of 1 were maintained. The chromosomes with the smallest numbers of chosen descriptors (total number of descriptors for each molecule reached 105) and the highest fitness were selected as the intended model. The predicted model was tested by leave-n-out cross-validation [27]. A leave-one-out cross-validation was triggered and the value of Q^2_{LOO} was obtained 0.850.

In GA-PLS, the resulted model with higher cross-validation statistics is reported in Equation 2 and the predicted values of pIC_{50} are shown in Table 1 and plotted against the experimental values in Figure 1B.

$$pIC_{50} = -12.589\ (\pm 1.208) + 6.363\ (\pm 0.394)\ IC1 + 2.119\ (\pm 0.485)\ Mor24m - 0.665\ (\pm 0.189)\ Mor15e - 0.784\ (\pm 0.370)\ Mor32e \qquad (2)$$

$$N = 24 \quad R^2_c = 0.932 \quad S.E = 0.328 \quad Q^2_{LOO} = 0.900 \quad RMSCV = 0.391$$

This equation has three MLR descriptors (IC1, Mor24m and Mor15e) with high calibration statistics and prediction ability. IC1 and Mor24m have a display positive effect and Mor15e and Mor32e have a display negative effect on inhibitory activity in GA-PLS. Unlike MLR, The radial distribution function (RDF) descriptors have no effect on inhibitory activity in GA-PLS.

As observed from Equation 2, the variables used in this equation can explain 93.2% of the variances in the inhibitory activity of the MMP-2 inhibitors used in this study.

The Y-randomization test was performed to evaluate the robustness of the created model in GA-PLS and 10 models were generated. All of the models were expected to have lower R^2 and Q^2_{LOO} values than the original GA-PLS model, as shown in Table 4.

Applicability domain of the model

A QSAR model is exploited to screen new compounds when its domain of application has been defined [28]. The prediction may be assumed reliable for only those

Table 4 R^2 and Q^2_{LOO} values after ten Y-randomization tests

Iteration	MLR		GA-PLS	
	R^2	Q^2_{LOO}	R^2	Q^2_{LOO}
1	0.204	0.001	0.319	0.102
2	0.048	0.265	0.048	0.244
3	0.314	0.068	0.206	0.016
4	0.075	0.260	0.040	0.235
5	0.118	0.022	0.097	0.028
6	0.106	0.069	0.132	0.020
7	0.256	0.010	0.394	0.194
8	0.096	0.099	0.038	0.296
9	0.068	0.175	0.062	0.175
10	0.191	0.007	0.177	0.002

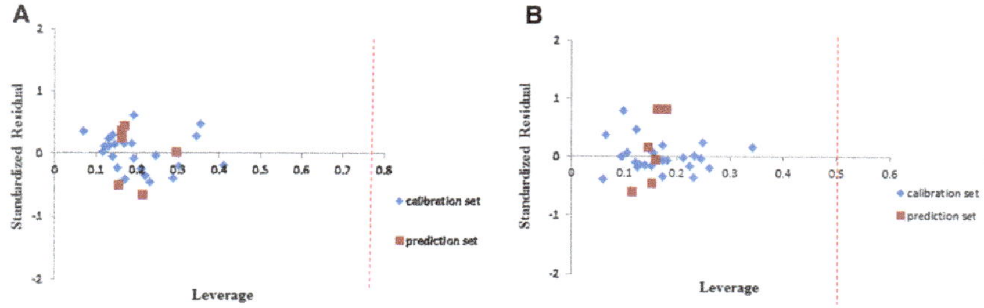

Figure 2 William's plot of generated MLR model **(A)**, and GA-PLS model **(B)**.

compounds which fall into this domain [29]. Standardized residuals of the activity were computed and were plotted versus leverage values (h). The value of leverage was calculated for every compound. Values are always between 0 and 1. A value of 0 is indicative of perfect prediction and usually is not accessible, and a value of 1 indicates very poor prediction. The lower the value, the higher confidence in the prediction. Warning leverage (h*) is another standard for explanation of the results and is, generally, fixed at 3 (k + 1)/ n, where k is the number of model parameters and n is the number of calibration set [29]. Calculated leverage for calibration set is useful for determining the compounds which affect the model and, in terms of validation set, useful for assigning the applicability domain of the model. The William's plot for the developed models in MLR and GA-PLS are shown in Figure 2.

Response outliers are compounds that have standard residual points higher than ± 2.0 standard deviation units and a leverage value higher than the warning leverage, which is 0.75 and 0.5 for MLR and GA-PLS respectively. As can be seen in Figure 2, all studied molecules in calibration and validation set lie with high degree of confidence in application domain of the developed models in both methods.

Molecular docking studies

To explore the ligand binding modes, and to find amino acids, which are essential in ligand binding to MMP-2, molecular docking was performed on a ligand-binding pocket. The way the compound was bound with the lowest free energy was studied. Interactions between MMP-2 and ligand N-4-[(1-hydroxycarbamoyl-2-methyl-propyl)-(2-morpholin-4-yl-ethyl)-sulfamoyl]-4- pentyl-benzamide (SC-74020) were obtained by Feng et al. and were reported. According to their results, the catalytic zinc is chelated by His120, His124, His130 and ligand, and the structural zinc is coordinated by His70, Asp72, His85 and His98. In addition, hydrogen bond was bound by Leu82 and Ala83 to a sulfoneoxygen atom of the inhibitor [30].

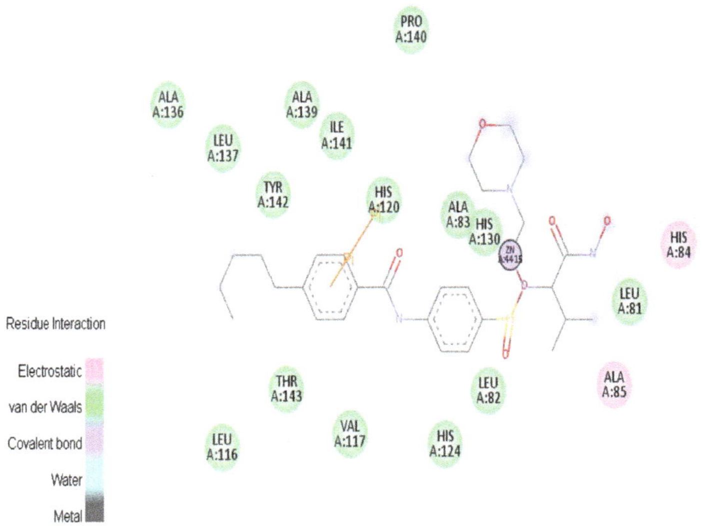

Figure 3 Interactions between ligand and MMP-2.

Table 5 The obtained binding energy by AutoDock

Compound	Binding energy (kcal/mol)	Compound	Binding energy (kcal/mol)
4a	−5.90	5f	−6.13
4b	−5.57	5 g	−6.34
4c	−5.96	5 h	−5.93
4d	−5.39	5i	−5.92
4e	−6.88	5j	−6.79
4f	−5.88	6a	−7.08
4 g	−5.67	6b	−7.07
4 h	−6.23	6c	−7.01
4i	−6.21	6d	−7.27
4j	−5.98	6e	−7.29
5a	−6.68	6f	−7.16
5b	−6.76	6 g	−6.92
5c	−6.85	6 h	−7.35
5d	−6.47	6i	−7.30
5e	−6.67	6j	−7.29

Initially, to assure binding mode of ligand and protein, ligand docking with MMP-2 protein has been validated by Feng. All of the interactions between the ligand and catalytic zinc with the protein from our results are shown in Figure 3. Root mean square deviation (RSMD) was lower than 1. Both of the prior cases proposed high reliability of docking program. Therefore, the AutoDock 4.2 could be used to find the binding mode of other inhibitors of MMP-2.

All of the 30 compounds were docked into the binding site of protein by AutoDock 4.2 and were studied. The binding energy of all the compounds is reported in Table 5. The obtained energies were compared with the experimental IC_{50}, and the 6a-6j compounds have the lowest binding energy. This means that based on the binding energy of the active site, these compounds, especially compound (6 h), are the best L-tyrosine scaffold based inhibitors. The binding orientation of compound (6 h) and hydrogen bond of the ligand with Leu82 and Ala83 are depicted in Figure 4. This compound was fitted into the active site of MMP-2. In all of the compounds, the oxygen of carbonyl and sulfonyl groups are important for hydrogen bond of the ligand with Leu82 and Ala83. R_2 and R_3 substituents have the main role for hydrogen bonding interactions. In 4a-4j compounds, IC_{50} is higher than 5a-5j and 6a-6j compounds. When R_3 is OH and NHOH groups, hydrogen bond can be created better than when R_3 is $-OCH_3$. Moreover, when R_2 is sulfonyl, because of two oxygen groups, a stronger hydrogen bond can be created than that of carbonyl.

R_1 is sited in hydrophobic pocket. Methylene group can help the ligand to be fitted in lipophilic pocket, so two Methylene groups are better than one. Phenyl group can create a π- π interaction with Phe86. Therefore, phenethyl ($C_6H_5CH_2CH_2$) is better than benzyl ($C_6H_5CH_2$).

To design L-tyrosine based inhibitors and prediction of their activity against MMP-2 based on AutoDock 4.2 and QSAR studies, addition to a higher value of molecular size, degree of branching, flexibility, shape and three-dimensional coordination of the different atoms in a molecule, hydrophobicity and hydrophilicity of R_1, R_2 and R_3 are highly important. When R_1 is more hydrophobic, and R_2, is more hydrophilic, there is a stronger inhibition against MMP-2.

Conclusion

In this study, quantitative relationships between molecular structure and inhibitory effect of L-tyrosine scaffold based

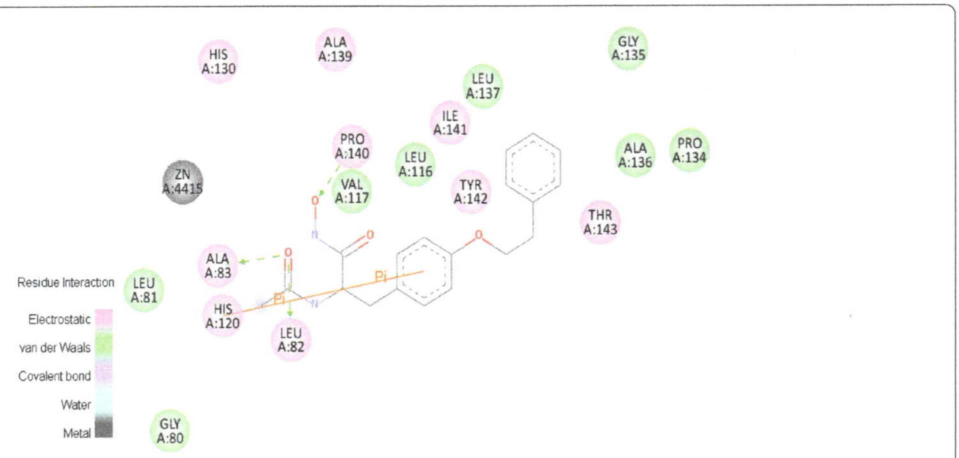

Figure 4 The best orientation of 6 h ligand.

MMP-2 inhibitors were investigated by MLR and GA-PLS. In MLR, A combined data splitting-feature selection method (CDFS) was offered to develop a quantitative structure–activity relationship model. It was found that topological parameter (IC1) has a main effect on the inhibitory activity of the compounds, among the different QSAR models. By this simple procedure, a multilinear 5-parametric model was created out of 22 descriptors. This method yielded acceptable results for the prediction set which was measured by cross-validation and Y-randomization. The findings indicate that the linear model produced by CDFS methodology could reproduce more than 92% of variances in the inhibitory activity. In addition to MLR, genetic algorithms, which demonstrated much better outcomes in comparison with stepwise regression, were used. By GA-PLS, the model with higher cross-validation statistics was created and the results indicated that IC1, Mor24m, Mor15e and Mor32e are main descriptors. It can be concluded from the two methods that higher values of molecular size, degree of branching, flexibility, shape and three-dimensional coordination of the different atoms in a molecule are particularly important

The docking study revealed that two hydrogen bonds between all of the inhibitors and the active site of MMP-2 (Leu82 and Ala83) are formed, as well as a π-π interaction between phenyl group and Phe86.

The information above could be used to design new inhibitors, and to show higher inhibitory activities and chemical synthesis of new inhibitors.

Abbreviations

MMP: Matrix metalloproteinase; QSAR: Quantitative structure activity relationship; MLR: Multiple linear regression; ECM: Extracellular matrix; CDFS: Combined data splitting-feature selection; Q^2_{LOO}: Square correlation coefficient for leave-one-out cross-validation; R^2_C: Calibration correlation coefficient; R^2_P: Prediction correlation coefficient; RSMD: Root-mean-square deviation; S.E: standard error of calibration; RMS_{CV}: root mean square error of cross-validation; RDF: radial distribution function descriptors; GA-PLS: Genetic algorithm partial least squares.

Competing interests

The authors declare that they have no competing interests.

Authors' contributions

MA: Participated in the design of the study, carried out the QSAR study, performed molecular docking and drafted the manuscript. FR: Carried out the QSAR study and drafted the manuscript. ME: Helped the QSAR analysis. HAS: Participated in the design of the study drafted the manuscript. MA: Was responsible for the study registration, financial and administrative support, and also gave final approval of the version to be published. All authors read and approved the final manuscript.

Author details

[1]Department of Medicinal Chemistry, Faculty of Pharmacy, Pharmaceutical Science Research Center, Tehran University of Medical Science, Tehran, Iran. [2]Department of Medicinal Chemistry, Faculty of Pharmacy, Isfahan University of Medical Sciences, 81746-73461 Isfahan, Iran. [3]Medicinal & Natural Product Chemistry Research Center, Shiraz University of Medical Sciences, Shiraz, Iran.

References

1. Cheng X-C, Wang R-L, Dong Z-K, Li J, Li Y-Y, Li R-R. Design, synthesis and evaluation of novel metalloproteinase inhibitors based on L-tyrosine scaffold. Bioorg Med Chem. 2012;20:5738–44.
2. Lerchenberger M, Uhl B, Stark K, Zuchtriegel G, Eckart A, Miller M, et al. Matrix metalloproteinases modulate ameboid-like migration of neutrophils through inflamed interstitial tissue. Blood. 2013;122:770–80.
3. Page-McCaw A, Ewald AJ, Werb Z. Matrix metalloproteinases and the regulation of tissue remodelling. Nat Rev Mol Cell Bio. 2007;8:221–33.
4. Sapna G, Gokul S, Bagri-Manjrekar K. Matrix metalloproteinases and periodontal diseases. Oral Dis. 2013;20:538–50.
5. Bouloumié A, Sengenès C, Portolan G, Galitzky J, Lafontan M. Adipocyte produces matrix metalloproteinases 2 and 9 involvement in adipose differentiation. Diabetes. 2001;50:2080–6.
6. Visse R, Nagase H. Matrix metalloproteinases and tissue inhibitors of metalloproteinases structure, function, and biochemistry. Circ Res. 2003;92:827–39.
7. Hu Q, Yu L, Liao Q. Methylation of matrix metalloproteinases-2 promoter in endometrial cancer invasion. Beijing Da Xue Xue Bao. 2012;44:911–5.
8. Wang Y, Hu C, Dong R, Huang X, Qiu H. Platelet-derived growth factor-D promotes ovarian cancer invasion by regulating matrix metalloproteinases 2 and 9. Asian Pac J Cancer Prev. 2011;12:3367–70.
9. Maskos K. Crystal structures of MMPs in complex with physiological and pharmacological inhibitors. Biochimie. 2005;87:249–63.
10. Zucker S, Cao J. Selective matrix metalloproteinase (MMP) inhibitors in cancer therapy. Cancer Biol Ther. 2009;8:2371–3.
11. Di Pizio A, Laghezza A, Tortorella P, Agamennone M. Probing the S1' Site for the Identification of Non-Zinc-Binding MMP-2 Inhibitors. Chem Med Chem. 2013;8:1475–82.
12. Wojtowicz-Praga SM, Dickson RB, Hawkins MJ. Matrix metalloproteinase inhibitors. Invest New Drugs. 1997;15:61–75.
13. Cheng X-C, Wang Q, Fang H, Tang W, Xu W-F. Design, synthesis and evaluation of novel sulfonyl pyrrolidine derivatives as matrix metalloproteinase inhibitors. Bioorg Med Chem. 2008;16:5398–404.
14. Hansch C, Hoekman D, Gao H. Comparative QSAR: toward a deeper understanding of chemicobiological interactions. Chem Rev. 1996;96:1045–76.
15. Hansch C, Kurup A, Garg R, Gao H. Chem-bioinformatics and QSAR: a review of QSAR lacking positive hydrophobic terms. Chem Rev. 2001;101:619–72.
16. Sabet R, Mohammadpour M, Sadeghi A, Fassihi A. QSAR study of isatin analogues as in vitro anti-cancer agents. Eur J Med Che. 2010;45:1113–8.
17. Frisch M, Trucks G, Schlegel H, Scuseria G, Robb M, Cheeseman J, et al. Gaussian 98, revision A. 7. Pittsburgh, Pa: Gaussian, Inc; 1998. p. 12.
18. Thanikaivelan P, Subramanian V, Raghava Rao J, Unni Nair B. Application of quantum chemical descriptor in quantitative structure activity and structure property relationship. Chem Phys Lett. 2000;323:59–70.
19. Hemmateenejad B, Shamsipur M, Miri R, Elyasi M, Foroghinia F, Sharghi H. Linear and nonlinear quantitative structure–property relationship models for solubility of some anthraquinone, anthrone and xanthone derivatives in supercritical carbon dioxide. Anal Chim Acta. 2008;610:25–34.
20. Morris GM, Huey R, Lindstrom W, Sanner MF, Belew RK, Goodsell DS, et al. AutoDock4 and AutoDockTools4: Automated docking with selective receptor flexibility. J Comput Chem. 2009;30:2785–91.
21. Hashimoto H, Takeuchi T, Komatsu K, Miyazaki K, Sato M, Higashi S. Structural basis for matrix metalloproteinase-2 (MMP-2)-selective inhibitory action of β-amyloid precursor protein-derived inhibitor. J Biol Chem. 2011;286:33236–43.
22. Singh UC, Kollman PA. An approach to computing electrostatic charges for molecules. J Comput Chem. 1984;5:129–45.
23. Azizian H, Bahrami H, Pasalar P, Amanlou M. Molecular modeling of Helicobacter pylori arginase and the inhibitor coordination interactions. J Mol Graph Model. 2010;28:626–35.
24. Shahlaei M, Madadkar-Sobhani A, Saghaie L, Fassihi A. Application of an expert system based on Genetic Algorithm–Adaptive Neuro-Fuzzy Inference System (GA–ANFIS) in QSAR of cathepsin K inhibitors. Expert Syst Appl. 2012;39:6182–91.
25. Barros A, Rutledge D. Genetic algorithm applied to the selection of principal components. Chemometr Intell Lab Syst. 1998;40:65–81.
26. Liu S-S, Liu H-L, Yin C-S, Wang L-S. VSMP: a novel variable selection and modeling method based on the prediction. J Chem Inform Comput Sci. 2003;43:964–9.
27. Fernández M, Caballero J. Modeling of activity of cyclic urea HIV-1 protease inhibitors using regularized-artificial neural networks. Bioor Med Chem. 2006;14:280–94.

28. Tropsha A, Gramatica P, Gombar VK. The importance of being earnest: validation is the absolute essential for successful application and interpretation of QSPR models. QSAR Comb Sci. 2003;22:69–77.
29. Mansourian M, Fassihi A, Saghaie L, Madadkar-Sobhani A, Mahnam K, Abbasi M. QSAR and docking analysis of A_{2B} adenosine receptor antagonists based on non-xanthine scaffold. Med Chem Res. 2015;24:394–407.
30. Feng Y, Likos JJ, Zhu L, Woodward H, Munie G, McDonald JJ, et al. Solution structure and backbone dynamics of the catalytic domain of matrix metalloproteinase-2 complexed with a hydroxamic acid inhibitor. BBA Proteins Proteom. 2002;1598:10–23.

Permissions

All chapters in this book were first published in JPS, by BioMed Central; hereby published with permission under the Creative Commons Attribution License or equivalent. Every chapter published in this book has been scrutinized by our experts. Their significance has been extensively debated. The topics covered herein carry significant findings which will fuel the growth of the discipline. They may even be implemented as practical applications or may be referred to as a beginning point for another development.

The contributors of this book come from diverse backgrounds, making this book a truly international effort. This book will bring forth new frontiers with its revolutionizing research information and detailed analysis of the nascent developments around the world.

We would like to thank all the contributing authors for lending their expertise to make the book truly unique. They have played a crucial role in the development of this book. Without their invaluable contributions this book wouldn't have been possible. They have made vital efforts to compile up to date information on the varied aspects of this subject to make this book a valuable addition to the collection of many professionals and students.

This book was conceptualized with the vision of imparting up-to-date information and advanced data in this field. To ensure the same, a matchless editorial board was set up. Every individual on the board went through rigorous rounds of assessment to prove their worth. After which they invested a large part of their time researching and compiling the most relevant data for our readers.

The editorial board has been involved in producing this book since its inception. They have spent rigorous hours researching and exploring the diverse topics which have resulted in the successful publishing of this book. They have passed on their knowledge of decades through this book. To expedite this challenging task, the publisher supported the team at every step. A small team of assistant editors was also appointed to further simplify the editing procedure and attain best results for the readers.

Apart from the editorial board, the designing team has also invested a significant amount of their time in understanding the subject and creating the most relevant covers. They scrutinized every image to scout for the most suitable representation of the subject and create an appropriate cover for the book.

The publishing team has been an ardent support to the editorial, designing and production team. Their endless efforts to recruit the best for this project, has resulted in the accomplishment of this book. They are a veteran in the field of academics and their pool of knowledge is as vast as their experience in printing. Their expertise and guidance has proved useful at every step. Their uncompromising quality standards have made this book an exceptional effort. Their encouragement from time to time has been an inspiration for everyone.

The publisher and the editorial board hope that this book will prove to be a valuable piece of knowledge for researchers, students, practitioners and scholars across the globe.

List of Contributors

Ghodsi Mohammadi Ziarani, Sakineh Faramarzi and Shima Asadi
Department of Chemistry, Alzahra University, Vanak Square, P.O. Box 19938939973, Tehran, Iran

Alireza Badiei
School of Chemistry, College of Science, University of Tehran, Tehran, Iran

Roya Bazl and Massoud Amanlou
Drug Design and Development Research Center and Department of Medicinal Chemistry, Faculty of Pharmacy, Tehran University of Medical Sciences, Tehran, Iran

Pooneh Salari
Medical Ethics and History of Medicine Research Center, Tehran University of Medical Sciences, 23# 16 Azar Ave, Keshavarz Blvd, 1417633114 Tehran, Iran

Mohammad Abdollahi
Faculty of Pharmacy and Pharmaceutical Sciences Research Center, Tehran University of Medical Sciences, Tehran, Iran

Ramin Heshmat, Hamidreza Aghaei Meybodi and Farideh Razi
Endocrinology and Metabolism Research Institute, Tehran University of Medical Sciences, Tehran, Iran

Khosrou Abdi
Department Radiopharmacy, Tehran University of Medical Sciences, Tehran, 14174, Iran
Department of Medicinal Chemistry, Tehran University of Medical Sciences, Tehran 14174, Iran

Ali Khalaj
Department of Medicinal Chemistry, Tehran University of Medical Sciences, Tehran 14174, Iran
Drug Design & Development Research Center, Tehran University of Medical Sciences, Tehran 14174, Iran

Seyed Nasser Ostad
Department of Toxicology & Pharmacology, Tehran University of Medical Sciences, Tehran 14174, Iran

Navid Lamei
Drug Design & Development Research Center, Tehran University of Medical Sciences, Tehran 14174, Iran

Mohammad Reza Khoshayand
Department of Drug and Food Control, Faculty of Pharmacy, Tehran University of Medical Sciences, Tehran 14174, Iran

Gilda Kianimehr
Psychiatric Research Center, Roozbeh Hospital, Tehran University of Medical Sciences, Tehran 13337, Iran

Farzad Fatehi
Shariati Hospital, Neurology Department, Tehran University of medical Sciences, Tehran, Iran

Sara Hashempoor and Mohammad-Reza Khodaei-Ardakani
Razi Psychiatric Hospital, University of Social Welfare and Rehabilitation, Tehran, Iran

Farzin Rezaei and Ali Nazari
Qods Hospital, Kurdistan University of Medical Sciences, Sanandaj, Iran

Ladan Kashani
Infertility WardArash Hospital, Tehran University of Medical Sciences, Tehran, Iran

Shahin Akhondzadeh
Psychiatric Research Center, Roozbeh Psychiatric Hospital, Tehran University of Medical Sciences, South Kargar Street 13337, Tehran, Iran

Atabak Najafi and Arezoo Ahmadi
Department of Anesthesiology and Critical Care Medicine, Sina Hospital, Faculty of Medicine, Tehran University of Medical Sciences, Tehran, Iran

Keyvan Haji Ahmadi and Farhad Najmeddin
Department of Clinical Pharmacy, Faculty of Pharmacy, Tehran University of Medical Sciences, Tehran, Iran

Legese Chelkeba
Department of Clinical Pharmacy, Faculty of Pharmacy, Tehran University of Medical Sciences, Tehran, Iran
Faculty of Pharmacy and Pharmaceutical Sciences Research Center, Tehran University of Medical Sciences, Tehran, Iran

Mojtaba Mojtahedzadeh
Department of Anesthesiology and Critical Care Medicine, Sina Hospital, Faculty of Medicine, Tehran University of Medical Sciences, Tehran, Iran
Department of Clinical Pharmacy, Faculty of Pharmacy, Tehran University of Medical Sciences, Tehran, Iran
Faculty of Pharmacy and Pharmaceutical Sciences Research Center, Tehran University of Medical Sciences, Tehran, Iran

Mohammad Abdollahi
Faculty of Pharmacy and Pharmaceutical Sciences Research Center, Tehran University of Medical Sciences, Tehran, Iran

Maryam Mousavi
Department of Clinical Pharmacy, Faculty of Pharmacy, Mashhad University of Medical sciences, Mashhad, Iran

Ahmad Mohammadi-Farani
Department of Pharmacology, Toxicology and Medical Services, Faculty of Pharmacy, Kermanshah University of Medical Sciences, Kermanshah, Iran

Aram Ahmadi
Students Research Committee, Kermanshah University of Medical Sciences, Kermanshah, Iran
Department of MedicinalChemistry, Faculty of Pharmacy, Kermanshah University of Medical Sciences, Kermanshah, Iran

Hamid Nadri
Neurobiomedical Research Center, Shahid Sadoughi University of Medical Sciences, Yazd, Iran

Alireza Aliabadi
Department of MedicinalChemistry, Faculty of Pharmacy, Kermanshah University of Medical Sciences, Kermanshah, Iran

Abbas Azadmehr
Immunology Department, Qazvin University of Medical Sciences, Qazvin, Iran

Robabeh latifi, Sahar Mosalla and Mojtaba Shahnazi
Parasitology Department, Qazvin University of Medical Sciences, Qazvin, Iran

Reza Hajiaghaee
Pharmacognosy and Pharmaceutics department of Medicinal Plants Research Center, Institute of Medicinal Plants, (ACECR), Karaj, Iran

Araz Mohammad Davoodipoor
Department of Pharmacognosy and Medicinal Plants Research Center, Faculty of Pharmacy, Tehran University of Medical Sciences, Tehran 14155-6451, Iran

Mahnaz Khanavi and Mohammad Reza Shams Ardekani
Department of Pharmacognosy and Medicinal Plants Research Center, Faculty of Pharmacy, Tehran University of Medical Sciences, Tehran 14155-6451, Iran
Department of Traditional Pharmacy, School of Traditional Iranian Medicine and Traditional Iranian Medicine and Pharmacy Research Center, Tehran University of Medical Sciences, Tehran, Iran

Seyede Nargess Sadati
Department of Traditional Pharmacy, School of Traditional Iranian Medicine and Traditional Iranian Medicine and Pharmacy

Research Center, Tehran University of Medical Sciences, Tehran, Iran

Mohammad Sharifzadeh
Department of Pharmacology and Toxicology, Faculty of Pharmacy, Tehran University of Medical Sciences, Tehran, P.O. Box 14155-6451, Iran

Monia Deghrigue and Abderrahman Bouraoui
Laboratoire de développement chimique, galénique et pharmacologique des médicaments (LR12ES09). Equipe de Pharmacologie marine, Faculté de pharmacie de Monastir, Université de Monastir, Monastir, Tunisie

Carmen Festa, Maria Valeria D'auria and Simona de Marino
Department of Pharmacy, University of Naples "Federico II", via D. Montesano 49, I- 80131 Napoli, Italy

Hichem Ben Jannet and Lotfi Ghribi
Laboratoire de chimie hétérocyclique, produits naturels et réactivité. Equipe de chimie médicinale et produits naturels (LR11ES39), Faculté des sciences de Monastir, Université de Monastir, Monastir, Tunisie

Rafik Ben Said
Institut National des Sciences et Technologie de la Mer (INSTM), Salambo, Tunis, Tunisie

Afshin Gharekhani
Resident of Clinical Pharmacy, Faculty of Pharmacy, Tehran University of Medical Sciences, Tehran 1417614411, Iran

Mohammad-Reza Khatami and Effat Razeghi
Nephrology Research Center, Tehran University of Medical Sciences, Tehran 1417614411, Iran

Simin Dashti-Khavidaki
Nephrology Research Center, Tehran University of Medical Sciences, Tehran 1417614411, Iran
Faculty of Pharmacy, Tehran University of Medical Sciences, Tehran 1417614411, Iran

Alireza Abdollahi
Vali-e-Asr Hospital, Tehran University of Medical Sciences, Tehran 1417614411, Iran

Seyed-Saeed Hashemi-Nazari
Department of Epidemiology, School of Public Health, Shahid Beheshti University of Medical Sciences, Tehran 1417614411, Iran

Mohammad-Ali Mansournia
Department of Epidemiology and Biostatistics, School of Public Health, Tehran University of Medical Sciences, Tehran 1417614411, Iran

Mehdi Khoshneviszadeh
Medicinal and Natural Products Chemistry Research Center, Shiraz University of Medical Sciences, PO Box 3288-71345, Shiraz, Iran

Ahmad Ebadi, Nima Razzaghi-Asl, and Ramin Miri
Medicinal and Natural Products Chemistry Research Center, Shiraz University of Medical Sciences, PO Box 3288-71345, Shiraz, Iran
Department of Medicinal Chemistry, School of Pharmacy, Shiraz University of Medical Sciences, PO Box 1583-71345, Shiraz, Iran

Nasrin Maleki-Dizaji and Alireza Garjani
Department of Pharmacology and Toxicology, Faculty of Pharmacy, Tabriz University of Medical Sciences, Tabriz, Iran

Arash Khorrami
Department of Pharmacology and Toxicology, Faculty of Pharmacy, Tabriz University of Medical Sciences, Tabriz, Iran
Student Research Committee, Tabriz University of Medical Sciences, Tabriz, Iran

Mojtaba Hammami and Mehraveh Garjani
Student Research Committee, Tabriz University of Medical Sciences, Tabriz, Iran

Zahra Daman, Abdolhossein Rouholamini Najafabadi and Hamid Reza Eftekhari
Aerosol Research Laboratory, Department of Pharmaceutics, School of Pharmacy, Tehran University of Medical Sciences, Tehran, Iran

Kambiz Gilani
Aerosol Research Laboratory, Department of Pharmaceutics, School of Pharmacy, Tehran University of Medical Sciences, Tehran, Iran
Medicinal Plants Research Center, Tehran University of Medical Sciences, Tehran, Iran

Mohammad Ali Barghi
XRD Research Laboratory, School of Sciences, Tehran University, Tehran, Iran

Saeed Manoochehri and Behrad Darvishi
Department of Pharmaceutics, Faculty of Pharmacy, Tehran University of Medical Sciences, Tehran 1417614411, Iran

Fatemeh Atyabi and Rassoul Dinarvand
Department of Pharmaceutics, Faculty of Pharmacy, Tehran University of Medical Sciences, Tehran 1417614411, Iran
Nanotechnology Research Centre, Tehran University of Medical Sciences, Tehran, Iran

Golnaz Kamalinia
Nanotechnology Research Centre, Tehran University of Medical Sciences, Tehran, Iran

Mohsen Amini
Department of Medicinal Chemistry, Faculty of Pharmacy, Tehran University of Medical Sciences, Tehran, Iran

Mahdieh Fallah
Arash Hospital, Faculty of Medicine, Tehran University of Medical Sciences, Tehran, Iran

Seyed Naser Ostad
Department of Toxicology and Pharmacology, Faculty of Pharmacy, Tehran University of Medical Sciences, Tehran, Iran

Mehdi Mogharabi and Mohammad Ali Faramarzi
Department of Pharmaceutical Biotechnology, Faculty of Pharmacy & Biotechnology Research Center, Tehran University of Medical Sciences, Tehran 1417614411, Iran
Department of Toxicology and Pharmacology, Faculty of Pharmacy and Pharmaceutical Sciences Research Center, Tehran University of Medical Sciences, Tehran 1417614411, Iran

Mohammad Abdollahi
Department of Toxicology and Pharmacology, Faculty of Pharmacy and Pharmaceutical Sciences Research Center, Tehran University of Medical Sciences, Tehran 1417614411, Iran

Niusha Sharifi and Effat Souri
Department of Medicinal Chemistry, Faculty of Pharmacy, Tehran University of Medical Sciences, Tehran, Iran

Seyed Ali Ziai
Department of Pharmacology, Faculty of Medicine, Shahid Beheshti University of Medical Sciences, Tehran, Iran

Gholamreza Amin
Department of Pharmacognosy, Faculty of Pharmacy, Tehran University of Medical Sciences, Tehran, Iran

Massoud Amanlou
Department of Medicinal Chemistry, Faculty of Pharmacy, Tehran University of Medical Sciences, Tehran, Iran
Medicinal Plants Research Center, Faculty of Pharmacy, Tehran University of Medical Sciences, Tehran, Iran

Massoud Amanlou
Department of Medicinal Chemistry, Faculty of Pharmacy and Pharmaceutical Sciences Research Center, Tehran University of Medical Sciences, Tehran, Iran

Anahita Johari
Department of Medicinal Chemistry, Faculty of Pharmacy and Pharmaceutical Sciences Research Center, Tehran University of Medical Sciences, Tehran, Iran
Institute of Biochemistry and Biophysics, University of Tehran, Tehran, Iran

Ali Akbar Moosavi-Movahedi
Institute of Biochemistry and Biophysics, University of Tehran, Tehran, Iran

Alessio Di Luca, Michael Henry and Paula Meleady
National Institute for Cellular Biotechnology, DCU, Glasnevin, Dublin 9, Dublin, Ireland

Robert O'Conno
National Institute for Cellular Biotechnology, DCU, Glasnevin, Dublin 9, Dublin, Ireland
School of Nursing and Human Sciences, DCU, Glasnevin, Dublin 9, Dublin, Ireland

Shaghayegh Norouzi, Mahnaz Norouzi, Mohamad Nabiuni and Saeed Irian
Department of Cell and Molecular Biology, Faculty of Biological Sciences, Kharazmi University, P.O. Box 1481765544 Tehran, Iran

Mohsen Amini
Department of Medicinal Chemistry, School of Pharmacy, Tehran University of Medical Sciences, Tehran, Iran

Amir Amanzadeh
National Cell Bank of Iran, Pasteur Institute of Iran, Tehran, Iran

Mona Salimi
Department of Physiology and Pharmacology, Pasteur Institute of Iran, P.O. Box 13164 Tehran, Iran

Hwan Hee Lee, Seulki Lee and Hyosun Cho
College of Pharmacy, Duksung Women's University, Seoul 132-714, Republic of Korea
Innovative Drug Center, Duksung Women's University, Seoul 132-714, Republic of Korea

Kanghyo Lee
Mushroom Research Division, National Institute of Horticultural and Herbal Science, Rural Development Administration, Eumseong 369-873, Republic of Korea

Yu Su Shin
Department of Medicinal Crop Research, National Institute of Horticultural and Herbal Science, Rural Development Administration, Eumseong 369-873, Republic of Korea

Hyojeung Kang
College of Pharmacy, Research Institute of Pharmaceutical Sciences and Institute for Microorganisms, Kyungpook National University, Daegu 702-701, Republic of Korea

Wen-Bi Xiong, Zhen-Jun Shao, Yao Xiong, Jian Chen, Yun Sun, Ling Zhu and Li-Ming Zhou
Department of Pharmacology, West China Medical Center, Preclinical and Forensic Medical College, Sichuan University, Chengdu 610041, P.R. China

Leila Vali, Ali A. Dashti, Mehrez M. Jadaon and Sherief El-Shazly
Department of Medical Laboratory Sciences, Faculty of Allied Health, Sciences, Kuwait University, P.O. Box 31470-Sulaibekhat, 90805 Sulaibekhat, Kuwait

Amir Ghaderi
Department of Addiction studies, School of Medical Kashan University of Medical Sciences, Kashan, Iran

Naser Vahdati-Mashhadian and Valiallah Moradi
Departments of Pharmacodynamics and Toxicology, School of Pharmacy, Mashhad University of Medical Sciences, Mashhad, Iran

Zohreh Oghabian
Department of Clinical Toxicology, Kerman University of Medical Sciences, Kerman, Iran

Reza Afshari
Addiction Research Centre, Mashhad University of Medical Sciences, Imam Reza Hospital, Ibn-e-Sina Street, Mashhad 91735-348, Iran
British Columbia Center for Disease Control, Vancouver, Canada

Omid Mehrpour
Atherosclerosis and Coronary Artery Research Center, Birjand University of Medical Science, Birjand, Iran

Alireza Aliabadi
Pharmaceutical Sciences Research Center, School of Pharmacy, Kermanshah University of Medical Sciences, Kermanshah, Iran
Department of Medicinal Chemistry, Faculty of Pharmacy, Kermanshah University of Medical Sciences, Kermanshah, Iran

Ahmad Mohammadi-Farani, and Farahnaz Ahmadi
Pharmaceutical Sciences Research Center, School of Pharmacy, Kermanshah University of Medical Sciences, Kermanshah, Iran
Department of Pharmacology, Toxicology and Medical Services, Faculty of Pharmacy, Kermanshah University of Medical Sciences, Kermanshah, Iran

Zeinab Hosseinzadeh
Department of Medicinal Chemistry, Faculty of Pharmacy, Kermanshah University of Medical Sciences, Kermanshah, Iran
Students Research Committee, Kermanshah University of Medical Sciences, Kermanshah, Iran

Hamid Nadri and Alireza Moradi
Neurobiomedical Research Center, Yazd Shahid Sadoughi University of Medical Sciences, Yazd, Iran

Hossein Ali Ebrahimi
Biotechnology Research Center, Tabriz University of Medical Sciences, Tabriz, Iran
Department of Pharmaceutics, Faculty of Pharmacy, Tabriz University of Medical Sciences, Tabriz, Iran
Zanjan Pharmaceutical Nanotechnology Research Center (ZPNRC), Zanjan University of Medical Sciences, Zanjan, Iran

Yousef Javadzadeh
Biotechnology Research Center, Tabriz University of Medical Sciences, Tabriz, Iran
Department of Pharmaceutics, Faculty of Pharmacy, Tabriz University of Medical Sciences, Tabriz, Iran

Mohammad Barzegar Jalali
Department of Pharmaceutics, Faculty of Pharmacy, Tabriz University of Medical Sciences, Tabriz, Iran

Mehrdad Hamidi
Zanjan Pharmaceutical Nanotechnology Research Center (ZPNRC), Zanjan University of Medical Sciences, Zanjan, Iran
Department of Pharmaceutics, School of Pharmacy, Zanjan University of Medical Sciences, Zanjan, Iran

Mohammadreza Mobinizadeh, Amir Ashkan Nasiripour and Seyed Jamaleddin Tabibi
Department of Health Services Management, Science and Research Branch, Islamic Azad University, Tehran, Iran

Pouran Raeissi
Department of Health Services Management, School of Management and Medical Information Science, Iran University of Medical Sciences, Tehran, Iran

Alireza Olyaeemanesh
National Institute for Health Research, Tehran University of Medical Sciences, Tehran, Iran

Fatemeh Ramezani and Massoud Amanlou
Department of Medicinal Chemistry, Faculty of Pharmacy, Pharmaceutical Science Research Center, Tehran University of Medical Science, Tehran, Iran

Hojjat Sadeghi-Aliabadi
Department of Medicinal Chemistry, Faculty of Pharmacy, Isfahan University of Medical Sciences, 81746-73461 Isfahan, Iran

Maryam Abbasi
Department of Medicinal Chemistry, Faculty of Pharmacy, Pharmaceutical Science Research Center, Tehran University of Medical Science, Tehran, Iran
Department of Medicinal Chemistry, Faculty of Pharmacy, Isfahan University of Medical Sciences, 81746-73461 Isfahan, Iran

Maryam Elyasi
Medicinal & Natural Product Chemistry Research Center, Shiraz University of Medical Sciences, Shiraz, Iran

Index